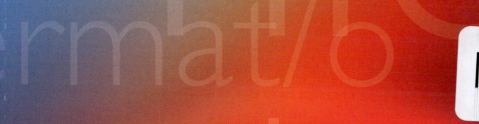

D0226292

A GUIDE TO...

Medical Terminology Systems
A Body Systems Approach, SEVENTH EDITION

+ The Medical Language Lab

Master the language of medicine with ease!
Whatever your learning style—looking, listening, doing, or a little bit of each—this popular word-building and body-systems approach is designed just for you.

Increase your knowledge and retention.
A clear, concise word-building approach guides you step-by-step through the parts of words—roots, combining forms, suffixes, and prefixes—*before* you learn the vocabulary, avoiding tedious memorization.

Explore captivating detail.
Brilliant, full-color photographs and precise illustrations bring important concepts to life.

Sharpen your skills.
Find handy mnemonic devices, crossword puzzles, word scrambles, and drag-and-drop games on the Term*Plus* CD-ROM* to build your confidence.

* The Term*Plus* CD-ROM can be purchased separately at www.FADavis.com.

Access even MORE online at

- Study Questions
- Audio Tutorials and Pronunciations
- Medical Record Activities
- Animations

Just log onto **Davis*Plus*.FADavis.com** today!

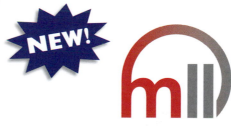

Medical Language Lab
Turning terminology into language

Join the new, interactive online experience!

Build your speaking confidence with **The Medical Language Lab!** Learn the language of medicine as you progress through critical listening, speaking, and writing activities. Look for the access code on the previous page to gain exclusive access today.

www.MedicalLanguageLab.com

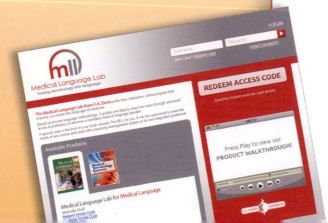

A unique blend of words, art, and technology...

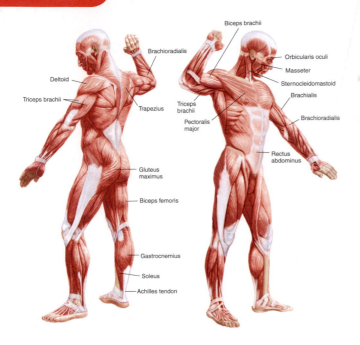

INCREASE YOUR PROFICIENCY

A proven **word-building approach** in the text combined with detailed depictions of the body make every concept crystal clear.

VISUALIZE MUST-KNOW VOCABULARY

Brilliant, **full-color illustrations** and **precise labels** leap from the pages to build your understanding.

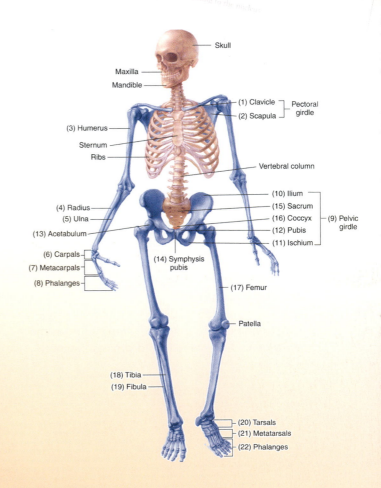

Term*Plus* CD-ROM

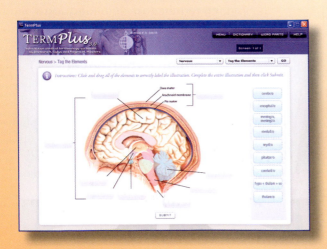

PLAY GAMES

Crossword puzzles, word scrambles, drag-and-drop activities, and much more on the Term*Plus* CD-ROM* make learning fun.

*The Term*Plus* CD-ROM can be purchased separately at www.FADavis.com.

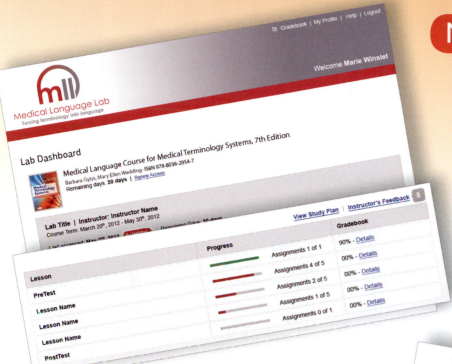

Medical Language Lab

STAY ON TRACK

Progress Bars in **The Medical Language Lab** let you know exactly how many exercises you've completed in each lesson.

STUDY SMART

Your personal **Study Plan** in **The Medical Language Lab** shows you the content areas in which you need to devote the most study time to master the language of medicine.

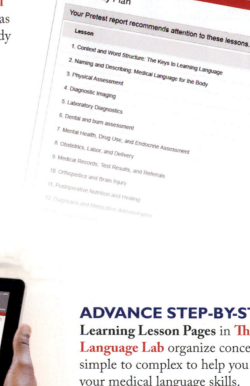

ADVANCE STEP-BY-STEP

Learning Lesson Pages in **The Medical Language Lab** organize concepts from simple to complex to help you develop your medical language skills.

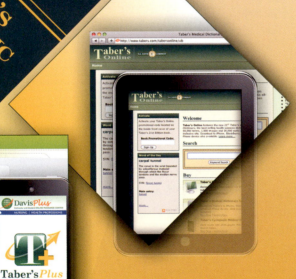
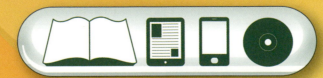
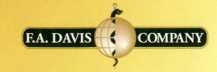

Medical Terminology Systems

A BODY SYSTEMS APPROACH

SEVENTH EDITION

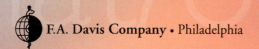

F.A. Davis Company • Philadelphia

Medical Terminology Systems

A BODY SYSTEMS APPROACH

SEVENTH EDITION

Barbara A. Gylys, MEd, CMA-A (AAMA)

Professor Emerita
College of Health and Human Services
Coordinator of Medical Assisting Technology
University of Toledo
Toledo, Ohio

Mary Ellen Wedding, MEd, MT(ASCP), CMA (AAMA), CPC (AAPC)

Professor of Health Education
Judith Herb College of Education, Health
    Science, and Human Service
University of Toledo
Toledo, Ohio

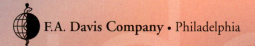

F.A. Davis Company • Philadelphia

F. A. Davis Company
1915 Arch Street
Philadelphia, PA 19103
www.fadavis.com

Printed in the United States of America

Last digit indicates print number: 10 9 8 7 6 5 4 3

Acquisitions Editor: T. Quincy McDonald
Developmental Editor: Brenna Mayer
Manager of Content Development: George Lang
Art and Design Manager: Carolyn O'Brien

As new scientific information becomes available through basic and clinical research, recommended treatments and drug therapies undergo changes. The author(s) and publisher have done everything possible to make this book accurate, up to date, and in accord with accepted standards at the time of publication. The author(s), editors, and publisher are not responsible for errors or omissions or for consequences from application of the book, and make no warranty, expressed or implied, in regard to the contents of the book. Any practice described in this book should be applied by the reader in accordance with professional standards of care used in regard to the unique circumstances that may apply in each situation. The reader is advised always to check product information (package inserts) for changes and new information regarding dose and contraindications before administering any drug. Caution is especially urged when using new or infrequently ordered drugs.

Library of Congress Cataloging-in-Publication Data

Gylys, Barbara A.
  Medical terminology systems : a body systems approach / Barbara A.
Gylys, Mary Ellen Wedding. — 7th ed.
    p. ; cm.
  Includes indexes.
  ISBN 978-0-8036-2954-7
  I. Wedding, Mary Ellen. II. Title.
  [DNLM: 1. Terminology as Topic—Problems and Exercises. W 15]

  610.1'4—dc23
                    2012037210

This Book Is Dedicated with Love

To my best friend, colleague, and husband, Dr. Julius A. Gylys, and to my children, Regina Maria and Dr. Julius Anthony, and to my grandchildren, Andrew Masters, Dr. Julia Halm, Caitlin Masters, Anthony Bishop-Gylys, Matthew Bishop-Gylys, and the little one, Liam Halm

B.A.G.

To my loving grandchildren, Andrew Arthur Kurtz, Katherine Louise Kurtz, Daniel Keith Wedding II, Carol Ann Estelle Wedding, Jonathan Michael Kurtz, Donald Keith Wedding III, Emily Michelle Wedding, Katelyn Christine Wedding, and David Michael Wedding

M.E.W.

Acknowledgments

The authors would like to acknowledge the valuable contributions of F.A. Davis's editorial and production team who were responsible for this project:

- **Quincy McDonald, Senior Acquisitions Editor,** who provided the overall design and layout for the seventh edition. His vision and guidance focused the authors at the onset of the project, and his support throughout this endeavor provided cohesiveness.
- **Brenna H. Mayer, Developmental Editor,** whose careful and conscientious edits and suggestions for the manuscript are evident throughout the entire work. Her enthusiasm and untiring assistance and support during this project are deeply appreciated and the authors extend their sincerest gratitude.
- **George W. Lang, Manager of Content of Development,** who meticulously guided the manuscript through the developmental and production phases of the textbook.
- **Margaret Biblis, Publisher,** once again provided her support and efforts for the quality of the finished product.

In addition, we wish to acknowledge the many exceptionally dedicated publishing partners that helped in this publication:

- Samantha Luceri, Administrative Assistant
- Liz Schaeffer, Ancillary Developmental Editor
- Kate Margeson, Illustrations Coordinator
- Bob Butler, Production Manager
- Carolyn O'Brien, Art and Design Manager
- Linda Van Pelt, Managing Editor
- Kirk Pedrick, Electronic Product Development Manager, Electronic Publishing
- Elizabeth Y. Stepchin, Developmental Associate

We also extend our sincerest appreciation to Neil Kelly, Executive Director of Sales, and his staff of sales representatives whose continued efforts have undoubtedly contributed to the success of this textbook.

Reviewers

The authors extend a special thanks to the clinical reviewers who read and edited the manuscript and provided detailed evaluations and ideas for improving the textbook.

Algie LaKesa Bond, MHA, RHIA, PMP
Clinical Assistant Professor
Health Information Management Program
Temple University
Philadelphia, Pennsylvania

Margaret J. Bower, BS, AMA
Adjunct Instructor
Allied Health Division
Central Pennsylvania College
Summerdale, Pennsylvania

Bonnie L. Deister, EdD, BSN, RN, CMA-C, CLNC
Professor
Medical Assisting Program
College of the Redwoods
Eureka, California

Cynthia Ferguson, RHIT
Instructor
Health Information Technology Program
Texas State Technical College
Sweetwater, Texas

Heather M. Grable, MS, RRT
Online Instructor
Health Sciences Program
Globe Education Network/Minnesota School of
Business and Ivy Tech Community College of Indiana
Greencastle, Indiana

Kim O'Connell-Brock, MS, ATC/L
Director of Clinical Rehabilitation
Human Performance Dance and Recreation Program
New Mexico State University
Las Cruces, New Mexico

Leata Rigg, RN, BScN, MN
Professor
Nursing Program
Northern College of Applied Arts & Technology
Timmins, Ontario, Canada

Wren Stratton, BSN, RN
Instructor
Health Careers Program
Indian Capital Technology Center
Muskogee, Oklahoma

Timothy A. Tolbert, PhD, ATC
Assistant Professor, Clinical Coordinator
Athletic Training Program
Marshall University
Huntington, West Virginia

Preface

As medical terminology educators, we face common challenges. First, we must present a vast amount of fairly complex information to students of various learning levels and abilities. Second, we need to impress upon them the importance of medical terminology as an essential tool of communication in the health-care industry. Finally, we must help them apply what they have learned to the "real world of medicine."

Building on the success of the sixth edition, which received the prestigious McGuffey Longevity and Excellence Award from the Textbook Authors' Association (TAA), *Medical Terminology Systems: A Body Systems Approach,* 7th edition, continues to live up to its well-established track record of presenting medical word-building principles based on competency-based curricula. Because of the pedagogical success of previous editions, the seventh edition continues its structural design as a textbook–workbook that complements all teaching formats, including traditional lecture, distance learning, and independent or self-paced study. The popular, basic features of the previous edition have been enhanced and expanded. The body systems chapters have been updated to include new diagnostic and therapeutic procedures as well as new pharmaceutical agents in current use. Many new, visually impressive, full-color illustrations have been added to this edition. Artwork throughout the book is specifically designed to present accurate and aesthetically pleasing representations of anatomical structures, disease conditions, and medical procedures. Illustrations augment course content in new and interesting ways and help make difficult concepts clear. Two new learning activities have been incorporated in each body-system chapter.

All modifications and additions in the seventh edition are designed to aid in the learning process and improve retention of medical terms. The following is a brief summary of chapter content:

- **Chapter 1** explains the techniques of medical word-building using basic word elements.
- **Chapter 2** categorizes major surgical, diagnostic, symptomatic, and grammatical suffixes.
- **Chapter 3** presents major prefixes of position, number and measurement, direction, and other parameters.
- **Chapter 4** introduces anatomical, physiological, and pathological terms. It also presents combining forms denoting cellular and body structure, body position and direction, regions of the body, and additional combining forms related to diagnostic methods and pathology. General diagnostic and therapeutic terms are described and provide a solid foundation for specific terms addressed in the body-system chapters that follow.
- **Chapters 5 through 16** are organized according to specific body systems and may be taught in any sequence. These chapters include key anatomical and physiological terms; basic anatomy and physiology; a body systems connections table; combining forms, suffixes, and prefixes; pathology; diagnostic, symptomatic, and related terms; diagnostic and therapeutic procedures; pharmacology; abbreviations; learning activities; and medical record

activities. All activities allow self-assessment and evaluation of competency.

- **Appendix A:** The Answer Key contains answers to each learning activity to validate proficiency and provide immediate feedback for student assessment. Although the answer key for the terminology section of each medical record is not included in this appendix, it is available to adopters in the Activity Pack.
- **Appendix B:** Common Abbreviations and Symbols include an updated, comprehensive list of medical abbreviations and their meanings, an updated summary of common symbols, and an updated list of "do-not-use" abbreviations.
- **Appendix C:** The Glossary of Medical Word Elements contains alphabetical lists of medical word elements and their meanings. This appendix presents two methods for word–element indexing—first by medical word element, then by English term.
- **Appendix D:** The Index of Genetic Disorders lists genetic disorders presented in the textbook.
- **Appendix E:** The Index of Clinical, Laboratory, and Imaging Procedures lists radiographic and other diagnostic imaging procedures presented in the textbook.

• **Appendix F:** The Index of Pharmacology lists medications presented in the textbook.

• **Appendix G:** The Index of Oncological Disorders lists oncological disorders presented in the textbook.

Medical Language Lab

Now included in every new copy of *Medical Terminology Systems: A Body Systems Approach*, 7th edition, is access to the ultimate online medical terminology resource for students. The Medical Language Lab is a rich learning environment utilizing proven language development methods to help students become effective users of medical language. To access the Medical Language Lab, students simply go to http://www.medicallanguagelab.com and redeem the access code provided in their new copies of *Medical Terminology Systems: A Body Systems Approach*, 7th edition.

Each lesson in the Medical Language Lab teaches the student how to listen critically for important terms, respond to others using medical terminology, and generate their own terminology-rich writing and speech. By following the activities in each lesson, students graduate from simple memorization to becoming stronger users of medical language.

In addition to critical listening, response, and generation exercises for each lesson, students are supplied with a wide variety of practice activities, which help them to solidify their recall of key terms from the chapter, as well as audio glossary features where students can hear words pronounced and used properly in context.

Designed to work seamlessly with *Medical Terminology Systems: A Body Systems Approach*, 7th edition, each activity in the Medical Language Lab has been crafted with content specific to the textbook. Every chapter in *Medical Terminology Systems: A Body Systems Approach*, 7th edition, has a corresponding lesson in the Medical Language Lab. These pedagogical features help students develop confidence, and every activity on the Medical Language Lab is relevant and useful in helping them understand their textbook.

Instructors benefit from a powerful, yet easy to understand instructor's page, which allows them to decide which chapters and activities will be available to their students. Instructors also control how student scores are reported to them, either through the native Medical Language Lab grade book, or reported to their own BlackBoard, Angel, Moodle, or SCORM-compliant course management solution.

DavisPlus Online Resource Center

Although the study of medical terminology demands hard work and discipline, various self-paced activities offer interest and variety to the learning process. A multiplicity of activities and resources are available to adopters of the textbook on Davis*Plus* Instructor and Student Online Resource Center. The Online Resource Center is designed to help teachers teach and students learn medical terminology in an exciting, challenging, and effective fashion. Visit http://davisplus.fadavis.com for the Instructor and Student Online Resource Center to explore the various ancillaries available for instructors and students.

Instructor Online Resource Center

The Davis*Plus* Instructor Online Resource Center provides many updated, innovative instructional activities. These activities make teaching medical terminology easier and more effective. Teachers can use the supplemental activities in various educational settings—traditional classroom, distance learning, or independent or self-paced studies. The many ancillaries help instructors maximize the benefits of the textbook and include the following:

- Electronic test bank with *ExamView Pro* test-generating software
- PowerPoint presentations for each chapter
- Searchable image bank
- Printable Activity Pack
- Resources in Blackboard, Angel, Moodle, and SCORM formats

Electronic Test Bank

This edition offers a powerful *ExamView Pro* test-generating program that allows you to create custom-made or randomly generated tests in a printable or online format from a test bank of more than 2,500 test items. This expanded test bank contains over twice as many questions as in the previous edition.

PowerPoint Presentations

Bring the book to life in the classroom with the accompanying *Lecture Note* PowerPoint presentations. Each chapter has an outline-based presentation consisting of a chapter overview; main functions of the body system; and selected pathology, vocabulary, and procedures. Full-color illustrations from the book and in-class assessment activities are included.

Image Bank

The image bank contains all illustrations from the textbook. It is fully searchable and allows users to zoom in and out and display a JPG image of an illustration that can be copied into a Microsoft Word document or PowerPoint presentation.

Activity Pack

The Activity Pack has been expanded to meet today's instructional needs and now includes the following:

- *Suggested Course Outlines.* Course outlines are provided to help you plan the best method of covering material presented in the textbook. A newly designed course outline is provided for textbooks packaged with Term*Plus,* the completely revised and updated interactive software. Now it will be easy to correlate instructional software with textbook chapters.
- *Student and Instructor-Directed Activities.* These comprehensive teaching aids have been updated, and new ones have been added for this edition. They offer an assortment of activities for each body-system chapter. Instructors can use these activities as course requirements or supplemental material. In addition, they can assign activities as individual or collaborative projects. For group projects, peer evaluation forms are included.
- *Community and Internet Resources.* This resources section provides an expanded list of resources, including technical journals, community organizations, and Internet sites to complement course content.

- *Supplemental Medical Record Activities.* The supplemental medical record activities have been updated and include student activities that complement and expand information presented in the body-system chapters. As in the textbook, these activities use common clinical scenarios to show how medical terminology is used to document patient care. Medical terms, their pronunciations, and a medical record analysis are provided for each record, along with an answer key. In addition, each medical record highlights a specific body system and correlates it with a medical specialty. Medical records can be used for various activities, including oral reports, medical coding, medical transcribing, or individual assignments.
- *Pronunciations and Answer Keys.* We've continued to provide an answer key for the medical record research activities in the textbook. This key should prove helpful for grading or for class presentations.

Student Online Resource Center

The Davis*Plus* Student Online Resource Center includes many user-friendly activities to help students reinforce material covered in the textbook. At the same time, it is structured to make learning medical terminology an exciting, challenging activity. Resources include medical record activities, audio tutorials, and animations.

Medical Record Activities

Health-care providers in hospitals, medical centers, and private practice facilities dictate various types of medical reports that become part of the medical record. Included are chart notes, history and physical examinations, progress notes, consultation reports, operative reports, discharge summaries, and diagnostic studies. Samples of these types of reports are included in the medical records activities found in the body-system chapters (Chapters 5 to 16). To reinforce these activities, the student online resource center includes a medical records activities section in which the key terms in each report are underlined. As students click the underlined terms, they hear the correct pronunciation of each term. All reports are styled following the guidelines established by the American Association of Medical Transcription (AAMT). This formatting provides an opportunity for students to learn correct styling of various types of medical reports.

Audio Tutorials

The audio tutorials are developed from the "Medical Word Elements" sections of the body-system chapters (Chapters 5 to 16). It is designed to strengthen spelling, pronunciation, and understanding of selected medical terms. In addition to teaching combining forms and pronunciations, it is also useful for students in beginning transcription and medical secretarial courses. They can develop transcription skills by typing each word as it is pronounced. After typing the words, the student can correct spelling by referring to the textbook or a medical dictionary.

Animations

Several animations are included to help students better visualize complex concepts. For example, one animation explores the pathology of gastroesophageal reflux disease (GERD). Another shows the various stages of pregnancy and delivery. These innovative tools help students better understand important processes and procedures as they learn the associated medical terminology.

Other Student Ancillaries
Term*Plus*

Term*Plus* continues to be a powerful, interactive CD-ROM program offered with some texts, depending on the version that has been selected. Term*Plus* is a competency-based, self-paced, multimedia program that includes graphics, audio, and a dictionary culled from *Taber's Cyclopedic Medical Dictionary,* 22nd edition. Help menus provide navigational support. The software comes with numerous interactive learning activities, including:

- Anatomy Focus
- Tag the Elements (drag-and-drop)
- Spotlight the Elements
- Concentration
- Build Medical Words
- Programmed Learning
- Medical Vocabulary
- Chart Notes
- Spelling
- Crossword Puzzles
- Word Scramble

All activities can be graded and the results printed or e-mailed to the instructor. This feature makes Term*Plus* especially valuable as a distance-learning tool, because it provides evidence of student drill and practice completions in various learning activities.

Taber's Cyclopedic Medical Dictionary

The world-famous *Taber's Cyclopedic Medical Dictionary* is the recommended companion reference for this book. Virtually all terms in *Systems* may be found in *Taber's*. In addition, *Taber's* contains etymologies for nearly all main entries presented in this textbook.

We hope you enjoy this new edition as much as we enjoyed preparing it. We think you will find this the best edition ever.

Barbara A. Gylys
Mary Ellen Wedding

Contents at a Glance

Contents

CHAPTER **5**   **Integumentary System**   77

CHAPTER 10   **Musculoskeletal System**   *297*

CHAPTER 13   **Male Reproductive System**   *427*

CHAPTER 14   **Endocrine System**   *459*

Basic Elements of a Medical Word

Objectives

Upon completion of this chapter, you will be able to:

- Identify the four word elements used to build medical words.
- Divide medical words into their component parts.
- Apply the basic rules to define and build medical words.
- Locate the pronunciation guidelines chart and interpret pronunciation marks.
- Pronounce medical terms presented in this chapter.
- Demonstrate your knowledge of this chapter by completing the learning activities.

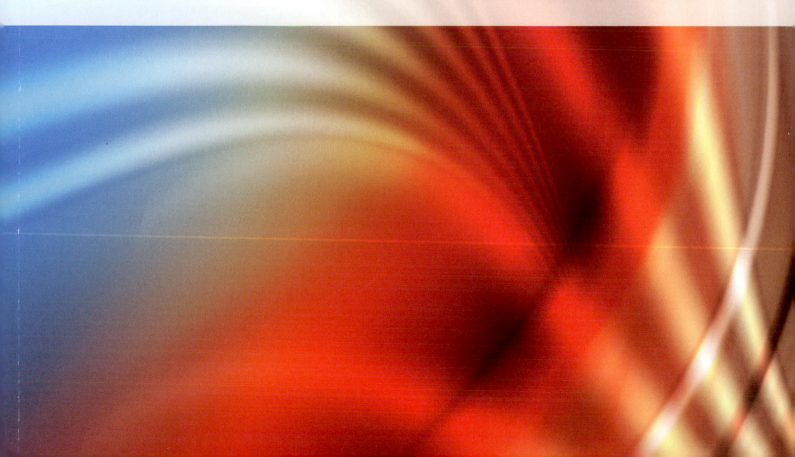

Medical Word Elements

The language of medicine is a specialized vocabulary used by health care providers. Many current medical word elements originated as early as the 4th century B.C., when Hippocrates practiced medicine. With technological and scientific advancements in medicine, new terms have evolved to reflect these innovations. For example, radiographic terms, such as magnetic resonance imaging (MRI) and ultrasound (US), are now commonly used to describe current diagnostic procedures.

A medical word consists of some or all of the following elements:

• word root
• combining form
• suffix
• prefix

How these elements are combined, and whether all or some of them are present in a medical term, determines the meaning of a word. To understand the meaning of medical words, it is important to learn how to divide them into their basic elements. The purpose of this chapter is to cover the basic principles of medical word building and learn how to pronounce the terms correctly. Thus, pronunciations are provided throughout the textbook with the medical terms. In addition, pronunciation guidelines are located on the inside front cover of this book. They can be used as a convenient reference to help pronounce terms correctly.

Word Roots

A **word root** is the foundation of a medical term and contains its primary meaning. All medical terms have at least one word root. Most word roots are derived from Greek or Latin language. Thus, two different roots may have the same meaning. For example, the Greek word *dermatos* and the Latin word *cutane* both refer to the skin. As a general rule, Greek roots are used to build words that describe a disease, condition, treatment, or diagnosis. Latin roots are used to build words that describe anatomical structures. Consequently, the Greek root *dermat* is used primarily in terms that describe a disease, condition, treatment, or diagnosis of the skin; the Latin root *cutane* is used primarily to describe an anatomical structure. (See Table 1-1.)

Table I-I	Examples of Word Roots		

This table lists examples of word roots as well as their phonetic pronunciations. Begin learning the pronunciations as you review the information below.

English Term	Greek or Latin Term*	Word Root	Word Analysis
skin	dermatos (Gr)	dermat	**dermat**/itis (dĕr-mă-TĪ-tĭs): inflammation of the skin *A term that identifies a skin disease*
	cutis (L)	cutane	**cutane**/ous (kū-TĀ-nē-ŭs): pertaining to the skin *A term that identifies an anatomical structure*
kidney	nephros (Gr)	nephr	**nephr**/oma (nĕ-FRŌ-mă): tumor of the kidney *A term that describes a kidney disease*
	renes (L)	ren	**ren**/al (RĒ-năl): pertains to the kidney *A term that identifies an anatomical structure*

Table 1-1	Examples of Word Roots—cont'd			
English Term	**Greek or Latin Term***	**Word Root**	**Word Analysis**	
mouth	stomatos (Gr)	stomat	**stomat**/itis (stō-mă-TĪ-tĭs): inflammation of the mouth *A term that describes an inflammatory condition of the mouth*	
	oris (L)	or	**or**/al (OR-ăl): pertaining to the mouth *A term that identifies an anatomical structure*	

*It is not important to know the origin of a medical word. This information is provided here to help avoid confusion and illustrate that there may be two different word roots for a single term.

Combining Forms

A **combining form** is created when a word root is combined with a vowel. The vowel, known as a **combining vowel**, is usually an *o*, but sometimes it is an *i*. The combining vowel has no meaning of its own but enables two or more word elements to be connected. Like a word root, a combining form is the basic foundation to which other word elements are added to build a complete medical word. In this text, a combining form will be listed as *word root/vowel* (such as *gastr/o*), as illustrated in Table 1-2.

Table 1-2	Examples of Combining Forms				
*This table illustrates how word roots and vowels create combining forms. Learning combining forms rather than word roots makes pronunciations a little easier because of the terminal vowel. For example, in the table below, the word roots **gastr** and **nephr** are difficult to pronounce, whereas their combining forms **gastr/o** and **nephr/o** are easier to pronounce.*					
Word Root	**+**	**Vowel**	**=**	**Combining Form**	**Meaning**
erythr/	+	o	=	erythr/o	red
gastr/	+	o	=	gastr/o	stomach
hepat/	+	o	=	hepat/o	liver
immun/	+	o	=	immun/o	immune, immunity, safe
nephr/	+	o	=	nephr/o	kidney
oste/	+	o	=	oste/o	bone

Suffixes

A **suffix** is a word element placed at the end of a word that changes the meaning of the word. In the terms tonsill/*itis*, and tonsill/*ectomy*, the suffixes are *-itis* (inflammation) and *-ectomy* (excision, removal). Changing the suffix changes the meaning of the word. In medical terminology, a suffix usually describes a pathology (disease or abnormality), symptom, surgical or diagnostic procedure, or part of speech. Many suffixes are derived from Greek or Latin words. (See Table 1-3.)

Table 1-3	**Examples of Suffixes**

This table lists examples of pathological suffixes as well as their phonetic pronunciations. Begin learning the pronunciations as you review the information below.

Combining Form	+	Suffix	=	Medical Word	Meaning
	+	-itis (inflammation)	=	gastritis găs-TRĪ-tĭs	inflammation of the stomach
gastr/o (stomach)	+	-megaly (enlargement)	=	gastromegaly găs-trō-MĔG-ă-lē	enlargement of the stomach
	+	-oma (tumor)	=	gastroma găs-TRŌ-mă	tumor of the stomach
	+	-itis (inflammation)	=	hepatitis hĕp-ă-TĪ-tĭs	inflammation of the liver
hepat/o (liver)	+	-megaly (enlargement)	=	hepatomegaly hĕp-ă-tō-MĔG-ă-lē	enlargement of the liver
	+	-oma (tumor)	=	hepatoma hĕp-ă-TŌ-mă	tumor of the liver

Prefixes

A **prefix** is a word element attached to the beginning of a word or word root. However, not all medical terms have a prefix. Adding or changing a prefix changes the meaning of the word. The prefix usually indicates a number, time, position, direction, or negation. Many of the same prefixes used in medical terminology are also used in the English language. (See Table 1-4.)

Table 1-4	**Examples of Prefixes**

This table lists examples of prefixes as well as their phonetic pronunciations. Begin learning the pronunciations as you review the information below.

Prefix	+	Word Root	+	Suffix	=	Medical Word	Meaning
an- (without, not)	+	esthes (feeling)	+	-ia (condition)	=	anesthesia ăn-ĕs-THĒ-zē-ă	condition of not feeling
hyper- (excessive, above normal)	+	therm (heat)	+	-ia (condition)	=	hyperthermia hī-pĕr-THĔR-mē-ă	condition of excessive heat
intra- (in, within)	+	muscul (muscle)	+	-ar (pertaining to)	=	intramuscular ĭn-tră-MŬS-kū-lăr	pertaining to within the muscle
para- (near, beside; beyond)	+	nas (nose)	+	-al (pertaining to)	=	paranasal păr-ă-NĀ-săl	pertaining to (area) near the nose
poly- (many, much)	+	ur (urine)	+	-ia (condition)	=	polyuria pŏl-ē-Ū-rē-ă	condition of much urine
pre- (before)	+	nat (birth)	+	-al (pertaining to)	=	prenatal prē-NĀ-tăl	pertaining to (the period) before birth

Basic Guidelines

Defining and building medical words are crucial skills in mastering medical terminology. Following the basic guidelines for each will help you develop these skills.

Defining Medical Words

Here are three steps for defining medical words using gastroenteritis as an example.

- **Step 1.** Define the suffix, or last part of the word. In this case, the suffix *–itis* means *inflammation.*
- **Step 2.** Define the first part of the word (which may be a word root, combining form, or prefix). In this case, the combining form *gastr/o* means *stomach.*
- **Step 3.** Define the middle parts of the word. In this case, the word root *enter* means *intestine.*

When you analyze **gastroenteritis** following the three previous rules, the meaning is:

1. inflammation (of)
2. stomach (and)
3. intestine.

Thus, the meaning of **gastroenteritis** is *inflammation (of) stomach (and) intestine.* Table 1-5 further illustrates this process.

Table 1-5	**Defining Gastroenteritis**	
This table illustrates the three steps of defining a medical word using the example gastroenteritis.		
Combining Form	**Middle**	**Suffix**
gastr/o	enter/	-itis
stomach	intestine	inflammation
(step 2)	(step 3)	(step 1)

Building Medical Words

There are three basic rules for building medical words.

Rule #1

A word root links a suffix that begins with a vowel.

Word Root	**+**	**Suffix**	**=**	**Medical Word**	**Meaning**
hepat	+	-itis	=	hepatitis	inflammation of the liver
(liver)		(inflammation)		hĕp-ă-TĪ-tĭs	

Rule #2

A combining form (root + o) links a suffix that begins with a consonant.

Combining Form	+	Suffix	=	Medical Word	Meaning
hepat/o (liver)	+	-cyte (cell)	=	hepatocyte HĔP-ă-tō-sīt	liver cell

Rule #3

A combining form links one root to another root to form a compound word. This rule holds true even if the second root begins with a vowel, as in **osteoarthritis**. Keep in mind that the rules for linking multiple roots to each other are slightly different from the rules for linking roots and combining forms to suffixes.

Combining Form	+	Word Root	+	Suffix	=	Medical Word	Meaning
oste/o (bone)	+	chondr (cartilage)	+	-itis (inflammation)	=	osteochondritis ŏs-tē-ō-kŏn-DRĪ-tĭs	inflammation of bone and cartilage
	+	arthr (joint)	+	-itis (inflammation)	=	osteoarthritis ŏs-tē-ō-ăr-THRĪ-tĭs	inflammation of bone and joint

 It is time to review medical word elements by completing Learning Activities 1–1 and 1–2 on page 7–8.

Pronunciation Guidelines

Although pronunciation of medical words usually follows the same rules that govern pronunciations of English words, some medical words may be difficult to pronounce when first encountered. Therefore, selected terms in this book include phonetic pronunciation. Also, pronunciation guidelines can be found on the inside back cover of this book and at the end of selected tables. Use them whenever you need help with pronunciation of medical words.

 It is time to review pronunciations, analysis of word elements, and defining medical terms by completing Learning Activities 1–3, 1–4, and 1–5 on page 9–12.

LEARNING ACTIVITIES

The following activities provide a review of the basic medical word elements introduced in this chapter. Complete each activity and review your answers to evaluate your understanding of this chapter.

Learning Activity 1-1
Understanding Medical Word Elements

Fill in the following blanks to complete the sentences correctly.

1. The four elements used to form words are _____.

2. A root is the main part or foundation of a word. In the words arthritis, arthrectomy, and arthroscope, the root is _____.

Identify the following statements as true or false. If false, rewrite the statement correctly on the line provided.

3. A combining vowel is usually an e.	True	False
4. A word root links a suffix that begins with a consonant.	True	False
5. A combining form links multiple roots to each other.	True	False
6. A combining form links a suffix that begins with a consonant.	True	False
7. To define a medical word, first define the prefix.	True	False
8. In the term *intramuscular, intra* is the prefix.	True	False

Underline the word root in each of following combining forms.

9. splen/o (spleen)

10. hyster/o (uterus)

11. enter/o (intestine)

12. neur/o (nerve)

13. ot/o (ear)

14. dermat/o (skin)

15. hydr/o (water)

✓ *Check your answers in Appendix A. Review material that you did not answer correctly.*

Correct Answers _____ X 6.67 = _____ % Score

Learning Activity 1-2
Identifying Word Roots and Combining Forms

Underline the word roots in the following medical words.

Medical Word   Meaning

1. nephritis   inflammation of the kidney

2. arthrodesis   fixation of a joint

3. dermatitis   inflammation of the skin

4. dentist   specialist in teeth

5. gastrectomy   excision of the stomach

6. chondritis   inflammation of cartilage

7. hepatoma   tumor of the liver

8. muscular   pertaining to muscle

9. gastric   pertaining to the stomach

10. osteoma   tumor of the bone

Underline the combining forms below.

11. nephr   kidney

12. hepat/o   liver

13. arthr   joint

14. oste/o/arthr   bone, joint

15. cholangi/o   bile vessel

Check your answers in Appendix A. Review material that you did not answer correctly.

Correct Answers _____ X 6.67 = _____ % Score

Learning Activity 1-3
Understanding Pronunciations

Review the pronunciation guidelines (located inside the front cover of this book) and then underline the correct answer in each of the following statements.

1. The diacritical mark ¯ is called a (breve, macron).

2. The diacritical mark ˘ is called a (breve, macron).

3. The ¯ indicates the (short, long) sound of vowels.

4. The ˘ indicates the (short, long) sound of vowels.

5. The combination *ch* is sometimes pronounced like (k, chiy). Examples are *cholesterol, cholemia.*

6. When *pn* is at the beginning of a word, it is pronounced only with the sound of (p, n). Examples are *pneumonia, pneumotoxin.*

7. When *pn* is in middle of a word, the *p* (is, is not) pronounced. Examples are *orthopnea, hyperpnea.*

8. When *i* is at the end of a word, it is pronounced like (eye, ee). Examples are *bronchi, fungi, nuclei.*

9. For *ae* and *oe*, only the (first, second) vowel is pronounced. Examples are *bursae, pleurae.*

10. When *e* and *es* form the final letter or letters of a word, they are commonly pronounced as (combined, separate) syllables. Examples are *syncope, systole, nares.*

Check your answers in Appendix A. Review material that you did not answer correctly.

Correct Answers _____ X 10 = _____ % Score

Learning Activity 1-4
Identifying Suffixes and Prefixes

Pronounce the following medical terms. Then analyze each term and write the suffix in the right-hand column. The first suffix is completed for you.

Term	Suffix
1. thoracotomy thōr-ă-KŎT-ō-mē	*-tomy*
2. gastroscope GĂS-trō-skōp	
3. tonsillitis tŏn-sĭl-Ī-tĭs	
4. gastric GĂS-trĭk	
5. tonsillectomy tŏn-sĭl-ĔK-tō-mē	

Pronunciation Help	Long Sound	ā — rate	ē — rebirth	ī — isle	ō — over	ū — unite
	Short Sound	ă — alone	ĕ — ever	ĭ — it	ŏ — not	ŭ — cut

Pronounce the following medical terms. Then analyze each term and write the element that is a prefix in the right-hand column. The first prefix is completed for you.

Term	Prefix
6. anesthesia ăn-ĕs-THĒ-zē-ă	*an-*
7. hyperthermia hī-pĕr-THĔR-mē-ă	
8. intramuscular ĭn-tră-MŬS-kū-lăr	
9. paranasal păr-ă-NĀ-săl	
10. polyuria pŏl-ē-Ū-rē-ă	

Check your answers in Appendix A. Review material that you did not answer correctly.

Correct Answers _____ X 10 = _____ % Score

Defining Medical Words

The three steps for defining medical words are:

1. Define the last part of the word, or **suffix**.

2. Define the first part of the word, or **prefix, word root,** or **combining form**.

3. Define the **middle** of the word.

First, pronounce the term aloud. Then apply the above three steps to define the terms in the following table. If you are not certain of a definition, refer to Appendix C, Part 1, of this textbook, which provides an alphabetical list of word elements and their meanings.

Term	Definition
1. gastritis găs-TRĪ-tĭs	_____
2. nephritis nĕf-RĪ-tĭs	_____
3. gastrectomy găs-TRĔK-tō-mē	_____
4. osteoma ŏs-tē-Ō-mă	_____
5. hepatoma hĕp-ă-TŌ-mă	_____
6. hepatitis hĕp-ă-TĪ-tĭs	_____

Refer to the section "Building Medical Words" on pages 5-6 to complete this activity. Write the number for the rule that applies to each listed term as well as a short summary of the rule. Use the abbreviation WR to designate *word root*, CF to designate *combining form*. The first one is completed for you.

Term	Rule	Summary of the Rule
7. arthr/itis ăr-THRĪ-tĭs	1	*A WR links a suffix that begins with a vowel.*
8. scler/osis sklĕ-RŌ-sĭs	____	_____
9. arthr/o/centesis ăr-thrō-sĕn-TĒ-sĭs	____	_____
10. colon/o/scope kō-LŎN-ō-skōp	____	_____
11. chondr/itis kŏn-DRĪ-tĭs	____	_____

12. chondr/oma   _____   _____
    kŏn-DRŌ-mă

13. oste/o/chondr/itis   _____   _____
    ŏs-tē-ō-kŏn-DRĪ-tĭs

14. muscul/ar   _____   _____
    MŬS-kū-lăr

15. oste/o/arthr/itis   _____   _____
    ŏs-tē-ō-ăr-THRĪ-tĭs

✔ *Check your answers in Appendix A. Review material that you did not answer correctly.*

Correct Answers _____ X 6.67 = _____ % Score

Suffixes

Chapter Outline

Objectives
Suffix Linking
Suffix Types
    Surgical, Diagnostic, Pathological, and Related Suffixes
    Grammatical Suffixes
    Plural Suffixes
Learning Activities

Objectives

Upon completion of this chapter, you will be able to:

- Define and provide examples of surgical, diagnostic, pathological, and related suffixes.
- Link combining forms and word roots to suffixes.
- Identify surgical, diagnostic, pathological, and related suffixes.
- Identify adjective, noun, and diminutive suffixes.
- Locate and apply guidelines for pluralizing terms.
- Pronounce medical terms presented in this chapter.
- Demonstrate your knowledge of the chapter by completing the learning activities.

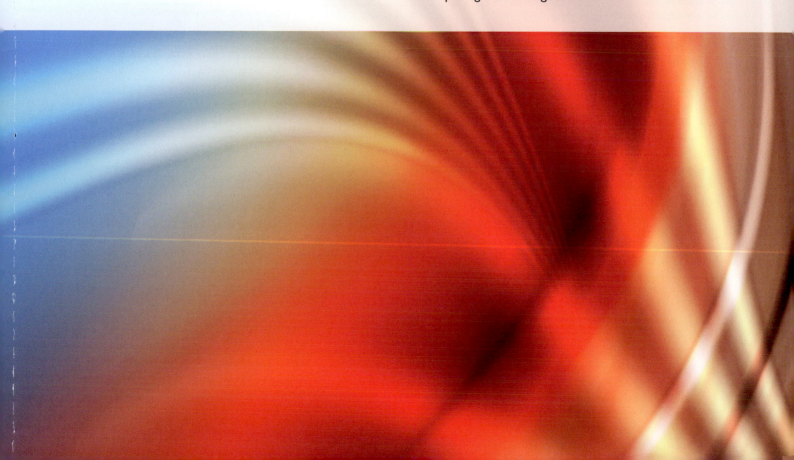

Suffix Linking

In medical words, a suffix is added to the end of a word root or combining form to change its meaning. For example, the combining form *gastr/o* means *stomach*. The suffix *-megaly* means *enlargement*, and *-itis* means *inflammation*. *Gastr/o/megaly* is an enlargement of the stomach. *Gastr/itis* is an inflammation of the stomach.

Whenever you change the suffix, you change the meaning of the word. Suffixes are also used to denote singular and plural forms of a word as well as a part of speech. The following tables provide additional examples to reinforce the rules you learned in Chapter 1. (See Tables 2-1 and 2-2.)

Words that contain more than one word root are known as **compound words.** Multiple roots within a compound word are joined together with a vowel, regardless of whether the second root begins with a vowel or a consonant. Notice that a vowel is used in Table 2-2 between **gastr** and **enter,** even though the second root, **enter,** begins with a vowel.

Keep in mind that the rule for linking multiple roots is slightly different from the rules for linking roots to suffixes. As reinforced from examples in the above table, suffixes that begin

Table 2-1	**Word Roots and Combining Forms With Suffixes**				

This table provides examples of word roots linking a suffix that begins with a vowel. It also provides examples of combining forms (root + o) linking a suffix that begins with a consonant.

Element	+	Suffix	=	Medical Word	Meaning
Word Roots					
gastr (stomach)	+	-itis (inflammation)	=	gastritis găs-TRĪ-tĭs	inflammation of the stomach
hemat (blood)	+	-emesis (vomiting)	=	hematemesis hĕm-ăt-ĔM-ĕ-sĭs	vomiting blood
arthr (joint)	+	-itis (inflammation)	=	arthritis ăr-THRĪ-tĭs	inflammation of a joint
Combining Forms					
gastr/o (stomach)	+	-dynia (pain)	=	gastrodynia găs-trō-DĬN-ē-ă	pain in the stomach
hemat/o (blood)	+	-logy (study of)	=	hematology hē-mă-TŎL-ō-jē	study of blood
arthr/o (joint)	+	-centesis (surgical puncture)	=	arthrocentesis ăr-thrō-sĕn-TĒ-sĭs	surgical puncture of a joint

Table 2-2	**Compound Words With Suffixes**					

This table provides examples of medical terms with more than one word root as well as suffixes linked together with roots when the suffix begins with a vowel.

Combining Form	+	Word Root	+	Suffix	=	Medical Word	Meaning
gastr/o (stomach)	+	enter (intestine)	+	-itis (inflammation)	=	gastroenteritis găs-trō-ĕn-tĕr-Ī-tĭs	inflammation of stomach and intestine
oste/o (bone)	+	arthr (joint)	+	-itis (inflammation)	=	osteoarthritis ŏs-tē-ō-ăr-THRĪ-tĭs	inflammation of bone and joint
encephal/o (brain)	+	mening (meninges)	+	-itis (inflammation)	=	encephalomeningitis ĕn-sĕf-ă-lō-mĕn-ĭn-JĪ-tĭs	inflammation of brain and meninges

with a vowel are linked with a root; suffixes that begin with a consonant are linked with a combining form.

Suffix Types

An effective method in mastering medical terminology is to learn the major types of suffixes in categories. By grouping the surgical, diagnostic, pathological, related, and grammatical suffixes, they will be easier to remember.

Surgical, Diagnostic, Pathological, and Related Suffixes

Surgical suffixes describe a type of invasive procedure performed on a body part. (See Table 2-3.) Diagnostic suffixes describe a procedure performed to identify the cause and nature of an illness. Pathological suffixes describe an abnormal condition or disease. (See Table 2-4.)

Table 2-3	Common Surgical Suffixes

This table lists commonly used surgical suffixes along with their meanings and word analyses.

Suffix	Meaning	Word Analysis
-centesis	surgical puncture	arthr/o/**centesis** (ăr-thrō-sĕn-TĒ-sĭs): puncture of a joint space with a needle and the withdrawal of fluid *arthr/o:* joint *Arthrocentesis may also be performed to obtain samples of synovial fluid for diagnostic purposes, instill medications, and remove fluid from joints to relieve pain.*
-clasis	to break; surgical fracture	oste/o/**clasis** (ŏs-tē-ŎK-lă-sĭs): surgical fracture of a bone to correct a deformity *oste/o:* bone
-desis	binding, fixation (of a bone or joint)	arthr/o/**desis** (ăr-thrō-DĒ-sĭs): binding together of a joint *arthr/o:* joint *Arthrodesis fuses bones across the joint space in a degenerated, unstable joint.*
-ectomy	excision, removal	append/**ectomy** (ăp-ĕn-DĔK-tō-mē): excision of the appendix *append:* appendix
-lysis	separation; destruction; loosening	thromb/o/**lysis** (thrŏm-BŎL-ĭ-sĭs): destruction of a blood clot *thromb/o:* blood clot *Drug therapy is usually used to dissolve a blood clot.*
-pexy	fixation (of an organ)	mast/o/**pexy** (MĂS-tō-pĕks-ē): fixation of the breast(s) *mast/o:* breast *Mastopexy, an elective surgery, affixes sagging breasts in a more elevated position, commonly improving their shape.*
-plasty	surgical repair	rhin/o/**plasty** (RĪ-nō-plăs-tē): surgical repair of the nose *rhin/o:* nose *Rhinoplastic is a type of plastic surgery that changes the size or shape of the nose.*
-rrhaphy	suture	my/o/**rrhaphy** (mī-OR-ă-fē): suture of a muscle *my/o:* muscle

(continued)

Table 2-3	Common Surgical Suffixes—cont'd		
Suffix	**Meaning**	**Word Analysis**	
-stomy	forming an opening (mouth)	trache/o/**stomy** (tră-kē-ŎS-tō-mē): forming an opening into the trachea 　*trache/o:* trachea (windpipe) *A tracheostomy is an artificial opening created to bypass an obstructed upper airway.*	
-tome	instrument to cut	oste/o/**tome** (ŎS-tē-ō-tōm): instrument to cut bone 　*oste/o:* bone *An osteotome is a surgical chisel used to cut through bone.*	
-tomy	incision	trache/o/**tomy** (tră-kē-ŎT-ō-mē): incision (through the neck) into the trachea 　*trache/o:* trachea (windpipe) *Tracheotomy is performed to gain access to an airway below a blockage.*	
-tripsy	crushing	lith/o/**tripsy** (LĬTH-ō-trĭp-sē): crushing a stone 　*lith/o:* stone, calculus *Lithotripsy is a surgical procedure for eliminating a stone in the kidney, ureter, bladder, or gallbladder.*	

It is time to review surgical suffixes by completing Learning Activities 2–1, 2–2, and 2–3.

Table 2-4	Diagnostic, Pathological, and Related Suffixes		
This table lists commonly used diagnostic, pathological, and related suffixes along with their meanings and word analyses.			
Suffix	**Meaning**	**Word Analysis**	
Diagnostic			
-gram	record, writing	electr/o/cardi/o/**gram** (ē-lĕk-trō-KĂR-dē-ō-grăm): record of the electrical activity of the heart 　*electr/o:* electricity 　*cardi/o:* heart	
-graph	instrument for recording	cardi/o/**graph** (KĂR-dē-ō-grăf): instrument for recording electrical activity of the heart 　*cardi/o:* heart	
-graphy	process of recording	angi/o/**graphy** (ăn-jē-ŎG-ră-fē): process of recording blood vessels 　*angi/o:* vessel (usually blood or lymph) *Angiography is the radiographic imaging of blood vessels after injection of a contrast medium.*	
-meter	instrument for measuring	**pelv/i/meter*** (pĕl-VĬM-ĕ-ter): instrument for measuring the pelvis 　*pelv/i:* pelvis	
-metry	act of measuring	pelv/i/**metry*** (pĕl-VĬM-ĕ-trē): act or process of measuring the dimensions of the pelvis 　*pelv/i:* pelvis	

*The *i* in *pelv/i/meter* and *pelv/i/metry* and the *e* in *chol/e/lithiasis* and *chol/e/lith* are exceptions to the rule of using the connecting vowel *o.*

Table 2-4	Diagnostic, Pathological, and Related Suffixes—cont'd	
Suffix	**Meaning**	**Word Analysis**
-scope	instrument for examining	endo/**scope** (ĔN-dō-skōp): instrument for examining within *endo-*: in, within *An endoscope is a flexible or rigid instrument consisting of a tube and optical system for observing the inside of a hollow organ or cavity.*
-scopy	visual examination	endo/**scopy** (ĕn-DŎS-kō-pē): visual examination within *endo-*: in, within *Endoscopy is performed to visualize a body cavity or canal using a specialized lighted instrument called an endoscope.*
Pathological and Related		
-algia	pain	neur/**algia** (nū-RĂL-jē-ă): pain of a nerve *neur*: nerve *The pain of neuralgia usually occurs along the path of a nerve.*
-dynia		ot/o/**dynia** (ō-tō-DĬN-ē-ă): pain in the ear; also called earache *ot/o*: ear
-cele	hernia, swelling	hepat/o/**cele** (hĕ-PĂT-ō-sēl): hernia of the liver *hepat/o*: liver
-ectasis	dilation, expansion	bronchi/**ectasis** (brŏng-kē-ĔK-tă-sĭs): dilation or expansion of one or more bronchi *bronchi*: bronchus (plural, bronchi) *Bronchiectasis is associated with various lung conditions and is commonly accompanied by chronic infection.*
-edema	swelling	lymph/**edema** (lĭmf-ĕ-DĒ-mă): swelling and accumulation of tissue fluid *lymph*: lymph *Lymphedema may be caused by a blockage of the lymph vessels.*
-emesis	vomiting	hyper/**emesis** (hī-pĕr-ĔM-ĕ-sĭs): excessive vomiting *hyper-*: excessive, above normal
-emia	blood condition	an/**emia** (ă-NĒ-mē-ă): blood condition caused by a decrease in red blood cells (erythrocytes) *an-*: without, not
-gen	forming, producing, origin	carcin/o/**gen** (kăr-SĬN-ō-jĕn): forming, producing, or origin of cancer *carcin/o*: cancer *A carcinogen is a substance or agent, such as a cigarette, that causes the development or increases the incidence of cancer.*
-genesis		carcin/o/**genesis** (kăr-sĭ-nō-JĔN-ĕ-sĭs): forming, producing, or origin of cancer *carcin/o*: cancer *Carcinogenesis is the transformation of normal cells into cancer cells, commonly as a result of chemical, viral, or radioactive damage to genes.*

(continued)

Table 2-4	Diagnostic, Pathological, and Related Suffixes—cont'd

Suffix	Meaning	Word Analysis
-iasis	abnormal condition (produced by something specified)	chol/e/lith/iasis* (kō-lē-lĭ-THĪ-ă-sĭs): abnormal condition of gallstones *chol/e:* bile, gall *lith:* stone, calculus *Cholelithasis is the presence or formation of gallstones in the gallbladder or common bile duct.*
-itis	inflammation	gastr/itis (găs-TRĪ-tĭs): inflammation of the stomach *gastr:* stomach
-lith	stone, calculus	chol/e/lith* (KŌ-lē-lĭth): gallstone *chol/e:* bile, gall
-malacia	softening	chondr/o/malacia (kŏn-drō-măl-Ā-shē-ă): softening of the articular cartilage, usually involving the patella *chondr/o:* cartilage
-megaly	enlargement	cardi/o/megaly (kăr-dē-ō-MĔG-ă-lē): enlargement of the heart *cardi/o:* heart
-oma	tumor	neur/oma (nū-RŌ-mă): tumor composed of nerve tissue *neur:* nerve *A neuroma is a benign tumor composed chiefly of neurons and nerve fibers, usually arising from nerve tissue. It may also be a swelling of a nerve that usually results from compression.*
-osis	abnormal condition; increase (used primarily with blood cells)	cyan/osis (sī-ă-NŌ-sĭs): dark blue or purple discoloration of the skin and mucous membrane *cyan:* blue *Cyanosis indicates a deficiency of oxygen in the blood.*
-pathy	disease	my/o/pathy (mī-ŎP-ă-thē): disease of muscle *my/o:* muscle
-penia	decrease, deficiency	erythr/o/penia (ĕ-rĭth-rō-PĒ-nē-ă): decrease in red blood cells *erythr/o:* red
-phagia	eating, swallowing	dys/phagia (dĭs-FĀ-jē-ă): inability or difficulty in swallowing *dys-:* bad; painful; difficult
-phasia	speech	a/phasia (ă-FĀ-zē-ă): absence or impairment of speech *a-:* without, not
-phobia	fear	hem/o/phobia (hē-mō-FŌ-bē-ă): fear of blood *hem/o:* blood
-plasia	formation, growth	dys/plasia (dĭs-PLĀ-zē-ă): abnormal formation or growth of cells, tissues, or organs *dys-:* bad; painful; difficult *Dysplasia is a general term for abnormal formation of an anatomic structure.*

Table 2-4	**Diagnostic, Pathological, and Related Suffixes—cont'd**	
Suffix	**Meaning**	**Word Analysis**
-plasm		neo/**plasm** (NĒ-ō-plăzm): new formation or growth of tissue *neo-*: new *A neoplasm is an abnormal formation of new tissue, such as a tumor or growth.*
-plegia	paralysis	hemi/**plegia** (hĕm-ē-PLĒ-jē-ă): paralysis of one side of the body *hemi-*: one half *Hemiplegia affects the right or left side of the body and is usually caused by a brain injury or stroke.*
-ptosis	prolapse, downward displacement	blephar/o/**ptosis** (blĕf-ă-rō-TŌ-sĭs): drooping of the upper eyelid *blephar/o*: eyelid
-rrhage	bursting forth (of)	hem/o/**rrhage** (HĔM-ĕ-rĭj): bursting forth (of) blood *hem/o*: blood *Hemorrhage refers to a loss of a large amount of blood within a short period, either externally or internally.*
-rrhagia		men/o/**rrhagia** (mĕn-ō-RĀ-jē-ă): profuse discharge of blood during menstruation *men/o*: menses, menstruation
-rrhea	discharge, flow	dia/**rrhea** (dī-ă-RĒ-ă): abnormally frequent discharge or flow of fluid fecal matter from the bowel *dia-*: through, across
-rrhexis	rupture	arteri/o/**rrhexis** (ăr-tē-rē-ō-RĔK-sĭs): rupture of an artery *arteri/o*: artery
-sclerosis	abnormal condition of hardening	arteri/o/**sclerosis** (ăr-tē-rē-ō-sklĕ-RŌ-sĭs): abnormal condition of hardening of an artery *arteri/o*: artery
-spasm	involuntary contraction, twitching	blephar/o/**spasm** (BLĔF-ă-rō-spăsm): twitching of the eyelid *blephar/o*: eyelid
-stenosis	narrowing, stricture	arteri/o/**stenosis** (ăr-tē-rē-ō-stĕ-NŌ-sĭs): abnormal narrowing of an artery *arteri/o*: artery
-toxic	poison	hepat/o/**toxic** (HĔP-ă-tō-tŏk-sĭk): pertaining to an agent (poison) that damages the liver *hepat/o*: liver *Alcohol and drugs are examples of agents that have destructive effects on the liver.*
-trophy	nourishment, development	dys/**trophy** (DĬS-trō-fē): bad nourishment *dys-*: bad; painful; difficult *Dystrophy is an abnormal condition caused by improper nutrition or altered metabolism.*

It is time to review diagnostic, pathological, and related suffixes by completing Learning Activities 2–4 and 2–5.

Grammatical Suffixes

Grammatical suffixes are attached to word roots to form parts of speech, such as adjectives and nouns. They are also used to denote a diminutive form, or smaller version, of a word—for example, *tubule*, which means a small tube. Many of these same suffixes are used in the English language. (See Table 2-5.)

Table 2-5	Adjective, Noun, and Diminutive Suffixes

This table lists adjective, noun, and diminutive suffixes along with their meanings and word analyses.

Suffix	Meaning	Word Analysis
Adjective		
-ac	pertaining to	cardi/**ac** (KĂR-dē-ăk): pertaining to the heart *cardi*: heart
-al		neur/**al** (NŪ-răl): pertaining to a nerve *neur*: nerve
-ar		muscul/**ar** (MŬS-kū-lăr): pertaining to muscle *muscul*: muscle
-ary		pulmon/**ary** (PŬL-mō-nĕr-ē): pertaining to the lungs *pulmon*: lung
-eal		esophag/**eal** (ē-sŏf-ă-JĒ-ăl): pertaining to the esophagus *esophag*: esophagus
-ic		thorac/**ic** (thō-RĂS-ĭk): pertaining to the chest *thorac*: chest
-ical*		path/o/log/**ical** (păth-ō-LŎJ-ĭ-kăl): pertaining to the study of disease *path/o*: disease *log*: study of
-ile		pen/**ile** (PĒ-nīl): pertaining to the penis *pen*: penis
-ior		poster/**ior** (pŏs-TĒ-rē-or): pertaining to the back of the body *poster*: back (of body), behind, posterior
-ous		cutane/**ous** (kū-TĀ-nē-ŭs): pertaining to the skin *cutane*: skin
-tic		acous/**tic** (ă-KOOS-tĭk): pertaining to hearing *acous*: hearing
Noun		
-esis	condition	di/ur/**esis** (dī-ū-RĒ-sĭs): abnormal secretion of large amounts of urine *di-*: double *ur*: urine
-ia		pneumon/**ia** (nū-MŌ-nē-ă): infection of the lung usually caused by bacteria, viruses, or diseases *pneumon*: air; lung
-ism		hyper/thyroid/**ism** (hī-pĕr-THĪ-royd-ĭzm): condition characterized by overactivity of the thyroid gland *hyper-*: excessive, above normal *thyroid*: thyroid gland

*The suffix *-ical* is a combination of *-ic* and *-al*.

Table 2-5	**Adjective, Noun, and Diminutive Suffixes—cont'd**

Suffix	Meaning	Word Analysis
Noun		
-iatry	medicine; treatment	pod/**iatry** (pō-DĪ-ă-trē): specialty concerned with treatment and prevention of conditions of the feet *pod:* foot
-ician	specialist	obstetr/**ician** (ŏb-stĕ-TRĬSH-ăn): physician who specializes in the branch of medicine concerned with pregnancy and childbirth *obstetr:* midwife
-ist		hemat/o/log/**ist** (hē-mă-TŎL-ō-jĭst): physician who specializes in the treatment of disorders of blood and blood-forming tissues *hemat/o:* blood *log:* study of
-y	condition; process	neur/o/path/**y** (nū-RŎP-ă-thē): condition of the nerves (related to a) disease *neur/o:* nerve *path:* disease
Diminutive		
-icle	small, minute	ventr/**icle** (VĔN-trĭ-kl): small cavity, as of the brain or heart *ventr:* belly, belly side
-ole		arteri/**ole** (ăr-TĒ-rē-ōl): the smallest of the arteries; also called a minute artery *arteri:* artery ***Arteries narrow to form arterioles (minute arteries), which branch into capillaries (microscopic blood vessels).***
-ule		ven/**ule** (VĔN-ūl): small vein continuous with a capillary *ven:* vein

 It is time to review grammatical suffixes by completing Learning Activity 2–6.

Plural Suffixes

Many medical words have Greek or Latin origins and follow the rules of these languages in building singular and plural forms. Once you learn these rules, you will find that they are easy to apply. You will also find that some English endings have also been adopted for commonly used medical terms. When a word changes from a singular to a plural form, the suffix of the word is the part that changes. A summary of the rules for changing a singular word into its plural form is located on the inside back cover of this textbook. Use it to complete Learning Activity 2-7 and whenever you need help forming plural words.

 It is time to review the rules for forming plural words by completing Learning Activity 2-7.

LEARNING ACTIVITIES

The following activities provide review of the suffixes introduced in this chapter. Complete each activity and review your answers to evaluate your understanding of the chapter.

Learning Activity 2-1
Building Surgical Words

Use the meanings in the right column to complete the surgical words in the left column. The first one is completed for you. Note: The word roots are underlined in the left column.

Incomplete Word	Meaning
1. episi/o/ t o m y	incision of the perineum
2. col _ _ _ _ _ _	excision (of all or part)* of the colon
3. arthr/o/ _ _ _ _ _ _ _ _	surgical puncture of a joint (to remove fluid)
4. splen _ _ _ _ _ _	excision of the spleen
5. col/o/ _ _ _ _ _	forming an opening (mouth) into the colon
6. oste/o/ _ _ _ _	instrument to cut bone
7. tympan/o/ _ _ _ _	incision of the tympanic membrane
8. trache/o/ _ _ _ _ _	forming an opening (mouth) into the trachea
9. mast _ _ _ _ _ _	excision of a breast
10. lith/o/ _ _ _ _	incision to remove a stone or calculus
11. hemorrhoid _ _ _ _ _ _	excision of hemorrhoids

Build a surgical word that means

12. forming an opening (mouth) into the colon: _____

13. excision of the colon: _____

14. instrument to cut bone: _____

15. surgical puncture of a joint: _____

16. incision to remove a stone: _____

17. excision of a breast: _____

18. incision of the tympanic membrane: _____

19. forming an opening (mouth) into the trachea: _____

20. excision of the spleen: _____

✔ *Check your answers in Appendix A. Review any material that you did not answer correctly.*

Correct Answers _____ X 5 = _____ % Score

---

*Information in parentheses is used to clarify the meaning of the word but not to build the medical term.

Learning Activity 2-2

Building More Surgical Words

Use the meanings in the right column to complete the surgical words in the left column. The word roots are underlined in the left column.

Incomplete Word

Meaning

1. <u>arthr</u>/o/ _ _ _ _ _   fixation or binding of a joint
2. <u>rhin</u>/o/ _ _ _ _ _ _   surgical repair of the nose
3. <u>ten</u>/o/ _ _ _ _ _ _   surgical repair of tendons
4. <u>my</u>/o/ _ _ _ _ _ _ _   suture of a muscle
5. <u>mast</u>/o/ _ _ _ _   fixation of a (pendulous)* breast
6. <u>cyst</u>/o/ _ _ _ _ _ _ _   suture of the bladder
7. <u>oste</u>/o/ _ _ _ _ _ _   surgical fracture of a bone
8. <u>lith</u>/o/ _ _ _ _ _ _   crushing of a stone
9. <u>enter</u>/o/ _ _ _ _ _   separation of intestinal (adhesions)
10. <u>neur</u>/o/ _ _ _ _ _ _   crushing a nerve

Build a surgical word that means

11. surgical repair of the nose: _____
12. fixation of a joint: _____
13. suture of a muscle: _____
14. fixation of a (pendulous) breast: _____
15. suture of the bladder: _____
16. repair of tendons: _____
17. surgical fracture of a bone: _____
18. crushing stones: _____
19. separation of intestinal (adhesions): _____
20. crushing a nerve: _____

Check your answers in Appendix A. Review any material that you did not answer correctly.

Correct Answers _____ X 5 = _____ % Score

*Information in parentheses is used to clarify the meaning of the word but not to build the medical term.

Learning Activity 2-3
Selecting a Surgical Suffix

Use the suffixes listed below to build surgical words in the right column that reflect the meanings in the left column. You may use the same suffix more than one time.

-centesis	-ectomy	-plasty	-tome
-clasis	-lysis	-rrhaphy	-tomy
-desis	-pexy	-stomy	-tripsy

1. crushing of a stone: lith/o/ _____
2. puncture of a joint (to remove fluid)*:   arthr/o/ _____
3. excision of the spleen: splen/ _____
4. forming an opening (mouth) into the colon: col/o/ _____
5. instrument to cut skin: derma/ _____
6. forming an opening (mouth) into the trachea: trache/o/ _____
7. incision to remove a stone or calculus: lith/ _____ / _____
8. excision of a breast: mast/ _____
9. excision of hemorrhoids: hemorrhoid/ _____
10. incision of the trachea: trache/ _____ / _____
11. fixation of a breast: mast/ _____ / _____
12. excision of the colon: col/ _____
13. suture of the stomach (wall):   gastr/ _____ / _____
14. fixation of the uterus: hyster/ _____ / _____
15. surgical repair of the nose: rhin/ _____ / _____
16. fixation or binding of a joint: arthr/ _____ / _____
17. to break or surgically fracture a bone: oste/ _____ / _____
18. loosening of nerve (tissue):   neur/ _____ / _____
19. suture of muscle: my/o/ _____
20. incision of the tympanic membrane: tympan/ _____ / _____

 Check your answers in Appendix A. Review any material that you did not answer correctly.

Correct Answers _____ X 5 = _____ % Score

---

*Information in parentheses is used to clarify the meaning of the word but not to build the medical term.

Learning Activity 2-4

Selecting Diagnostic, Pathological, and Related Suffixes

Use the suffixes in this list to build diagnostic, pathological, and related words in the right column that reflect the meanings in the left column.

-algia	-graph	-metry	-penia	-rrhage
-cele	-iasis	-oma	-phagia	-rrhea
-ectasis	-malacia	-osis	-phasia	-rrhexis
-emia	-megaly	-pathy	-plegia	-spasm
-genesis				

1. tumor of the liver: hepat/ _____
2. pain (along the course) of a nerve: neur/ _____
3. dilation of a bronchus: bronchi/ _____
4. producing or forming cancer: carcin/o/ _____
5. abnormal condition of the skin: dermat/ _____
6. enlargement of the kidney: nephr/o/ _____
7. discharge or flow from the ear: ot/ _____ / _____
8. rupture of the uterus: hyster/ _____ / _____
9. twitching of the eyelid: blephar/ _____ / _____
10. herniation of the bladder: cyst/ _____ / _____
11. bursting forth (of) blood: hem/o/ _____
12. abnormal condition of a stone or calculus: lith/ _____
13. paralysis affecting one side (of the body):   hemi/ _____
14. disease of muscle (tissue):   my/ _____ / _____
15. difficult or painful swallowing or eating: dys/ _____
16. softening of the bones: oste/ _____ / _____
17. without (or absence of) speech: a/ _____
18. white blood condition: leuk/ _____
19. deficiency in red (blood) cells: erythr/ _____ / _____
20. measuring the pelvis: pelv/i/ _____

Check your answers in Appendix A. Review any material that you did not answer correctly.

Correct Answers _____ X 5 = _____ % Score

Learning Activity 2-5

Building Pathological and Related Words

Use the meanings in the right column to complete the pathological and related words in the left column.

Incomplete Word	Meaning
1. bronchi/ _____	dilation of a bronchus
2. chole/ _____	gallstone
3. carcin/o/ _____	forming or producing cancer
4. oste/ _____ / _____	softening of bone
5. hepat/ _____ / _____	enlargement of the liver
6. cholelith/ _____	abnormal condition of gallstones
7. hepat/ _____ / _____	herniation of the liver
8. neur/o/ _____	disease of the nerves
9. dermat/ _____	abnormal condition of the skin
10. hemi/ _____	paralysis of one half of the body
11. dys/ _____	difficult swallowing
12. a/ _____	without (or absence of) speech
13. cephal/o/ _____	pain in the head; headache
14. blephar/ _____ / _____	twitching of the eyelid
15. hyper/ _____	excessive formation (of an organ or tissue)

✓ *Check your answers in Appendix A. Review any material that you did not answer correctly.*

Correct Answers _____ X 6.67 = _____ Score

Selecting Adjective, Noun, and Diminutive Suffixes

Use the adjective suffixes in the following list to create a medical term. The first one is completed for you. Note: When in doubt about the validity of a word, refer to a medical dictionary.

-ac	-ary	-ic	-tic
-al	-eal	-ous	-tix

Element	Medical Term	Meaning
1. thorac/	*thoracic*	pertaining to the chest
2. gastr/		pertaining to the stomach
3. bacteri/		pertaining to bacteria
4. aqua/		pertaining to water
5. axill/		pertaining to the armpit
6. cardi/		pertaining to the heart
7. spin/		pertaining to the spine
8. membran/		pertaining to a membrane

Use the noun suffixes in the following list to create a medical term.

-er	-ism	-iatry
-ia	-ist	
-is	-y	

Element	Medical Term	Meaning
9. intern/		specialist in internal medicine
10. leuk/em/		condition of "white" blood
11. sigmoid/o/scop/		visual examination of the sigmoid colon
12. alcohol/		condition of (excessive) alcohol
13. pod/		treatment of the feet
14. allerg/		specialist in treating allergic disorders
15. man/		condition of madness

Use the diminutive suffixes in the following list to create a medical term.

-icle	-ole	-ula	-ule

Element	Medical Term	Meaning
16. arteri/		minute artery
17. ventr/		small cavity
18. ven/		small vein

Check your answers in Appendix A. Review any material that you did not answer correctly.

Correct Answers _____ X 5.6 = _____ % Score

Learning Activity 2-7
Forming Plural Words

Review the guidelines for plural suffixes (located inside the back cover of this book). Then write the plural form for each of the following singular terms and briefly state the rule that applies. The first one is completed for you.

Singular	Plural	Rule
1. diagnosis	*diagnoses*	*Drop the* is *and add* es.
2. fornix		
3. vertebra		
4. keratosis		
5. bronchus		
6. spermatozoon		
7. septum		
8. coccus		
9. ganglion		
10. prognosis		
11. thrombus		
12. appendix		
13. bacterium		
14. testis		
15. nevus		

 Check your answers in Appendix A. Review any material that you did not answer correctly.

Correct Answers _____ X 6.67 = _____ % Score

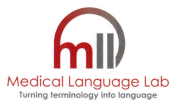

Medical Language Lab
Turning terminology into language

Visit the Medical Language Lab at the web site: medicallanguagelab.com. Use it to enhance your study and reinforcement of suffixes with the flash-card activity related to suffixes. We recommend you complete the flash-card activity before moving on to Chapter 3.

Prefixes

Chapter Outline

Objectives

Upon completion of this chapter, you will be able to:

- Define common prefixes used in medical terminology.
- Describe how a prefix changes the meaning of a medical word.
- Recognize and define prefixes of position, number and measurement, and direction.
- Demonstrate your knowledge of this chapter by completing the learning activities.

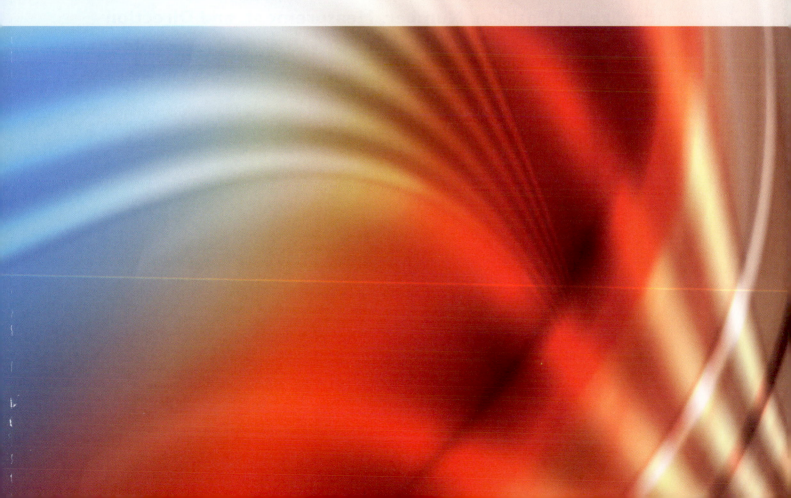

Prefix Linking

Most medical words contain a root or combining form with a suffix. Some of them also contain prefixes. A prefix is a word element located at the beginning of a word. Substituting one prefix for another alters the meaning of the word. For example, in the term *macro/cyte*, *macro-* is a prefix meaning large; *-cyte* is a suffix meaning cell. A **macrocyte** is a large cell. By changing the prefix *macro-* (large) to *micro-* (small), the meaning of the word changes. A **microcyte** is a small cell. See Table 3-1 for three other examples of how a prefix changes the meaning of a word.

Table 3-1	**Changing Prefixes and Meanings**

In this table, each word has the same root, nat (birth), and suffix, -al (pertaining to). By substituting different prefixes, new words with different meanings are formed.

Prefix	+	Word Root	+	Suffix	=	Medical Word	Meaning
pre- (before)	+		+		=	prenatal prē-NĀ-tăl	pertaining to (the period) before birth
peri- (around)	+	nat (birth)	+	-al (pertaining to)	=	perinatal pĕr-ĭ-NĀ-tăl	pertaining to (the period) around birth
post- (after)	+		+		=	postnatal pōst-NĀ-tăl	pertaining to (the period) after birth

Prefix Types

Learning the major types of prefixes, such as prefixes of position, number and measurement, and direction, as well as some others, will help you master medical terminology.

Prefixes of Position, Number, Measurement, and Direction

Prefixes are used in medical terms to denote position, number and measurement, and direction. Prefixes of position describe a place or location. (See Table 3-2.) Prefixes of number and measurement describe an amount, size, or degree of involvement. (See Table 3-3.) Prefixes of direction indicate a pathway or route. (See Table 3-4.)

Table 3-2	**Prefixes of Position**

This table lists commonly used prefixes of position along with their meanings and word analyses.

Prefix	Meaning	Word Analysis
epi-	above, upon	**epi**/gastr/ic (ĕp-ĭ-GĂS-trĭk): pertaining to above the stomach *gastr*: stomach *-ic*: pertaining to
hypo-	under, below, deficient	**hypo**/derm/ic (hī-pō-DĔR-mĭk): pertaining to under the skin *derm*: skin *-ic*: pertaining to *Hypodermic injections are given under the skin.*
infra-	under, below	**infra**/cost/al (ĭn-fră-KŎS-tăl): below the ribs *cost*: ribs *-al*: pertaining to
sub-		**sub**/nas/al (sŭb-NĀ-săl): under the nose *nas*: nose *-al*: pertaining to

Table 3-2	**Prefixes of Position—cont'd**		

Prefix	Meaning	Word Analysis	
inter-	between	**inter**/cost/al (ĭn-tĕr-KŎS-tăl): between the ribs *cost*: ribs *-al*: pertaining to	
post-	after, behind	**post**/nat/al (pōst-NĀ-tăl): pertaining to (the period) after birth *nat*: birth *-al*: pertaining to	
pre-	before, in front of	**pre**/nat/al (prē-NĀ-tăl): pertaining to (the period) before birth *nat*: birth *-al*: pertaining to	
pro-		**pro**/gnosis (prŏg-NŌ-sĭs): knowing before *-gnosis*: knowing *Prognosis is the prediction of the course and end of a disease and the estimated chance of recovery.*	
retro-	backward, behind	**retro**/version (rĕt-rō-VĔR-shŭn): turning backwards *-version*: turning *Retroversion refers to tipping backward of an organ (such as the uterus) from its normal position.*	

Table 3-3	**Prefixes of Number and Measurement**		

This table lists commonly used prefixes of number and measurement along with their meanings and word analyses.

Prefix	Meaning	Word Analysis	
bi-	two	**bi**/later/al (bī-LĂT-ĕr-ăl): pertaining to two sides *later*: side *-al*: pertaining to	
dipl-	double	**dipl**/opia (dĭp-LŌ-pē-ă): double vision *-opia*: vision	
diplo-		**diplo**/bacteri/al (dĭp-lō-băk-TĒR-ē-ăl): bacteria linked together in pairs *bacteri*: bacteria *-al*: pertaining to *Diplobacteria reproduce in such a manner that they are joined together in pairs.*	
hemi-	one half	**hemi**/plegia (hĕm-ē-PLĒ-jē-ă): paralysis of one half of the body *-plegia*: paralysis	
hyper-	excessive, above normal	**hyper**/calc/emia (hī-pĕr-kăl-SĒ-mē-ă): excessive calcium in the blood *calc*: calcium *-emia*: blood condition	
macro-	large	**macro**/cyte (MĂK-rō-sīt): large cell *-cyte*: cell	
micro-	small	**micro**/scope (MĪ-krō-skōp): instrument for examining small (objects) *-scope*: instrument for examining *The microscope is an optical instrument that greatly magnifies minute objects.*	

(continued)

Table 3-3	**Prefixes of Number and Measurement—cont'd**	
Prefix	**Meaning**	**Word Analysis**
mono-	one	**mono**/therapy (MŎN-ō-thĕr-ă-pē): one treatment *-therapy:* treatment *An example of monotherapy is treatment using only a single drug or a single treatment modality.*
uni-		**uni**/nucle/ar (ū-nĭ-NŪ-klē-ăr): pertaining to one nucleus *nucle:* nucleus *-ar:* pertaining to
multi-	many, much	**multi**/gravida (mŭl-tĭ-GRĂV-ĭ-dă): woman who has been pregnant more than once *-gravida:* pregnant woman
poly-		**poly**/phobia (pŏl-ē-FŌ-bē-ă): fear of many things *-phobia:* fear
nulli-	none	**nulli**/gravida (nŭl-ĭ-GRĂV-ĭ-dă): woman who has not been pregnant *-gravida:* pregnant woman
primi-	first	**primi**/gravida (prī-mĭ-GRĂV-ĭ-dă): woman during her first pregnancy *-gravida:* pregnant woman
quadri-	four	**quadri**/plegia (kwŏd-rĭ-PLĒ-jē-ă): paralysis of four limbs *-plegia:* paralysis
tri-	three	**tri**/ceps (TRĪ-cĕps): three heads *-ceps:* head *Triceps describes a muscle having three heads with a single insertion, as the tricep muscle of the posterior arm.*

Table 3-4	**Prefixes of Direction**	
This table lists commonly used prefixes of direction as well as their meanings and word analyses.		
Prefix	**Meaning**	**Word Analysis**
ab-	from, away from	**ab**/duction (ăb-DŬK-shŭn): movement of a limb away from (an axis of) the body *-duction:* act of leading, bringing, conducting
ad-	toward	**ad**/duction (ă-DŬK-shŭn): movement of a limb toward (an axis of) the body *-duction:* act of leading, bringing, conducting
circum-	around	**circum**/ren/al (sĕr-kŭm-RĒ-năl): pertaining to around the kidney *ren:* kidney *-al:* pertaining to
peri-		**peri**/odont/al (pĕr-ē-ō-DŎN-tăl): pertaining to around a tooth *odont:* teeth *-al:* pertaining to
dia-	through, across	**dia**/rrhea (dī-ă-RĒ-ă): flow through *-rrhea:* discharge, flow *Diarrhea is a condition of abnormally frequent discharge or flow of fluid fecal matter from the bowel.*
trans-		**trans**/vagin/al (trăns-VĂJ-ĭn-ăl): pertaining to across or through the vagina *vagin:* vagina *-al:* pertaining to

Table 3-4	**Prefixes of Direction—cont'd**	
Prefix	**Meaning**	**Word Analysis**
ecto-	outside, outward	**ecto**/gen/ous (ĕk-TŎJ-ĕ-nŭs): forming outside the body or structure *gen:* forming, producing, origin *-ous:* pertaining to *An ectogenous infection is one that originates outside of the body.*
exo-		**exo**/tropia (ĕks-ō-TRŌ-pē-ă): turning outward (of one or both eyes) *-tropia:* turning
extra-		**extra**/crani/al (ĕks-tră-KRĀ-nē-ăl): pertaining to outside the skull *crani:* cranium (skull) *-al:* pertaining to
endo-	in, within	**endo**/crine (ĔN-dō-krĭn): secrete within *-crine:* secrete *Endocrine describes a gland that secretes directly into the bloodstream.*
intra-		**intra**/muscul/ar (ĭn-tră-MŬS-kū-lăr): within the muscle *muscul:* muscle *-ar:* pertaining to
para-*	near, beside; beyond	**para**/nas/al (păr-ă-NĀ-săl): beside the nose *nas:* nose *-al:* pertaining to
super-	upper, above	**super**/ior (soo-PĒ-rē-or): pertaining to the upper part of a structure *-ior:* pertaining to
supra-	above; excessive; superior	**supra**/ren/al (soo-pră-RĒ-năl): pertaining to above the kidney *ren:* kidney *-al:* pertaining to
ultra-	excess, beyond	**ultra**/son/ic (ŭl-tră-SŎN-ĭk): pertaining to sound beyond (that which can be heard by the human ear) *son:* sound *-ic:* pertaining to

*Para- may also be used as a suffix meaning *to bear (offspring).*

Other Common Prefixes

Many other common prefixes may also be used to change the meaning of a word. See Table 3-5 for a list of some other common prefixes.

Table 3-5	**Other Common Prefixes**	
	This table lists other commonly used prefixes along with their meanings and word analyses.	
Prefix	**Meaning**	**Word Analysis**
a-*	without, not	**a**/mast/ia (ă-MĂS-tē-ă): without a breast *mast:* breast *-ia:* condition *Amastia may be the result of a congenital defect, an endocrine disorder, or mastectomy.*
an-**		**an**/esthesia (ăn-ĕs-THĒ-zē-ă): without feeling *-esthesia:* feeling *Anesthesia may be a partial or complete loss of sensation with or without loss of consciousness.*

(continued)

*The prefix a- is usually used before a consonant.

** The prefix an- is usually used before a vowel.

Table 3-5 Other Common Prefixes—cont'd

Prefix	Meaning	Word Analysis
anti-	against	anti/bacteri/al (ăn-tĭ-băk-TĒR-ē-ăl): against bacteria *bacteri*: bacteria *-al*: pertaining to *Antibacterials are substances that kill bacteria or inhibit their growth or replication.*
contra-		contra/ception (kŏn-tră-SĔP-shŭn): against conception or impregnation *-ception*: conceiving *Contraceptive techniques prevent pregnancy by means of medication, a device, or a method that blocks or alters one or more of the processes of reproduction.*
brady-	slow	brady/cardia (brăd-ē-KĂR-dē-ă): slow heart rate *-cardia*: heart
dys-	bad; painful; difficult	dys/tocia (dĭs-TŌ-sē-ă): difficult childbirth *-tocia*: childbirth, labor
eu-	good, normal	eu/pnea (ūp-NĒ-ă): normal breathing *-pnea*: breathing
hetero-	different	hetero/graft (HĔT-ĕ-rō-grăft): different transplant; also called heteroplasty or xenograft *-graft*: transplantation *Heterograft is a type of tissue graft in which the donor and recipient are of different species. It is used as a temporary graft when tissue cannot be obtained from the patient or from a tissue bank.*
homo-	same	homo/graft (HŌ-mō-grăft): same transplant; also called allograft *-graft*: transplantation *A homograft is a transplant of tissue obtained from a member of the patient's own species. Commonly transplanted organs include bone, kidney, lung, and heart. Recipients take immunosuppressive drugs to prevent tissue rejection.*
homeo-		homeo/plasia (hō-mē-ō-PLĀ-zē-ă): formation of new tissue similar to that already existing in a part *-plasia*: formation, growth
mal-	bad	mal/nutrition (măl-nū-TRĬ-shŭn): bad nutrition *Malnutrition refers to any disorder resulting from an inadequate or excessive intake of food.*
pan-	all	pan/arthr/itis (păn-ăr-THRĪ-tĭs): inflammation of all (or many) joints *arthr*: joint *-itis*: inflammation
pseudo-	false	pseudo/cyesis (soo-dō-sī-Ē-sĭs): false pregnancy *-cyesis*: pregnancy *Pseudocyesis is a condition in which a woman believes she is pregnant when she is not and begins to develop all the physical characteristics associated with pregnancy.*

Table 3-5	Other Common Prefixes—cont'd	

Prefix	Meaning	Word Analysis
syn-***	union, together, joined	syn/dactyl/ism (sĭn-DĂK-tĭl-ĭzm): condition of joined fingers or toes *dactyl:* fingers; toes *-ism:* condition *Syndactylism varies in degree of severity from incomplete webbing of the skin of two digits to complete union of digits and fusion of the bones and nails.*
tachy-	rapid	tachy/pnea (tăk-ĭp-NĒ-ă): rapid breathing *-pnea:* breathing

*** The prefix *syn-* appears as *sym-* before *b, p, ph,* or *m.*

 It is time to review prefixes by completing Learning Activities 3–1, 3–2, and 3–3.

LEARNING ACTIVITIES

The following activities provide review of the prefixes introduced in this chapter. Complete each activity and review your answers to evaluate your understanding of the chapter. You can also enhance your study and reinforcement of prefixes with the power of Davis*Plus*.

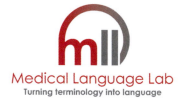

Visit the Medical Language Lab at the web site: medicallanguagelab.com. Use it to enhance your study and reinforcement of prefixes with the flash-card activity related to prefixes. We recommend you complete the flash-card activity before moving on to Chapter 4.

Learning Activity 3-1
Identifying and Defining Prefixes

Place a slash after each of the following prefixes and then define the prefix. The first one is completed for you.

Word	Definition of Prefix
1. inter/dental	*between*
2. hypodermic	
3. epidermis	
4. retroversion	
5. sublingual	
6. quadriplegia	
7. microscope	
8. triceps	
9. anesthesia	
10. intramuscular	
11. suprapelvic	
12. diarrhea	
13. periodontal	
14. bradycardia	
15. tachypnea	
16. dystocia	
17. eupnea	
18. heterograft	
19. malnutrition	
20. pseudocyesis	

✓ *Check your answers in Appendix A. Review any material that you did not answer correctly.*

Correct Answers _____ X 5 = _____ % Score

Learning Activity 3-2

Matching Prefixes of Position, Number and Measurement, and Direction

Match the following terms with the definitions in the numbered list.

diarrhea	macrocyte	pseudocyesis
ectogenous	periodontal	quadriplegia
hemiplegia	polyphobia	retroversion
hypodermic	postoperative	subnasal
intercostal	prenatal	suprarenal

1. _____ tipping back of an organ

2. _____ pertaining to under the skin

3. _____ before birth

4. _____ pertaining to under the nose

5. _____ after surgery

6. _____ pertaining to between the ribs

7. _____ false pregnancy

8. _____ pertaining to around the teeth

9. _____ flow through (watery bowel movement)

10. _____ pertaining to an origin outside (the body or structure)

11. _____ above the kidney

12. _____ paralysis of one half (of the body)

13. _____ paralysis of four (limbs)

14. _____ (abnormally) large blood cell

15. _____ many fears

Check your answers in Appendix A. Review any material that you did not answer correctly.

Correct Answers _____ X 6.67 = _____ % Score

Learning Activity 3-3
Matching Other Prefixes

Match the following terms with the definitions in the numbered list.

amastia	dyspepsia	homograft
anesthesia	dystocia	malnutrition
antibacterial	eupnea	panarthritis
bradycardia	heterograft	syndactylism
contraception	homeoplasia	tachycardia

1. _____ difficult digestion

2. _____ tissue transplant from a different species

3. _____ inflammation of many joints

4. _____ against bacteria

5. _____ slow heartbeat

6. _____ poor or bad nutrition

7. _____ without a breast

8. _____ without sensation

9. _____ good or normal breathing

10. _____ condition of fused fingers and toes

11. _____ rapid heartbeat

12. _____ against conception

13. _____ tissue transplant from the same species

14. _____ difficult childbirth

15. _____ formation of the same tissue

 Check your answers in Appendix A. Review any material that you did not answer correctly.

Correct Answers _____ X 6.67 = _____ % Score

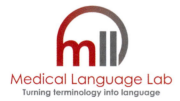
Medical Language Lab
Turning terminology into language

Visit the Medical Language Lab at the web site: medicallanguagelab.com. Use it to enhance your study and reinforcement of prefixes with the flash-card activity related to prefixes. We recommend you complete the flash-card activity before moving on to Chapter 4.

Body Structure

CHAPTER

4

Chapter Outline

Objectives

Upon completion of this chapter, you will be able to:

- List the levels of organization of the body.
- Define and identify three planes of the body.
- Identify the cavities, quadrants, and regions of the body.
- List and identify terms related to direction, position, and planes of the body.
- Recognize, pronounce, spell, and build words related to body structure.
- Describe diseases, conditions, and procedures related to body structure.
- Demonstrate your knowledge of this chapter by completing the learning and medical record activities.

Introduction

This chapter is the basic foundation for understanding the body system chapters that follow. First, the structural and functional organization of the body—from the cellular level to the organism level—is introduced. Second, terms used to describe anatomical positions, planes of the body, body cavities, quadrants and regions of the abdominal cavity, and divisions of the spinal column are included. Third, diseases and conditions associated with the disease process as well as medical, surgical, and diagnostic procedures that are commonly used in most medical specialties are introduced. All of these terms are an essential part of medical terminology and are used in all body systems.

Body Structure Key Terms

This section introduces important terms associated with body structure, along with their definitions and pronunciations. Word analyses are also provided for selected terms.

Term	Definition
chromatin KRŌ-mă-tĭn	Structural component of the nucleus, composed of nucleic acids and proteins *Chromatin condenses to form chromosomes during cell division.*
chromosome KRŌ-mō-sōm	Threadlike structures within the nucleus composed of deoxyribonucleic acid (DNA) that carries hereditary information encoded in genes *Each sperm and each egg has 23 unpaired chromosomes. After fertilization, each cell of the embryo then has 46 chromosomes (23 pairs). In each pair of chromosomes, one chromosome is provided by the father and the other by the mother.*
deoxyribonucleic acid (DNA) dē-ŏk-sē-rĪ-bō-noo-KLĒ-ĭk ĂS-ĭd	Molecule that holds genetic information capable of replicating and producing an exact copy whenever the cell divides
diaphragm DĪ-ă-frăm	Muscular wall that divides the thoracic cavity from the abdominopelvic cavity *Alternating contraction and relaxation of the diaphragm is essential to the breathing process.*
metabolism mĕ-TĂB-ō-lĭzm	Sum of all physical and chemical changes that take place in a cell or an organism *Metabolism includes the building up (anabolism) and breaking down (catabolism) of body constituents.*
organelle or-găn-ĔL	Cellular structure that provides a specialized function, such as the nucleus (reproduction), ribosomes (protein synthesis), Golgi apparatus (removal of material from the cell), and lysosomes (digestion) *The membranes of many organelles act as sites of chemical reactions.*

Pronunciation Help	Long Sound	ā — rate	ē — rebirth	ī — isle	ō — over	ū — unite
	Short Sound	ă — alone	ĕ — ever	ĭ — it	ŏ — not	ŭ — cut

Levels of Organization

The body is made up of several levels of structure and function. Each of these levels builds on the previous level, and contributes to the structure and function of the entire organism. (See Figure 4-1.) The levels of organization from least to most complex are:

- cell
- tissue
- organ
- system
- organism.

Cell

The cell is the smallest structural and functional unit of life. Body cells perform all activities associated with life, including utilizing food, eliminating waste, and reproducing. Cells have many shapes and sizes, but they share three main parts: **cell membrane, cytoplasm,** and the **nucleus.** The study of the body at the cellular level is called **cytology.**

Cell Membrane and Cytoplasm

The cell membrane acts as a barrier that supports and protects the intracellular contents. Within the cell membrane is a jellylike matrix of proteins, salts, water, dissolved gases, and nutrients called **cytoplasm.** Inside the cytoplasm are specialized structures called **organelles**. These organelles perform specific functions of the cell, such as reproduction and movement. The largest cell organelle is the nucleus, which directs the cell's activities and contains chromosomes.

Nucleus

The nucleus is responsible for **metabolism,** growth, and reproduction. It also carries the genetic blueprint of the organism. This blueprint is found in a complex molecule called **deoxyribonucleic acid (DNA)** that is organized into a threadlike structure called **chromatin**. When the cell is ready to divide, chromatin forms **chromosomes**, which carry thousands of genes that make up our genetic blueprint. In the human, there are about 31,000 genes that determine unique human characteristics. Genes pass biological information from one generation to the next. This biological information includes such traits as hair color, body structure, and metabolic activity. In the human, all cells except sperm and eggs cells contain 23 pairs, or 46 chromosomes.

Tissue

Groups of cells that perform a specialized activity are called **tissues.** The study of tissues is called **histology.** Between the cells that make up tissues are varying amounts and types of nonliving, intercellular substances that provide pathways for cellular interaction. More than 200 cell types compose four major tissues of the body:

- **Epithelial tissue** covers surfaces of organs, lines cavities and canals, forms tubes and ducts, provides the secreting portions of glands, and makes up the epidermis of the skin. It is composed of cells arranged in a continuous sheet consisting of one or more layers.
- **Connective tissue** supports and connects other tissues and organs. It is made up of diverse cell types, including fibroblasts, fat cells, and blood.
- **Muscle tissue** provides the contractile tissue of the body, which is responsible for movement.
- **Nervous tissue** transmits electrical impulses as it relays information throughout the entire body.

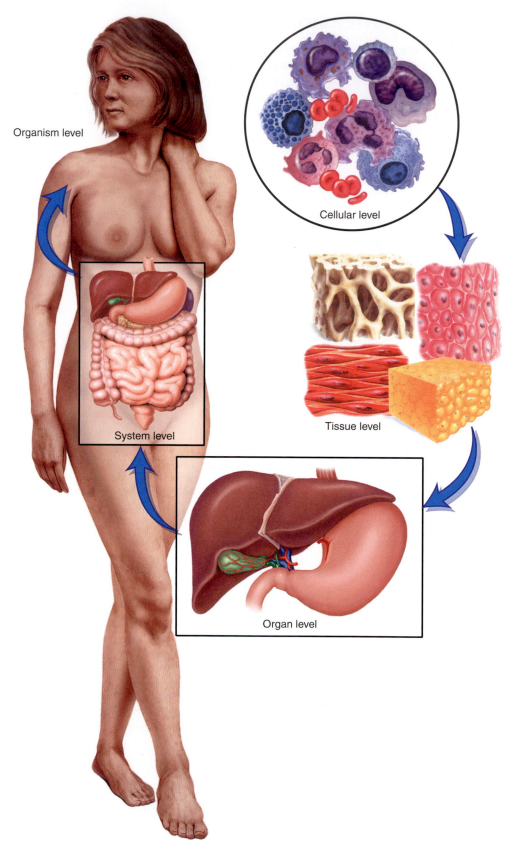

Organism level

Cellular level

Tissue level

System level

Organ level

Figure 4-1 Levels of organization of the human body.

Organ

Organs are body structures that perform specialized functions. They are composed of two or more tissue types. For example, the stomach is made up of connective tissue, muscle tissue, epithelial tissue, and nervous tissue. Muscle and connective tissue form the wall of the stomach. Epithelial and connective tissue cover the inner and outer surfaces of the stomach. Nervous tissue penetrates the epithelial lining of the stomach and its muscular wall to stimulate the release of chemicals for digestion.

System

A body system is composed of varying numbers of organs and accessory structures that have similar or related functions. For example, organs of the gastrointestinal system include the esophagus, stomach, small intestine, and bowel. Some of its accessory structures include the liver, gallbladder, and pancreas. The purpose of this system is to digest food, remove and use its nutrients, and expel waste products. Other body systems include the reproductive, respiratory, urinary, and cardiovascular systems.

Organism

The highest level of organization is the organism. An organism is a complete living entity capable of independent existence. All complex organisms, including humans, are made up of several body systems that work together to sustain life.

Anatomical Position

The **anatomical position** is a body posture used to locate anatomical parts or divisions. It is used by health care providers and other members of the scientific community to ensure uniformity and accuracy in descriptions. In the anatomical position, the body is standing erect and the face forward. The arms are at the sides, with the palms facing forward. No matter how the body is actually positioned—standing or lying down, facing forward or backward—or how the limbs are actually placed, the positions and relationships of a structure are always described as if the body were in the anatomical position. (See Figure 4-2.)

Planes of the Body

A **plane** is an imaginary flat surface that divides the body into two sections. When the body is in anatomical position, the planes serve as points of reference to identify the different sections of the body. The most commonly used planes are **midsagittal** (median), **coronal** (frontal), and **transverse** (horizontal). (See Table 4-1.) The section is named for the plane along which it is cut. Thus, a cut along a transverse plane divides the body into top and bottom sections.

Before the development of modern imaging techniques, standard x-ray images showed only a single plane, and many body abnormalities were difficult, if not impossible, to see. Current imaging procedures, such as magnetic resonance imaging (MRI) and computed tomography (CT), produce three-dimensional images on more than one plane. Thus, structural abnormalities and body masses that were previously not found using a standard single plane x-ray are now detected with scanning devices that show images taken in several body planes.

Body Cavities

Body cavities are spaces within the body that help protect, separate, and support internal organs. The cavities are used by clinicians to locate structures and also to identify abnormalities within the cavities. (See Figure 4-3.) Each of the two major cavities consist of two smaller cavities:

- dorsal (posterior), including the cranial and spinal cavities
- ventral (anterior), including the thoracic and abdominopelvic cavities. (See Table 4-2.)

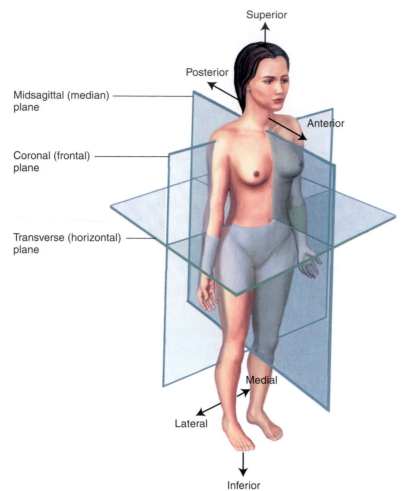

Figure 4-2 Body planes and directional terms. Note the body is in the anatomical position.

Table 4-1	**Planes of the Body**	
This table lists planes of the body and their anatomical divisions.		
Plane	**Anatomical Division**	
Midsagittal (median)	Right and left halves	
Coronal (frontal)	Anterior (ventral) and posterior (dorsal) aspects	
Transverse (horizontal)	Superior (upper) and inferior (lower) aspects	

Abdominopelvic Quadrants and Regions

To describe the location of the many abdominal and pelvic organs more easily, anatomists and clinicians use two methods of dividing the abdominopelvic cavity into smaller areas. These two divisions are known as **quadrants** and **regions.**

Quadrants

The abdominopelvic cavity is divided into four **quadrants** with two imaginary lines that form a cross in the midsection of the lower torso. (See Figure 4-4 A.)

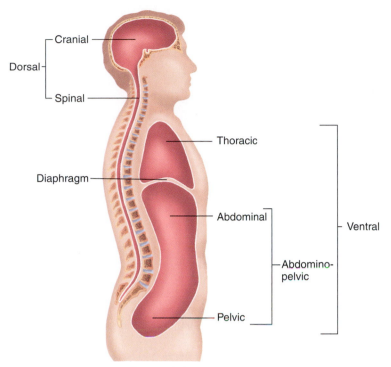

Figure 4-3 Body cavities.

Table 4-2	Body Cavities	
This table lists the body cavities and some of the major organs found within them. The thoracic cavity is separated from the abdominopelvic cavity by a muscular wall called the diaphragm.		
Cavity	**Major Organ(s) in the Cavity**	
Dorsal		
Cranial	Brain	
Spinal	Spinal cord	
Ventral		
Thoracic	Heart, lungs, and associated structures	
Abdominopelvic	Digestive, excretory, and reproductive organs and structures	

The quadrants provide a means of locating specific sites of the abdomen for descriptive and diagnostic purposes. (See Table 4-3.) They are also used as a point of reference in clinical examinations and medical reports. Pain, lesions, abrasions, punctures, and burns are commonly described as located in a specific quadrant. Incision sites are also identified by using body quadrants as the method of location.

Regions

Anatomists and clinicians divide the abdominopelvic cavity into nine **abdominopelvic regions** The regions are used primarily to identify the location of underlying body structures and visceral organs. (See Table 4-4.) For example, the stomach is located in the left hypochondriac and epigastric region; the appendix is located in the hypogastric region. (See Figure 4-4 B.)

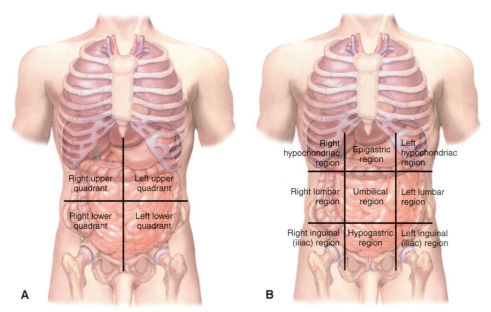

Figure 4-4 Quadrants and regions. **(A)** Four quadrants of the abdomen. **(B)** Nine regions of the abdomen.

Table 4-3	Abdominopelvic Quadrants

This table lists the abdominopelvic quadrants, their corresponding abbreviations, and the major structures located within the quadrant.

Quadrant	Abbreviation	Major Structures
Right upper	RUQ	Right lobe of the liver, the gallbladder, part of the pancreas, and part of the small and large intestines
Left upper	LUQ	Left lobe of the liver, the stomach, the spleen, part of the pancreas, and part of the small and large intestines
Right lower	RLQ	Part of the small and large intestines, the appendix, the right ovary, the right fallopian tube, and the right ureter
Left lower	LLQ	Part of the small and large intestines, the left ovary, the left fallopian tube, and the left ureter

Table 4-4	Abdominopelvic Regions

This table lists the divisions of the abdominopelvic regions and their location.

Region	Location
Right hypochondriac	Upper right lateral region beneath the ribs
Epigastric	Upper middle region
Left hypochondriac	Upper left lateral region beneath the ribs
Right lumbar	Middle right lateral region
Umbilical	Region of the navel
Left lumbar	Middle left lateral region
Right inguinal (iliac)	Lower right lateral region
Hypogastric	Lower middle region
Left inguinal (iliac)	Lower left lateral region

Directional Terms

Directional terms are used to locate the position of structures, surfaces, and regions of the body. These terms are always relative to the anatomical position. The terms also identify the position of a structure in relation to another structure. For example, the kidneys are superior to the urinary bladder. The directional term **superior** denotes *above*. This means that the kidneys are located above the urinary bladder. (See Table 4-5.)

Table 4-5	Directional Terms	

This table lists directional terms along with their definitions. In this list, opposing terms are presented consecutively to aid memorization.

Term	Definition
Abduction	Movement away from the midsagittal (median) plane of the body or one of its parts
Adduction	Movement toward the midsagittal (median) plane of the body
Medial	Pertaining to the midline of the body or structure
Lateral	Pertaining to a side
Superior (cephalad)	Toward the head or upper portion of a structure
Inferior (caudal)	Away from the head, or toward the tail or lower part of a structure
Proximal	Nearer to the center (trunk of the body) or to the point of attachment to the body
Distal	Further from the center (trunk of the body) or from the point of attachment to the body
Anterior (ventral)	Front of the body
Posterior (dorsal)	Back of the body
Parietal	Pertaining to the outer wall of the body cavity
Visceral	Pertaining to the viscera, or internal organs, especially the abdominal organs
Prone	Lying on the abdomen, face down
Supine	Lying horizontally on the back, face up
Inversion	Turning inward or inside out
Eversion	Turning outward
Palmar	Pertaining to the palm of the hand
Plantar	Pertaining to the sole of the foot
Superficial	Toward the surface of the body (external)
Deep	Away from the surface of the body (internal)

Anatomy Review: Body Planes

To review the body planes and directional terms, label the illustration using the terms below.

anterior	lateral	posterior
coronal (frontal) plane	medial	superior
inferior	midsagittal (median) plane	transverse (horizontal) plane

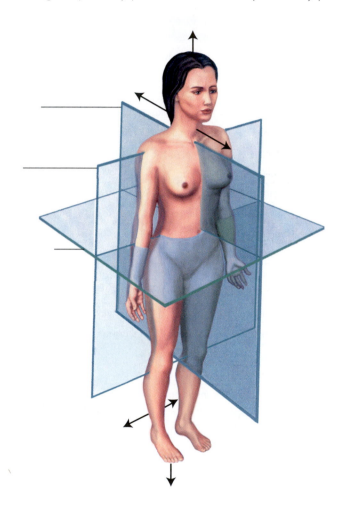

 Check your answers by referring to Figure 4–2 on page 44. Review material that you did not answer correctly.

Anatomy Review: Quadrants and Regions

To review quadrants and regions, label the quadrants on Figure A and regions on Figure B using the terms below.

epigastric region

hypogastric region

left hypochondriac region

left iliac region

left lower quadrant

left lumbar region

left upper quadrant

right hypochondriac region

right iliac region

right lower quadrant

right lumbar region

right upper quadrant

umbilical region

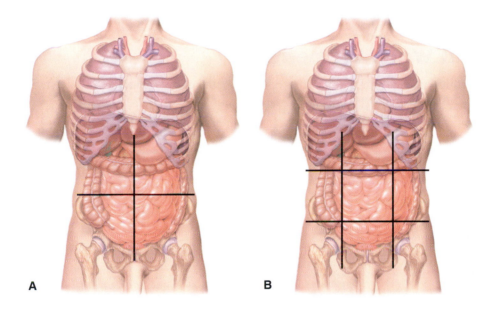

A   B

 Check your answers by referring to Figures 4–4A and 4–4B on page 46. Review material that you did not answer correctly.

Spine

The **spine**, also called the **vertebral column** or **backbone**, is composed of a series of bones called vertebrae (singular: **vertebra**). It is formed from 26 irregular bones and connective tissue in such a way that a flexible, curved structure results. The spine is divided into sections corresponding to the vertebrae located in the spinal column. These divisions are:

- cervical (neck)
- thoracic (chest)
- lumbar (loin)
- sacral (lower back)
- coccyx (tailbone).

 It is time to review body cavities, the spine, and directional terms by completing Learning Activity 4–1.

Medical Word Elements

This section introduces combining forms, suffixes, and prefixes related to body structure. Word analyses are also provided.

Element	Meaning	Word Analysis
Combining Forms		
Cellular Structure		
cyt/o	cell	**cyt/o**/logist (sī-TŎL-ō-jĭst): specialist in the study of cells *-logist:* specialist in the study of *Cytologists study the formation, structure, and function of cells.*
hist/o	tissue	**hist/o**/logy (hĭs-TŎL-ō-jē): study of tissues *-logy:* study of *Histology is the branch of science that investigates the microscopic structures and functions of tissues.*
kary/o	nucleus	**kary/o**/lysis (kăr-ē-ŎL-ĭ-sĭs): destruction of the nucleus *-lysis:* separation; destruction; loosening *Karyolysis results in death of the cell.*
nucle/o		**nucle/**ar (NŪ-klē-ăr): pertaining to the nucleus *-ar:* pertaining to
Position and Direction		
anter/o	anterior, front	**anter/**ior (ăn-TĒR-ē-or): pertaining to the front *-ior:* pertaining to
caud/o	tail	**caud/**ad (KAW-dăd): toward the tail *-ad:* toward *Caudad is opposite of craniad.*

Element	Meaning	Word Analysis
cephal/o	head	**cephal**/ad: (SĔF-ă-lăd): toward the head *-ad:* toward
dist/o	far, farthest	**dist**/al (DĬS-tăl): pertaining to the farthest (point of attachment) *-al:* pertaining to *Distal refers to the point furthest from the center (trunk) of the body or from the point of attachment to the body. Thus, the fingers are distal to the wrist.*
dors/o	back (of body)	**dors**/al (DOR-săl): pertaining to the back (of the body) *-al:* pertaining to
infer/o	lower, below	**infer**/ior (ĭn-FĒR-rē-or): pertaining to a lower (structure or surface) *-ior:* pertaining to *The inferior surface is the undersurface of a structure or organ, or a place below a structure or organ.*
later/o	side, to one side	**later**/al (LĂT-ĕr-ăl): pertaining to a side *-al:* pertaining to
medi/o	middle	**medi**/ad (MĒ-dē-ăd): toward the middle *-ad:* toward
poster/o	back (of body), behind, posterior	**poster**/ior (pōs-TĒR-ē-or): pertaining to the back (of the body) *-ior:* pertaining to
proxim/o	near, nearest	**proxim**/al (PRŎK-sĭm-ăl): pertaining to the nearest (point of attachment) *-al:* pertaining to *Proximal refers to the point closest to the center (trunk) of the body or to the point of attachment to the body. Thus, the elbow is proximal to the wrist.*
ventr/o	belly, belly side	**ventr**/al (VĔN-trăl): pertaining to the belly side (front of the body) *-al:* pertaining to
Regions of the Body		
abdomin/o	abdomen	**abdomin**/al (ăb-DŎM-ĭ-năl): pertaining to the abdomen *-al:* pertaining to
cervic/o	neck; cervix uteri (neck of uterus)	**cervic**/al (SĔR-vĭ-kăl): pertaining to the neck *-al:* pertaining to
crani/o	cranium (skull)	**crani**/al (KRĀ-nē-ăl): pertaining to the cranium *-al:* pertaining to
gastr/o	stomach	hypo/**gastr**/ic (hī-pō-GĂS-trĭk): pertaining to (the area) below the stomach *hypo-:* under, below *-ic:* pertaining to

(continued)

Element	Meaning	Word Analysis
ili/o	ilium (lateral, flaring portion of hip bone)	**ili**/ac (ĬL-ē-ăk): pertaining to the ilium *-ac:* pertaining to
inguin/o	groin	**inguin**/al (ĬNG-gwĭ-năl): pertaining to the groin *-al:* pertaining to *The groin is the depression located between the thigh and trunk.*
lumb/o	loins (lower back)	**lumb**/ar (LŬM-băr): pertaining to the loins (lower back) *-ar:* pertaining to
pelv/i	pelvis	**pelv/i**/meter* (pĕl-VĬM-ĕ-tĕr): instrument for measuring the pelvis *-meter:* instrument for measuring
pelv/o		**pelv**/ic (PĔL-vĭk): pertaining to the pelvis *-ic:* pertaining to
spin/o	spine	**spin**/al (SPĪ-năl): pertaining to the spine *-al:* pertaining to
thorac/o	chest	**thorac**/ic (thō-RĂS-ĭk): pertaining to the chest *-ic:* pertaining to
umbilic/o	umbilicus, navel	**umbilic**/al (ŭm-BĬL-ĭ-kăl): pertaining to the navel *-al:* pertaining to
Color		
albin/o	white	**albin**/ism (ĂL-bĭn-ĭzm): condition of whiteness *-ism:* condition *Albinism is characterized by a partial or total lack of pigment in the skin, hair, and eyes.*
leuk/o		**leuk/o**/cyte (LOO-kō-sīt): white cell *-cyte:* cell *A leukocyte is a white blood cell.*
chlor/o	green	**chlor**/opia (klō-RŌ-pē-ă): green vision *-opia:* vision *Chloropia is a disorder in which viewed objects appear green. It is associated with a toxic reaction to digitalis.*
chrom/o	color	hetero/**chrom**/ic (hĕt-ĕr-ō-KRŌ-mĭk): pertaining to different colors *hetero-:* different *-ic:* pertaining to *Heterochromia is associated with the iris or sections of the iris of the eyes. Thus, the individual with heterochromia may have one brown iris and one blue iris.*

*The *i* in *pelv/i/meter* is an exception to the rule of using the connecting vowel *o.*

Element	Meaning	Word Analysis
cirrh/o	yellow	**cirrh**/osis (sĭr-RŌ-sĭs): abnormal yellowing *-osis:* abnormal condition; increase (used primarily with blood cells) *In cirrhosis, the skin, sclera of the eyes, and mucous membranes take on a yellow color. Cirrhosis of the liver is usually associated with alcoholism or chronic hepatitis.*
jaund/o		**jaund**/ice (JAWN-dĭs): yellowing *-ice:* noun ending *Jaundice is associated with obstruction in the bile passageways causing bile to back flow into the liver. Bile is than absorbed by the blood causing abnormal yellowing of body tissues.*
xanth/o		**xanth**/osis (ZĂN-thō-sĭs): abnormal condition of yellow(ness) *-osis:* abnormal condition; increase (used primarily with blood cells) *Xanthosis is a yellow discoloration commonly associated with cancerous tumors.*
cyan/o	blue	**cyan/o**/tic (sī-ăn-ŎT-ĭk): pertaining to blueness *-tic:* pertaining to *Cyanosis is associated with lack of oxygen in the blood.*
erythr/o	red	**erythr/o**/cyte (ĕ-RĬTH-rō-sīt): red cell *-cyte:* cell *An erythrocyte is a red blood cell.*
melan/o	black	**melan**/oma (mĕl-ă-NŌ-mă): black tumor *-oma:* tumor *Melanoma is a malignancy that arises from melanocytes.*
poli/o	gray; gray matter (of brain or spinal cord)	**poli/o**/myel/itis (pō-lē-ō-mĭ-ĕ-LĬ-tĭs): inflammation of the gray matter of the spinal cord *myel:* bone marrow; spinal cord *-itis:* inflammation
Other		
acr/o	extremity	**acr/o**/cyan/osis (ăk-rō-sī-ă-NŌ-sĭs): abnormal condition in which the extremities are blue *cyan:* blue *-osis:* abnormal condition; increase (used primarily with blood cells)
eti/o	cause	**eti/o**/logy (ē-tē-ŎL-ō-jē): study of the causes of disease *-logy:* study of
idi/o	unknown, peculiar	**idi/o**/path/ic (ĭd-ē-ō-PĂTH-ĭk): pertaining to an unknown (cause of) disease *path:* disease *-ic:* pertaining to
morph/o	form, shape, structure	**morph/o**/logy (mor-FŎL-ō-jē): study of form, shape, or structure *-logy:* study of

(continued)

Element	Meaning	Word Analysis
path/o	disease	**path/o**/logist (pă-THŎL-ō-jĭst): specialist in the study of disease *-logist:* specialist in the study of *Pathologists examine tissues, cells, and body fluids for evidence of disease.*
radi/o	radiation, x-ray; radius (lower arm bone on thumb side)	**radi/o**/logist (rā-dē-ŎL-ŏ-jĭst): specialist in the study of radiation *-logist:* specialist in the study of *Radiologists are physicians who employ imaging techniques for diagnosing and treating disease.*
somat/o	body	**somat**/ic (sō-MĂT-ĭk): pertaining to the body *-ic:* pertaining to
son/o	sound	**son/o**/graphy (sō-NŎG-ră-fē): process of recording sound; also called ultrasonography *-graphy:* process of recording *Sonography employs ultrasound (inaudible sound) to produce images. It is a painless, noninvasive imaging technique that does not use x-rays.*
tom/o	to cut	**tom/o**/graphy (tō-MŎG-ră-fē): process of recording a cut (or slice) *-graphy:* process of recording *Tomography is an imaging procedure that employs a computer to produce images that appear as "slices" of an organ or structure.*
viscer/o	internal organs	**viscer**/al (VĬS-ĕr-ăl): pertaining to internal organs *-al:* pertaining to
xer/o	dry	**xer**/osis (zē-RŌ-sĭs): abnormal condition of dryness *-osis:* abnormal condition; increase (used primarily with blood cells) *Xerosis refers to abnormal dryness of the skin, mucous membranes, or conjunctiva.*

Suffixes		
-genesis	forming, pro-ducing, origin	path/o/**genesis** (păth-ō-JĔN-ĕ-sĭs): origin of disease *path/o:* disease
-gnosis	knowing	pro/**gnosis** (prŏg-NŌ-sĭs): knowing before *pro-:* before, in front of *Prognosis is the prediction of the course and end of a disease and the estimated chance of recovery.*
-gram	record, writing	arteri/o/**gram** (ăr-TĒ-rē-ō-grăm): record of an artery *arteri/o:* artery *An arteriogram is a radiological image of an artery taken after injection of a radiopaque contrast medium.*

Element	Meaning	Word Analysis
-graph	instrument for recording	radi/o/**graph** (RĀ-dē-ō-grăf): instrument for recording x-rays *radi/o:* radiation, x-rays; radius (lower arm bone on thumb side)
-graphy	process of recording	arthr/o/**graphy** (ăr-THRŎG-ră-fē): process of recording a joint *arthr/o:* joint *Arthrography is the process of recording an image of a joint, such as the knee, shoulder, or elbow, usually with the use of a contrast medium.*
-logist	specialist in the study of	dermat/o/**logist** (dĕr-mă-TŎL-ō-jĭst): specialist in the study of skin *dermat/o:* skin
-logy	study of	hemat/o/**logy** (hē-mă-TŎL-ō-jē): study of blood *hemat/o:* blood
-meter	instrument for measuring	therm/o/**meter** (thĕr-MŎM-ĕ-tĕr): instrument for measuring heat *therm/o:* heat
-metry	act of measuring	ventricul/o/**metry** (vĕn-trĭk-ū-LŎM-ĕ-trē): act of measuring the ventricles *ventricul/o:* ventricle (of heart or brain)
-pathy	disease	gastr/o/**pathy** (găs-TRŎP-ă-thē): disease of the stomach *gastr/o:* stomach
Prefixes		
ab-	from, away from	**ab**/duction (ăb-DŬK-shŭn): act of bringing away from (midline of the body) *-duction:* act of leading, bringing, conducting *Abduction is the movement of a limb or body part away from the midline of the body.*
ad-	toward	**ad**/duction (ă-DŬK-shŭn): act of bringing toward (the midline of the body) *-duction:* act of leading, bringing, conducting *Adduction is the movement of a limb toward the midline of the body.*
hetero-	different	**hetero**/morph/ous (hĕt-ĕr-ō-MOR-fŭs): different form or shape *morph:* form, shape, structure *-ous:* pertaining to *Heteromorphous refers to any deviation from a normal type or shape.*
homeo-	same, alike	**homeo**/plasia (hō-mē-ō-PLĀ-zē-ă): formation of same (tissue) *-plasia:* formation, growth *Homeoplasia is the formation of new tissue similar to that already existing in a part.*
infra-	below, under	**infra**/cost/al (ĭn-fră-KŎS-tăl): pertaining to (the area) below the ribs *cost:* ribs *-al:* pertaining to

(continued)

Element	Meaning	Word Analysis
peri-	around	**peri**/umbilic/al (pĕr-ē-ŭm-BĬL-ĭ-kăl): pertaining to (the area) around the umbilicus *umbilic:* umbilicus, navel *-al:* pertaining to
super-	upper, above	**super**/ior (soo-PĒ-rē-or): pertaining to the upper (area) *-ior:* pertaining to
trans-	across, through	**trans**/abdomin/al (trăns-ăb-DŎM-ĭ-năl): pertaining to (a direction) across or through the abdomen *abdomin:* abdomen *-al:* pertaining to
ultra-	excess, beyond	**ultra**/son/ic (ŭl-tră-SŎN-ĭk): pertaining to beyond (audible) sound *son:* sound *-ic:* pertaining to *Ultrasound includes sound frequencies too high to be perceived by the human ear.*

 It is time to review medical word elements by completing Learning Activities 4-2 and 4-3.

Pathology

All body cells require oxygen and nutrients for survival. They also need a stable internal environment that provides a narrow range of temperature, water, acidity, and salt concentration. This stable internal environment is called **homeostasis.** When homeostasis is disrupted and cells, tissues, organs, or systems are unable to function effectively, the condition is called **disease.** From a clinical point of view, disease is a **pathological,** or **morbid,** condition that presents a group of signs, symptoms, and clinical findings. **Signs** are objective indicators that are observable. A rash, tissue redness, and swelling are examples of signs. In Figure 4-5, the rash is a sign of rubella (German measles), which is an acute infectious disease. A **symptom (Sx)** is a subjective indicator of disease. As such it is experienced only by the patient. Dizziness, pain, and nausea are examples of symptoms. Clinical findings are the results of radiologic, laboratory, and other medical procedures performed on the patient or his specimens.

Etiology is the study of the cause or origin of a disease or disorder. Some possible causes of diseases include:

- metabolic (such as diabetes)
- infectious (such as measles and mumps)
- congenital (such as cleft lip)
- hereditary (such as hemophilia)
- environmental (such as burns and trauma)
- neoplastic (such as cancer).

Establishing the cause and nature of a disease is called **diagnosis (Dx).** Determining a diagnosis helps in the selection of a treatment (Tx). A **prognosis** is the prediction of the course of a disease and its probable outcome. Any disease whose cause is unknown is said to be **idiopathic.**

Some diseases, injuries, or treatments cause complications that arise directly from disease, injury, or treatment. These complications are referred to as **sequelae.** For example, paralysis may be the sequela of a head injury.

A variety of diagnostic procedures are used to identify a disease and to determine its extent or involvement in the body. (See Figure 4-6.) Many diagnostic tests listed in this text are categorized as surgical, clinical, endoscopic, laboratory, and imaging procedures and some may include more than one testing modality.

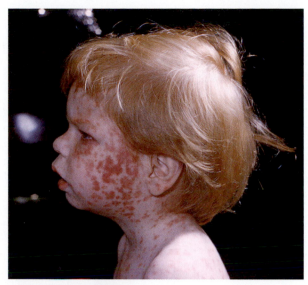

Figure 4-5 Skin rash (a sign of disease). From Tamparo: *Diseases of the Human Body,* 5th ed. FA Davis, Philadelphia, 2011, p 82, with permission.

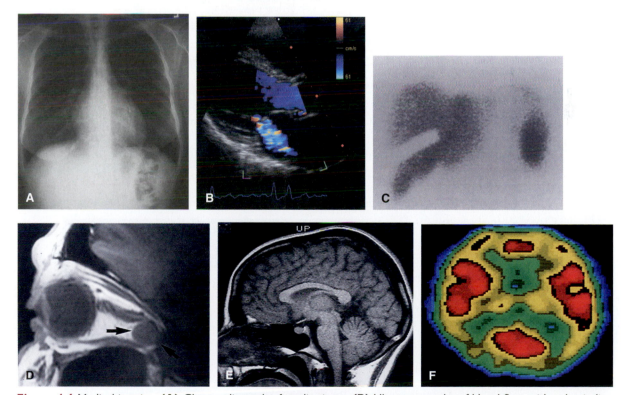

Figure 4-6 Medical imaging. **(A)** Chest radiograph of mediastinum. **(B)** Ultrasonography of blood flow with color indicating direction. **(C)** Nuclear scan of liver and spleen. **(D)** CT scan of the eye in lateral view showing a tumor (*arrows*). **(E)** MRI scan of midsagittal section of the head. **(F)** PET scan of the brain in transverse section (frontal lobes at top).

Diseases and Conditions

This section introduces diseases and conditions along with their meanings and their pronunciations. These terms are applicable to one or more of the body system chapters that follow. Word analyses for selected terms are also provided.

Term	Definition
adhesion ăd-HĒ-zhŭn	Abnormal fibrous band that holds or binds together tissues that are normally separated *Adhesions may occur within body cavities as a result of surgery. (See Figure 4-7.)* **Figure 4-7** Abdominal adhesions.
ascites ă-SĪ-tēz	Abnormal accumulation of fluid in the abdominal cavity
edema ĕ-DĒ-mă	Abnormal accumulation of fluid within tissue spaces (See Figure 4-8.) **Figure 4-8** Pitting edema. Indentation or pit shown from application of pressure over a bony area, which displaces the excess fluid. From Williams and Hopper: *Understanding Medical-Surgical Nursing,* 4th edition. FA Davis, Philadelphia, 2011, p 397, with permission.

Term	Definition
febrile FĔ-brĭl	Pertaining to a fever; also called *pyretic*
gangrene GĂNG-grēn	Death and decay of soft tissue, usually caused by circulatory obstruction, trauma, or infection
hernia HĔR-nē-ă	Protrusion of any organ through the structure that normally contains it
inflammation ĭn-flă-MĀ-shŭn	Body defense against injury, infection, or allergy marked by redness, swelling, heat, pain and, sometimes, loss of function *Inflammation is one mechanism used by the body to protect against invasion by foreign organisms and to repair injured tissue.*
mycosis mī-KŌ-sĭs *myc:* fungus (plural, fungi) *-osis:* abnormal condition; increase (used primarily with blood cells)	Any fungal infection in or on the body
perforation pĕr-fŏ-RĀ-shŭn	Hole that completely penetrates a structure *A perforation in the gastrointestinal tract is a medical emergency because gastrointestinal contents may flow into the abdominal cavity and infect the peritoneum.*
peritonitis pĕr-ĭ-tŏ-NĪ-tĭs *periton:* peritoneum *-itis:* inflammation	Inflammation of the peritoneum, the serous membrane that surrounds the abdominal cavity and covers its organs
rupture RŬP-chūr	Sudden breaking or bursting of a structure or organ
sepsis SĔP-sĭs	Pathological state, usually febrile, resulting from the presence of microorganisms or their products in the bloodstream
suppuration sŭp-ū-RĀ-shŭn	Producing or associated with the generation of pus

It is time to review pathology, diseases, and conditions by completing Learning Activity 4–4.

Medical, Surgical, and Diagnostic Procedures

This section introduces medical, surgical and diagnostic procedures that are applicable in the body systems chapters. Descriptions are provided as well as pronunciations and word analyses for selected terms.

Procedure	Description
Medical	
infusion therapy	Delivery of fluids directly into the blood stream via a vein for treating various disorders; also called IV therapy
	This procedure is commonly used for antibiotic therapy and to treat electrolyte imbalance, dehydration, cancer, and pain.
Surgical	
ablation ăb-LĀ-shŭn	Removal of a part, pathway, or function by surgery, chemical destruction, electrocautery, freezing, or radio frequency (RF)
anastomosis ă-năs-tō-MŌ-sĭs	Surgical joining of two ducts, vessels, or bowel segments to allow flow from one to another (See Figure 4-9.)

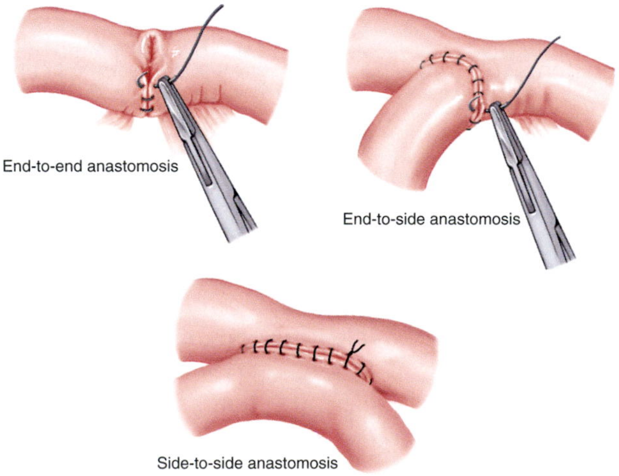

Figure 4-9 Anastomoses.

Procedure	Description
cauterize KAW-tĕr-īz	Destruction of tissue by electricity, freezing, heat, or corrosive chemicals
curettage kū-rĕ-TĂZH	Scraping of a body cavity with a spoon-shaped instrument called a curette (curet)
incision and drainage (I&D) ĭn-SĬZH-ŭn, DRĀN-ĭj	Incision made to allow the free flow or withdrawal of fluids from a wound or cavity
laser surgery LĀ-zĕr SŬR-jĕr-ē	Use of a high intensity laser light beam to remove diseased tissues, stop bleeding blood vessels, or for cosmetic purposes
	Laser surgery is used to remove lesions, scars, tattoos, wrinkles, sunspots, or birthmarks.

Procedure	Description
resection rē-SĔK-shŭn	Removal of part or all of a structure, organ, or tissue
revision	Surgical procedure used to replace or compensate for a previously implanted device or correct an undesirable result or effect of a previous surgery

Diagnostic

Clinical

assessment techniques	Sequence of procedures designed to evaluate the health status of a patient
inspection	General observation of the patient as a whole, progressing to specific body areas
palpation păl-PĀ-shŭn	Gentle application of the hands to a specific structure or body area to determine size, consistency, texture, symmetry, and tenderness of underlying structures
percussion pĕr-KŬSH-ŭn	Tapping a structure with the hand or fingers to assess consistency and the presence or absence of fluids within the underlying structure *Percussion is especially helpful in assessing the lung and abdomen.*
auscultation aws-kŭl-TĀ-shŭn	Listening to the heart, bowel, and lungs with or without a stethoscope to assess the presence and quality of sounds

Endoscopic

endoscopy ĕn-DŎS-kō-pē *endo-:* in, within *-scopy:* visual examination	Visual examination of a body cavity or canal using a specialized lighted instrument called an endoscope *Endoscopy is used for biopsy, surgery, aspirating fluids, and coagulating bleeding areas. The endoscope is usually named for the organ, cavity, or canal being examined, such as gastroscope and sigmoidoscope. (See Figure 4-10.) A camera and video recorder are commonly used during the procedure to provide a permanent record.*

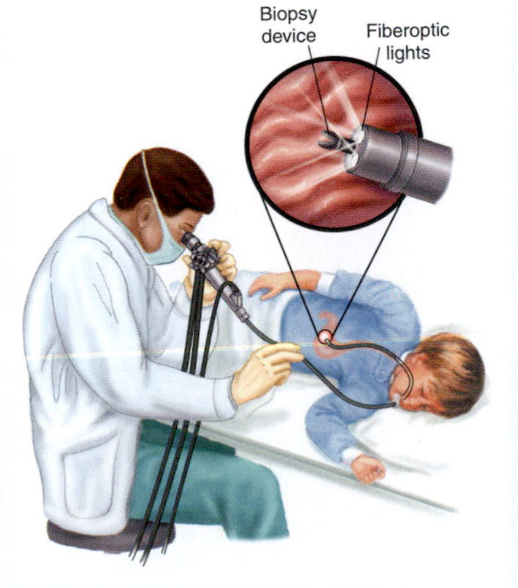

Biopsy device   Fiberoptic lights

Figure 4-10 Endoscopy (gastroscopy).

(continued)

Procedure	Description
Laboratory	
blood chemistry analysis ă-NĂL-ĭ-sĭs	Laboratory test, usually performed on serum, to evaluate various substances to determine whether they fall within a normal range *An example of a blood chemistry test is a cholesterol test. In this test, cholesterol is the substance being analyzed.*
complete blood count (CBC)	Panel of blood tests used as a broad screening test for anemias, infections, and other diseases *The CBC is usually performed as part of routine physical examinations to determine general health status.*
organ-disease panels	Series of blood tests used to evaluate a specific organ (liver panel) or disease (anemia panel)
Imaging	
computed tomography (CT) kŏm-PŪ-tĕd tō-MŎG-ră-fē *tom/o:* to cut *-graphy:* process of recording	Imaging technique in which an x-ray emitter rotates around the area to be scanned and a computer measures the intensity of transmitted x-rays from different angles; formerly called computerized axial tomography *In a CT scan, the computer generates a detailed cross-sectional image that appears as a slice. (See Figure 4-6 D.) Tumor masses, bone displacement, and accumulations of fluid may be detected. This technique may be used with or without a contrast medium.*
fluoroscopy floo-or-ŎS-kō-pē *fluor/o:* luminous, fluorescent *-scopy:* visual examination	Technique in which x-rays are directed through the body to a fluorescent screen that displays internal structures in continuous motion *Fluoroscopy is used to view the motion of organs, such as the digestive tract, heart, and joints, or to aid in the placement of catheters or other devices.*
magnetic resonance imaging (MRI) măg-NĔT-ĭk RĔZ-ĕn-ăns ĬM-ăj-ĭng	Technique that uses radio waves and a strong magnetic field, rather than an x-ray beam, to produce highly detailed, multiplanar, cross-sectional views of soft tissues (See Figure 4-6 E.) *MRI is used to diagnose a growing number of diseases because it provides superior soft tissue contrast. It commonly proves superior to CT scan for most central nervous system images, musculoskeletal images, and images of the pelvic areas. The procedure usually does not require a contrast medium.*
nuclear scan NŪ-klē-ăr	Technique in which a radioactive material (radiopharmaceutical) called a tracer is introduced into the body (inhaled, ingested, or injected) and a specialized camera (gamma camera) is used to produce images of organs and structures (See Figure 4-6 C.) *A nuclear scan is the reverse of a conventional radiograph. Rather than being directed into the body, radiation comes from inside the body and is then detected by a specialized camera to produce an image.*

Procedure	Description
positron emission tomography (PET) PŎZ-ĭ-trŏn ē-MĬSH-ŭn tō-MŎG-rǎ-fē	Computed tomography records the positrons (positive charged particles) emitted from a radiopharmaceutical to produce a cross-sectional image of metabolic activity of body tissues to determine the presence of disease (See Figure 4-6 F.) *PET is particularly useful in scanning the brain and nervous system to diagnose disorders that involve abnormal tissue metabolism, such as schizophrenia, brain tumors, epilepsy, stroke, and Alzheimer disease, as well as cardiac and pulmonary disorders.*

radiography
rā-dē-ŎG-rǎ-fē
   radi/o: radiation, x-ray, radius (lower arm bone on thumb side)
   -graphy: process of recording
	Technique in which x-rays are passed through the body or area and captured on a film to generate an image; also called x-ray (See Figure 4-6 A.)
	Radiography of soft tissue usually requires the use of a contrast medium to enhance images. Commonly used x-ray contrast media are barium and iodine compounds.

single photon emission computed tomography (SPECT)
FŌ-tŏn ē-MĬ-shŭn tō-MŎG-rǎ-fē
   tom/o: to cut
   -graphy: process of recording
	Radiological technique that integrates computed tomography (CT) and a radioactive material (tracer) injected into the bloodstream to visualize blood flow to tissues and organs
	
	SPECT differs from a PET scan in that the tracer remains in the blood stream rather than being absorbed by surrounding tissue. It is especially useful to visualize blood flow through arteries and veins in the brain.

ultrasonography (US)
ŭl-trǎ-sŏn-ŎG-rǎ-fē
   ultra-: excess, beyond
   son/o: sound
   -graphy: process of recording
	High-frequency sound waves (ultrasound) are directed at soft tissue and reflected as "echoes" to produce an image on a monitor of an internal body structure; also called *ultrasound, sonography,* and *echo* (See Figure 4-6 B.)
	US, unlike most other imaging methods, creates real-time moving images to view organs and functions of organs in motion. A computer analyzes the reflected echoes and converts them into an image on a video monitor. Because this procedure does not utilize ionizing radiation (x-ray), it is used during pregnancy to observe fetal growth and also to study other internal organs for possible pathologies or lesions.

Surgical	
biopsy (bx) BĪ-ŏp-sē	Removal of a representative tissue sample from a body site for microscopic examination, usually to establish a diagnosis
excisional ĕk-SĬ-zhŭn-ǎl	Biopsy in which the entire lesion is removed
incisional ĭn-SĬZH-ŭn-ǎl	Biopsy in which only a small sample of the lesion is removed

Abbreviations

This section introduces body structure abbreviations and their meanings.

Abbreviation	Meaning	Abbreviation	Meaning
AP	anteroposterior	MRI	magnetic resonance imaging
Bx, bx	biopsy	PET	positron emission tomography
CBC	complete blood count	RF	rheumatoid factor; radio frequency
CT	computed tomography	RLQ	right lower quadrant
DNA	deoxyribonucleic acid	RUQ	right upper quadrant
Dx	diagnosis	SPECT	single photon emission computed tomography
I&D	incision and drainage	Sx	symptom
LAT, lat	lateral	Tx	treatment
LLQ	left lower quadrant	U&L, U/L	upper and lower
LUQ	left upper quadrant	US	ultrasound, ultrasonography

It is time to review procedures and abbreviations by completing Learning Activity 4–5.

LEARNING ACTIVITIES

The following activities provide review of the body structure terms introduced in this chapter. Complete each activity and review your answers to evaluate your understanding of the chapter.

Learning Activity 4-1

Matching Body Cavity, Spine, and Directional Terms

Match each term on the left with its meaning on the right.

1. _____ abdominopelvic	a. pertaining to the sole of the foot
2. _____ adduction	b. tail bone
3. _____ cervical	c. ventral cavity that contains heart, lungs, and associated structures
4. _____ coccyx	d. toward the surface of the body (external)
5. _____ deep	e. lying horizontal with face downward
6. _____ eversion	f. turning outward
7. _____ inferior (caudal)	g. nearer to the center (trunk of the body)
8. _____ inversion	h. ventral cavity that contains digestive, reproductive, and excretory structures
9. _____ lumbar	i. turning inward or inside out
10. _____ plantar	j. part of the spine known as the neck
11. _____ posterior (dorsal)	k. movement toward the median plane
12. _____ prone	l. away from the head; toward the tail or lower part of a structure
13. _____ proximal	m. away from the surface of the body (internal)
14. _____ superficial	n. part of the spine known as the loin
15. _____ thoracic	o. near the back of the body

 Check your answers in Appendix A. Review any material that you did not answer correctly.

Correct Answers _____ X 6.67 = _____ % Score

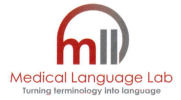

Medical Language Lab
Turning terminology into language

Visit the Medical Language Lab at the web site: medicallanguagelab.com. Use it to enhance your study and reinforcement of this chapter with the flash-card activity. We recommend you complete the flash-card activity before starting Learning Activities 4-2 and 4-3.

Learning Activity 4-2
Matching Word Elements

Match the following word elements with the definitions in the numbered list.

Combining Forms		Suffixes	Prefixes
caud/o	kary/o	-genesis	ad-
dist/o	leuk/o	-gnosis	infra-
dors/o	morph/o	-graphy	ultra-
eti/o	poli/o		
hist/o	somat/o		
idi/o	viscer/o		
jaund/o	xer/o		

1. nucleus _____
2. far, farthest _____
3. process of recording _____
4. knowing _____
5. white _____
6. internal organs _____
7. yellow _____
8. tissue _____
9. forming, producing, origin _____
10. below, under _____
11. excess, beyond _____
12. tail _____
13. back (of body) _____
14. gray _____
15. cause _____
16. form, shape, structure _____
17. dry _____
18. unknown, peculiar _____
19. toward _____
20. body _____

✔ *Check your answers in Appendix A. Review any material that you did not answer correctly.*

Correct Answers _____ X 5.0 = _____ % Score

Learning Activity 4-3
Combining Forms, Suffixes, and Prefixes

Use the elements listed in the table to build medical words. You may use the elements more than once.

Combining Forms		Suffixes		Prefixes
abdomin/o	eti/o	-al	-megaly	dia-
cirrh/o	gastr/o	-algia	-meter	infra-
cost/o	leuk/o	-gnosis	-oma	super-
crani/o	melan/o	-graphy	-osis	trans-
cyt/o	son/o	-ior	-plasty	
dors/o		-logy	-rrhea	
erythr/o		-lysis		

  1. instrument to measure cells _____
  2. pertaining to across the abdomen _____
  3. discharge of white (material) _____
  4. surgical repair of the cranium (skull) _____
  5. pain in the back (of the body) _____
  6. enlargement of the stomach _____
  7. tumor of black (cells) _____
  8. pertaining to below the ribs _____
  9. destruction of the a cell _____
10. pertaining to (the area) above _____
11. abnormal condition of red(ness) _____
12. study of the cause (of disease) _____
13. knowing through (examination) _____
14. process of recording sound _____
15. abnormal condition of yellow(ness) _____

 Check your answers in Appendix A. Review any material that you did not answer correctly.

Correct Answers _____ X 6.67 = _____ % Score

Learning Activity 4-4
Pathology, Diseases and Conditions

Match the following terms with the definitions in the numbered list.

adhesion	gangrene	perforation
ascites	hernia	prognosis
diagnosis	idiopathic	rupture
edema	inflammation	sign
etiology	mycosis	symptom

1. study of the cause or origin of a disease _____

2. establishing the cause and nature of a disease _____

3. fibrous band that binds together tissues that are normally separated _____

4. death and decay of soft tissue _____

5. protrusion of any organ through the structure that normally contains it _____

6. abnormal accumulation of fluid in the abdominal cavity _____

7. objective indicator of a disease _____

8. disease whose cause is unknown _____

9. prediction of the course of a disease and its probable outcome _____

10. body defense against injury, infection, or allergy, marked by redness, heat, pain, and swelling _____

11. sudden breaking or bursting of a structure or organ _____

12. subjective indicator of a disease _____

13. abnormal accumulation of fluid in tissue spaces _____

14. fungal infection in or on the body _____

15. hole made through a structure or a body part _____

✓ *Check your answers in Appendix A. Review any material that you did not answer correctly.*

Correct Answers _____ X 6.67 = _____ % Score

Learning Activity 4-5

Matching Procedures and Abbreviations

Match the following terms with the definitions in the numbered list.

ablation	*Dx*	*nuclear scan*
anastomosis	*endoscopy*	*palpation*
cauterize	*excisional*	*percussion*
CBC	*fluoroscopy*	*resection*
computed tomography	*MRI*	*revision*

1. assessment technique that involves the gentle tapping of a structure _____

2. type of biopsy in which the entire lesion is removed _____

3. panel of blood tests used as a broad screening test for anemias, infections, and other diseases _____

4. removal of a part, pathway, or function by surgery, chemical destruction, or other techniques _____

5. visual examination of a cavity or canal using a special lighted instrument _____

6. imaging technique that directs x-rays to a fluorescent screen and displays "live" images on a monitor _____

7. establishing the nature and cause of a disease _____

8. destroy tissue by electricity, freezing, heat, or corrosive chemicals _____

9. surgery to compensate or correct a previously performed surgery _____

10. imaging procedure that uses radio waves and a strong magnetic field to produce images _____

11. surgical joining of two ducts, vessels, or bowel segments _____

12. imaging procedure that uses a radioactive material introduced into the body to produce an image _____

13. gentle application of hands to evaluate a specific structure of the body _____

14. removal of part or all of a structure _____

15. imaging procedure that generates detailed cross-sectional images that appear as a slice _____

✔ *Check your answers in Appendix A. Review any material that you did not answer correctly.*

Correct Answers _____ X 6.67 = _____ % Score

MEDICAL RECORD ACTIVITIES

The two medical records included in the following activities use common clinical scenarios to show how medical terminology is used to document patient care. Complete the terminology and analysis sections for each activity to help you recognize and understand terms related to body structure.

Medical Record Activity 4-1

Radiological Consultation Letter: Cervical and Lumbar Spine

Terminology

Terms listed in the following table are taken from *Radiology Report: Cervical and Lumbar Spine* that follows. Use a medical dictionary such as *Taber's Cyclopedic Medical Dictionary;* the appendices of *Systems,* 7th ed.; or other resources to define each term. Then review pronunciations for each term and practice by reading the medical record aloud.

Term	Definition
AP	
atlantoaxial ăt-lăn-tō-ĂK-sē-ăl	
cervical SĔR-vĭ-kăl	
lateral LĂT-ĕr-ăl	
lumbar LŬM-băr	
lumbosacral junction lŭm-bō-SĀ-krăl	
odontoid ō-DŎN-toyd	
sacral SĀ-krăl	
scoliosis skō-lē-Ō-sĭs	
spasm SPĂZM	

Term	Definition
spina bifida occulta SPĪ-nă BĬF-ĭ-dă ŏ-KŬL-tă	
vertebral bodies VĔR-tĕ-brăl	

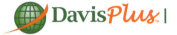 | Visit the *Medical Terminology Systems* online resource center at Davis*Plus* to practice pronunciation and reinforce the meanings of the terms in this medical report.

RADIOLOGICAL CONSULTATION LETTER: CERVICAL AND LUMBAR SPINE

Physician Center

2422 Rodeo Drive ■■ Sun City, USA 12345 ■■ (555) 333-2427

May 3, 20xx

John Roberts, MD
1115 Forest Ave
Sun City, USA 12345

Dear Doctor Roberts:

Thank you for referring Chester Bowen to our office. Mr. Bowen presents with neck and lower back pain of more than 2 years' duration. Radiographic examination of June 14, 20xx reveals the following: AP, lateral, and odontoid views of the cervical spine demonstrate some reversal of normal cervical curvature, as seen on lateral projection. There is some right lateral scoliosis of the cervical spine. The vertebral bodies, however, appear to be well maintained in height; the intervertebral spaces are well maintained. The odontoid is visualized and appears to be intact. The atlantoaxial joint appears symmetrical.

Impression: Films of the cervical spine demonstrate some reversal of normal cervical curvature and a minimal scoliosis, possibly secondary to muscle spasm, without evidence of recent bony disease or injury. AP and lateral films of the lumbar spine, with spots of the lumbosacral junction, demonstrate an apparent minimal spina bifida occulta of the first sacral segment. The vertebral bodies, however, are well maintained in height; the intervertebral spaces appear well maintained.

Pathological Diagnosis: Right lateral scoliosis with some reversal of normal cervical curvature.

If you have any further questions, please feel free to contact me.

Sincerely yours,

Adrian Jones, MD
Adrian Jones, MD

aj:bg

Analysis

Review the medical record *Radiological Consultation Letter: Cervical and Lumbar Spine* to answer the following questions.

1. What was the presenting problem?

_____

2. What were the three views of the radiological examination of June 14, 20xx?

_____

3. Was there evidence of recent bony disease or injury?

_____

4. Which cervical vertebrae form the atlantoaxial joint?

_____

5. Was the odontoid fractured?

_____

6. What did the AP and lateral films of the lumbar spine demonstrate?

_____

Radiology Report: Injury of Left Wrist, Elbow, and Humerus

Terminology

Terms listed in the following table are taken from *Radiology Report: Injury of Left Wrist, Elbow, and Humerus* that follows. Use a medical dictionary such as *Taber's Cyclopedic Medical Dictionary;* the appendices of *Systems,* 7th ed.; or other resources to define each term. Then review the pronunciations for each term and practice by reading the medical record aloud.

Term	Definition
AP	
anterior	
distal DĬS-tăl	
dorsal DOR-săl	
epicondyle ĕp-ĭ-KŎN-dīl	
humerus HŪ-mĕr-ŭs	
lucency LOO-sĕnt-sē	
medial MĒ-dē-ăl	
mm	
posterior	
radius RĀ-dē-ŭs	
ulna ŬL-nă	
ventral-lateral VĔN-trăl-LĂT-ĕr-ăl	

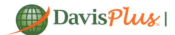

Visit the *Medical Terminology Systems* online resource center at Davis*Plus* to practice pronunciation and reinforce the meanings of the terms in this medical report.

RADIOLOGY REPORT: INJURY OF LEFT WRIST, ELBOW, AND HUMERUS

General Hospital

1511 Ninth Avenue ■■ Sun City, USA 12345 ■■ (555) 802-1887

RADIOLOGY REPORT

Date:	June 5, 20xx	Patient:	Hill, Joan
Physician:	Adrian Jones, MD	DOB:	5/25/19xx
Examination:	Left wrist, left elbow, and left humerus	X-ray No:	43201

LEFT WRIST: Images obtained with the patient's arm taped to an arm board. There are fractures through the distal shafts of the radius and ulna. The radial fracture fragments show approximately 8-mm overlap with dorsal displacement of the distal radial fracture fragment. The distal ulnar shaft fracture shows ventral-lateral angulation at the fracture apex. There is no overriding at this fracture. No additional fracture is seen. Soft-tissue deformity is present, correlating with the fracture sites.

LEFT ELBOW AND LEFT HUMERUS: Single view of the left elbow was obtained in the lateral projection. AP view of the humerus was obtained to include a portion of the elbow. A third radiograph was obtained but is not currently available for review. There is lucency through the distal humerus on the AP view along its medial aspect. It would be difficult to exclude fracture just above the medial epicondyle. On the lateral view, there is elevation of the anterior and posterior fat pad. These findings are of some concern. Repeat elbow study is recommended.

Jason Skinner, MD
Jason Skinner, MD

JS: bg

D: 6-05-20xx
T: 6-05-20xx

Analysis

Review the medical record *Radiology Report: Injury of Left Wrist, Elbow, and Humerus* to answer the following questions.

1. Where are the fractures located?

_____

2. What caused the soft-tissue deformity?

_____

3. Did the radiologist take any side views of the left elbow?

_____

4. In the AP view of the humerus, what structure was also visualized?

_____

5. What findings are causes for concern to the radiologist?

_____

Integumentary System

Chapter Outline

Objectives

Upon completion of this chapter, you will be able to:

- Locate the major organs of the integumentary system and describe their structure and function.
- Describe the functional relationship between the integumentary system and other body systems.
- Pronounce, spell, and build words related to the integumentary system.
- Describe diseases, conditions, and procedures related to the integumentary system.
- Explain pharmacology associated with the treatment of skin disorders.
- Demonstrate your knowledge of this chapter by completing the learning and medical record activities.

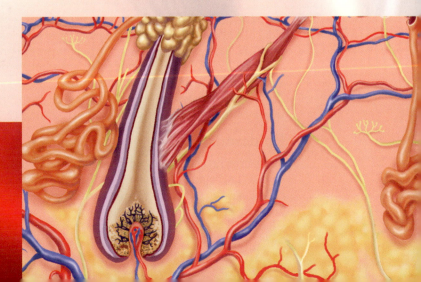

Anatomy and Physiology

The skin, also called **integument,** is the largest organ in the body. Together with its accessory organs (hair, nails, and glands), the skin makes up the **integumentary system.** This elaborate system of distinct tissues includes glands that produce several types of secretions, nerves that transmit impulses, and blood vessels that help regulate body temperature. The skin covers and protects all outer surfaces of the body and performs many vital functions, including the sense of touch. (See Figure 5-1.)

Anatomy and Physiology Key Terms

This section introduces important terms, along with their definitions and pronunciations. Word analyses for selected terms are also provided.

Term	Definition
androgen ĂN-drō-jĕn	Generic term for an agent (usually a hormone, such as testosterone and androsterone) that stimulates development of male characteristics *Androgens also regulate production of sebum.*
ductule DŬK-tūl *duct:* to lead; carry *-ule:* small, minute	Very small duct
homeostasis hō-mē-ō-STĀ-sĭs *homeo-:* same, alike *-stasis:* standing still	State in which the regulatory mechanisms of the body maintain an internal environment within tolerable levels, despite changes in the external environment *The regulatory mechanisms of the body control temperature, acidity, and the concentration of salt, food, and waste products.*
synthesize SĬN-thĕ-sīz	Forming a complex substance by the union of simpler compounds or elements *Skin synthesizes vitamin D (needed by bones for calcium absorption).*

Pronunciation Help	Long Sound	ā — rate	ē — rebirth	ī — isle	ō — over	ū — unite
	Short Sound	ă — alone	ĕ — ever	ĭ — it	ŏ — not	ŭ — cut

Skin

The skin protects underlying structures from injury and provides sensory information to the brain. Beneath the skin's surface is an intricate network of nerve fibers that register sensations of temperature, pain, and pressure. Other important functions of the skin include protecting the body against ultraviolet rays, regulating body temperature, and preventing dehydration. The skin also acts as a reservoir for food and water. It also **synthesizes** vitamin D when exposed to sunlight. The skin consists of two distinct layers: the epidermis and the dermis. A subcutaneous layer of tissue binds the skin to underlying structures.

Epidermis

The outer layer, the (1) **epidermis,** is relatively thin over most areas but is thickest on the palms of the hands and the soles of the feet. Although the epidermis is composed of several sublayers called **strata,** the (2) **stratum corneum** and the (3) **basal layer,** which is the deepest layer, are of greatest importance.

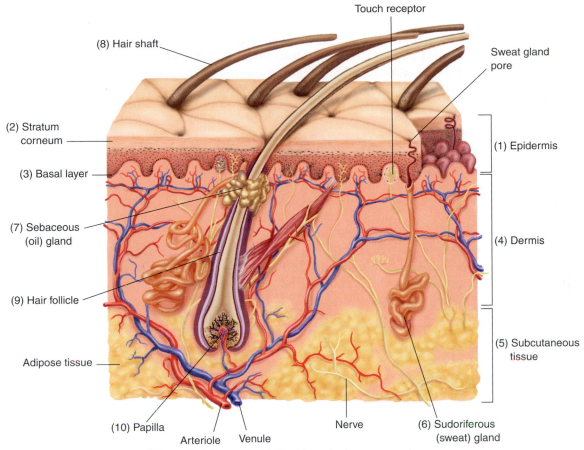

Figure 5-1 Structure of the skin and subcutaneous tissue.

The stratum corneum is composed of dead, flat cells that lack a blood supply and sensory receptors. Its thickness is related to normal wear of the area it covers. The basal layer is the only layer of the epidermis that is composed of living cells where new cells are formed. As these cells move toward the stratum corneum to replace the cells that have been sloughed off, they die and become filled with a hard protein material called **keratin.** The relatively waterproof characteristic of keratin prevents body fluids from evaporating and moisture from entering the body. The entire process by which a cell forms in the basal layer, rises to the surface, becomes keratinized, and sloughs off takes about 1 month.

In the basal layer, special cells called **melanocytes** produce a black pigment called **melanin.** Melanin provides a protective barrier from the damaging effects of the sun's ultraviolet radiation, which can cause skin cancer. Moderate sun exposure increases the rate of melanin production and results in a suntan. However, overexposure results in sunburn due to melanin's inability to absorb sufficient ultraviolet rays to prevent the burn.

Differences in skin color are attributed to the amount of melanin in each cell. Dark-skinned people produce large amounts of melanin and are less likely to have wrinkles or skin cancer. Production of melanocytes is genetically regulated and, thus, inherited. Local accumulations of melanin are seen in pigmented moles and freckles. An absence of pigment in the skin, eyes, and hair is most likely due to an inherited inability to produce melanin. An individual who cannot produce melanin, known as an **albino,** has a marked deficiency of pigment in the eyes, hair, and skin.

Dermis

The second layer of the skin, the (4) **dermis,** also called **corium,** lies directly beneath the epidermis. It is composed of living tissue and contains numerous capillaries, lymphatic vessels, and nerve endings. Hair follicles, **sebaceous** (oil) glands, and **sudoriferous** (sweat) glands are also located in the dermis.

The (5) **subcutaneous layer,** also called **hypodermis,** binds the dermis to underlying structures. It is composed primarily of loose connective tissue and **adipose** (fat) tissue interlaced with blood vessels. The subcutaneous layer stores fats, insulates and cushions the body, and regulates temperature. The amount of fat in the subcutaneous layer varies with the region of the body and sex, age, and nutritional state.

Accessory Organs of the Skin

The accessory organs of the skin consist of integumentary glands, hair, and nails. The glands play an important role in defending the body against disease and maintaining **homeostasis**, whereas the hair and nails have more limited functional roles.

Glands

Two important glands located in the dermis produce secretions: The (6) **sudoriferous (sweat) glands** produce sweat and the (7) **sebaceous (oil) glands** produce oil. These two glands are **exocrine glands** because they secrete substances through ducts to an outer surface of the body rather than directly into the bloodstream.

The sudoriferous glands secrete perspiration, or sweat, onto the surface of the skin through pores. Pores are most plentiful on the palms, soles, forehead, and **axillae** (armpits). The main functions of the sudoriferous glands are to cool the body by evaporation, excrete waste products, and moisten surface cells.

The sebaceous glands are filled with cells, the centers of which contain fatty droplets. As these cells disintegrate, they yield an oily secretion called **sebum.** The acidic nature of sebum helps destroy harmful organisms on the skin, thus preventing infection. When **ductules** of the sebaceous glands become blocked, acne may result. Congested sebum causes formation of pimples or whiteheads. If the sebum is dark, it forms blackheads. Sex hormones, particularly **androgens**, regulate production and secretion of sebum. During adolescence, secretions increase; as the person ages, secretions diminish. The loss of sebum, which lubricates the skin, may be one of the reasons for the formation of wrinkles that accompany old age. Sebaceous glands are present over the entire body except on the soles of the feet and the palms of the hands. They are especially prevalent on the scalp and face; around such openings as the nose, mouth, external ear, and anus; and on the upper back.

Hair

Hair is found on nearly all parts of the body except for the lips, nipples, palms of the hands, soles of the feet, and parts of the external genitalia. The visible part of the hair is the (8) **hair shaft;** the part that is embedded in the dermis is the hair root. The root, together with its coverings, forms the (9) **hair follicle.** At the bottom of the follicle is a loop of capillaries enclosed in a covering called the (10) **papilla.** The cluster of epithelial cells lying over the papilla reproduces and is responsible for the eventual formation of the hair shaft. As long as these cells remain alive, hair will regenerate even if it is cut, plucked, or otherwise removed. Alopecia (baldness) occurs when the hairs of the scalp are not replaced because of death of the papillae (singular, papilla).

Like skin color, hair color is related to the amount of pigment produced by epidermal melanocytes. Melanocytes are found at the base of the hair follicle. Melanin ranges in color from yellow to reddish brown to black. Varying amounts of melanin produce hair ranging in color from blond to brunette to black; the more abundant the melanin, the darker the hair. Heredity and aging affect melanin levels. A decrease or an absence of melanin causes loss of hair color.

Nails

Nails protect the tips of the fingers and toes from bruises and injuries. (See Figure 5-2.) Each nail is formed in the (1) **nail root** and is composed of keratinized, stratified, squamous epithelial cells producing a very tough covering. As the nail grows, it stays attached and slides forward over the layer of epithelium called the (2) **nail bed.** This epithelial layer is continuous with the epithelium

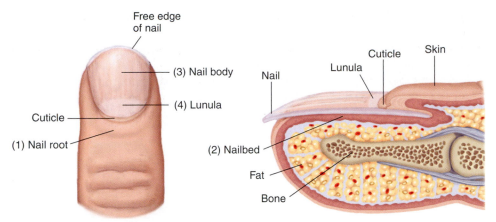

Figure 5-2 Structure of a fingernail.

of the skin. Most of the (3) **nail body** appears pink because of the underlying vascular tissue. The half-moon–shaped area at the base of the nail, the (4) **lunula,** is the region where new growth occurs. The lunula has a whitish appearance because the vascular tissue underneath does not show through.

Anatomy Review

To review the anatomy of the integumentary system, label the illustration using the terms below.

dermis

epidermis

hair follicle

hair shaft

papilla

sebaceous (oil) gland

stratum corneum

stratum germinativum

subcutaneous tissue

sudoriferous (sweat) gland

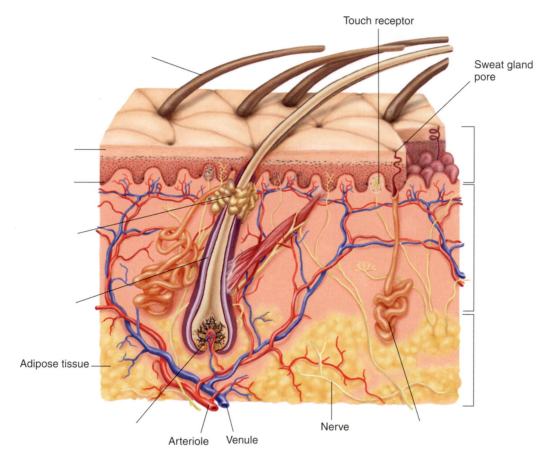

Touch receptor

Sweat gland pore

Adipose tissue

Arteriole   Venule

Nerve

 Check your answers by referring to Figure 5–1 on page 79. Review material that you did not answer correctly.

CONNECTING BODY SYSTEMS—INTEGUMENTARY SYSTEM

The main function of the skin is to protect the entire body, including all of its organs, from the external environment. Specific functional relationships between the skin and other body systems are summarized below.

Blood, Lymph, and Immune
- Skin is the first line of defense against the invasion of pathogens into the body.

Cardiovascular
- Cutaneous blood vessels dilate and constrict to help regulate body temperature.

Digestive
- Skin absorbs vitamin D (produced when skin is exposed to sunlight) needed for intestinal absorption of calcium.
- Excess calories are stored as subcutaneous fat.

Endocrine
- Subcutaneous layer of the skin stores adipose tissue when insulin secretions cause excess carbohydrate intake to fat storage.

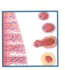

Female Reproductive
- Subcutaneous receptors provide pleasurable sensations associated with sexual behavior.
- Skin stretches to accommodate the growing fetus during pregnancy.

Male Reproductive
- Receptors in the skin respond to sexual stimuli.

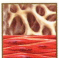

Musculoskeletal
- Skin synthesizes the vitamin D needed for absorption of calcium, which is essential for muscle contraction.
- Skin also synthesizes the vitamin D needed for growth, repair, and maintenance of bones.

Nervous
- Cutaneous receptors detect stimuli related to touch, pain, pressure, and temperature.

Respiratory
- Skin temperature may influence respiratory rate. As temperature increases, respiratory rate may also increase.
- Hairs of the nasal cavity filter particles from inspired air before it reaches the lower respiratory tract.

Urinary
- Skin provides an alternative route for excreting salts and nitrogenous wastes in the form of perspiration.

Medical Word Elements

This section introduces combining forms, suffixes, and prefixes related to the integumentary system. Word analyses are also provided.

Element	Meaning	Word Analysis
Combining Forms		

adip/o	fat	**adip**/osis (ăd-ĭ-PŌ-sĭs): abnormal condition of fat
		  -*osis:* abnormal condition; increase (used primarily with blood cells)
		  Adiposis is an abnormal accumulation of fatty tissue in the body.

lip/o		**lip/o**/cele (LĬP-ō-sēl): hernia containing fat -*cele:* hernia, swelling
steat/o		**steat**/itis (stē-ă-TĪ-tĭs): inflammation of fatty (adipose) tissue -*itis:* inflammation

(continued)

Element	Meaning	Word Analysis
cutane/o	skin	sub/**cutane**/ous (sŭb-kū-TĀ-nē-ŭs): pertaining to beneath the skin *sub-:* under, below *-ous:* pertaining to
dermat/o		**dermat/o**/plasty (DĔR-mă-tō-plăs-tē): surgical repair of the skin *-plasty:* surgical repair
derm/o		hypo/**derm**/ic (hī-pō-DĔR-mĭk): pertaining to under the skin *hypo-:* under, below *-ic:* pertaining to *A hypodermic injection is one in which the needle is inserted under the skin.*
hidr/o	sweat	**hidr**/aden/itis (hī-drăd-ĕ-NĪ-tĭs): inflammation of the sweat glands *aden:* gland *-itis:* inflammation *Do not confuse* hidr/o *(sweat) with* hydr/o *(water).*
sudor/o		**sudor**/esis (soo-dō-RĒ-sĭs): profuse sweating; also called *hyperhidrosis* *-esis:* condition
ichthy/o	dry, scaly	**ichthy**/osis (ĭk-thē-Ō-sĭs): abnormal condition of dry or scaly skin *-osis:* abnormal condition; increase (used primarily with blood cells) *Ichthyosis can be any of several dermatological conditions in which the skin is dry and hardened (hyperkeratotic), resembling fish scales. A mild form of ichthyosis, called winter itch, is commonly seen on the legs of older patients, especially during the winter months.*
kerat/o	horny tissue; hard; cornea	**kerat**/osis (kĕr-ă-TŌ-sĭs): abnormal condition of horny tissue *-osis:* abnormal condition; increase (used primarily with blood cells) *Keratosis is a thickened area of the epidermis or any horny growth on the skin, such as a callus or wart.*
melan/o	black	**melan**/oma (mĕl-ă-NŌ-mă): black tumor *-oma:* tumor *Melanoma is a malignant tumor of melanocytes that commonly begins in a darkly pigmented mole and can metastasize widely.*
myc/o	fungus (plural, fungi)	dermat/o/**myc**/osis (dĕr-mă-tō-mī-KŌ-sĭs): fungal infection of the skin *dermat/o:* skin *-osis:* abnormal condition; increase (used primarily with blood cells)
onych/o	nail	**onych/o**/malacia (ŏn-ĭ-kō-mă-LĀ-shē-ă): softening of the nails *-malacia:* softening
ungu/o		**ungu**/al (ŬNG-gwăl): pertaining to the nails *-al:* pertaining to

Element	Meaning	Word Analysis
pil/o	hair	**pil/o**/nid/al (pī-lō-NĬ-dăl): pertaining to hair in a nest *nid:* nest *-al:* pertaining to *A pilonidal cyst commonly develops in the skin at the base of the spine. It develops as a growth of hair in a dermoid cyst.*
trich/o		**trich/o**/pathy (trĭk-ŎP-ă-thē): disease involving the hair *-pathy:* disease
scler/o	hardening; sclera (white of eye)	**scler/o**/derma (sklĕ-rō-DĔR-mă): hardening of the skin *-derma:* skin *Scleroderma is an autoimmune disorder that causes the skin and internal organs to become progressively hardened due to deposits of collagen. It may occur as a localized form or as a systemic disease.*
seb/o	sebum, sebaceous	**seb/o**/rrhea (sĕb-ō-RĒ-ă): discharge of sebum *-rrhea:* discharge, flow *Seborrhea is an excessive secretion of sebum from the sebaceous glands.*
squam/o	scale	**squam**/ous (SKWĀ-mŭs): pertaining to scales (or covered with scales) *-ous:* pertaining to
xen/o	foreign, strange	xen/o/graft (ZĔN-ō-grăft): skin transplantation from a foreign donor (usually a pig) for a human; also called heterograft. *-graft:* transplantation *Xenografts are used as a temporary graft to protect the patient against infection and fluid loss.*
xer/o	dry	**xer/o**/derma (zē-rō-DĔR-mă): dry skin *-derma:* skin *Xeroderma is a chronic skin condition characterized by dryness and roughness and is a mild form of ichthyosis.*

Suffixes

Element	Meaning	Word Analysis
-cyte	cell	lip/o/**cyte** (LĬP-ō-sīt): fat cell *lip/o:* fat
-derma	skin	py/o/**derma** (pī-ō-DĔR-mă): pus in the skin *py/o:* pus *Pyoderma is an acute, inflammatory, purulent bacterial dermatitis. It may be primary, such as impetigo, or secondary to a previous skin condition.*
-logist	specialist in the study of	dermat/o/**logist** (dĕr-mă-TŎL-ō-jĭst): specialist in the study of skin disorders *dermat/o:* skin

(continued)

Element	Meaning	Word Analysis
-logy	study of	dermat/o/**logy** (dĕr-mă-TŎL-ō-jē): study of the skin (and its diseases) *dermat/o:* skin
-therapy	treatment	cry/o/**therapy** (krī-ō-THĔR-ă-pē): use of cold in the treatment (of disease) *cry/o:* cold *Cryotherapy is used to destroy tissue by freezing with liquid nitrogen. Cutaneous warts and actinic keratosis are common skin disorders that respond well to cryotherapy treatment.*
Prefixes		
an-	without, not	**an**/hidr/osis (ăn-hī-DRŌ-sĭs): abnormal condition of not sweating *hidr:* sweat *-osis:* abnormal condition; increase (used primarily with blood cells)
dia-	through, across	**dia**/phoresis (dī-ă-fă-RĒ-sĭs): excessive or profuse sweating; also called sudoresis or hyperhidrosis *-phoresis:* carrying; transmission
epi-	above, upon	**epi**/derm/is (ĕp-ĭ-DĔR-mĭs): above the skin *derm:* skin *-is:* noun ending *Epidermis is the outermost layer of the skin.*
homo-	same	**homo**/graft (HŌ-mō-grăft): transplantation of tissue between individuals of the same species; also called allograft *-graft:* transplantation
hyper-	excessive, above normal	**hyper**/hidr/osis (hī-pĕr-hī-DRŌ-sĭs): excessive or profuse sweating; also called diaphoresis or sudoresis *hidr:* sweat *-osis:* abnormal condition; increase (used primarily with blood cells)
sub-	under, below	**sub**/ungu/al (sŭb-ŬNG-gwăl): pertaining to beneath the nail of a finger or toe *ungu:* nail *-al:* pertaining to

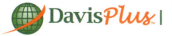 **DavisPlus** | Visit the *Medical Terminology Systems* online resource center at Davis*Plus* for an audio exercise of the terms in this table. Other activities are also available to reinforce content.

⊕ *It is time to review medical word elements by completing Learning Activities 5-1 and 5-2.*

Pathology

General appearance and condition of the skin are clinically important because they may provide clues to body conditions or dysfunctions. Pale skin may indicate shock; red, flushed, very warm skin may indicate fever and infection. A rash may indicate allergies or local infections. Even chewed fingernails may be a clue to emotional problems. For diagnosis, treatment, and management of skin disorders, the medical services of a specialist may be warranted. **Dermatology** is the medical specialty concerned with diseases that directly affect the skin and systemic diseases that manifest their effects on the skin. The physician who specializes in diagnosis and treatment of skin diseases is known as a **dermatologist.**

Skin Lesions

Lesions are areas of tissue that have been pathologically altered by injury, wound, or infection. Lesions may affect tissue over an area of a definite size **(localized)** or may be widely spread throughout the body **(systemic).** Evaluation of skin lesions, injuries, or changes to tissue helps establish the diagnosis of skin disorders.

Lesions are described as primary or secondary. **Primary skin lesions** are the initial reaction to **pathologically** altered tissue and may be flat or elevated. **Secondary skin lesions** are changes that take place in the primary lesion due to infection, scratching, trauma, or various stages of a disease. Lesions are also described by their appearance, color, location, and size as measured in centimeters. Some of the major primary and secondary skin lesions are described and illustrated in Figure 5-3.

 It is time to review skin lesions by completing Learning Activity 5–3.

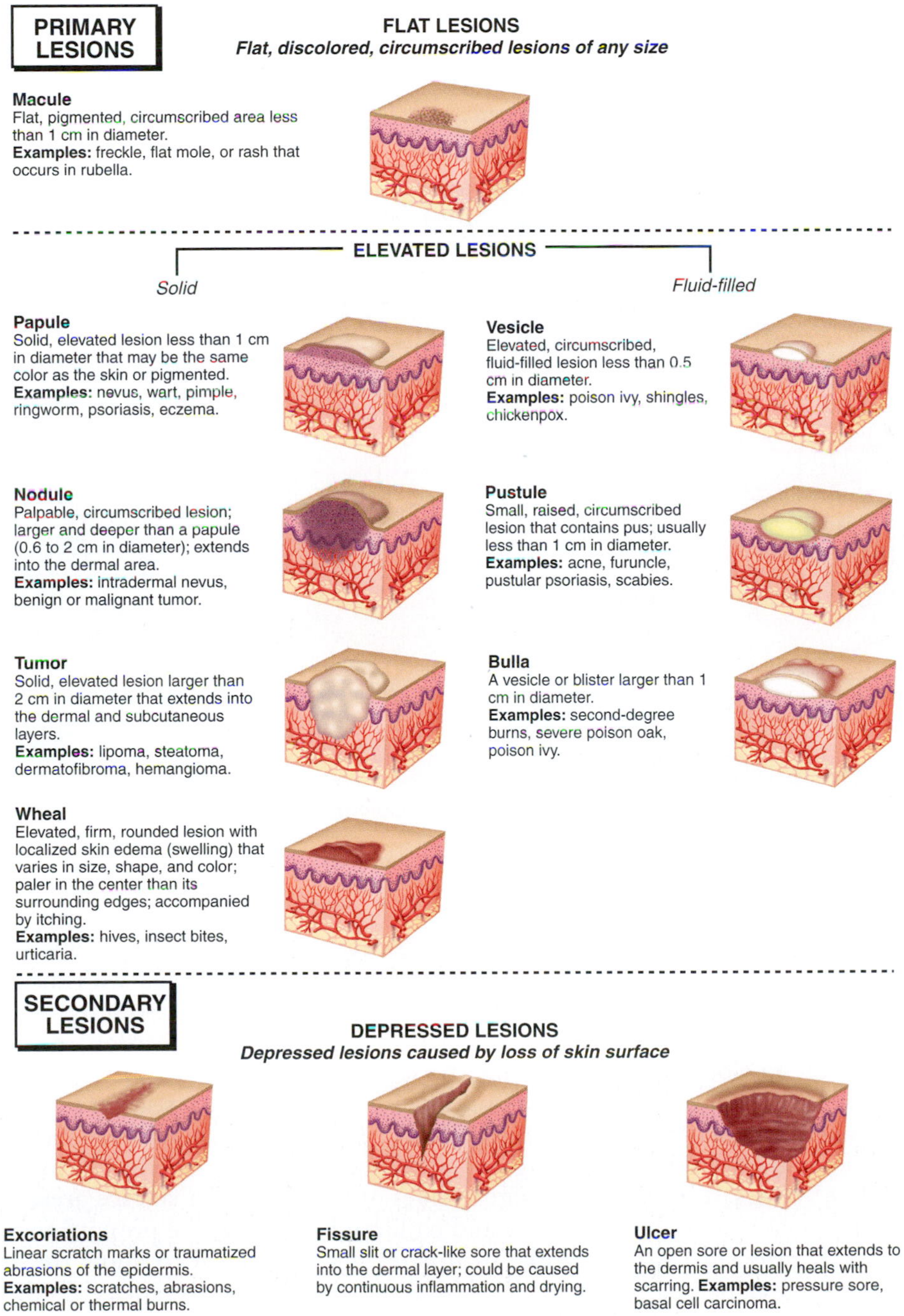

PRIMARY LESIONS

FLAT LESIONS
Flat, discolored, circumscribed lesions of any size

Macule
Flat, pigmented, circumscribed area less than 1 cm in diameter.
Examples: freckle, flat mole, or rash that occurs in rubella.

ELEVATED LESIONS

Solid

Fluid-filled

Papule
Solid, elevated lesion less than 1 cm in diameter that may be the same color as the skin or pigmented.
Examples: nevus, wart, pimple, ringworm, psoriasis, eczema.

Vesicle
Elevated, circumscribed, fluid-filled lesion less than 0.5 cm in diameter.
Examples: poison ivy, shingles, chickenpox.

Nodule
Palpable, circumscribed lesion; larger and deeper than a papule (0.6 to 2 cm in diameter); extends into the dermal area.
Examples: intradermal nevus, benign or malignant tumor.

Pustule
Small, raised, circumscribed lesion that contains pus; usually less than 1 cm in diameter.
Examples: acne, furuncle, pustular psoriasis, scabies.

Tumor
Solid, elevated lesion larger than 2 cm in diameter that extends into the dermal and subcutaneous layers.
Examples: lipoma, steatoma, dermatofibroma, hemangioma.

Bulla
A vesicle or blister larger than 1 cm in diameter.
Examples: second-degree burns, severe poison oak, poison ivy.

Wheal
Elevated, firm, rounded lesion with localized skin edema (swelling) that varies in size, shape, and color; paler in the center than its surrounding edges; accompanied by itching.
Examples: hives, insect bites, urticaria.

SECONDARY LESIONS

DEPRESSED LESIONS
Depressed lesions caused by loss of skin surface

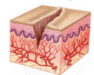

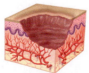

Excoriations
Linear scratch marks or traumatized abrasions of the epidermis.
Examples: scratches, abrasions, chemical or thermal burns.

Fissure
Small slit or crack-like sore that extends into the dermal layer; could be caused by continuous inflammation and drying.

Ulcer
An open sore or lesion that extends to the dermis and usually heals with scarring. **Examples:** pressure sore, basal cell carcinoma.

Figure 5-3 Primary and secondary lesions.

Burns

Burns are tissue injuries caused by contact with thermal, chemical, electrical, or radioactive agents. Although burns generally occur on the skin, they can also affect the respiratory and digestive tract linings. Burns that have a local effect are not as serious as those that have a systemic effect. Systemic effects are life threatening and may include dehydration, shock, and infection.

Burns are usually classified as first-, second-, or third-degree burns. The extent of injury and degree of severity determine a burn's classification. **First-degree (superficial) burns** are the least serious type of burn because they injure only the top layers of the skin, the epidermis. These burns are most commonly caused by brief contact with dry or moist heat **(thermal burn),** spending too much time in the sun **(sunburn),** or exposure to chemicals **(chemical burn).** Injury is restricted to local effects, such as skin redness **(erythema)** and acute sensitivity to such sensory stimuli as touch, heat, or cold **(hyperesthesia).** Generally, blisters do not form and the burn heals without scar formation. **Second-degree (partial-thickness)** burns are deep burns that damage the epidermis and part of the dermis. These burns may be caused by contact with flames, hot liquids, or chemicals. Symptoms mimic those of first-degree burns, but fluid-filled blisters **(vesicles** or **bullae)** form and the burn may heal with little or no scarring. (See Figure 5-4.)

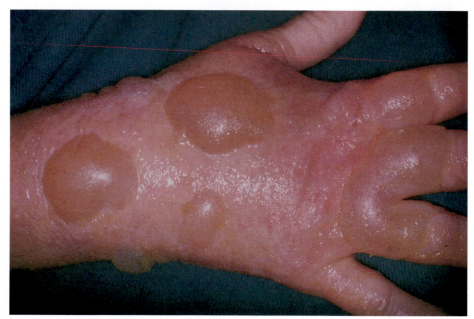

Figure 5-4 Second-degree burn of the hand. From Goldsmith, Lazarus, and Tharp: *Adult and Pediatric Dermatology: A Color Guide to Diagnosis and Treatment.* FA Davis, Philadelphia, 1997, p 318, with permission.

In **third-degree (full-thickness) burns,** the epidermis and dermis are destroyed and some of the underlying connective tissue is damaged, leaving the skin waxy and charred with insensitivity to touch. The underlying bones, muscles, and tendons may also be damaged. These burns may be caused by corrosive chemicals, flames, electricity, or extremely hot objects; immersion of the body in extremely hot water; or clothing that catches fire. Because of the extensiveness of tissue destruction, ulcerating wounds develop and the body attempts to heal itself by forming scar tissue. Skin grafting **(dermatoplasty)** is commonly required to protect the underlying tissue and assist in recovery.

A formula for estimating the percentage of adult body surface area affected by burns is to apply the Rule of Nines. This method assigns values of 9% or 18% of surface areas to specific regions. The formula is modified in infants and children because of the proportionately larger head size. (See Figure 5-5.) To determine treatment, it is important to know the amount of the burned surface area because IV fluids for hydration are required to replace fluids lost from tissue damage.

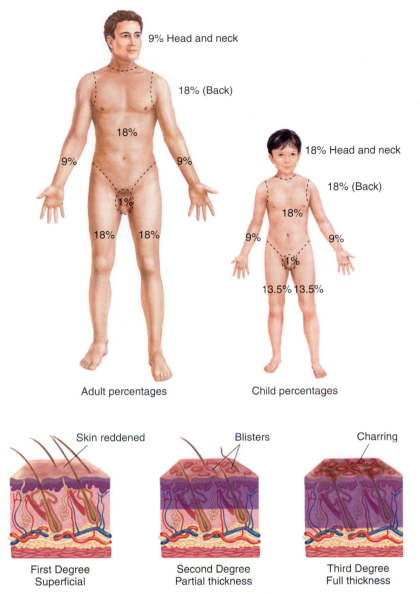

9% Head and neck

18% (Back)

18%

9%   9%

1%

18%   18%

Adult percentages

18% Head and neck

18% (Back)

18%

9%   9%

1%

13.5% 13.5%

Child percentages

Skin reddened

Blisters

Charring

First Degree
Superficial

Second Degree
Partial thickness

Third Degree
Full thickness

Figure 5-5 Rule of Nines and burn classification.

Oncology

Neoplasms are abnormal growths of new tissue that are classified as benign or malignant. **Benign neoplasms** are noncancerous growths composed of the same type of cells as the tissue in which they are growing. They harm the individual only insofar as they place pressure on surrounding structures. If the benign neoplasm remains small and places no pressure on adjacent structures, it commonly is not removed. When the tumor becomes excessively large, causes pain, or places pressure on other organs or structures, excision is necessary. **Malignant neoplasms,** also called **cancer,** are composed of cells that tend to become invasive and spread to remote regions of the body **(metastasis)**. Once the malignant cells from the primary tumor invade surrounding tissues, they tend to enter blood and lymph vessels and travel to remote regions of the body to form secondary tumor sites. If left untreated, cancer tends to be progressive and generally fatal.

Cancer treatment includes surgery, chemotherapy, immunotherapy, and radiation therapy. **Immunotherapy,** also called **biotherapy,** is a newer treatment that stimulates the body's own immune defenses to fight tumor cells. To provide the most effective treatment, the physician may prescribe one of the above treatments or use a combination of them **(combined modality treatment).**

Grading and Staging Cancer

Pathologists grade and stage tumors to help in diagnosis and treatment planning, provide a possible prognosis, and aid comparison of treatment results when different treatment methods are used.

Tumor Grading

In tumor **grading,** cells from the tumor site are evaluated to determine the degree of loss of cellular differentiation and function **(anaplasia).** Pathologists commonly describe these changes using four grades of severity based on the microscopic appearance of the cells. (See Table 5-1.) A grade I tumor shows cells that closely resemble the tissue of origin. In other words, most of the cells are well differentiated and able to carry on the function of the tissue. A patient with a grade I tumor has a good prognosis for full recovery. On the other hand, a patient with a grade IV tumor shows cells that are very poorly differentiated and grow rapidly. These cells spread to surrounding tissue and are incapable of carrying on the normal function of the tissue. A patient with a grade IV tumor has the poorest prognosis.

Table 5-1	Tumor Grading
The table below defines the four tumor grades and their characteristics.	
Grading	**Tumor Characteristics**
Grade I Tumor cells well differentiated	• Close resemblance to tissue of origin and, thus, retaining some specialized functions
Grade II Tumor cells moderately or poorly differentiated	• Less resemblance to tissue of origin • More variation in size and shape of tumor cells • Increased mitoses
Grade III Tumor cells poorly differentiated	• Increased abnormality in appearance with only remote resemblance to the tissue of origin • Marked variation in shape and size of tumor cells • Greatly increased mitoses
Grade IV Tumor cells very poorly differentiated	• Abnormal appearance to the extent that recognition of the tumor's tissue origin is difficult • Extreme variation in size and shape of tumor cells

Tumor Staging

The most common system used for staging tumors is the **tumor-node-metastasis (TNM) system.** It is an international system that allows comparison of statistics among cancer centers. The TNM staging system classifies solid tumors by size and degree of spread according to three basic criteria:

- **T**—size and invasiveness of the primary tumor
- **N**—area lymph nodes involved
- **M**—invasiveness (metastasis) of the primary tumor.

Numbers are used to indicate size or spread of the tumor. The higher the number, the greater the extent or spread of the malignancy. For example, T2 designates a small tumor; M0 designates no evidence of metastasis. (See Table 5-2.) As with grading, staging provides valuable information to guide treatment plans.

Basal Cell Carcinoma

Basal cell carcinoma, the most common type of skin cancer, is a malignancy of the basal layer of the epidermis, or hair follicles. This type of cancer is commonly caused by overexposure to sunlight. The tumors are locally invasive but rarely metastasize. (See Figure 5-6). Basal cell

Table 5-2	**TNM System of Staging**

The table below outlines the tumor, node, metastasis (TNM) system of staging, including designations, stages, and degrees of tissue involvement.

Designation	Stage	Tissue Involvement
Tumor		
TX		Primary tumor that cannot be evaluated
T0		No evidence of tumor
Tis	Stage I	Carcinoma in situ, which indicates that the tumor is in a defined location and shows no invasion into surrounding tissues
T1, T2, T3, T4	Stage II	Primary tumor size and extent of local invasion, where T1 is small with minimal invasion and T4 is large with extensive local invasion into surrounding organs and tissues
Node		
NX		Regional lymph nodes that cannot be evaluated
N0		Regional lymph nodes that show no abnormalities
N1, N2, N3, N4	Stage III	Degree of lymph node involvement and spread to regional lymph nodes, where N1 is less involvement with minimal spreading and N4 is more involvement with extensive spreading
Metastasis		
MX		Distant metastasis that cannot be evaluated
M0		No evidence of metastasis
M1	Stage IV	Presence of metastasis

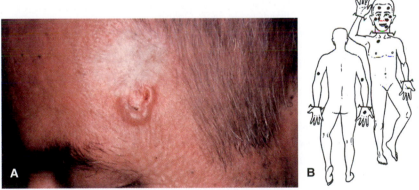

Figure 5-6 (A) Basal cell carcinoma with pearly, flesh-colored papule with depressed center and rolled edge. **(B)** Common sites of basal cell carcinoma. From Goldsmith, Lazarus, and Tharp: *Adult and Pediatric Dermatology: A Color Guide to Diagnosis and Treatment.* FA Davis, Philadelphia, 1997, p 157, with permission.

carcinoma is most prevalent in blond, fair-skinned men and is the most common malignant tumor affecting white people. Although these tumors grow slowly, they commonly ulcerate as they increase in size and develop crusting that is firm to the touch. Metastases are uncommon with this type of cancer; however, the disease can invade the tissue sufficiently to destroy an ear, nose, or eyelid. Depending on the location, size, and depth of the lesion, treatment may include curettage and electrodesiccation, chemotherapy, surgical excision, irradiation, or chemosurgery.

Squamous Cell Carcinoma

Squamous cell carcinoma arises from skin that undergoes pathological hardening **(keratinizing)** of epidermal cells. It is an invasive tumor with potential for metastasis and occurs most commonly in fair-skinned white men over age 60. (See Figure 5-7) Repeated overexposure to the sun's ultraviolet rays greatly increases the risk of squamous cell carcinoma. Other predisposing factors associated with this type of cancer include radiation therapy, chronic skin irritation and inflammation, exposure to cancer-causing agents **(carcinogens),** including tar and oil, hereditary diseases (such as **xeroderma pigmentosum** and **albinism**), and the presence of premalignant lesions (such as **actinic keratosis** or **Bowen disease**).

There are two types of squamous cell carcinoma: those that are confined to the original site **(in situ)** and those that penetrate the surrounding tissue **(invasive).** Treatment may consist of surgical excision; curettage and electrodesiccation, which provide good cosmetic results for smaller lesions; radiation therapy, usually for older or debilitated patients; and chemotherapy, depending on the location, size, shape, degree of invasion, and condition of underlying tissue. A combination of these treatment methods may be required for a deeply invasive tumor.

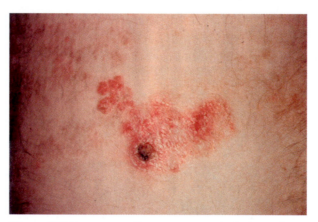

Figure 5-7 Squamous cell carcinoma, in which the surface is fragile and bleeds easily. From Goldsmith, Lazarus, and Tharp: *Adult and Pediatric Dermatology: A Color Guide to Diagnosis and Treatment.* FA Davis, Philadelphia, 1997, p 237, with permission.

Malignant Melanoma

Malignant melanoma, as the name implies, is a malignant growth of melanocytes. (See Figure 5-8.) This tumor is highly metastatic, with a higher mortality rate than basal or squamous cell carcinomas. It is the most lethal of the skin cancers and can metastasize extensively to the liver, lungs, or brain.

Several factors may influence the development of melanoma, but persons at greatest risk have fair complexions, blue eyes, red or blonde hair, and freckles. Excessive exposure to sunlight and severe sunburn during childhood are believed to increase the risk of melanoma in later life. Avoiding the sun and using sunscreen have proved effective in preventing the disease.

Melanomas are diagnosed by **biopsy** along with histological examination. Treatment requires surgery to remove the primary cancer, along with adjuvant therapies to reduce the risk of metastasis. The extent of surgery depends on the size and location of the primary tumor and is determined by staging the disease.

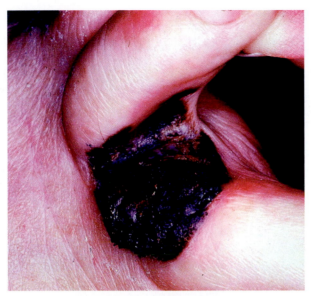

Figure 5-8 Malignant melanoma, in which the lesion appears between the fingers as is an irregularly pigmented blue-black papule with flecks of brown, red, and white pigment. The borders of the lesions are irregular and may be notched. From Goldsmith, Lazarus, and Tharp: *Adult and Pediatric Dermatology: A Color Guide to Diagnosis and Treatment.* FA Davis, Philadelphia, 1997, p 137, with permission.

 It is time to review burn and oncology terms by completing Learning Activity 5-4.

Diseases and Conditions

This section introduces diseases and conditions of the integumentary system with their meanings and pronunciations. Word analyses for selected terms are also provided.

Term	Definition
abscess ĂB-sĕs	Localized collection of pus at the site of an infection (characteristically a staphylococcal infection) *When a localized abscess originates in a hair follicle, it is called a furuncle, or boil. A cluster of furuncles in the subcutaneous tissue results in the formation of a carbuncle. (See Figure 5-9.)*

Figure 5-9 Dome-shaped abscess that has formed a furuncle in hair follicles of the neck. Large furuncles with connecting channels to the skin surface form a carbuncle.

(continued)

Term	Definition
acne ĂK-nē	Inflammatory disease of the sebaceous glands and hair follicles of the skin with characteristic lesions that include blackheads (comedos), inflammatory papules, pustules, nodules, and cysts and usually associated with seborrhea; also called *acne vulgaris* (See Figure 5-10.) *Acne results from thickening of the follicular opening, increased sebum production, and the presence of bacteria. It is associated with an inflammatory response. The face, neck, and shoulders are common sites for this condition.* **Figure 5-10** Acne vulgaris. From Goldsmith, Lazarus, and Tharp: *Adult and Pediatric Dermatology: A Color Guide to Diagnosis and Treatment.* FA Davis, Philadelphia, 1997, p 227, with permission.
alopecia al-ō-PĒ-shē-ă	Partial or complete loss of hair resulting from normal aging, an endocrine disorder, a drug reaction, anticancer medication, or a skin disease; commonly called *baldness*
Bowen disease BŌ-ĕn	Form of intraepidermal carcinoma (squamous cell) characterized by red-brown scaly or crusted lesions that resemble a patch of psoriasis or dermatitis; also called *Bowen precancerous dermatosis* *Treatment for Bowen disease includes curettage and electrodesiccation.*
cellulitis sĕl-ū-LĪ-tĭs	Diffuse (widespread), acute infection of the skin and subcutaneous tissue *Cellulitis is characterized by a light glossy appearance of the skin, localized heat, redness, pain, swelling and, occasionally, fever, malaise, and chills.*
chloasma klō-ĂZ-mă	Pigmentary skin discoloration usually occurring in yellowish brown patches or spots
comedo KŎM-ē-dō	Typical small skin lesion of acne vulgaris caused by accumulation of keratin, bacteria, and dried sebum plugging an excretory duct of the skin *The closed form of comedo, called a whitehead, consists of a papule from which the contents are not easily expressed.*
dermatomycosis dĕr-mă-tō-mī-KŌ-sĭs *dermat/o:* skin *myc:* fungus *-osis:* abnormal condition; increase (used primarily with blood cells)	Infection of the skin caused by fungi *A common type of dermatomycosis is called ringworm.*

Term	Definition
ecchymosis ĕk-ĭ-MŌ-sĭs	Skin discoloration consisting of a large, irregularly formed hemorrhagic area with colors changing from blue-black to greenish brown or yellow; commonly called a *bruise* (See Figure 5-11.) **Figure 5-11** Ecchymosis.
eczema ĔK-zĕ-mă	Chronic inflammatory skin condition that is characterized by erythema, papules, vesicles, pustules, scales, crusts, and scabs and accompanied by intense itching (pruritis); also called *atopic dermatitis* *Eczema most commonly occurs during infancy and childhood, with decreasing incidence in adolescence and adulthood. Statistics support a convincing genetic component in that it tends to occur in patients with a family history of allergic conditions.*
erythema ĕr-ĭ-THĒ-mă	Redness of the skin caused by swelling of the capillaries *An example of erythema is a mild sunburn or nervous blushing.*
eschar ĔS-kăr	Dead matter that is sloughed off from the surface of the skin, especially after a burn *Eschar material is commonly crusty or scabbed.*
impetigo ĭm-pĕ-TĪ-gō	Bacterial skin infection characterized by isolated pustules that become crusted and rupture
keratosis kĕr-ă-TŌ-sĭs *kerat:* horny tissue, hard; cornea *-osis:* abnormal condition; increase (used primarily with blood cells)	Thickened area of the epidermis or any horny growth on the skin (such as a callus or wart)
lentigo lĕn-TĪ-gō	Small brown macules, especially on the face and arms, brought on by sun exposure, usually in a middle-aged or older person *Lentigo are benign pigmented lesions of the skin that require no treatment unless cosmetic repair is desired.*
pallor PĂL-or	Unnatural paleness or absence of color in the skin
pediculosis pĕ-dĭk-ū-LŌ-sĭs *pedicul:* lice *-osis:* abnormal condition; increase (used primarily with blood cells)	Infestation with lice, transmitted by personal contact or common use of brushes, combs, or headgear

(continued)

Term	Definition
petechia p ē-TĔ-kē-ă	Minute, pinpoint hemorrhage under the skin *A petechia(plural, petechiae) is a smaller version of an ecchymosis.*
pressure ulcer ŬL-sĕr	Inflammation, sore, or skin deterioration caused by prolonged pressure from lying in one position that prevents blood flow to the tissues, usually in elderly bedridden persons; also known as *decubitus ulcer* (See Figure 5-12.) *Pressure ulcers are most commonly found in skin overlying a bony projection, such as the hip, ankle, heel, shoulder, and elbow. The wounds are categorized from stage 1 to stage 4. (See Figure 5-13.)*

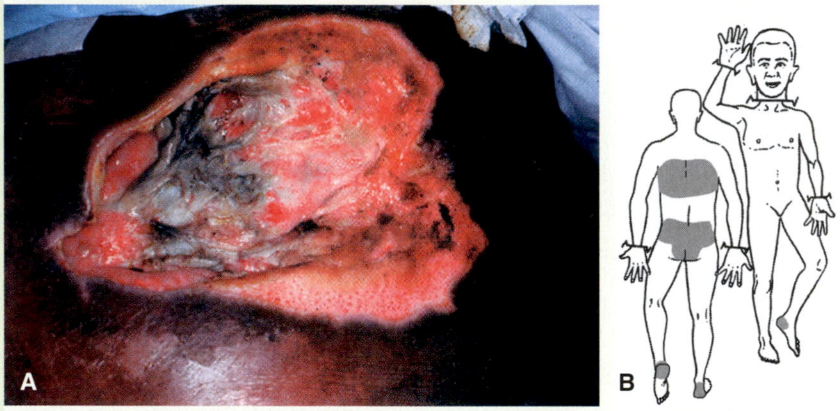

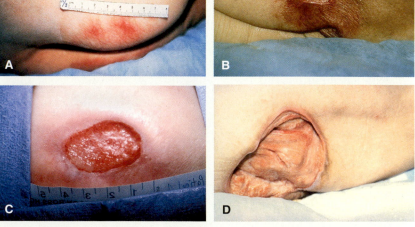

Figure 5-12 Pressure ulcer. **(A)** Deep pressure ulcer over a bony prominence in a bedridden patient. **(B)** Common sites of pressure ulcers. From Goldsmith, Lazarus, and Tharp: *Adult and Pediatric Dermatology: A Color Guide to Diagnosis and Treatment.* FA Davis, Philadelphia, 1997, p 445, with permission.

Figure 5-13 Stages of pressure ulcer. **(A)** Stage 1, with shiny, reddened skin that usually appears over a bony prominence. **(B)** Stage 2, untreated stage 1 ulcer that becomes more serious when skin is swollen and shows a blister. **(C)** Stage 3, in which a craterlike ulcer goes deeper into the skin. **(D)** Stage 4 ulcer that goes into a muscle or bone. From Dillon: *Nursing Health Assessment,* 2nd ed. FA Davis, Philadelphia, 2007, p 239, with permission.

Term	Definition
pruritus proo-RĪ-t ŭs	Intense itching
psoriasis sō-RĪ-ă-sĭs	Chronic skin disease characterized by circumscribed red patches covered by thick, dry, silvery, adherent scales and caused by excessive development of the basal layer of the epidermis (See Figure 5-14.) *New psoriasis lesions tend to appear at sites of trauma. They may be found in any location but commonly on the scalp, knees, elbows, umbilicus, and genitalia. Treatment includes topical application of various medications, keratolytics, phototherapy, and ultraviolet light therapy in an attempt to slow hyperkeratosis.* **Figure 5-14** Psoriasis. From Goldsmith, Lazarus, and Tharp: *Adult and Pediatric Dermatology: A Color Guide to Diagnosis and Treatment.* FA Davis, Philadelphia, 1997, p 381, with permission.
purpura PŬR-pŭ-ră	Any of several bleeding disorders characterized by hemorrhage into the tissues, particularly beneath the skin or mucous membranes, producing ecchymoses or petechiae *Hemorrhage into the skin shows red darkening into purple and then brownish yellow and finally disappearing in 2 to 3 weeks. Areas of discoloration do not disappear under pressure.*
scabies SKĀ-bēz	Contagious skin disease transmitted by the itch mite, commonly through sexual contact *Scabies manifests as papules, vesicles, pustules, and burrows and causes intense itching, commonly resulting in secondary infections. The axillae, genitalia, inner aspect of the thighs, and areas between the fingers are most commonly affected.*
tinea TĬN-ē-ăh	Fungal skin infection whose name commonly indicates the body part affected; also called *ringworm* *Examples of tinea include tinea barbae (beard), tinea corporis (body), tinea pedis (athlete's foot), tinea versicolor (skin), and tinea cruris (jock itch).*

(continued)

Term	Definition
urticaria ŭr-tĭ-KĂR-ē-ă	Allergic reaction of the skin characterized by the eruption of pale red, elevated patches called *wheals* or *hives* (See Figure 5-15.) **Figure 5-15** Urticaria. From Goldsmith, Lazarus, and Tharp: *Adult and Pediatric Dermatology: A Color Guide to Diagnosis and Treatment.* FA Davis, Philadelphia, 1997, p 381, with permission.
verruca vĕr-ROO-kă	Epidermal growth caused by a virus; also known as *warts.* Types include plantar warts, juvenile warts, and venereal warts (See Figure 5-16.) *Verrucae may be removed by cryosurgery, electrocautery, or acids; however, they may regrow if the virus remains in the skin.* **Figure 5-16** Verruca. From Goldsmith, Lazarus, and Tharp: *Adult and Pediatric Dermatology: A Color Guide to Diagnosis and Treatment.* FA Davis, Philadelphia, 1997, p 241, with permission.

Term	Definition
vitiligo vĭt-ĭl-Ī-gō	Localized loss of skin pigmentation characterized by milk-white patches (See Figure 5-17.) **Figure 5-17** Vitiligo. From Goldsmith, Lazarus, and Tharp: *Adult and Pediatric Dermatology: A Color Guide to Diagnosis and Treatment.* FA Davis, Philadelphia, 1997, p 121, with permission.

✦ *It is time to review pathology, diseases, and conditions by completing Learning Activity 5-5.*

Medical, Surgical, and Diagnostic Procedures

This section introduces medical, surgical, and diagnostic procedures used to treat and diagnose skin disorders. Descriptions are provided as well as pronunciations and word analyses for selected terms.

Procedure	Description
Medical	
chemical peel	Chemical removal of the outer layers of skin to treat acne scarring and general keratoses; also called chemabrasion *Chemical peels are also commonly used for cosmetic purposes to remove fine wrinkles on the face.*
cryosurgery krī-ō-SĔR-jĕr-ē	Use of subfreezing temperature (commonly liquid nitrogen) to destroy or eliminate abnormal tissue, such as tumors, warts, and unwanted, cancerous, or infected tissue
debridement dĭ-BRĒD-mĕnt	Removal of necrotized tissue from a wound by surgical excision, enzymes, or chemical agents *Debridement is used to promote healing and prevent infection.*
dermabrasion DĔRM-ă-brā-zhŭn	Rubbing (abrasion) using wire brushes or sandpaper to mechanically scrape away (abrade) the epidermis *This procedure is commonly used to remove acne scars, tattoos, and scar tissue.*

(continued)

Procedure	Description
fulguration fŭl-gū-RĀ-shŭn	Tissue destruction by means of high-frequency electric current; also called *electrodesiccation* *This procedure is used to remove tumors and lesions in and on the body.*
photodynamic therapy (PDT)	Procedure in which cells selectively treated with an agent called a *photo-sensitizer* are exposed to light to produce a reaction that destroys the cells *Various forms of photodynamic therapy are used in treatment of cancer, actinic keratosis, and macular degeneration.*
Surgical	
biopsy (Bx, bx) BĪ-ŏp-sē	Representative tissue sample removed from a body site for microscopic examination *Skin biopsies are used to establish or confirm a diagnosis, estimate prognosis, or follow the course of disease. Any lesion suspected of malignancy is removed and sent to the pathology laboratory for evaluation.*
frozen section (FS)	Ultrathin slice of tissue from a frozen specimen for immediate pathological examination *FS is commonly used for rapid diagnosis of malignancy after the patient has been anesthetized to determine treatment options.*
needle	Removal of a small tissue sample for examination using a hollow needle, usually attached to a syringe
punch	Removal of a small core of tissue using a hollow punch
shave	Removal of elevated lesions using a surgical blade
Mohs MŌZ	Layers of cancer-containing skin are progressively removed and examined until only cancer-free tissue remains
skin graft	Transplantation of healthy tissue to an injured site *Human, animal, or artificial skin can be used to provide a temporary covering or permanent layer of skin over a wound or burn.*
allograft ĂL-ō-grăft	Transplantation of healthy tissue from one person to another person; also called *homograft* *In an allograft, the skin donor is usually a cadaver. This type of skin graft is temporary and is used to protect the patient against infection and fluid loss. The allograft is frozen and stored in a skin bank until needed.*
autograft AW-tō-grăft	Transplantation of healthy tissue from one site to another site in the same individual
synthetic sĭn-THĔT-ĭk	Transplantation of artificial skin produced from collagen fibers arranged in a lattice pattern *The recipient's body does not reject synthetic skin (produced artificially) and healing skin grows into it as the graft gradually disintegrates.*
xenograft ZĔN-ō-grăft	Transplantation (dermis only) from a foreign donor (usually a pig) and transferred to a human; also called *heterograft* *A xenograft is used as a temporary graft to protect the patient against infection and fluid loss.*

Procedure	Description
Diagnostic	
allergy skin test	Any test in which a suspected allergen or sensitizer is applied to or injected into the skin to determine the patient's sensitivity to it
	Most commonly used skin tests are the intradermal, patch, and scratch tests. The intensity of the response is determined by the wheal-and-flare reaction after the suspected allergen is applied. Positive and negative controls are used to verify normal skin reactivity (See Figure 5-8.)
intradermal ĭn-tră-dĕr-măl	Skin test that identifies suspected allergens by subcutaneously injecting small amounts of extracts of the suspected allergens and observing the skin for a subsequent reaction
	Intradermal skin tests are used to determine immunity to diphtheria (Schick test) or tuberculosis (Mantoux test).
patch	Skin test that identifies allergic contact dermatitis by applying a suspected allergen to a patch which is then taped on the skin, usually the forearm, and observing the area 24 hours later for an allergic response
	After the patch is removed, a lack of noticeable reaction indicates a negative result; skin reddening or swelling indicates a positive result and means the person is allergic to the suspected allergen.
scratch	Skin test that identifies suspected allergens by placing a small quantity of the suspected allergen on a lightly scratched area of the skin; also called *puncture or prick test*
	Redness or swelling at the scratch sites within 10 minutes indicates an allergy to the substance, or a positive test result. If no reaction occurs, the test result is negative.
	  Figure 5-18 Allergy skin tests. **(A)** Intradermal allergy test reactions. **(B)** Scratch (prick) skin test kit for allergy testing.
culture & sensitivity (C&S)	Laboratory test that grows a colony of bacteria removed from an infected area (such as an ulcer, wound, or pus from an infection) in order to identify the specific infecting bacterium and then determine its sensitivity to antibiotic drugs

Pharmacology

Various medications are available to treat skin disorders. (See Table 5-3.) Because of their superficial nature and location, many skin disorders respond well to topical drug therapy. Such mild, localized skin disorders as contact dermatitis, acne, poison ivy, and diaper rash can be effectively treated with topical agents available as over-the-counter products.

Widespread or particularly severe dermatological disorders may require systemic treatment. For example, poison ivy with large areas of open, weeping lesions may be difficult to treat with topical medication and may require a prescription-strength drug. In such a case, an oral steroid or antihistamine might be prescribed to relieve inflammation and severe itching.

Table 5-3	**Drugs Used to Treat Skin Disorders**

This table lists common drug classifications used to treat skin disorders, their therapeutic actions, and selected generic and trade names.

Classification	Therapeutic Action	Generic and *Trade* Names
antifungals ăn-tĭ-FŬNG-găls	Alter the cell wall of fungi or disrupt enzyme activity, resulting in cell death *Antifungals are used to treat ringworm (tinea corporis), athlete's foot (tinea pedis), and fungal infection of the nail (onychomycosis). When topical antifungals are not effective, oral or intravenous antifungal drugs may be necessary.*	**nystatin** NĬS-tă-tĭn *Mycostatin, Nyston* **itraconazole** ĭt-ră-KŎN-ă-zōl *Sporanox*
antihistamines ăn-tĭ-HĬS-tă-mĭns	Inhibit allergic reactions of inflammation, redness, and itching caused by the release of histamine *In a case of severe itching, antihistamines may be given orally. As a group, these drugs are also known as antipruritics (because pruritus means itching).*	**diphenhydramine** dī-fĕn-HĪ-dră-mēn *Benadryl* **loratadine** lor-ĂH-tă-dēn *Claritin*
antiparasitics ăn-tĭ-păr-ă-SĬT-ĭks	Kills insect parasites, such as mites and lice *Parasiticides are used to treat scabies (mites) and pediculosis (lice). The drug is applied as a cream or lotion to the body and as a shampoo to treat the scalp.*	**lindane** LĬN-dān *Kwell, Thion* **permethrin** pĕr-MĔTH-rĭn *Nix*
antiseptics ăn-tĭ-SĔP-tĭks	Topically applied agents that inhibit growth of bacteria, thus preventing infections in cuts, scratches, and surgical incisions	**ethyl or isopropyl alcohol** ĔTH-ĭl, ī-sō-PRŌ-pĭl **hydrogen peroxide** HĪ-drō-jĕn pĕ-RŎK-sīd
corticosteroids kor-tĭ-kō-STĔR-oyds	Decrease inflammation and itching by suppressing the immune system's inflammatory response to tissue damage *Topical corticosteroids are used to treat contact dermatitis, poison ivy, insect bites, psoriasis, seborrhea, and eczema. Oral corticosteroids may be prescribed for systemic treatment of severe or widespread inflammation or itching.*	**hydrocortisone*** HĪ-drō-KOR-tĭ-sōn *Certacort, Cortaid* **triamcinolone** trī-ăm-SĬN-ō-lōn *Azmacort, Kenalog*

Table 5-3	Drugs Used to Treat Skin Disorders—cont'd		
Classification	**Therapeutic Action**		**Generic and *Trade* Names**
keratolytics kĕr-ă-tō-LĬT-ĭks	Destroy and soften the outer layer of skin so that it is sloughed off or shed *Strong keratolytics remove warts and corns and aid in penetration of antifungal drugs. Milder keratolytics promote shedding of scales and crusts in eczema, psoriasis, seborrheic dermatitis, and other dry, scaly conditions. Weak keratolytics irritate inflamed skin, acting as a tonic to accelerate healing.*		**tretinoin** TRĔT-ĭ-noyn *Retin-A, Vesanoid*
protectives prŏ-TĔK-tĭvs	Cover, cool, dry, or soothe inflamed skin *Protectives do not penetrate the skin or soften it. Rather, they allow the natural healing process to occur by forming a long-lasting film that protects the skin from air, water, and clothing.*		**lotions** *Cetaphil moisturizing lotion* **ointments** *Vaseline*
topical anesthetics ăn-ĕs-THĔT-ĭks	Block sensation of pain by numbing the skin layers and mucous membranes *These topical drugs are administered directly by means of sprays, creams, gargles, suppositories, and other preparations. They provide temporary symptomatic relief of minor burns, sunburns, rashes, and insect bites.*		**lidocaine** LĪ-dō-kān *Xylocaine* **procaine** PRŌ-kān *Novocain*

*The suffixes *-sone*, *-olone*, and *-onide* are common to generic corticosteroids.

Abbreviations

This section introduces integumentary-related abbreviations and their meanings.

Abbreviation	Meaning	Abbreviation	Meaning
Bx, bx	biopsy	**I&D**	incision and drainage
BCC	basal cell carcinoma	**IMP**	impression (synonymous with diagnosis)
C&S	culture and sensitivity	**IV**	intravenous
CA	cancer; chronological age; cardiac arrest	**TNM**	tumor-node-metastasis
FS	frozen section	**ung**	ointment
ID	intradermal	**XP, XDP**	xeroderma pigmentosum

 It is time to review procedures, pharmacology, and abbreviations by completing Learning Activities 5–6 and 5–7.

LEARNING ACTIVITIES

The following activities provide review of the integumentary system terms introduced in this chapter. Complete each activity and review your answers to evaluate your understanding of the chapter.

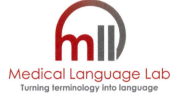

Medical Language Lab
Turning terminology into language

Visit the Medical Language Lab at the web site: medicallanguagelab.com. Use it to enhance your study and reinforcement of this chapter with the flash-card activity. We recommend you complete the flash-card activity before starting Learning Activities 5-1 and 5-2 below.

Learning Activity 5-1
Combining Forms, Suffixes, and Prefixes

Use the elements listed in the table to build medical words. You may use the elements more than once.

Combining Forms		Suffixes		Prefixes
derm/o	myc/o	-al	-osis	an-
dermat/o	py/o	-cyte	-pathy	homo-
hidr/o	scler/o	-derma	-plasty	hypo-
ichthy/o	seb/o	-graft	-rrhea	
kerat/o	trich/o	-ic		
lip/o	xer/o	-logist		
melan/o		-oma		

1. tumor (that is) black _____
2. pertaining to under the skin _____
3. surgical repair of the skin _____
4. cell (composed of) fat _____
5. skin (containing) pus _____
6. specialist in the study of skin disorders _____
7. skin that is dry _____
8. abnormal condition without sweat _____
9. graft from the same (species) _____
10. abnormal condition of dry or scaly skin _____
11. skin (that has) hardened _____
12. abnormal condition of a fungus _____
13. discharge or flow of sebum _____
14. disease of the hair _____
15. abnormal condition of horny tissue _____

Check your answers in Appendix A. Review any material that you did not answer correctly.

Correct Answers _____ X 6.67 = _____ % Score

Building Medical Words

Use *adip/o* or *lip/o* (fat) to build words that mean:

1. tumor consisting of fat _____
2. hernia containing fat _____
3. resembling fat _____
4. fat cell _____

Use *dermat/o* (skin) to build words that mean:

5. inflammation of the skin _____
6. abnormal condition of a skin fungus _____

Use *onych/o* (nail) to build words that mean:

7. tumor of the nails _____
8. softening of the nails _____
9. abnormal condition of the nails _____
10. abnormal condition of the nails caused by a fungus _____
11. abnormal condition of a hidden (ingrown) nail _____
12. disease of the nails _____

Use *trich/o* (hair) to build words that mean:

13. disease of the hair _____
14. abnormal condition of hair caused by a fungus _____

Use *–logy* or *–logist* to build words that mean:

15. study of the skin _____
16. specialist in the study of skin (diseases) _____

Build surgical words that mean:

17. excision of fat (adipose tissue) _____
18. removal of a nail _____
19. incision of a nail _____
20. surgical repair (plastic surgery) of the skin _____

✓ *Check your answers in Appendix A. Review material that you did not answer correctly.*

Correct Answers _____ X 5 = _____ % Score

Learning Activity 5-3

Identifying Skin Lesions

Label the following skin lesions on the lines provided, using the terms listed below.

bulla	*macule*	*pustule*	*vesicle*
excoriations	*nodule*	*tumor*	*wheal*
fissure	*papule*	*ulcer*	

PRIMARY LESIONS

FLAT LESIONS
Flat, discolored, circumscribed lesions of any size

Flat, pigmented, circumscribed area less than 1 cm in diameter.
Examples: freckle, flat mole, or rash that occurs in rubella.

ELEVATED LESIONS

Solid   *Fluid-filled*

Solid, elevated lesion less than 1 cm in diameter that may be the same color as the skin or pigmented. **Examples:** nevus, wart, pimple, ringworm, psoriasis, eczema.

Elevated, circumscribed, fluid-filled lesion less than 0.5 cm in diameter.
Examples: poison ivy, shingles, chickenpox.

Palpable, circumscribed lesion; larger and deeper than a papule (0.6 to 2 cm in diameter); extends into the dermal area.
Examples: intradermal nevus, benign or malignant tumor.

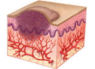

Small, raised, circumscribed lesion that contains pus; usually less than 1 cm in diameter.
Examples: acne, furuncle, pustular psoriasis, scabies.

Solid, elevated lesion larger than 2 cm in diameter that extends into the dermal and subcutaneous layers.
Examples: lipoma, steatoma, dermatofibroma, hemangioma.

A vesicle or blister larger than 1 cm in diameter.
Examples: second-degree burns, severe poison oak, poison ivy.

Elevated, firm, rounded lesion with localized skin edema (swelling) that varies in size, shape, and color; paler in the center than its surrounding edges; accompanied by itching.
Examples: hives, insect bites, urticaria.

SECONDARY LESIONS

DEPRESSED LESIONS
Depressed lesions caused by loss of skin surface

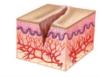

Linear scratch marks or traumatized abrasions of the epidermis.
Examples: scratches, abrasions, chemical or thermal burns.

Small slit or crack-like sore that extends into the dermal layer; could be caused by continuous inflammation and drying.

An open sore or lesion that extends to the dermis and usually heals with scarring. **Examples:** pressure sore, basal cell carcinoma.

 Check your answers by referring to Figure 5–3 on page 87. Review material that you did not answer correctly.

Learning Activity 5-4
Matching Burn and Oncology Terms

Match each term on the left with its meaning on the right.

1. _____ erythema
2. _____ T0
3. _____ malignant
4. _____ first-degree burn
5. _____ grading
6. _____ squamous cell carcinoma

7. _____ benign
8. _____ T1
9. _____ M0
10. _____ third-degree burns

a. develops from keratinizing epidermal cells
b. noncancerous
c. no evidence of metastasis
d. extensive damage to underlying connective tissue
e. no evidence of primary tumor
f. determines degree of abnormal cancer cells compared with normal cells
g. burn that heals without scar formation
h. cancerous; may be life-threatening
i. redness of skin
j. primary tumor size, small with minimal invasion

Check your answers in Appendix A. Review any material that you did not answer correctly.

Correct Answers _____ X 10 = _____ % Score

Learning Activity 5-5
Pathology, Diseases, and Conditions

Match the following terms with the definitions in the numbered list.

abscess	eschar	scabies
alopecia	impetigo	tinea
chloasma	pediculosis	urticaria
ecchymosis	petechiae	verruca
erythema	pruritus	vitiligo

1. infestation with lice _____

2. skin depigmentation characterized by milk-white patches _____

3. fungal skin infection, also called ringworm _____

4. contagious skin disease transmitted by the itch mite _____

5. bacterial skin infection characterized by pustules that become crusted and rupture _____

6. allergic reaction of the skin, characterized by elevated red patches called hives _____

7. hyperpigmentation of the skin, characterized by yellowish brown patches or spots _____

8. hemorrhagic spot or bruise on the skin _____

9. minute or small hemorrhagic spots on the skin _____

10. loss or absence of hair _____

11. localized collection of pus at the site of infection (staphylococcal) _____

12. redness of the skin caused by swelling of the capillaries _____

13. damaged tissue following a severe burn _____

14. intense itching _____

15. epidermal growth caused by a virus; also known as *wart* _____

✓ *Check your answers in Appendix A. Review material that you did not answer correctly.*

Correct Answers _____ X 6.67 = _____ % Score

Learning Activity 5-6

Procedures, Pharmacology, and Abbreviations

Match the following terms with the definitions in the numbered list.

antifungals	*fulguration*	*parasiticides*
autograft	*intradermal test*	*patch test*
corticosteroids	*keratolytics*	*xenograft*
dermabrasion		

1. topical agents to treat athlete's foot and onychomycosis _____
2. tissue destruction by means of high-frequency electric current _____
3. agents that decrease inflammation or itching _____
4. use of wire brushes or other abrasive materials to remove scars, tattoos, or fine wrinkles _____
5. agents that kill parasitic skin infestations _____
6. agents that soften the outer layer of skin so that it sloughs off _____
7. procedure in which extracts of suspected allergens are injected subcutaneously _____
8. procedure in which allergens are applied topically, usually on the forearm _____
9. skin graft taken from one site and applied to another site of the patient's body _____
10. skin graft taken from another species (usually a pig) to a human _____

✓ *Check your answers in Appendix A. Review material that you did not answer correctly.*

Correct Answers _____ X 10 = _____ % Score

Learning Activity 5-7
Medical Scenarios

To construct chart notes, replace the italicized terms in each of the scenarios with one of the medical terms listed below.

asymptomatic   erythmatous   Mohs surgery

biopsy   lymphadenectomy   oncologist

chemotherapy   metastasize   pruritic

dermatologist

Mr. R. is concerned about a "patch" that developed on the back of his neck. Lately, the patch has become (1) *reddened* and is (2) *itchy*. Now that the patch is crusting and bleeding, his wife advises him to see a (3) *skin specialist.* After various tests are performed, the dermatologist identifies the patch as a basal cell carcinoma and explains that this type of cancer rarely (4) *spreads to other body sites.* The dermatologist advises to have the tumor removed next week at the outpatient facility. He also explains that he will perform (5) *removal of small slices of the tumor, layer after layer, and then examine each layer microscopically until a layer is reached that does not have malignant cells.*

1. _____
2. _____
3. _____
4. _____
5. _____

Miss M. noticed that a mole on her neck is increasing in size. Other than the increase in size, Miss M. is experiencing (6) *no other symptoms.* An appointment in the outpatient clinic is scheduled for the (7) *excision of the lesion for microscopic examination.* After evaluation of the biopsy, the pathology report indicates a diagnosis of melanoma. Miss M. is advised to see (8) *physician who specializes in tumors.* In addition to the melanoma, the surgeon discovers metastasis of adjacent lymph glands (nodes) and (9) *removes the lymph glands (nodes).* After her discharge, Miss M. will begin (10) *treatment using chemicals* to target and destroy any remaining cancer cells.

6. _____
7. _____
8. _____
9. _____
10. _____

✓ *Check your answers in Appendix A. Review any material that you did not answer correctly.*

Correct Answers _____ X 10 = _____ % Score

MEDICAL RECORD ACTIVITIES

The two medical records included in the following activities use common clinical scenarios to show how medical terminology is used to document patient care. Complete the terminology and analysis sections for each activity to help you recognize and understand terms related to the integumentary system.

Medical Record Activity 5-1

Pathology Report: Skin Lesion

Terminology

Terms listed in the following table are taken from *Pathology Report: Skin Lesion* that follows. Use a medical dictionary such as *Taber's Cyclopedic Medical Dictionary;* the appendices of *Systems,* 7th ed.; or other resources to define each term. Then review the pronunciations for each term and practice by reading the medical record aloud.

Term	Definition
atypia ā-TĬP-ē-ă	
atypical ā-TĬP-ĭ-kăl	
basal cell layer BĀ-săl	
Bowen disease BŌ-ĕn	
carcinoma kăr-sĭ-NŌ-mă	
dermatitis dĕr-mă-TĪ-tĭs	
dermis DĔR-mĭs	
dorsum DOR-sŭm	
epidermal hyperplasia ĕp-ĭ-DĔR-măl hī-pĕr-PLĀ-zē-ă	
fibroplasia fī-brō-PLĀ-sē-ă	

(continued)

Term	Definition
hyperkeratosis hī-pĕr-kĕr-ă-TŌ-sĭs	
infiltrate ĬN-fĭl-trāt	
keratinocytes kĕ-RĂT-ĭ-nō-sīts	
lymphocytic lĭm-fō-SĬT-ĭk	
neoplastic nē-ō-PLĂS-tĭk	
papillary PĂP-ĭ-lăr-ē	
pathological păth-ō-LŎJ-ĭk-ăl	
solar elastosis SŌ-lăr ĕ-lăs-TŌ-sĭs	
squamous SKWĀ-mŭs	

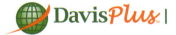

Visit the *Medical Terminology Systems* online resource center at Davis*Plus* to practice pronunciation and reinforce the meanings of the terms in this medical report.

PATHOLOGY REPORT: SKIN LESION

General Hospital

1511 Ninth Avenue ■■ Sun City, USA 12345 ■■ (555) 802-1887

PATHOLOGY REPORT

Date: April 14, 20xx   Pathology: 43022
Patient: Franks, Robert   Room: 910
Physician: Dante Riox, MD

Specimen: Skin from (a) dorsum left wrist and (b) left forearm, ulnar, near elbow.

Clinical Diagnosis: Bowen disease versus basal cell carcinoma versus dermatitis.

Microscopic Description: (a) There is mild hyperkeratosis and moderate epidermal hyperplasia with full-thickness atypia of squamous keratinocytes. Squamatization of the basal cell layer exists. A lymphocytic inflammatory infiltrate is present in the papillary dermis. Solar elastosis is present. (b) Nests, strands, and columns of atypical neoplastic basaloid keratinocytes grow down from the epidermis into the underlying dermis. Fibroplasia is present. Solar elastosis is noted.

Pathological Diagnosis: (a) Bowen disease of left wrist; (b) nodular and infiltrating basal cell carcinoma of left forearm, near elbow.

Samantha Roberts, MD
Samantha Roberts, MD

sr:bg

D: 4-16-xx
T: 4-16-xx

Analysis

Review the medical record *Pathology Report: Skin Lesion* to answer the following questions.

1. In the specimen section, what does "skin on dorsum left wrist" mean?

_____

_____

2. What was the inflammatory infiltrate?

_____

_____

3. What was the pathologist's diagnosis for the left forearm?

_____

_____

4. Provide a brief description of Bowen disease, the pathologist's diagnosis for the left wrist.

_____

_____

Patient Referral Letter: Onychomycosis

Terminology

Terms listed in the following table are taken from *Patient Referral Letter: Onychomycosis* that follows. Use a medical dictionary such as *Taber's Cyclopedic Medical Dictionary;* the appendices of *Systems,* 7th ed.; or other resources to define each term. Then review the pronunciations for each term and practice by reading the medical record aloud.

Term	Definition
alkaline phosphatase ĂL-kă-lĭn FŎS-fă-tās	
bilaterally bī-LĂT-ĕr-ăl-ē	
CA	
debridement dĭ-BRĒD-mĕnt	
hypertension hī-pĕr-TĔN-shŭn	
mastectomy măs-TĔK-tŏ-mē	
neurological noor-ō-LŎJ-ĭk-ăl	
onychomycosis ŏn-ĭ-kō-mī-KŌ-sĭs	
Sporanox* SPŎR-ă-nŏks	
vascular VĂS-kū-lăr	

*Refer to Table 5-3 to determine the drug classification and the generic name for Sporanox.

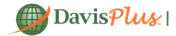

Visit the *Medical Terminology Systems* online resource center at Davis*Plus* to practice pronunciation and reinforce the meanings of the terms in this medical report.

PATIENT REFERRAL LETTER: ONYCHOMYCOSIS

Physician Center

2422 Rodeo Drive ■■ **Sun City, USA 12345** ■■ **(555)788-2427**

May 3, 20xx

John Roberts, MD
1115 Forest Ave
Sun City, USA 12345

Dear Doctor Roberts:

Thank you for referring Alicia Gonzoles to my office. Mrs. Gonzoles presents to the office for evaluation and treatment of onychomycosis with no previous treatment. Past pertinent medical history does reveal hypertension and breast CA. Pertinent surgical history does reveal mastectomy.

Examination of patient's feet does reveal onychomycosis, 1-5 bilaterally. Vascular and neurological examinations are intact. Previous laboratory work was within normal limits except for an elevated alkaline phosphatase of 100.

Tentative diagnosis: Onychomycosis, 1-5 bilaterally

Treatment consisted of debridement of mycotic nails, bilateral feet, as well as dispensing a prescription for Sporanox Pulse Pack to be taken for 3 months to treat the onychomycotic infection. I have also asked her to repeat her liver enzymes in approximately 4 weeks. Mrs. Gonzoles will make an appointment in 2 months for follow-up, and I will keep you informed of any changes in her progress. If you have any questions, please feel free to contact me.

Sincerely yours,

Juan Perez, MD
Juan Perez, MD

jp:az

Analysis

Review the medical record *Patient Referral Letter: Onychomycosis* to answer the following questions.

1. What pertinent disorders were identified in the past medical history?

_____

_____

2. What pertinent surgery was identified in the past surgical history?

_____

_____

3. Did the doctor identify any problems in the vascular system or nervous system?

_____

_____

4. What was the significant finding in the laboratory results?

_____

_____

5. What treatment did the doctor employ for the onychomycosis?

_____

_____

6. What did the doctor recommend regarding the abnormal laboratory finding?

_____

_____

Digestive System

CHAPTER

6

Chapter Outline

Objectives

Upon completion of this chapter, you will be able to:

- Locate the major organs of the digestive system and describe their structure and function.
- Describe the functional relationship between the digestive system and other body systems.
- Pronounce, spell, and build words related to the digestive system.
- Describe diseases, conditions, and procedures related to the digestive system.
- Explain pharmacology related to the treatment of digestive disorders.
- Demonstrate your knowledge of this chapter by completing the learning and medical record activities.

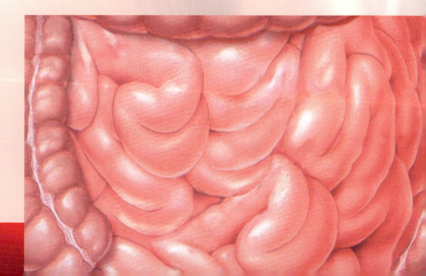

Anatomy and Physiology

The digestive system, also called the **gastrointestinal (GI)** system, consists of a digestive tube called the **GI tract (alimentary canal)**, and several accessory organs whose primary function is to break down food, prepare it for absorption, and eliminate waste. The GI tract, extending from the mouth to the anus, varies in size and structure in several distinct regions.

Food passing along the GI tract is mixed with digestive enzymes and broken down into nutrient molecules, which are absorbed in the bloodstream. Undigested waste materials not absorbed by the blood are then eliminated from the body through defecation. Included in the digestive system are the accessory organs of digestion: the liver, gallbladder, and pancreas. The process of digestion breaks down food into nutrients to nourish the body. (See Figure 6-1.)

Anatomy and Physiology Key Terms

This section introduces important terms, along with their definitions and pronunciations. Word analyses for selected terms are also provided.

Term	Definition
bilirubin bĭl-ĭ-ROO-bĭn	Orange-yellow pigment formed during destruction of erythrocytes that is taken up by liver cells to form bilirubin and eventually excreted in the feces *Elevated bilirubin in the blood produces yellowing of the skin (jaundice). It also indicates liver damage or disease.*
bolus BŌ-lŭs	Mass of masticated food ready to be swallowed

exocrine
ĔKS-ō-krĭn
  exo-: outside, outward
  -crine: secrete
	Gland that secretes its products through excretory ducts to the surface of an organ or tissue or into a vessel

sphincter SFĬNGK-tĕr	Circular band of muscle fibers that constricts a passage or closes a natural opening of the body *An example of a sphincter is the lower esophageal (cardiac) sphincter that constricts once food has passed into the stomach.*
triglycerides trī-GLĬS-ĕr-īd	Organic compound, a true fat, that is made of one glycerol and three fatty acids *In the blood, triglycerides combine with proteins to form lipoproteins. The liver synthesizes lipoproteins to transport fats to other tissues, where they are a source of energy. Fat in adipose tissue is stored energy.*
Pronunciation Help Long Sound ā — rate ē — rebirth ī — isle ō — over ū — unite Short Sound ă — alone ĕ — ever ĭ — it ŏ — not ŭ — cut	

Mouth

The process of digestion begins in the mouth. (See Figure 6-2.) The mouth, also known as the (1) **oral cavity,** is a receptacle for food. It is formed by the cheeks **(bucca),** lips, teeth, tongue, and hard and soft palates. Located around the oral cavity are three pairs of salivary glands that secrete saliva. Saliva contains important digestive enzymes that help begin the chemical breakdown of food. In the mouth, food is broken down mechanically (by the teeth) and chemically (by saliva), and then formed into a **bolus.**

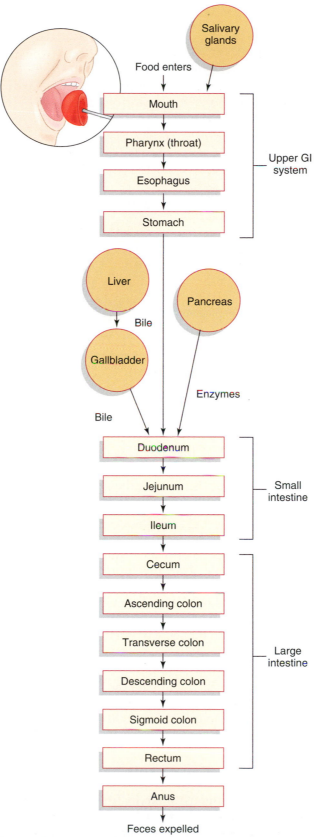

Figure 6-1 Pathway of food through the digestive system.

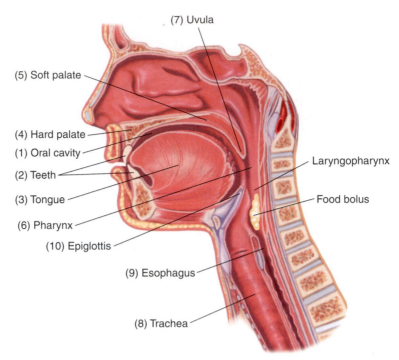

(7) Uvula

(5) Soft palate

(4) Hard palate
(1) Oral cavity
(2) Teeth
(3) Tongue
(6) Pharynx
(10) Epiglottis

Laryngopharynx

Food bolus

(9) Esophagus

(8) Trachea

Figure 6-2 Sagittal view of the head showing oral, nasal, and pharyngeal components of the digestive system.

Teeth

The (2) **teeth** play an important role in initial stages of digestion by mechanically breaking down food **(mastication)** into smaller pieces as they mix it with saliva. Teeth are covered by a hard enamel, giving them a smooth, white appearance. Beneath the enamel is **dentin,** the main structure of the tooth. The innermost part of the tooth is the **pulp,** which contains nerves and blood vessels. The teeth are embedded in pink, fleshy tissue known as **gums (gingiva).**

Tongue

The (3) **tongue** assists in the chewing process by manipulating the bolus of food during chewing and moving it to the back of the mouth for swallowing **(deglutition).** The tongue also aids in speech production and taste. Rough projections on the surface of the tongue called **papillae** contain taste buds. The four basic taste sensations registered by chemical stimulation of the taste buds are sweet, sour, salty, and bitter. All other taste perceptions are combinations of these four basic flavors. In addition, the sense of taste is intricately linked with the sense of smell, making taste perception very complex.

Hard and Soft Palates

The two structures forming the roof of the mouth are the (4) **hard palate** (anterior portion) and the (5) **soft palate** (posterior portion). The soft palate, which forms a partition between the mouth and the nasopharynx, is continuous with the hard palate. The entire oral cavity, like the rest of the GI tract, is lined with mucous membranes.

Pharynx, Esophagus, and Stomach

As the tongue pushes the bolus into the (6) **pharynx** (throat), it is guided by the soft, fleshy, V-shaped structure called the (7) **uvula.** The funnel-shaped pharynx serves as a passageway to the respiratory and GI tracts and provides a resonating chamber for speech sounds. The lowest portion of the pharynx divides into two tubes: one that leads to the lungs, called the (8) **trachea,** and one that leads to the stomach, called the (9) **esophagus.** A small flap of cartilage called the (10) **epiglottis** folds back to cover the trachea during swallowing, forcing food to enter the esophagus. At all other times, the epiglottis remains upright, allowing air to freely pass through the respiratory structures.

The **stomach,** a saclike structure located in the left upper quadrant (LUQ) of the abdominal cavity, serves as a food reservoir that continues mechanical and chemical digestion. (See Figure 6-3.) The stomach extends from the (1) **esophagus** to the first part of the small intestine, the (2) **duodenum.** The terminal portion of the esophagus, the (3) **lower esophageal (cardiac) sphincter,** is composed of muscle fibers that constrict once food has passed into the stomach. It prevents the stomach contents from regurgitating back into the esophagus. The (4) **body** of the stomach, the large central portion, together with the (5) **fundus,** the upper portion, are mainly storage areas. Most digestion takes place in the funnel-shaped terminal portion, the (6) **pylorus.** The interior lining of the stomach is composed of mucous membranes and contains numerous macroscopic longitudinal folds called (7) **rugae** that gradually unfold as the stomach fills. Located within the rugae, digestive glands produce hydrochloric acid (HCl) and enzymes. Secretions from these glands coupled with the mechanical churning of the stomach turn the bolus into a semiliquid form called **chyme** that slowly leaves the stomach through the (8) **pyloric sphincter** to enter the duodenum. This **sphincter** regulates the speed and movement of chyme into the small intestine and prohibits backflow. Food is propelled through the entire GI tract by coordinated, rhythmic muscle contractions called **peristalsis.**

Small Intestine

The small intestine is a coiled, 20-foot–long tube that begins at the pyloric sphincter and ends at the large intestine. (See Figure 6–4.) It consists of three parts:

- (1) **duodenum,** the uppermost segment, which is about 10 inches long
- (2) **jejunum,** which is approximately 8 feet long
- (3) **ileum,** which is about 12 feet long.

Digestion is completed in the small intestine with the help of additional enzymes and secretions from the (4) **pancreas** and (5) **liver.** Nutrients in chyme are absorbed through microscopic, fingerlike projections called **villi.** Nutrients enter the bloodstream and lymphatic system for distribution to the rest of the body. At the terminal end of the small intestine, a sphincter muscle

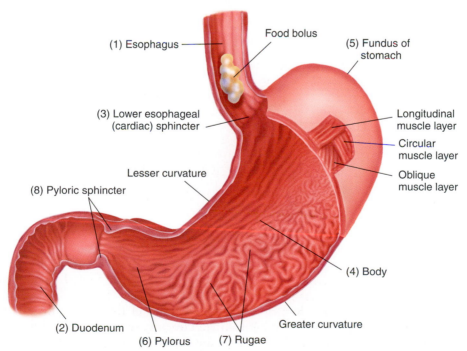

Figure 6-3 Anterior view of the stomach showing muscle layers and rugae of the mucosa.

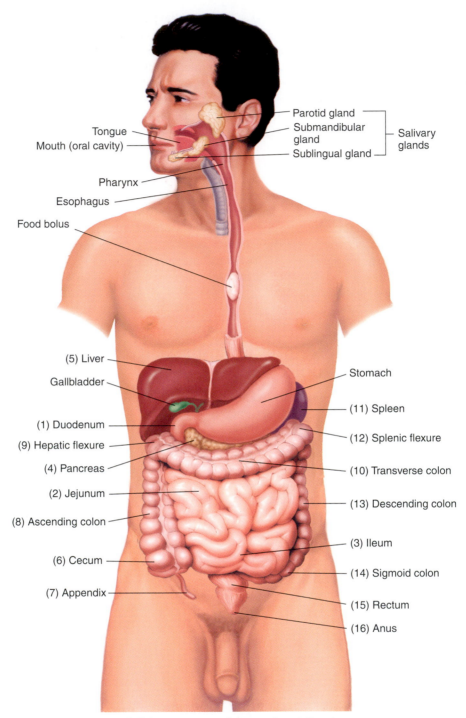

Tongue
Mouth (oral cavity)

Parotid gland
Submandibular gland
Sublingual gland

Salivary glands

Pharynx

Esophagus

Food bolus

(5) Liver

Gallbladder

Stomach

(11) Spleen

(1) Duodenum

(9) Hepatic flexure

(4) Pancreas

(12) Splenic flexure

(10) Transverse colon

(2) Jejunum

(8) Ascending colon

(13) Descending colon

(3) Ileum

(6) Cecum

(7) Appendix

(14) Sigmoid colon

(15) Rectum

(16) Anus

Figure 6-4 Anterior view of the trunk and digestive organs.

called the **ileocecal valve** allows undigested or unabsorbed material from the small intestine to pass into the large intestine and eventually be excreted from the body.

Large Intestine

The large intestine is about 5 feet long. It begins at the end of the ileum and extends to the anus. No digestion takes place in the large intestine. The only secretion is mucus in the colon, which lubricates fecal material so it can pass from the body. The large intestine has three main components: cecum, colon, and rectum. The first 2 or 3 inches of the large intestine is called the (6) **cecum,** a small pouch that hangs inferior to the ileocecal valve. Projecting downward from the cecum is a wormlike structure called the (7) **appendix.** The function of the appendix is unknown; however, it has an important structural shortcoming—its twisted structure provides an ideal location for enteric bacteria to accumulate and multiply. Inflammation of the appendix **(appendicitis)** may lead to ischemia and gangrene (**death** and **decay**) of the appendix. The cecum merges as it becomes the first part of the colon. The main functions of the colon are to absorb water and minerals and eliminate undigested material. The colon is divided into ascending, transverse, descending, and sigmoid portions:

- The (8) **ascending colon** extends from the cecum to the lower border of the liver and turns abruptly to form the (9) **hepatic flexure.**
- The colon continues across the abdomen to the left side as the (10) **transverse colon,** curving beneath the lower end of the (11) **spleen** to form the (12) **splenic flexure.**
- As the transverse colon turns downward, it becomes the (13) **descending colon.**
- The descending colon continues until it forms the (14) **sigmoid colon** and the (15) **rectum.** The rectum, the last part of the GI tract, terminates at the (16) **anus.**

Accessory Organs of Digestion

Although the liver, gallbladder, and pancreas lie outside the GI tract, they play a vital role in the proper digestion and absorption of nutrients. (See Figure 6-5.)

Liver

The (1) **liver,** the largest glandular organ in the body, weighs approximately 3 to 4 lb. It is located beneath the diaphragm in both the right upper quadrant (RUQ) and the left upper quadrant (LUQ) of the abdominal cavity. The liver performs many vital functions and death occurs if it ceases to function. Some of its important functions include:

- producing bile, which aids in the digestion of fat
- removing glucose (sugar) from blood to synthesize glycogen (starch) and retain it for later use
- storing vitamins, such as B_{12}, A, D, E, and K
- destroying or transforming toxic products into less harmful compounds
- maintaining normal glucose levels in the blood
- destroying old erythrocytes and releasing **bilirubin**
- synthesizing proteins that circulate in the blood, such as albumin for fluid balance and prothrombin and fibrinogen for coagulation (blood clotting).

Pancreas

The (2) **pancreas** is an elongated, somewhat flattened organ that lies posterior and slightly inferior to the stomach. It performs endocrine and exocrine functions. As an **endocrine** gland, the pancreas secretes insulin directly into the bloodstream to maintain normal blood glucose levels. For a comprehensive discussion of the endocrine function of the pancreas, review Chapter 13. As an **exocrine** gland, the pancreas produces digestive enzymes that pass into the duodenum through

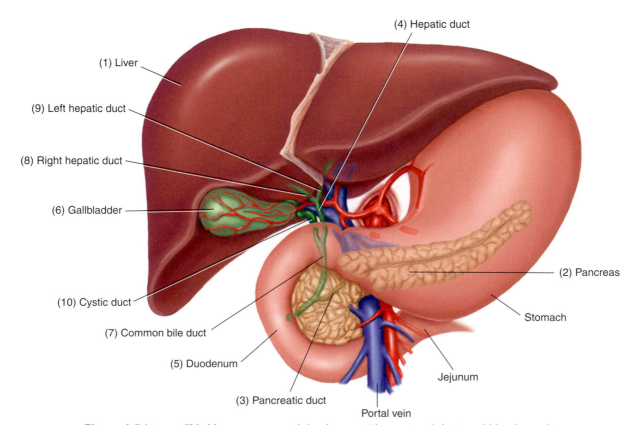

Figure 6-5 Liver, gallbladder, pancreas, and duodenum with associated ducts and blood vessels.

the (3) **pancreatic duct.** The pancreatic duct extends along the pancreas and, together with the (4) **hepatic duct** from the liver, enters the (5) **duodenum.** The pancreas produces enzymes, such as trypsin, which digests proteins; amylase, which digests starch; and lipase, which digests **triglycerides**. These pass into the duodenum through the pancreatic duct.

Gallbladder

The (6) **gallbladder,** a saclike structure on the inferior surface of the liver, serves as a storage area for bile, which is produced by the liver. When bile is needed for digestion, the gallbladder releases it into the duodenum through the (7) **common bile duct.** Bile is also drained from the liver through the (8) **right hepatic duct** and the (9) **left hepatic duct.** These two structures eventually form the hepatic duct. The (10) **cystic duct** of the gallbladder merges with the hepatic duct to form the common bile duct, which leads into the duodenum. Bile production is stimulated by hormone secretions, which are produced in the duodenum as soon as food enters the small intestine. Without bile, fat digestion is not possible.

Anatomy Review: Digestive System

To review the anatomy of the digestive system, label the illustration using the terms below.

anus	*hepatic flexure*	*rectum*
appendix	*ileum*	*sigmoid colon*
ascending colon	*jejunum*	*spleen*
cecum	*liver*	*splenic flexure*
descending colon	*pancreas*	*transverse colon*
duodenum		

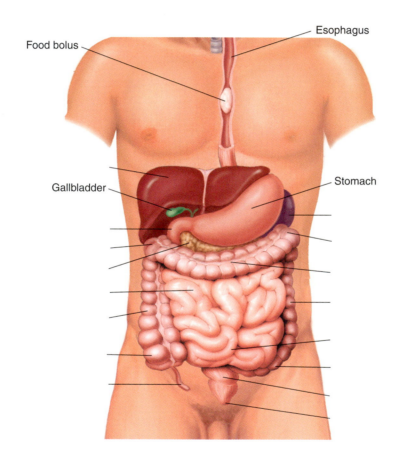

Food bolus —

Esophagus

Gallbladder —

Stomach

 Check your answers by referring to Figure 6–4 on page 124. Review material that you did not answer correctly.

Anatomy Review: Accessory Organs of Digestion

To review the anatomy of the accessory organs of digestion, label the following illustration using the terms listed below.

common bile duct	*hepatic duct*	*pancreas*
cystic duct	*left hepatic duct*	*pancreatic duct*
duodenum	*liver*	*right hepatic duct*
gallbladder		

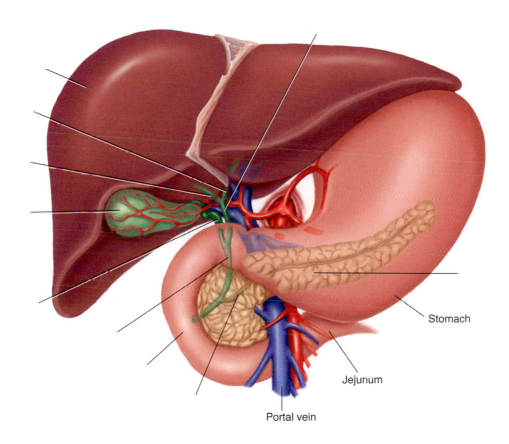

Stomach

Jejunum

Portal vein

Check your answers by referring to Figure 6–5 on page 126. Review material that you did not answer correctly.

CONNECTING BODY SYSTEMS—DIGESTIVE SYSTEM

The main function of the digestive system is to provide vital nutrients for growth, maintenance, and repair of all organs and body cells. Specific functional relationships between the digestive system and other body systems are discussed below.

Blood, Lymph, and Immune
- Liver regulates blood glucose levels.
- Digestive tract secretes acids and enzymes to provide a hostile environment for pathogens.
- Intestinal walls contain lymphoid nodules that help prevent invasion of pathogens.
- Digestive system absorbs vitamin K for blood clotting.

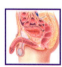

Cardiovascular
- Digestive system absorbs nutrients needed by the heart.

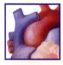

Endocrine
- Liver eliminates hormones from the blood to end their activity.
- Pancreas contains hormone-producing cells.

Female Reproductive
- Digestive system provides adequate nutrition, including fats, to make conception and normal fetal development possible.
- Digestive system provides nutrients for repair of the endometrium following menstruation.

Male Reproductive
- Digestive system provides adequate nutrients in the development of viable sperm.

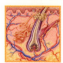

Integumentary
- Digestive system supplies fats that provide insulation in the dermis and subcutaneous tissue.
- Digestive system absorbs nutrients for maintenance, growth, and repair of the skin.

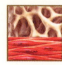

Musculoskeletal
- Digestive system provides nutrients needed for energy fuel.
- Digestive system absorbs calcium needed for bone salts and muscle contraction.
- Liver removes lactic acid (resulting from muscle activity) from the blood.

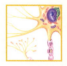

Nervous
- Digestive system supplies nutrients for normal neural functioning.
- Digestive system provides nutrients for synthesis of neurotransmitters and electrolytes for transmission of a nervous impulse.
- Liver plays a role in maintaining glucose levels for neural function.

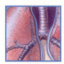

Respiratory
- Digestive system absorbs nutrients needed by cells in the lungs and other tissues in the respiratory tract.
- The pharynx is shared by the digestive and respiratory systems. The lowest portion of the pharynx divides into two tubes: one that leads to the lungs, called the trachea, and one that leads to the stomach, called the esophagus.

Urinary
- Liver metabolizes hormones, toxins, and drugs to forms that can be excreted in urine.

Medical Word Elements

This section introduces combining forms, suffixes, and prefixes related to the digestive system. Word analyses are also provided.

Element	Meaning	Word Analysis
Combining Forms		
Mouth		
or/o	mouth	**or**/al (OR-ăl): pertaining to the mouth *-al:* pertaining to
stomat/o		**stomat**/itis (stŏ-mă-TĪ-tĭs): inflammation of the mouth *-itis:* inflammation
gloss/o	tongue	**gloss**/ectomy (glŏs-ĔK-tō-mē): removal of all or part of the tongue *-ectomy:* excision, removal
lingu/o		**lingu**/al (LĬN-gwăl): pertaining to the tongue *-al:* pertaining to
bucc/o	cheek	**bucc**/al (BŬK-ăl): pertaining to the cheek *-al:* pertaining to
cheil/o	lip	**cheil/o**/plasty (KĪ-lō-plăs-tē): surgical repair of a defective lip *-plasty:* surgical repair
labi/o		**labi**/al (LĀ-bē-ăl): pertaining to the lips, particularly the lips of the mouth *-al:* pertaining to
dent/o	teeth	**dent**/ist (DĔN-tĭst): specialist who treats disorders of teeth *-ist:* specialist
odont/o		orth/**odont**/ist (or-thō-DŎN-tĭst): dentist who specializes in correcting and preventing irregularities of abnormally positioned or aligned teeth *orth:* straight *-ist:* specialist
gingiv/o	gum(s)	**gingiv**/ectomy (jĭn-jĭ-VĔK-tō-mē): excision of diseased gingival tissue *-ectomy:* excision, removal *Gingivectomy is performed as a surgical treatment for periodontal disease.*
sial/o	saliva, salivary gland	**sial/o**/lith (sī-ĂL-ō-lĭth): calculus formed in a salivary gland or duct *-lith:* stone, calculus
Esophagus, Pharynx, and Stomach		
esophag/o	esophagus	**esophag/o**/scope (ē-SŎF-ă-gō-skōp): instrument for examining the esophagus *-scope:* instrument for examining

(continued)

Element	Meaning	Word Analysis
pharyng/o	pharynx (throat)	**pharyng/o**/tonsill/itis (fă-rĭng-gō-tŏn-sĭ-LĪ-tĭs): inflammation of the pharynx and tonsils *tonsill:* tonsils *–itis:* inflammation
gastr/o	stomach	**gastr**/algia (găs-TRĂL-jē-ă): pain in the stomach; also called stomachache *–algia:* pain
pylor/o	pylorus	**pylor/o**/spasm (pī-LOR-ō-spăzm): involuntary contraction of the pyloric sphincter of the stomach, as in pyloric stenosis *–spasm:* involuntary contraction, twitching
Small Intestine		
duoden/o	duodenum (first part of small intestine)	**duoden/o**/scopy (dū-ŏd-ĕ-NŎS-kō-pē): visual examination of the duodenum *–scopy:* visual examination
enter/o	intestine (usually small intestine)	**enter/o**/pathy (ĕn-tĕr-ŎP-ă-thē): disease of the intestine *–pathy:* disease
jejun/o	jejunum (second part of small intestine)	**jejun/o**/rrhaphy (jĕ-joo-NOR-ă-fē): suture of the jejunum *–rrhaphy:* suture
ile/o	ileum (third part of small intestine)	**ile/o**/stomy (ĭl-ē-ŎS-tō-mē): creation of an opening between the ileum and the abdominal wall *–stomy*:* forming an opening (mouth) *An ileostomy creates an opening on the surface of the abdomen to allow feces to be discharged into a bag worn on the abdomen.*
Large Intestine		
append/o	appendix	**append**/ectomy (ăp-ĕn-DĔK-tō-mē): excision of the appendix *–ectomy:* excision, removal *Appendectomy is performed to remove a diseased appendix in danger of rupturing.*
appendic/o		**appendic**/itis (ă-pĕn-dĭ-SĪ-tĭs): inflammation of the appendix *–itis:* inflammation
col/o	colon	**col/o**/stomy (kō-LŎS-tō-mē): creation of an opening between the colon and the abdominal wall *–stomy*:* forming an opening (mouth) *A colostomy creates a place for fecal matter to exit the body other than through the anus.*
colon/o		**colon/o**/scopy (kō-lŏn-ŎS-kō-pē): visual examination of the colon *–scopy:* visual examination *Colonoscopy is performed with an elongated endoscope called a colonoscope.*

*When the suffix *-stomy* is used with a combining form that denotes an organ, it refers to a surgical opening to the outside of the body.

Element	Meaning	Word Analysis
sigmoid/o	sigmoid colon	**sigmoid/o**/tomy (sĭg-moyd-ŎT-ō-mē): incision of the sigmoid colon –*tomy:* incision
Terminal End of Large Intestine		
rect/o	rectum	**rect/o**/cele (RĔK-tŏ-sēl): herniation or protrusion of the rectum; also called proctocele –*cele:* hernia, swelling
proct/o	anus, rectum	**proct/o**/logist (prŏk-TŎL-ō-jĭst): physician who specializes in treating disorders of the colon, rectum, and anus –*logist:* specialist in the study of

an/o	anus	peri/**an**/al (pĕr-ē-Ā-năl): pertaining to the area around the anus
		  peri–: around
		  –*al:* pertaining to

Accessory Organs of Digestion		
hepat/o	liver	**hepat/o**/megaly (hĕp-ă-tō-MĔG-ă-lē): enlargement of the liver –*megaly:* enlargement
pancreat/o	pancreas	**pancreat/o**/lysis (păn-krē-ă-TŎL-ĭ-sĭs): destruction of the pancreas (caused by pancreatic enzymes) –*lysis:* separation; destruction; loosening
cholangi/o	bile vessel	**cholangi/o**le (kō-LĂN-jē-ōl): small terminal portion of the bile duct –*ole:* small, minute
chol/e**	bile, gall	**chol/e**/lith (KŌ-lē-lĭth): gallstone –*lith:* calculus, stone *Gallstones are solid masses composed of bile and cholesterol that form in the gallbladder and common bile duct.*
cholecyst/o	gallbladder	**cholecyst/o**ectomy (kō-lē-sĭs-TĔK-tō-mē): removal of the gallbladder –*ectomy:* excision, removal *Cholecystectomy is performed by laparoscopic or open surgery.*
choledoch/o	bile duct	**choledoch/o**/plasty (kō-LĔD-ō-kō-plăs-tē): surgical repair of the bile duct –*plasty:* surgical repair
Suffixes		
-emesis	vomit	hyper/**emesis** (hī-pĕr-ĔM-ĕ-sĭs): excessive vomiting *hyper–:* excessive, above normal

**The e in *chol/e* is an exception to the rule of using the connecting vowel o.

(continued)

Element	Meaning	Word Analysis
-iasis	abnormal condition (produced by something specified)	chol/e/lith/**iasis** (kō-lē-lĭ-THĪ-ă-sĭs): abnormal condition of gallstones *chol/e:* bile, gall *lith:* stone, calculus *When gallstones form in the common bile duct, the condition is called choledocholithiasis.*
-megaly	enlargement	hepat/o/**megaly** (hĕp-ă-tō-MĔG-ă-lē): enlargement of the liver *hepat/o:* liver *Hepatomegaly may be caused by hepatitis or infection, fatty infiltration (as in alcoholism), biliary obstruction, or malignancy.*
-orexia	appetite	an/**orexia** (ăn-ō-RĔK-sē-ă): without appetite *an-:* without, not *Anorexia can result from various conditions, such as adverse effects of drugs or various physical or psychological causes.*
-pepsia	digestion	dys/**pepsia** (dĭs-PĔP-sē-ă): difficult or painful digestion; also called *indigestion* *dys-:* bad; painful; difficult *Dyspepsia is an epigastric discomfort felt after eating.*
-phagia	swallowing, eating	aer/o/**phagia** (ĕr-ō-FĀ-jē-ă): swallowing air *aer/o:* air
-prandial	meal	post/**prandial** (pōst-PRĂN-dē-ăl): after a meal *post-:* after, behind
-rrhea	discharge, flow	steat/o/**rrhea** (stē-ă-tō-RĒ-ă): discharge of fat in fecal matter *-rrhea:* discharge, flow
Prefixes		
dia-	through, across	**dia**/rrhea (dī-ă-RĒ-ă): discharge or flow of fluid fecal matter through the bowel *-rrhea:* discharge, flow
peri-	around	**peri**/odent/itis (pĕr-ē-dĕn-TĪ-tĭs): inflammation (of tissue) around a tooth *odent-:* tooth *-itis:* inflammation
sub-	under, below	**sub**/lingu/al (sŭb-LĬN-gwăl): pertaining to the area under the tongue *lingu:* tongue *-al:* pertaining to

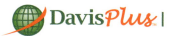 | Visit the *Medical Terminology Systems* online resource center at Davis*Plus* for an audio exercise of the terms in this table. Other activities are also available to reinforce content.

It is time to review medical word elements by completing Learning Activities 6-1, 6-2, and 6-3.

Pathology

Although some digestive disorders do not manifest symptoms **(asymptomatic),** many are associated with nausea, vomiting, bleeding, pain, and weight loss. Clinical signs, such as jaundice and edema, may indicate a hepatic disorder. Severe infection, drug toxicity, hepatic disease, and changes in fluid and electrolyte balance can cause behavioral abnormalities. Disorders of the GI tract or any of the accessory organs (liver, gallbladder, and pancreas) may result in far-reaching metabolic or systemic problems that can eventually threaten life itself. Assessment of a suspected digestive disorder includes a thorough history and physical examination. A range of diagnostic tests assist in identifying abnormalities of the GI tract, liver, gallbladder, and pancreas.

For diagnosis, treatment, and management of digestive disorders, the medical services of a specialist may be warranted. **Gastroenterology** is the branch of medicine concerned with digestive diseases. The physician who specializes in the diagnoses and treatment of digestive disorders is known as a **gastroenterologist.** Gastroenterologists do not perform surgeries; however, under the broad classification of surgery, they do perform such procedures as liver biopsy and endoscopic examination.

Peptic Ulcer Disease (PUD)

An **ulcer** is a circumscribed open sore on the skin or mucous membranes of the body. Peptic ulcer is one of the most common ulcer types that occur in the digestive system. It primarily develops in the stomach and duodenum but may also occur to a lesser extent in the lower esophagus. Ulcers are named by their location in the body: esophageal ulcer, gastric ulcer, or duodenal ulcer. (See Figure 6-6.)

A common cause of PUD is the erosion of the protective mucous membrane caused by infection with *H. pylori* bacteria. As the mucous membrane erodes, it exposes the tissue beneath to

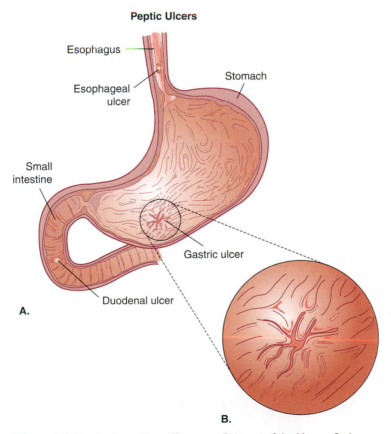

Peptic Ulcers

Esophagus

Esophageal ulcer

Stomach

Small intestine

Gastric ulcer

Duodenal ulcer

A.

B.

Figure 6-6 Peptic ulcers. From Tamparo: *Diseases of the Human Body,* 5th ed. FA Davis, Philadelphia, 2011, p. 403, with permission.

the strong acids and digestive enzymes of the stomach and, eventually, an ulcer forms. Some individuals have more rapid gastric emptying, which—combined with hypersecretion of acid—creates a large amount of acid moving into the duodenum. As a result, peptic ulcers occur more commonly in the duodenum.

Risk factors that contribute to PUD include smoking, chewing tobacco, stress, caffeine use, and such medications as steroids, aspirin, and nonsteroidal anti-inflammatory drugs (NSAIDs). Peptic ulcer development is influenced by smoking because smoking increases the harmful effects of *H. pylori*, alters protective mechanisms, and decreases gastric blood flow. Treatment includes antibiotics to destroy *H. pylori* and antacids to reduce stomach acids and allow the ulcer to heal. If left untreated, mucosal destruction produces a hole **(perforation)** in the wall lining with resultant bleeding from the damaged area. At worst, the hole penetrates the entire wall and gastric contents leak into the abdominal cavity, possibly leading to inflammation of the peritoneum **(peritonitis).**

Ulcerative Colitis

Ulcerative colitis, a chronic inflammatory disease of the colon, commonly begins in the rectum or sigmoid colon and extends upward into the entire colon. It is distinguished from other closely related bowel disorders by its characteristic inflammatory pattern. The inflammation involves only the mucosal lining of the colon, which exhibits erythema and numerous hemorrhagic ulcerations. The affected portion of the colon is uniformly involved, with no evidence of healthy mucosal tissue. Ulcerative colitis is characterized by profuse, watery diarrhea containing varying amounts of blood, mucus, and pus. Severe cases may require surgical creation of an opening **(stoma)** for bowel evacuation to a bag worn on the abdomen. Ulcerative colitis is associated with an increased risk of colon cancer.

Hernia

A **hernia** is a protrusion of any organ, tissue, or structure through the wall of the cavity in which it is naturally contained. (See Figure 6-7.) In general, though, the term is applied to protrusions of abdominal organs **(viscera)** through the abdominal wall.

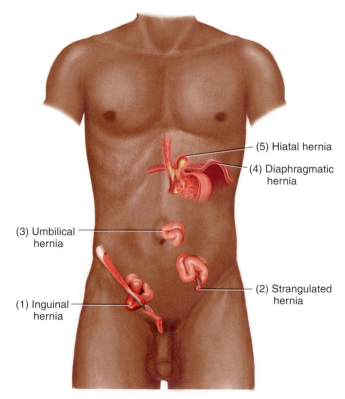

Figure 6-7 Common locations of hernia.

An (1) **inguinal hernia** develops in the groin where the abdominal folds of flesh meet the thighs. In initial stages, it may be hardly noticeable and appears as a soft lump under the skin, no larger than a marble. In early stages, an inguinal hernia is usually reducible; that is, it can be pushed gently back into its normal place. With this type of hernia, pain may be minimal. As time passes, pressure of the abdomen against the weak abdominal wall may increase the size of the opening as well as the size of the hernia lump. If the blood supply to the hernia is cut off because of pressure, a (2) **strangulated hernia** may develop leading to necrosis with gangrene. An (3) **umbilical hernia** is a protrusion of part of the intestine at the navel. It occurs more commonly in obese women and among those who have had several pregnancies. Hernias also occur in newborn infants **(congenital)** or during early childhood. If the defect has not corrected itself by age 2, the deformity can be surgically corrected. Treatment consists of surgical repair of the hernia **(hernioplasty)** with suture of the abdominal wall **(herniorrhaphy)**.

Although hernias most commonly occur in the abdominal region, they may develop in the diaphragm. Two forms of this type include (4) **diaphragmatic hernia,** a congenital disorder, and (5) **hiatal hernia,** in which the lower part of the esophagus and the top of the stomach slides through an opening **(hiatus)** in the diaphragm into the thorax. With hiatal hernia, stomach acid backs up into the esophagus, causing heartburn, chest pain, and swallowing difficulty. Although many hiatal hernias are asymptomatic, if the disease continues for a prolonged period, it may cause **gastroesophageal reflux disease (GERD).**

Intestinal Obstruction

Intestinal obstruction occurs when the flow of intestinal contents are blocked. The two types of intestinal obstruction are **mechanical** and **nonmechanical,** both of which can be either partial or complete. Complete obstruction in any part of the intestine constitutes a medical emergency and requires rapid diagnosis and treatment within a 24-hour period to prevent death.

Mechanical obstruction occurs when intestinal contents are prevented from moving forward due to an obstacle or barrier that blocks the lumen. **Nonmechanical obstruction** occurs when peristalsis is impaired and the intestinal contents cannot be propelled through the bowel. The severity of the obstruction depends on the area of bowel affected, the amount of occlusion within the lumen, and the amount of disturbance in blood flow to the bowel. Mechanical obstructions include tumors; scar tissue **(adhesions);** intestinal twisting **(volvolus);** intestinal "telescoping," where part of the intestine slips into another part just beneath it **(intussusceptions);** strangulated hernias; or the presence of foreign bodies, such as fruit pits and gallstones. Nonmechanical blockages commonly result after abdominal surgeries or with spinal cord lesions, and affect peristalsis or other neurogenic stimuli.

The primary medical treatment for an intestinal obstruction is to decompress the bowel by using a nasogastric tube, which relieves symptoms and may resolve the obstruction. An IV solution with electrolytes may also be initiated to correct the fluid and electrolyte imbalance. Sometimes the patient will also receive IV antibiotics. Complete mechanical obstruction requires surgical interventions, such as removal of tumors, release of adhesions, or bowel resection with anastomosis.

Hemorrhoids

Enlarged veins in the mucous membrane of the anal canal are called **hemorrhoids.** They commonly bleed, hurt, or itch. They may occur inside **(internal)** or outside **(external)** the rectal area. Hemorrhoids are usually caused by abdominal pressure, such as from straining during bowel movement, pregnancy, and standing or sitting for long periods. They may also be associated with some disorders of the liver or the heart.

A high-fiber diet as well as drinking plenty of water and juices plays a pivotal role in hemorrhoid prevention. Temporary relief from hemorrhoids can usually be obtained by cold compresses, sitz baths, stool softeners, or analgesic ointments. Treatment of an advanced condition involves surgical removal of the hemorrhoids **(hemorrhoidectomy).**

Hepatitis

Hepatitis is an inflammatory condition of the liver. The usual causes include exposure to toxic substances, especially alcohol; obstructions in the bile ducts; metabolic diseases; autoimmune diseases; and bacterial or viral infections. A growing public health concern is the increasing incidence of viral hepatitis. Even though its mortality rate is low, the disease is easily transmitted and can cause significant morbidity and prolonged loss of time from school or employment.

Although forms of hepatitis range from hepatitis A through hepatitis E, the three most common forms are hepatitis A, also called **infectious hepatitis;** hepatitis B, also called **serum hepatitis;** and hepatitis C. The most common causes of hepatitis A are ingestion of contaminated food, water, or milk. Hepatitis B and hepatitis C are usually transmitted by routes other than the mouth **(parenteral),** such as from blood transfusions and sexual contact. Because of patient exposure, health-care personnel are at increased risk for contracting hepatitis B, but a vaccine that provides immunity to hepatitis B is available. There is no vaccine available for hepatitis C. Patients with hepatitis C may remain asymptomatic for years or the disease may produce only mild, flulike symptoms. Treatment for hepatitis includes antiviral drugs; however, there is no cure. As the disease progresses, scarring of the liver may become so serious that liver transplantation is the only recourse.

One of the major symptoms of many liver disorders, including hepatitis and cirrhosis, is a yellowing of the skin, mucous membranes, and sclerae of the eyes (**jaundice** or **icterus**). This condition occurs because the liver is no longer able to remove **bilirubin,** a yellow compound formed when erythrocytes are destroyed. Jaundice may also result when the bile duct is blocked, causing bile to enter the bloodstream.

Diverticulosis

Diverticulosis is a condition in which small, blisterlike pockets **(diverticula)** develop in the inner lining of the large intestine and may balloon through the intestinal wall. These pockets occur most commonly in the sigmoid colon. They usually do not cause any problem unless they become inflamed **(diverticulitis).** (See Figure 6-8.) Symptoms of diverticulitis include pain, commonly in

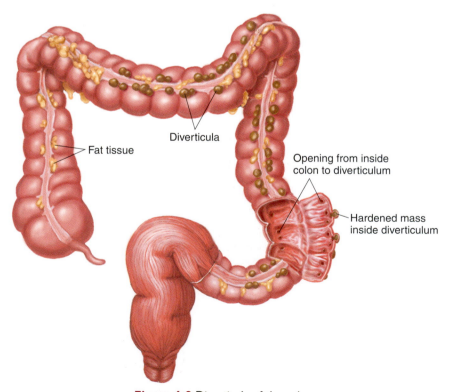

Fat tissue

Diverticula

Opening from inside
colon to diverticulum

Hardened mass
inside diverticulum

Figure 6-8 Diverticula of the colon.

the left lower quadrant (LLQ) of the abdomen; extreme constipation **(obstipation)** or diarrhea; fever; abdominal swelling; and occasional blood in bowel movements. Mild cases of diverticulitis can be treated with rest, antibiotics, and changes in diet. Severe cases, however, may require surgical intervention, such as excision of the affected segment of intestine.

Oncology

Although stomach cancer is rare in the United States, it is common in many parts of the world where food preservation is problematic. It is an important medical problem because of its high mortality rate. Men are more susceptible to stomach cancer than women. The neoplasm nearly always develops from the epithelial or mucosal lining of the stomach in the form of a cancerous glandular tumor **(gastric adenocarcinoma).** Persistent indigestion is one of the important warning signs of stomach cancer. Other types of GI carcinomas include **esophageal** carcinomas, **hepatocellular** carcinomas, and **pancreatic** carcinomas.

Colorectal cancer is one of the most common type of intestinal cancer in the United States. It originates in the epithelial lining of the colon or rectum and can occur anywhere in the large intestine. Symptoms of carcinoma of the colon depend largely on the location of the malignancy and include changes in bowel habits, passage of blood and mucus in stools, rectal or abdominal pain, anemia, weight loss, obstruction, and perforation. (See Figure 6-9.) An obstruction that develops suddenly may be the first symptom of cancer involving the colon between the cecum and the sigmoid colon. In this region, where bowel contents are liquid, a slowly developing obstruction will not become evident until the lumen is almost closed. Cancer of the sigmoid colon and rectum causes symptoms of partial obstruction with constipation alternating with diarrhea, lower abdominal cramping pain, and distention. Stages of colon cancer are illustrated in Figure 6-10.

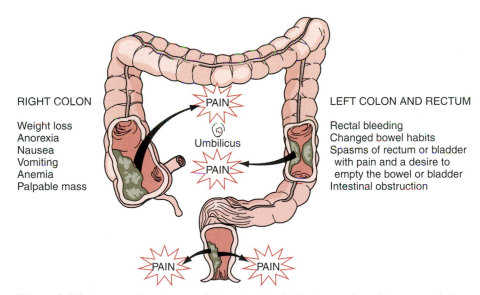

RIGHT COLON

Weight loss
Anorexia
Nausea
Vomiting
Anemia
Palpable mass

Umbilicus

PAIN
PAIN
PAIN
PAIN

LEFT COLON AND RECTUM

Rectal bleeding
Changed bowel habits
Spasms of rectum or bladder
 with pain and a desire to
 empty the bowel or bladder
Intestinal obstruction

Figure 6-9 Symptoms of carcinoma of the colon, in which pain usually radiates toward the umbilicus or perianal area. From Williams and Hopper: *Understanding Medical-Surgical Nursing,* 4th ed. FA Davis, Philadelphia, 2011, p 766, with permission.

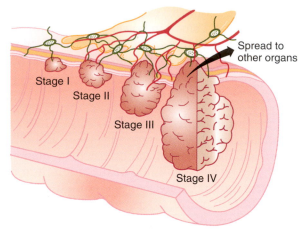

Figure 6-10 Stages of colon cancer. From Tamparo: *Diseases of the Human Body,* 5th ed. FA Davis, Philadelphia, 2011, p 425, with permission.

Diseases and Conditions

This section introduces diseases and conditions of the digestive system with their meanings and pronunciations. Word analyses for selected terms are also provided.

Term	Definition
anorexia ăn-ō-RĔK-sē-ă *an-:* without, not *-orexia:* appetite	Lack or loss of appetite, resulting in the inability to eat *Anorexia should not be confused with anorexia nervosa, which is a complex psychogenic eating disorder characterized by an all-consuming desire to remain thin.*
appendicitis ă-pĕn-dĭ-SĪ-tĭs *appendic:* appendix *-itis:* inflammation	Inflammation of the appendix, usually due to obstruction or infection *Treatment for appendicitis is appendectomy within 24 to 48 hours of the first symptoms, because delay usually results in rupture and peritonitis as fecal matter is released into the peritoneal cavity. (See Figure 6–11.)*

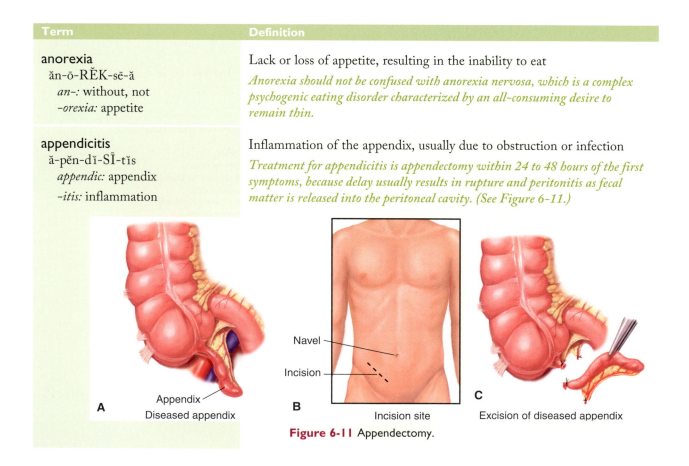

A
Appendix
Diseased appendix

B
Navel
Incision
Incision site

C
Excision of diseased appendix

Figure 6-11 Appendectomy.

Term	Definition
ascites ă-SĪ-tēz	Abnormal accumulation of fluid in the abdominal cavity, most commonly as a result of chronic liver disease (See Figure 6-12.) *Ascites is most commonly associated with cirrhosis of the liver, especially when caused by alcoholism. Failure of the liver to produce albumin (a protein that regulates the amount of fluid in the circulatory system), combined with portal hypertension, forces fluid to pass from the circulatory system and accumulate in the peritoneum.*

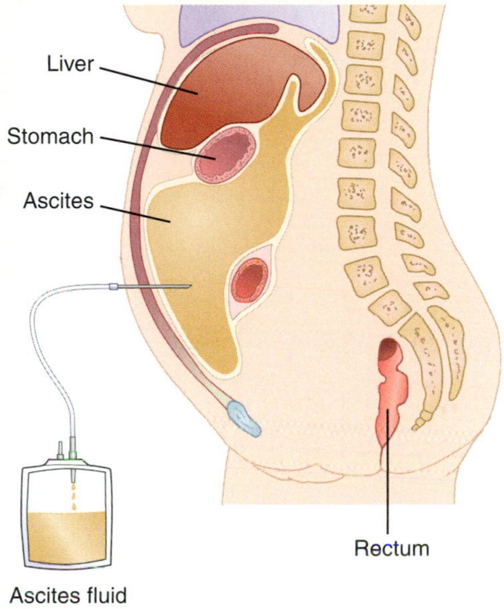

Figure 6-12 Ascites with removal of fluid from the abdominal cavity using a catheter.

Term	Definition
borborygmus bōr-bō-RĬG-mŭs	Rumbling or gurgling noises that are audible at a distance and caused by passage of gas through the liquid contents of the intestine
cachexia kă-KĔKS-ē-ă	Physical wasting that includes loss of weight and muscle mass and is commonly associated with acquired immune deficiency syndrome (AIDS) and cancer

(continued)

Term	Definition
cholelithiasis kō-lē-lĭ-THĬ-ă-sĭs *chol/e:* bile, gall *lith:* stone, calculus *-iasis:* abnormal condition (produced by something specified)	Presence or formation of gallstones in the gallbladder or common bile duct *Cholelithiasis may or may not produce symptoms. (See Figure 6-13.)* **Figure 6-13** Sites of gallstones.
cirrhosis sĭr-RŌ-sĭs	Scarring and dysfunction of the liver cause by chronic liver disease *Cirrhosis is most commonly caused by chronic alcoholism. It may also be caused by toxins, infectious agents, metabolic diseases, and circulatory disorders.*
colic KŎL-ĭk	Spasm in any hollow or tubular soft organ, especially in the colon, accompanied by pain
Crohn disease KRŌN	Form of inflammatory bowel disease (IBD), usually of the ileum but possibly affecting any portion of the intestinal tract; also called *regional enteritis* *Crohn disease is a chronic disease distinguished from closely related bowel disorders by its inflammatory pattern. It may cause fever, cramping, diarrhea, and weight loss.*
dysentery DĬS-ĕn-tĕr-ē	Inflammation of the intestine, especially the colon, that may be caused by ingesting water or food containing chemical irritants, bacteria, protozoa, or parasites and results in bloody diarrhea *Dysentery is common in underdeveloped countries and in times of disaster when sanitary living conditions, clean food, and safe water are not available.*
dysphagia dĭs-FĀ-jē-ă *dys-:* bad; painful; difficult *-phagia:* swallowing, eating	Inability or difficulty in swallowing; also called aphagia
eructation ĕ-rŭk-TĀ-shŭn	Producing gas from the stomach, usually with a characteristic sound; also called belching

Term	Definition
fecalith FĒ-kă-lĭth	Fecal concretion
flatus FLĀ-tŭs	Gas in the GI tract; expelling of air from a body orifice, especially the anus
gastroesophageal reflux disease (GERD) găs-trō-ĕ-sŏf-ă-JĒ-ăl RĒ-flŭks *gastr/o:* stomach *esophag:* esophagus *-eal:* pertaining to	Backflow of gastric contents into the esophagus due to a malfunction of the sphincter muscle at the inferior portion of the esophagus *GERD may occur whenever pressure in the stomach is greater than that in the esophagus and may be associated with heartburn, esophagitis, hiatal hernia, or chest pain.*
halitosis hăl-ĭ-TŌ-sĭs	Foul-smelling breath *Halitosis may result from poor oral hygiene; dental or oral infections; ingestion of certain foods, such as garlic or alcohol; use of tobacco; or a systemic disease, such as diabetes or liver disease.*
hematemesis hĕm-ăt-ĔM-ĕ-sĭs *hemat:* blood *-emesis:* vomiting	Vomiting of blood from bleeding in the stomach or esophagus *Hematemesis can be caused by an esophageal ulcer, esophageal varices (dilation of veins), or a gastric ulcer. Treatment requires correction of the underlying cause.*
irritable bowel syndrome (IBS)	Symptom complex marked by abdominal pain and altered bowel function (typically constipation, diarrhea, or alternating constipation and diarrhea) for which no organic cause can be determined; also called spastic colon *Contributing or aggravating factors of IBS include anxiety and stress.*
malabsorption syndrome măl-ăb-SORP-shŭn SĬN-drōm	Symptom complex of the small intestine characterized by the impaired passage of nutrients, minerals, or fluids through intestinal villi into the blood or lymph *Malabsorption syndrome may be associated with or due to a number of diseases, including those affecting the intestinal mucosa. It may also be due to surgery, such as gastric resection and ileal bypass, or antibiotic therapy.*
melena MĔL-ĕ-nă	Passage of dark-colored, tarry stools, due to the presence of blood altered by intestinal juices
obesity ō-BĒ-sĭ-tē	Excessive accumulation of fat that exceeds the body's skeletal and physical standards, usually an increase of 20 percent or more above ideal body weight *Obesity may be due to excessive intake of food (exogenous) or metabolic or endocrine abnormalities (endogenous).*
morbid obesity ō-BĒ-sĭ-tē	Body mass index (BMI) of 40 or greater, which is generally 100 pounds or more over ideal body weight *Morbid obesity is a disease with serious psychological, social, and medical ramifications and one that threatens necessary body functions such as respiration.*
obstipation ŏb-stĭ-PĀ-shŭn	Severe constipation, which may be caused by an intestinal obstruction

(continued)

Term	Definition
oral leukoplakia OR-ăl loo-kō-PLĀ-kē-ă *leuk/o:* white *-plakia:* plaque	Formation of white spots or patches on the mucous membrane of the tongue, lips, or cheek caused primarily by irritation *Oral leukoplakia is a precancerous condition usually associated with pipe or cigarette smoking or ill-fitting dentures.*
peristalsis pĕr-ĭ-STĂL-sĭs	Progressive, wavelike movement that occurs involuntarily in hollow tubes of the body, especially the GI tract
pyloric stenosis pī-LOR-ĭk stĕ-NŌ-sĭs *pylor:* pylorus *-ic:* pertaining to *sten:* narrowing, stricture *-osis:* abnormal condition; increase (used primarily with blood cells)	Stricture or narrowing of the pyloric sphincter (circular muscle of the pylorus) at the outlet of the stomach, causing an obstruction that blocks the flow of food into the small intestine
regurgitation rē-gŭr-jĭ-TĀ-shŭn	Backward flowing, as in the return of solids or fluids to the mouth from the stomach
steatorrhea stē-ă-tō-RĒ-ă *steat/o:* fat *-rrhea:* discharge, flow	Passage of fat in large amounts in the feces due to failure to digest and absorb it *Steatorrhea may occur in pancreatic disease when pancreatic enzymes are not sufficient. It also occurs in malabsorption syndrome.*

 It is time to review pathology, diseases, and conditions by completing Learning Activity 6-4.

Medical, Surgical, and Diagnostic Procedures

This section introduces medical, surgical, and diagnostic procedures used to treat and diagnose digestive system disorders. Descriptions are provided as well as pronunciations and word analyses for selected terms.

Procedure	Description
Medical	
nasogastric intubation nā-zō-GĂS-trĭk ĭn-tū-BĀ-shŭn *nas/o:* nose *gastr:* stomach *-ic:* pertaining to	Insertion of a nasogastric tube through the nose into the stomach to relieve gastric distention by removing gas, food, or gastric secretions; instill medication, food, or fluids; or obtain a specimen for laboratory analysis
Surgical	
anastomosis ă-năs-tō-MŌ-sĭs	Surgical joining of two ducts, vessels, or bowel segments to allow flow from one to another

ileorectal
  ĭl-ē-ō-RĔK-tăl
    ile/o: ileum
    rect: rectum
    -al: pertaining to
	Surgical connection of the ileum and rectum after total colectomy, as is sometimes performed in the treatment of ulcerative colitis

intestinal ĭn-TĔS-tĭ-năl	Surgical connection of two portions of the intestines; also called enteroenterostomy

Procedure	Description
bariatric surgery băr-ē-Ă-trĭk	Group of procedures that treat morbid obesity, a condition that arises from severe accumulation of excess weight as fatty tissue, and the resultant health problems *Commonly employed bariatric surgeries include vertical banded gastroplasty and Roux-en-Y gastric bypass. (See Figure 6-14.)*
vertical banded gastroplasty GĂS-trō-plăs-tē	Bariatric surgery that involves vertical stapling of the upper stomach near the esophagus to reduce it to a small pouch and insertion of a band that restricts food consumption and delays its passage from the pouch, causing a feeling of fullness
Roux-en-Y gastric bypass (RGB) rū-ĕn-WĪ GĂS-trĭk	Bariatric surgery that involves stapling the stomach to decrease its size and then shortening the jejunum and connecting it to the small stomach pouch, causing the base of the duodenum leading from the nonfunctioning portion of the stomach to form a Y configuration, which decreases the pathway of food through the intestine, thus reducing absorption of calories and fats *RGB can be performed laparoscopically or as an open procedure (laparotomy), depending on the health of the patient. RGB is the most commonly performed weight-loss surgery today.*

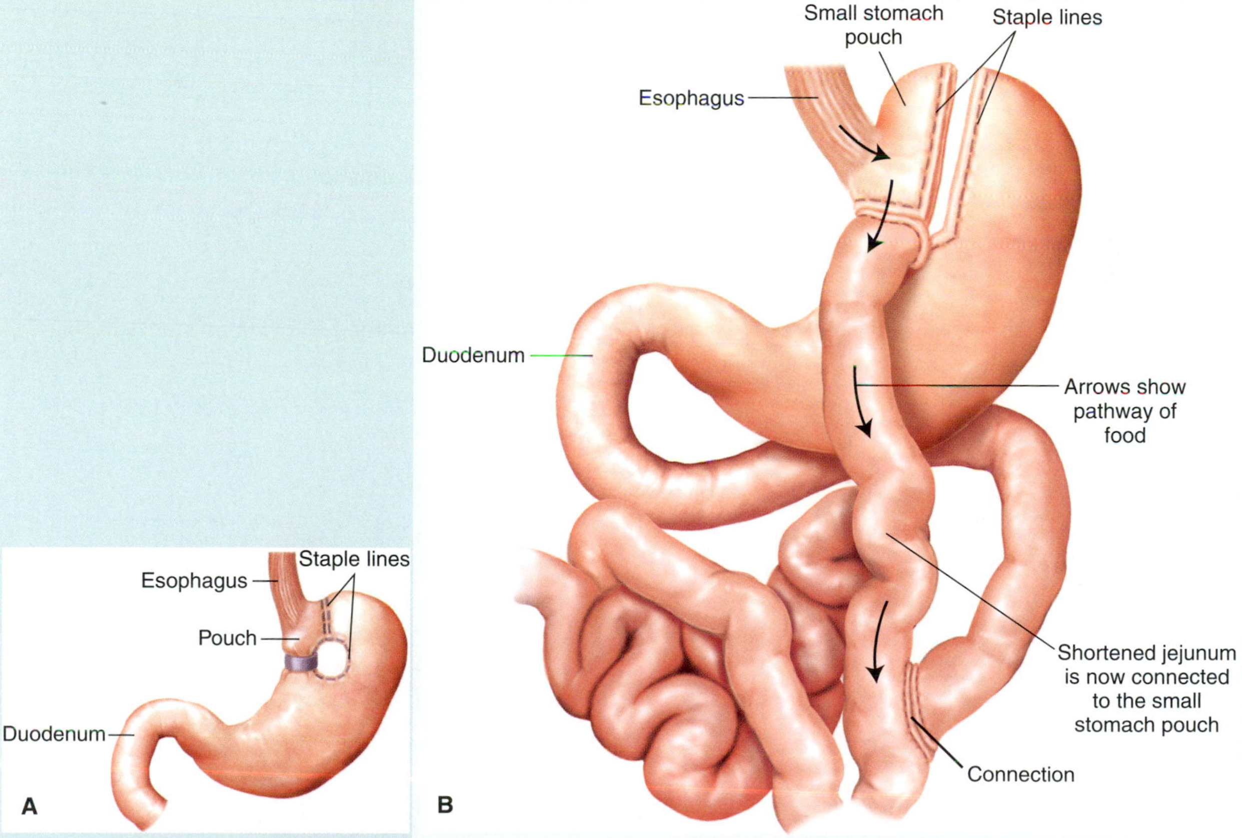

Figure 6-14 Bariatric surgery. **(A)** Vertical banded gastroplasty. **(B)** Roux-en-Y gastric bypass.

(continued)

Procedure	Description
colostomy kō-LŎS-tō-mē *col/o:* colon	Creation of an opening of a portion of the colon through the abdominal wall to its outside surface in order to divert fecal flow to a colostomy bag (See Figure 6-15.)

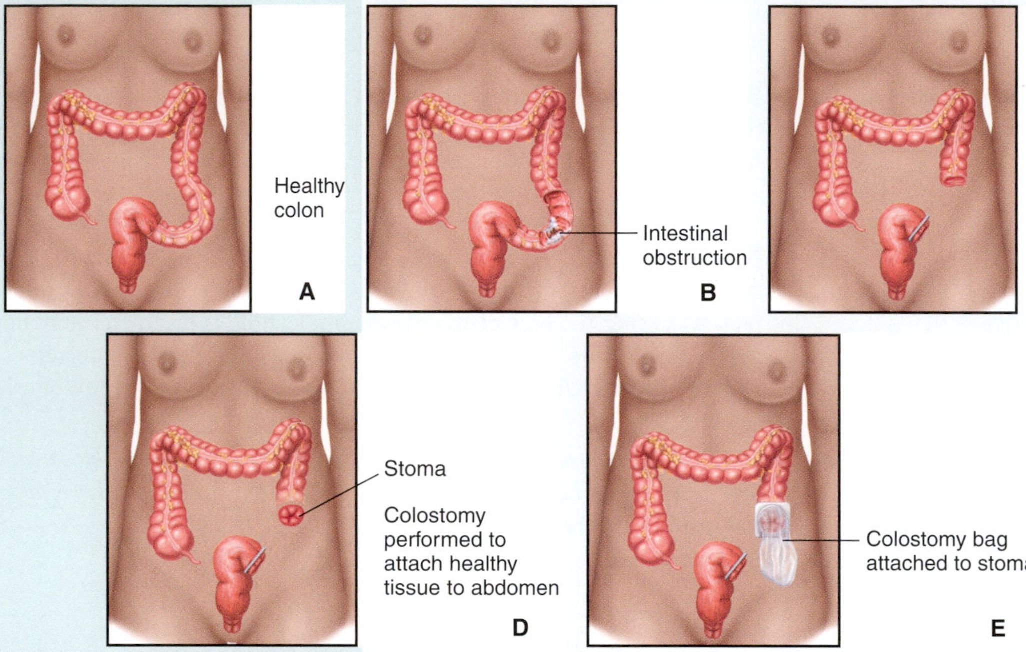

Healthy colon **A**

Intestinal obstruction **B**

Excision of diseased colon **C**

Stoma

Colostomy performed to attach healthy tissue to abdomen **D**

Colostomy bag attached to stoma **E**

Figure 6-15 Colostomy.

Procedure	Description
lithotripsy LĬTH-ō-trĭp-sē *lith/o:* stone, calculus *-tripsy:* crushing	Procedure for crushing a stone and eliminating its fragments surgically or using ultrasonic shock waves
extracorporeal shock-wave lithotripsy ĕks-tră-kor-POR-ē-ăl SHŎK-wāv	Use of shock waves as a noninvasive method to break up stones in the gallbladder or biliary ducts (See Figure 11-4.) *In extracorporeal shockwave lithotripsy (ESWL), ultrasound is used to locate the stone(s) and to monitor their destruction.*
polypectomy pŏl-ĭ-PĔK-tō-mē *polyp:* small growth *-ectomy:* excision, removal	Excision of a polyp *When polyps are discovered during sigmoidoscopy or colonoscopy, they are excised for microscopic tissue examination for abnormal or cancerous cells. (See Figure 6-16.)*

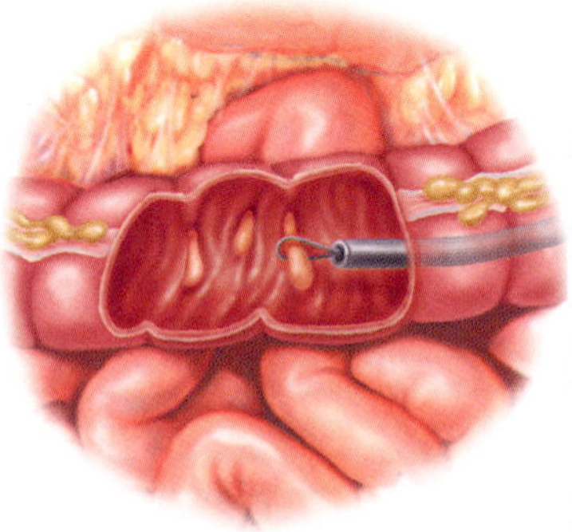

Polyps are removed from colon for examination
Figure 6-16 Polypectomy.

Procedure	Description

pyloromyotomy
pī-LŌ-rō-mī-ŏt-ō-mē
  pylor/o: pylorus
  my/o: muscle
  -tomy: incision
	Incision of the longitudinal and circular muscles of the pylorus, which is used to treat hypertrophic pyloric stenosis

Diagnostic

Endoscopic

gastrointestinal endoscopy
găs-trō-ĭn-TĔS-tĭn-ăl
ĕn-DŎS-kō-pē
  endo-: in, within
  -scopy: visual examination
	Visual examination of the gastrointestinal tract using a flexible fiberoptic instrument with a magnifying lens and a light source (endoscope) to identify abnormalities, including bleeding, ulcerations, and tumors
	
	In endoscopy of the esophagus (esophagoscopy), stomach (gastroscopy), and duodenum (duodenoscopy), the endoscope is inserted through the nose or mouth. In endoscopy of the colon (colonoscopy) and sigmoid colon (sigmoidoscopy) the endoscope is inserted through the rectum. (See Figure 6–17.)

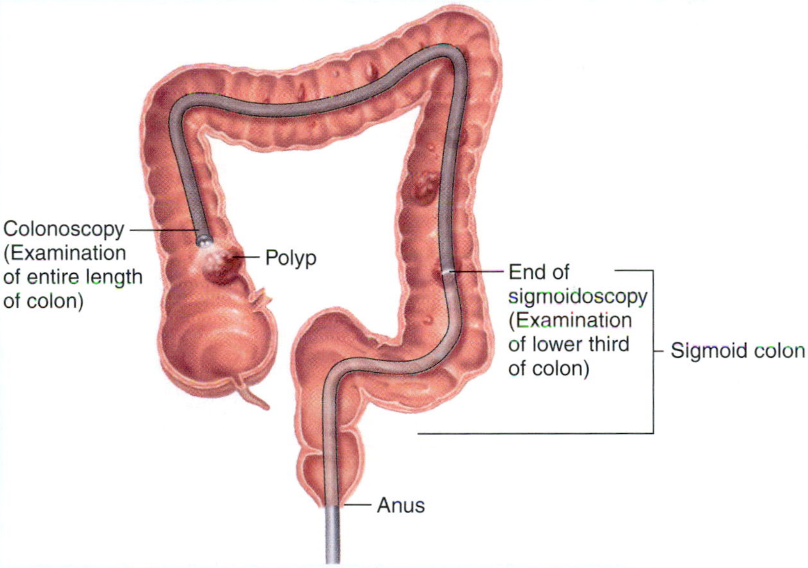

Figure 6-17 Colonoscopy and sigmoidoscopy.

Laboratory

hepatitis panel
hĕp-ă-TĪ-tĭs
  hepat: liver
  -itis: inflammation
	Panel of blood tests that identifies the specific virus—hepatitis A (HAV), hepatitis B (HBV), or hepatitis C (HCV)—that is causing hepatitis by testing serum using antibodies to each of these antigens

liver function tests (LFTs)	Group of blood tests that evaluate liver injury, liver function, and conditions commonly associated with the biliary tract *LFTs evaluate liver enzymes, bilirubin, and proteins produced by the liver.*
serum bilirubin SĔ-rŭm bĭl-ĭ-ROO-bĭn	Measurement of the level of bilirubin in the blood *Elevated serum bilirubin indicates excessive destruction of erythrocytes, liver disease, or biliary tract obstruction.*

(continued)

Procedure	Description
stool culture	Test to identify microorganisms or parasites present in feces that are causing a gastrointestinal infection *Feces are examined microscopically after being placed in a growth medium.*
stool guaiac GWĪ-ăk	Test that applies a substance called guaiac to a stool sample to detect the presence of occult (hidden) blood in the feces; also called Hemoccult (trade name of a modified guaiac test) *Stool guaiac test helps detect colon cancer and bleeding associated with digestive disorders.*

Imaging

computed tomography (CT)
kŏm-PŪ-tĕd tō-MŎG-ră-fē
  tom/o: to cut
  -graphy: process of recording
	Imaging technique achieved by rotating an x-ray emitter around the area to be scanned and measuring the intensity of transmitted rays from different angles
	
	In CT scanning, a computer is used to generate a detailed cross-sectional image that appears as a slice. (See Figure 4-5D.) In the digestive system, CT scans are used to view the gallbladder, bowel, liver, bile ducts, and pancreas. They are also used to diagnose tumors, cysts, inflammation, abscesses, perforation, bleeding, and obstruction.

lower gastrointestinal series GĂS-trō-ĭn-tĕs-tĭn-ăl, BĂ-rē-ŭm ĔN-ĕ-mă	Radiographic images of the rectum and colon following administration of barium into the rectum; also called *lower GI series* or *barium enema* *Barium is retained in the lower GI tract during fluoroscopic and radiographic studies. It is used for diagnosing obstructions, tumors, or other abnormalities of the colon. (See Figure 6-18.)*

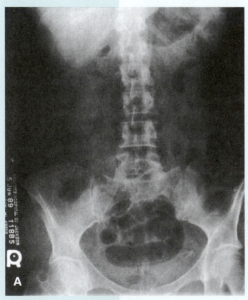 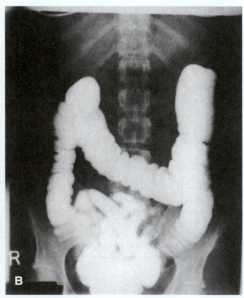

Figure 6-18 Barium enema done poorly **(A)** and correctly **(B).**

Procedure	Description
oral cholecystography (OCG) kō-lē-sĭs-TŎG-ră-fē *chol/e:* bile, gall *cyst/o:* bladder *-graphy:* process of recording	Radiographic images taken of the gallbladder after administration of a contrast material containing iodine, usually in the form of a tablet *OCG evaluates gallbladder function and identifies the presence of disease or gallstones.*
magnetic resonance cholangiopancreatography (MRCP) kō-lăn-jē-ō-păn-krē-ă-TŎG-ră-fē *cholangi/o:* bile vessel *pancreat/o:* pancreas *-graphy:* process of recording	Magnetic resonance imaging (MRI) is used to visualize the biliary and pancreatic ducts and gallbladder in a noninvasive manner *MRCP is a relatively new technique. Unlike other techniques, no contrast medium is required. MRCP can be used to determine if gallstones are lodged in any of the ducts surrounding the gallbladder. It may also detect tumors, inflammation, infection, or pancreatitis.*
sialography sī-ă-LŎG-ră-fē *sial/o:* saliva, salivary glands *-graphy:* process of recording	Radiologic examination of the salivary glands and ducts *Sialography may be performed with or without a contrast medium.*
ultrasonography (US) ŭl-tră-sŏn-ŎG-ră-fē *ultra-:* excess, beyond *son/o:* sound *-graphy:* process of recording	High-frequency sound waves (ultrasound) are directed at soft tissue and reflected as "echoes" to produce an image on a monitor of an internal body structure; also called *ultrasound, sonography,* and *echo* *US is a noninvasive procedure that does not require a contrast medium. It is used to detect diseases and abnormalities in the digestive organs, such as the gallbladder, liver, and pancreas. It is also used to locate abdominal masses outside the digestive organs.*

abdominal
    ăb-DŎM-ĭ-năl
    abdomin: abdomen
    -al: pertaining to
	Ultrasound visualization of the abdominal aorta, liver, gallbladder, bile ducts, pancreas, kidneys, ureters, and bladder
	An abdominal US is used to diagnose and locate cysts, tumors, and malformations as well as document the progression of various diseases and guide the insertion of instruments during surgical procedures.

endoscopic	Combines endoscopy and ultrasound to examine and obtain images of the digestive tract and the surrounding tissue and organs *In endoscopic US, a long, flexible tube (endoscope) inserted via the mouth or rectum emits high-frequency sound waves (ultrasound) that produce images of the organs and structures.*
upper gastrointestinal series (UGIS) GĂS-trō-ĭn-tĕs-tĭn-ăl	Radiographic images of the esophagus, stomach, and small intestine following oral administration of barium; also called *barium swallow* *Barium swallow is most commonly used in patients who are experiencing difficulty swallowing. It is also useful for identifying ulcers, tumors, or obstruction in the esophagus, stomach, and small intestine.*

Pharmacology

Various pharmaceutical agents are available to counteract abnormal conditions that occur in the GI tract. Antacids counteract or decrease excessive stomach acid, the cause of heartburn, gastric discomfort, and gastric reflux. Antidiarrheals and antiemetics are prescribed to preserve water and electrolytes, which are essential for body hydration and homeostasis. Medications that increase or decrease peristalsis are used to regulate the speed at which food passes through the GI tract. These drugs include agents that relieve "cramping" (**antispasmodics**) and those that help in the movement of material through a sluggish bowel (**laxatives**). (See Table 6-1.)

Table 6-1	**Drugs Used to Treat Digestive Disorders**	
This table lists common drug classifications used to treat digestive disorders, their therapeutic actions, and selected generic and trade names.		
Classification	**Therapeutic Action**	**Generic and *Trade* Names**
antacids ănt-ĂS-ĭds	Counteract or neutralize acidity, usually in the stomach *Antacids are used to treat and prevent heartburn and acid reflux.*	**calcium carbonate** KĂL-sē-ŭm KĂR-bŏn-āt *Mylanta, Rolaids, Tums*
antidiarrheals ăn-tĭ-dī-ă-RĒ-ăls	Control loose stools and relieve diarrhea by absorbing excess water in the bowel or slowing peristalsis in the intestinal tract	**loperamide** lō-PĔR-ă-mīd *Imodium*
		kaolin/pectin KĀ-ō-lĭn, PĔK-tĭn *Donnagel-MB, Kapectolin*
antiemetics ăn-tĭ-ē-MĔT-ĭks	Control nausea and vomiting by blocking nerve impulses to the vomiting center of the brain *Some emetics act by hastening movement of food through the digestive tract.*	**prochlorperazine** prō-klor-PĔR-ă-zēn *Compazine, Compro*
		ondansetron ŏn-DĂN-sĕ-trŏn *Zofran*
antispasmodics ăn-tē-spăz-MŎD-ĭks	Decrease gastrointestinal (GI) spasms by slowing peristalsis and motility throughout the GI tract *Antispasmodics are prescribed for irritable bowel syndrome (IBS), spastic colon, and diverticulitis.*	**glycopyrrolate** glī-kō-PĬR-rō-lāt *Robinul*
		dicyclomine dī-SĪ-klō-mēn *Bentyl*
laxatives LĂK-să-tĭvs	Treat constipation by increasing peristaltic activity in the large intestine or increasing water and electrolyte secretion into the bowel to induce defecation	**senna, sennosides** SĔN-ă, SĔN-ō-sīdz *Senokot, Senolax*
		psyllium SĬL-ē-ŭm *Metamucil, Natural Fiber Supplement*

Abbreviations

This section introduces digestive-related abbreviations and their meanings.

Abbreviation	Meaning	Abbreviation	Meaning
Common			
AIDS	acquired immune deficiency syndrome	**HCV**	hepatitis C virus
Ba	barium	**HDV**	hepatitis D virus
BaE, BE	barium enema	**HEV**	hepatitis E virus
BM	bowel movement	**IBS**	irritable bowel syndrome
BMI	body mass index	**LFT**	liver function test
CT	computed tomography	**MRCP**	magnetic resonance cholangiopancreatography
EGD	esophagogastroduodenoscopy lithotripsy	**NG**	nasogastric
ESWL	extracorporeal shock-wave	**OCG**	oral cholecystography
EUS	endoscopic ultrasonography (x-ray studies)	**PUD**	peptic ulcer disease
GBS	gallbladder series	**R/O**	rule out
GER	gastroesophageal reflux disease	**RGB**	Roux-en-Y gastric bypass
GERD	gastroesophageal reflux	**stat**	immediately
GI	gastrointestinal	**UGIS**	upper gastrointestinal series
HAV	hepatitis A virus	**US**	ultrasound; ultrasonography
HBV	hepatitis B virus		

⊕ *It is time to review procedures, pharmacology, and abbreviations by completing Learning Activity 6–5.*

LEARNING ACTIVITIES

The following activities provide review of the digestive system terms introduced in this chapter. Complete each activity and review your answers to evaluate your understanding of the chapter.

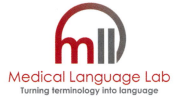

Medical Language Lab
Turning terminology into language

Visit the Medical Language Lab at the web site: medicallanguagelab.com. Use it to enhance your study and reinforcement of this chapter with the flash-card activity. We recommend you complete the flash-card activity before starting Learning Activities 6-1 and 6-2.

Learning Activity 6-1
Combining Forms, Suffixes, and Prefixes

Use the elements listed in the table to build medical words. You may use the elements more than once.

Combining Forms		Suffixes		Prefixes
an/o	jejun/o	-al	-pathy	an-
colon/o	pharyng/o	-emesis	-pepsia	dys-
dent/o	sial/o	-ic	-phagia	endo-
esophag/o	stomat/o	-ism	-plasty	hypo-
gastr/o	-itis	-rrhaphy	peri-	
gingiv/o	-lith	-scope		
hemat/o	-orexia	-scopy		

1. inflammation of the gum(s) _____

2. instrument to examine the colon _____

3. surgical repair of the stomach _____

4. pertaining to under or below the stomach _____

5. bad, painful, or difficult digestion _____

6. calculus in a salivary gland or duct _____

7. disease of the mouth _____

8. pertaining to around the anus _____

9. suture of the jejunum (second part of the small intestine) _____

10. inflammation of the pharynx _____

11. instrument to examine the esophaqus _____

12. without an appetite _____

13. vomiting blood _____

14. visual examination within _____

15. bad; painful; difficult swallowing or eating _____

✓ *Check your answers in Appendix A. Review any material that you did not answer correctly.*

Correct Answers _____ X 6.67 = _____ % Score

Learning Activity 6-2
Building Medical Words

Use *esophag/o* (esophagus) to build words that mean:

1. pain in the esophagus _____
2. spasm of the esophagus _____
3. stricture or narrowing of the esophagus _____

Use *gastr/o* (stomach) to build words that mean:

4. inflammation of the stomach _____
5. pain in the stomach _____
6. disease of the stomach _____

Use *duoden/o* (duodenum), *jejun/o* (jejunum), or *ile/o* (ileum) to build words that mean:

7. excision of all or part of the jejunum _____
8. relating to the duodenum _____
9. inflammation of the ileum _____
10. pertaining to the jejunum and ileum _____

Use *enter/o* (usually small intestine) to build words that mean:

11. inflammation of the small intestine _____
12. disease of the small intestine _____
13. inflammation of the small intestine and colon _____

Use *col/o* (colon) to build words that mean:

14. inflammation of the colon _____
15. pertaining to the colon and rectum _____
16. prolapse or downward displacement of the colon _____
17. disease of the colon _____

Use *proct/o* (anus, rectum) or *rect/o* (rectum) to build words that mean:

18. narrowing or constriction of the rectum _____
19. herniation of the rectum _____
20. paralysis of the anus (anal muscles) _____

Use *chol/e* (bile, gall) to build words that mean:

21. inflammation of the gallbladder _____
22. abnormal condition of a gallstone _____

Use *hepat/o* (liver) or *pancreat/o* (pancreas) to build words that mean:

23. tumor of the liver _____
24. enlargement of the liver _____
25. inflammation of the pancreas _____

Check your answers in Appendix A. Review material that you did not answer correctly.

Correct Answers _____ X 4 = _____ % Score

Learning Activity 6-3
Building Surgical Words

Build a surgical word that means:

1. excision of gums (tissue) _____

2. partial or complete excision of the tongue _____

3. repair of the esophagus _____

4. removal of part or all of the stomach _____

5. forming an opening between the stomach and jejunum _____

6. excision of (part of) the esophagus _____

7. forming an opening between the stomach, small intestine, and colon _____

8. surgical repair of the small intestine _____

9. fixation of the small intestine (to the abdominal wall) _____

10. suture of the bile duct _____

11. forming an opening into the colon _____

12. fixation of a movable liver (to the abdominal wall) _____

13. surgical repair of the anus or rectum _____

14. removal of the gallbladder _____

15. surgical repair of a bile duct _____

Check your answers in Appendix A. Review material that you did not answer correctly.

Correct Answers _____ X 6.67 = _____ % Score

Learning Activity 6-4
Pathology, Diseases, and Conditions

Match the following terms with the definitions in the numbered list.

anorexia	*dyspepsia*	*hematemesis*
ascites	*dysphagia*	*leukoplakia*
cachexia	*fecalith*	*lesion*
cirrhosis	*flatus*	*obstipation*
Crohn disease	*halitosis*	*steatorrhea*

1. vomiting blood _____
2. difficulty swallowing or inability to swallow _____
3. fecal concretion _____
4. foul-smelling breath _____
5. loss of appetite _____
6. poor digestion _____
7. yellowing of the skin due to liver disease _____
8. state of ill health, malnutrition, and wasting _____
9. intractable constipation _____
10. open sore _____
11. abnormal accumulation of fluid in the abdominal cavity _____
12. form of inflammatory bowel disease, usually of the ileum _____
13. passage of fat in large amounts in the feces _____
14. formation of white patches on the mucous membrane of the cheek _____
15. gas in the gastrointestinal tract _____

  Check your answers in Appendix A. Review any material that you did not answer correctly.

Correct Answers _____ X 6.67 = _____ % Score

Learning Activity 6-5
Procedures, Pharmacology, and Abbreviations

Match the following terms with the definitions in the numbered list.

anastomosis	*choledochoplasty*	*intubation*	*proctosigmoidoscopy*
antacids	*emetics*	*laxatives*	*stat*
antiemetics	*endoscopy*	*liver function tests*	*stool culture*
antispasmodics	*ESWL*	*lower GI series*	*stool guaiac*
bariatric	*gastroscopy*	*MRCP*	*upper GI series*

1. procedure to visualize biliary and pancreatic ducts by using magnetic resonance imaging _____
2. procedure in which shock waves are used to break up calculi in the biliary ducts _____
3. agents that produce vomiting _____
4. agents that alleviate muscle spasms _____
5. surgical reconstruction of a bile duct _____
6. administration of a barium enema while a series of radiographs are taken of the colon _____
7. visual examination of the stomach _____
8. agents that control nausea and vomiting _____
9. insertion of a tube into any hollow organ _____
10. surgical formation of a passage or opening between two hollow viscera or vessels _____
11. detects presence of blood in the feces; also called hemoccult _____
12. visual examination of a cavity or canal using a specialized lighted instrument _____
13. used to treat constipation _____
14. neutralize excess acid in the stomach and help to relieve gastritis and ulcer pain _____
15. test to identify microorganisms present in feces _____
16. measures the levels of certain enzymes, bilirubin, and various proteins _____
17. surgery that treats morbid obesity _____
18. immediately _____
19. endoscopic procedure for visualization of the rectosigmoid colon _____
20. radiographic imaging of the esophagus, duodenum, and stomach after ingestion of barium _____

Check your answers in Appendix A. Review material that you did not answer correctly.

Correct Answers _____ X 5 = _____ % Score

Learning Activity 6-6
Medical Scenarios

To construct chart notes, replace the italicized terms in each of the two scenarios with one of the medical terms listed below.

anorexia	gastric reflux	jaundice
antacids	hepatomegaly	nausea
dyspepsia	hiatal hernia	sclerae
dysphagia		

During her annual check-up, Mrs. L. complains that she has (1) *difficulty swallowing.* Also, she is awakened at night with a feeling of (2) *difficult or painful digestion.* She further complains of (3) *regurgitation of stomach acids* and has been taking Tums and Rolaids. She feels that the (4) *medications* to neutralize the backflow of acid from her stomach have not been effective. After a thorough examination along with some radiographic procedures, the doctor suspects her symptoms are due to a (5) *part of her stomach herniating up through the opening of the diaphragm.*

1. _____
2. _____
3. _____
4. _____
5. _____

Mr. K. recently returned from Haiti where he worked with other volunteers from his church. Their purpose was to help homeless families rebuild their communities. Lately, he complains of (6) *no appetite* and feeling feverish. He also complains of (7) *unpleasant queasy sensations of discomfort in the region of his stomach.* Today, he presents to the clinic and his doctor notes that the (8) *whites of his eyes* are now (9) *yellow in color.* After further examination and a series of blood tests, the doctor suspects that Mr. K. suffers from an (10) *enlarged liver* and will be further tested for hepatitis A.

6. _____
7. _____
8. _____
9. _____
10. _____

Check your answers in Appendix A. Review any material that you did not answer correctly.

Correct Answers _____ X 10 = _____ % Score

MEDICAL RECORD ACTIVITIES

The two medical records included in the following activities use common clinical scenarios to show how medical terminology is used to document patient care. Complete the terminology and analysis sections for each activity to help you recognize and understand terms related to the digestive system.

Medical Record Activity 6-1

Chart Note: GI Evaluation

Terminology

Terms listed in the following table are taken from *Chart Note: GI Evaluation* that follows. Use a medical dictionary such as *Taber's Cyclopedic Medical Dictionary;* the appendices of *Systems,* 7th ed.; or other resources to define each term. Then review the pronunciations for each term and practice by reading the medical record aloud.

Term	Definition
appendectomy* ăp-ĕn-DĚK-tō-mē	
cholecystectomy kō-lē-sĭs-TĚK-tō-mē	
cholecystitis kō-lē-sĭs-TĪ-tĭs	
cholelithiasis* kō-lē-lĭ-THĪ-ă-sĭs	
crescendo kră-SHĚN-dō	
decrescendo dā-kră-SHĚN-dō	
defecate DĚF-ĕ-kāt	
flatus FLĀ-tŭs	
heme-negative stool hēm-NĔG-ă-tĭv	
hepatomegaly hĕp-ă-tō-MĚG-ă-lē	

*Refer to Figure 6-11, p. 140 and Figure 6-13, p. 142 for a visual illustration of these terms.

Term	Definition
intermittent ĭn-tĕr-MĬT-ĕnt	
nausea NAW-sē-ă	
PMH	
postoperative pōst-ŎP-ĕr-ă-tĭv	
R/O	
splenomegaly splē-nō-MĔG-ă-lē	
tonsillectomy tŏn-sĭl-ĔK-tō-mē	

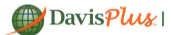 | Visit the *Medical Terminology Systems* online resource center at Davis*Plus* to practice pronunciation and reinforce the meanings of the terms in this medical report.

CHART NOTE: GI EVALUATION

Jones, Roberta   **March 15, 20xx**
Age: 50

HISTORY OF PRESENT ILLNESS: Patient's abdominal pain began 2 years ago when she first had intermittent, sharp epigastric pain. Each episode lasted 2 to 4 hours. Eventually, she was diagnosed as having cholecystitis with cholelithiasis and underwent cholecystectomy. Three to five large calcified stones were found.

POSTOPERATIVE COURSE: Her postoperative course was uneventful until 4 months ago when she began having continuous deep right-sided pain. This pain followed a crescendo pattern and peaked several weeks ago, at a time when family stress was also at its climax. Since then, the pain has been following a decrescendo pattern. It does not cause any nausea or vomiting, does not trigger any urge to defecate, and is not alleviated by passage of flatus. Her PMH is significant only for tonsillectomy, appendectomy, and the cholecystectomy. Her PE findings indicated that there was no hepatomegaly or splenomegaly. The rectal examination confirmed normal sphincter tone and heme-negative stool.

IMPRESSION: Abdominal pain. Rule out hepatomegaly and splenomegaly.

PLAN: Schedule a complete barium workup for possible obstruction.

Joseph Bogata, MD
Joseph Bogata, MD

bcg

Analysis

Review the medical record *Chart Note: GI Evaluation* to answer the following questions.

1. While referring to Figure 6-4, describe the location of the gallbladder in relation to the liver.

_____

2. Why did the patient undergo the cholecystectomy?

_____

3. List the patient's prior surgeries.

_____

4. How does the patient's most recent postoperative episode of discomfort (pain) differ from the initial pain she described?

_____

Medical Record Activity 6-2

Operative Report: Esophagogastroduodenoscopy with Biopsy

Terminology

Terms listed in the following table are taken from *Operative Report: Esophagogastroduo-denoscopy with Biopsy* that follows. Use a medical dictionary such as *Taber's Cyclopedic Medical Dictionary;* the appendices of *Systems,* 7th ed.; or other resources to define each term. Then review the pronunciations for each term and practice by reading the medical record aloud.

Term	Definition
Demerol DĔM-ĕr-ŏl	
duodenal bulb dū-ō-DĒ-năl bŭlb	
duodenitis dū-ŏd-ĕ-NĪ-tĭs	
erythema ĕr-ĭ-THĒ-mă	
esophageal varices ĕ-sŏf-ă-JĒ-ăl VĂR-ĭ-sēz	
esophagogastr- oduodenoscopy ĕ-sŏf-ă-gō-găs- trō-doo-ō-děn- ŎS-kō-pē	
etiology ē-tē-ŎL-ō-jē	
friability frī-ă-BĬL-ĭ-tē	
gastric antrum GĂS-trĭk ĂN-trŭm	
gastritis găs-TRĪ-tĭs	
hematemesis hĕm-ăt-ĔM-ĕ-sĭs	
lateral recumbent LĂT-ĕr-ăl rē-KŬM-bĕnt	

(continued)

Term	Definition
oximeter ŏk-SĬM-ĕ-tĕr	
punctate erythema PŬNK-tāt ĕr-ĭ-THĒ-mă	
tomography tō-MŎG-ră-fē	
Versed VĔR-sĕd	
videoendoscope vĭd-ē-ō-ĔND-ō- skōp	

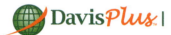

Visit the *Medical Terminology Systems* online resource center at Davis*Plus* to practice pronunciation and reinforce the meanings of the terms in this medical report.

OPERATIVE REPORT: ESOPHAGOGASTRODUODENOSCOPY WITH BIOPSY

OPERATIVE REPORT

Date:	May 14, 20xx	Physician:	Dante Riox, MD
Patient:	Franks, Roberta	Room:	703

PREOPERATIVE DIAGNOSIS: Hematemesis of unknown etiology.

POSTOPERATIVE DIAGNOSIS: Diffuse gastritis and duodenitis.

PROCEDURE: Esophagogastroduodenoscopy with biopsy.

SPECIMEN: Biopsies from gastric antrum and duodenal bulb.

ESTIMATED BLOOD LOSS: Nil.

COMPLICATIONS: None.   **TIME UNDER SEDATION:** 20 minutes.

PROCEDURE AND FINDINGS: After obtaining informed consent regarding the procedure, its risks, and its alternatives, the patient was taken to the GI lab, where she was placed on the examining table in the left lateral recumbent position. She was given nasal oxygen at 3 liters per minute and monitored with a pulse oximeter throughout the procedure. Through a previously inserted intravenous line, the patient was sedated with a total of 50 mg of Demerol intravenously plus 4 mg of Midazolam intravenously throughout the procedure. The Fujinon computed tomography scan videoendoscope was then readily introduced and the following organs evaluated.

Esophagus: The esophageal mucosa appeared normal throughout. No other abnormalities were seen. Specifically, there was prior evidence of esophageal varices.

Stomach: There was diffuse erythema with old blood seen within the stomach. No ulcerations, erosions, or fresh bleeding was seen. A representative biopsy was obtained from the gastric antrum and submitted to the pathology laboratory.

Duodenum: Punctate erythema was noted in the duodenal bulb. There was some friability. No ulcerations, erosions, or active bleeding was seen. A bulbar biopsy was obtained. The second portion of the duodenum appeared normal.

The patient tolerated the procedure well. Patient was transferred to the recovery room in stable condition.

Dante Riox, MD
Dante Riox, MD

dr:bg

D: 5-14-20xx; T: 5-14-20xx

Analysis

Review the medical report *Operative Report: Esophagogastroduodenoscopy with Biopsy* to answer the following questions.

1. What caused the hematemesis?

_____

2. What procedures were carried out to determine the cause of bleeding?

_____

3. How much blood did the patient lose during the procedure?

_____

4. Were any ulcerations or erosions found during the exploratory procedure that might account for the bleeding?

_____

5. What type of sedation was used during the procedure?

_____

6. What did the doctors find when they examined the stomach and duodenum?

_____

Respiratory System

Chapter Outline

Objectives

Upon completion of this chapter, you will be able to:

- Locate and describe the structures of the respiratory system.
- Describe the functional relationship between the respiratory system and other body systems.
- Pronounce, spell, and build words related to the respiratory system.
- Describe diseases, conditions, and procedures related to the respiratory system.
- Explain pharmacology related to the treatment of respiratory disorders.
- Demonstrate your knowledge of this chapter by completing the learning and medical record activities.

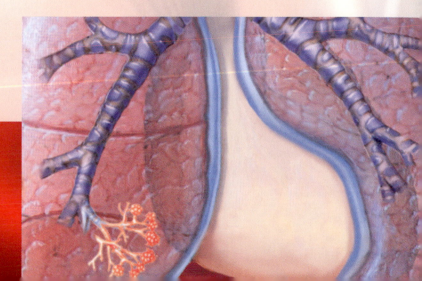

Anatomy and Physiology

The respiratory system is responsible for the exchange of **oxygen (O₂)** and **carbon dioxide (CO₂)**. Oxygen is essential for life. It is carried to all cells of the body in exchange for CO_2, a waste product. The lungs and airways transport oxygen-enriched air from the atmosphere to the lungs and carry waste CO_2 from the lungs to the atmosphere by a process called **breathing,** also known as **ventilation.** Breathing helps regulate the **pH** (acidity-alkalinity) of the blood, thereby maintaining homeostasis.

Anatomy and Physiology Key Terms

This section introduces important respiratory system terms and their definitions. Word analyses for selected terms are also provided.

Term	Definition
carbon dioxide (CO₂) KĂR-bŏn dī-ŎK-sīd	Tasteless, colorless, odorless gas produced by body cells during metabolism *The blood carries CO₂ to the lungs, which then exhale it.*
cartilage KĂR-tĭ-lĭj	Tough, elastic connective tissue that is more rigid than ligaments but less dense than bone *The tip of the nose and the outer ear are composed of cartilage.*
cilia SĬL-ē-ă	Hairlike structure *Cilia in the trachea move particles upward to the pharynx, where they are removed by coughing, sneezing, or swallowing. This mechanism is called the* cilia escalator. *Habitual smoking destroys the cilia escalator.*
diffuse dĭ-FŪZ	To move or spread out a substance at random, rather than by chemical reaction or application of external forces
mucous membrane MŪ-kŭs MĔM-brān *muc:* mucus *-ous:* pertaining to	Moist tissue layer lining hollow organs and cavities of the body that open to the environment; also called *mucosa*
oxygen (O₂) ŎK-sĭ-jĕn	Tasteless, odorless, colorless gas essential for human respiration *O₂ makes up about one-fifth (by volume) of the earth's atmosphere.*
pH	Symbol that indicates the degree of acidity or alkalinity of a substance *Increasing acidity is expressed as a number less than 7; increasing alkalinity as a number greater than 7, with 7 being neutral.*
septum SĔP-tŭm	Wall dividing two cavities *The nasal septum separates the two nostrils.*
serous membrane SĒR-ŭs MĔM-brān *ser:* serum *-ous:* pertaining to	Thin layer of tissue that covers internal body cavities and secretes a fluid that keeps the membrane moist; also called *serosa*

Pronunciation Help	Long Sound	ā — rate	ē — rebirth	ī — isle	ō — over	ū — unite
	Short Sound	ă — alone	ĕ — ever	ĭ — it	ŏ — not	ŭ — cut

Upper Respiratory Tract

The breathing process begins with inhalation. (See Figure 7-1.) Air is drawn into the (1) **nasal cavity,** a chamber lined with mucous membranes and tiny hairs called cilia. Here, air is filtered, heated, and moistened to prepare it for its journey to the lungs. The nasal cavity is divided into a right and left side by a vertical partition of cartilage called the **nasal septum.**

Olfactory neurons are receptors for the sense of smell. They are covered with a layer of mucus and located deep in the nasal cavity, embedded among the epithelial cells lining the nasal tract. Because they are located higher in the nasal passage than air normally travels during breathing, a person must sniff or inhale deeply to identify weak odors. Air passes from the nasal cavity to the throat **(pharynx),** a muscular tube that serves as a passageway for food and air. The pharynx consists of three sections: the (2) **nasopharynx,** posterior to the nose; the (3) **oropharynx,** posterior to the mouth; and the (4) **laryngopharynx,** superior to the larynx.

Within the nasopharynx is a collection of lymphoid tissue known as (5) **adenoids** (pharyngeal tonsils). The (6) **palatine tonsils,** more commonly known as **tonsils,** are located in the oropharynx. They protect the opening to the respiratory tract from microscopic organisms that may attempt entry by this route. The (7) **larynx** (voice box) contains the structures that make vocal sounds possible. A leaf-shaped structure on top of the larynx, the (8) **epiglottis,** seals off the air passage to the lungs during swallowing. This function ensures that food or liquids do not obstruct the flow of air to the lungs. The larynx is a short passage that joins the pharynx with the (9) **trachea** (windpipe). The trachea is composed of smooth muscle embedded with C-shaped rings of cartilage, which provide rigidity to keep the air passage open.

Lower Respiratory Tract

The trachea divides into two branches called (10) **bronchi** (singular, **bronchus**). One branch leads to the (11) **right lung** and the other to the (12) **left lung.** The inner walls of the trachea and bronchi are composed of **mucous membrane (mucosa)** embedded with cilia. This membrane traps incoming particles, and the cilia move the entrapped material upward into the pharynx, where it is expelled by coughing, sneezing, or swallowing. Like the trachea, bronchi contain C-shaped rings of cartilage.

Each bronchus divides into smaller and smaller branches, eventually forming (13) **bronchioles.** At the end of the bronchioles are tiny air sacs called (14) **alveoli** (singular, **alveolus**). An alveolus resembles a small balloon because it expands and contracts with inflow and outflow of air. The (15) **pulmonary capillaries** lie next to the thin tissue membranes of the alveoli. Carbon dioxide diffuses from the blood within the pulmonary capillaries and enters the alveolar spaces, while O_2 from the alveoli diffuses into the blood. After the exchange of gases, freshly oxygenated blood returns to the heart. Oxygen is now ready for delivery to all body tissues.

The lungs are divided into lobes: three lobes in the right lung and two lobes in the left lung. The space between the right and left lungs is called the (16) **mediastinum.** It contains the heart, aorta, esophagus, and bronchi. A serous membrane, the **pleura,** covers the lobes of the lungs and folds over to line the walls of the thoracic cavity. The membrane lying closest to the lung is the (17) **visceral pleura;** the membrane that lines the thoracic cavity is the (18) **parietal pleura.** The space between these two membranes is the (19) **pleural cavity.** It contains a small amount of lubricating fluid, which permits the visceral pleura to glide smoothly over the parietal pleura during breathing.

Ventilation depends on a pressure differential between the atmosphere and chest cavity. A large muscular partition, the (20) **diaphragm,** lies between the chest and abdominal cavities. The diaphragm assists in changing the volume of the thoracic cavity to produce the needed pressure differential for ventilation. When the diaphragm contracts, it partially descends into the abdominal cavity, thus decreasing the pressure within the chest and drawing air into the lungs **(inspiration).** When the diaphragm relaxes, it slowly reenters the thoracic cavity, thus increasing the

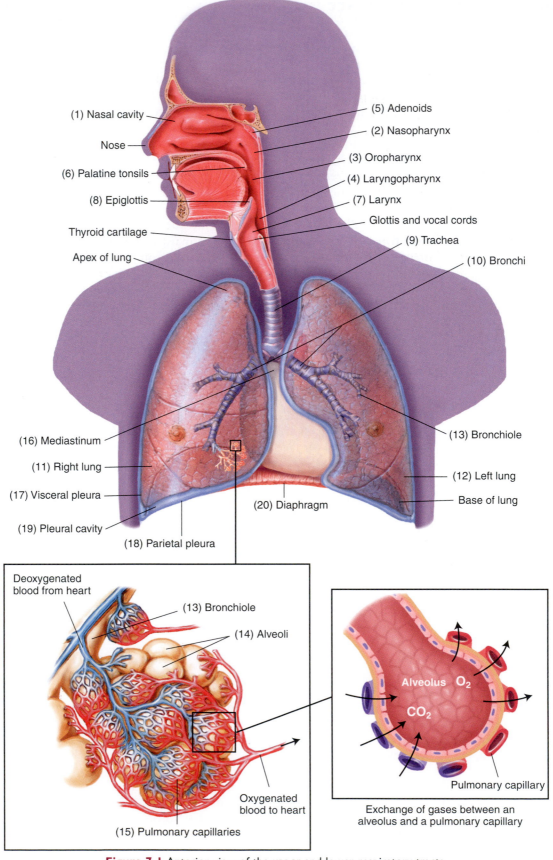

(1) Nasal cavity

(5) Adenoids

(2) Nasopharynx

Nose

(3) Oropharynx

(6) Palatine tonsils

(4) Laryngopharynx

(8) Epiglottis

(7) Larynx

Glottis and vocal cords

Thyroid cartilage

(9) Trachea

Apex of lung

(10) Bronchi

(16) Mediastinum

(13) Bronchiole

(11) Right lung

(12) Left lung

(17) Visceral pleura

Base of lung

(19) Pleural cavity

(20) Diaphragm

(18) Parietal pleura

Deoxygenated blood from heart

(13) Bronchiole

(14) Alveoli

Oxygenated blood to heart

(15) Pulmonary capillaries

Alveolus O$_2$

CO$_2$

Pulmonary capillary

Exchange of gases between an alveolus and a pulmonary capillary

Figure 7-1 Anterior view of the upper and lower respiratory tracts.

pressure within the chest. As pressure increases, air leaves the lungs **(expiration).** The intercostal muscles assist the diaphragm in changing the volume of the thoracic cavity by elevating and lowering the rib cage. (See Figure 7-2.)

Respiration

Respiration is the process by which O_2 is taken from air and carried to body cells for their use, while CO_2 and water, the waste products generated by these cells, are returned to the environment. Respiration includes four separate processes:

- **pulmonary ventilation,** more commonly called **breathing**, is a largely involuntary action that moves air into (inspiration) and out of (expiration) the lungs in response to changes in blood O_2 and CO_2 levels and nervous stimulation of the diaphragm and intercostal muscles
- **external respiration,** which is the exchange of O_2 and CO_2 between the alveoli and the blood in the pulmonary capillaries
- **transport of respiratory gases,** which occurs when blood, aided by the cardiovascular system, transports CO_2 to the lungs and O_2 to body cells
- **internal respiration,** which is the exchange of O_2 and CO_2 between body cells and the blood in systemic capillaries.

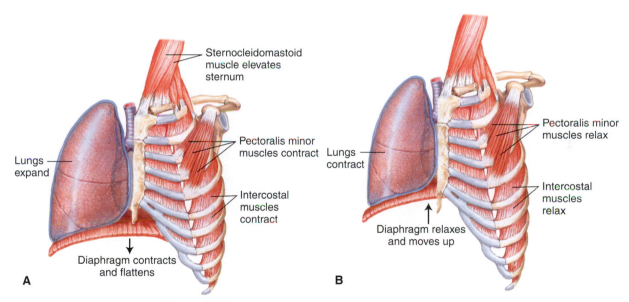

Figure 7-2 Breathing muscles. **(A)** Inspiration. **(B)** Expiration.

Anatomy Review

To review the anatomy of the respiratory system, label the illustration using the terms listed below.

adenoids	epiglottis	nasal cavity	pleural cavity
alveoli	laryngopharynx	nasopharynx	pulmonary capillaries
bronchi	larynx	oropharynx	right lung
bronchiole	left lung	palatine tonsils	trachea
diaphragm	mediastinum	parietal pleura	visceral pleura

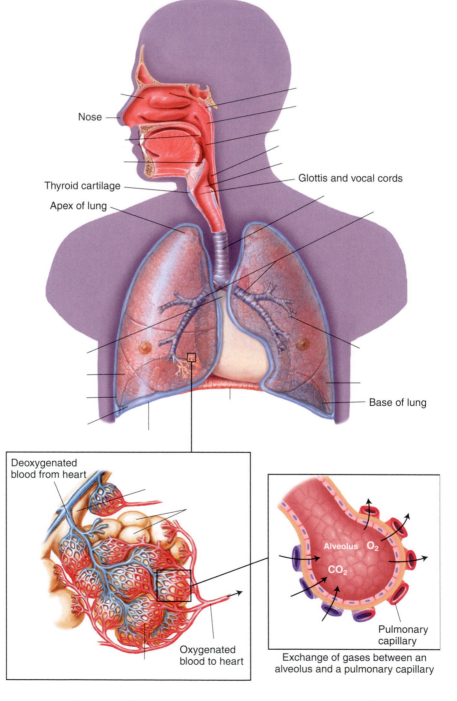

Nose

Thyroid cartilage

Apex of lung

Glottis and vocal cords

Base of lung

Deoxygenated blood from heart

Oxygenated blood to heart

Alveolus   O$_2$

CO$_2$

Pulmonary capillary

Exchange of gases between an alveolus and a pulmonary capillary

 Check your answers by referring to Figure 7-1 on page 168. Review material that you did not answer correctly.

CONNECTING BODY SYSTEMS—RESPIRATORY SYSTEM

The main function of the respiratory system is to provide oxygen to the entire body and expel carbon dioxide from the body. Specific functional relationships between the respiratory system and other body systems are summarized below.

Blood, Lymph, and Immune
- Tonsils, adenoids, and other immune structures in the respiratory tract protect against pathogens that enter through respiratory passageways.

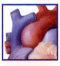
Cardiovascular
- Respiratory system provides O_2 and removes CO_2 from cardiac tissue.

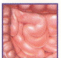
Digestive
- Respiratory system provides O_2 needed for digestive functions.
- Respiratory system removes CO_2 produced by the organs of digestion.
- Respiratory and digestive systems share the trachea, an anatomic structure of digestion.

Endocrine
- Respiratory system helps maintain a stable pH required for proper functioning of the endocrine glands.

Female Reproductive
- Respiratory rate increases in response to sexual activity.
- Fetal respiration occurs during pregnancy.

Integumentary
- Respiratory system furnishes O_2 and disposes of CO_2 to maintain healthy skin.

Male Reproductive
- Respiratory rate increases in response to sexual activity.
- Respiratory system helps maintain pH for gonadal hormone function.
- Oxygen is supplied to reproductive structures to maintain viable sperm.

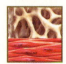
Musculoskeletal
- Respiratory system provides O_2 for muscle contraction.
- Respiratory system eliminates CO_2 produced by muscles.
- Respiratory system provides O_2 for bone development.

Nervous
- Respiratory system provides O_2 for brain, spinal cord, and sensory organ functions.
- Respiratory system helps maintain a stable pH for neural function.

Urinary
- Respiratory system supplies O_2 and removes CO_2 to maintain proper functioning of urinary structures.
- Respiratory system assists the urinary structures in regulating pH by removing CO_2.

Medical Word Elements

This section introduces combining forms, suffixes, and prefixes related to the respiratory system. Word analyses are also provided.

Element	Meaning	Word Analysis
Combining Forms		
Upper Respiratory Tract		
nas/o	nose	**nas/**al (NĀ-zl): pertaining to the nose *-al:* pertaining to
rhin/o		**rhin/**o/plasty (RĪ-nō-plăs-tē): surgical repair of the nose *-plasty:* surgical repair *Rhinoplasty is performed to correct birth defects or for cosmetic purposes.*
sept/o	septum	**sept/o/**plasty (SĔP-tō-plăs-tē): surgical repair of the septum *-plasty:* surgical repair *Septoplasty is commonly performed to correct a deviated septum.*
sinus/o	sinus, cavity	**sinus/o/**tomy (sī-nŭs-ŎT-ō-mē): incision of any of the sinuses *-tomy:* incision *Sinusotomy is performed to improve ventilation or drainage in unresponsive sinusitis.*
adenoid/o	adenoids	**adenoid/**ectomy (ăd-ě-noyd-ĔK-tō-mē): excision of adenoids *-ectomy:* excision, removal

tonsill/o	tonsils	peri/**tonsill/**ar (pěr-ĭ-TŎN-sĭ-lăr): pertaining to (the area) around the tonsils
		  peri-: around
		  -ar: pertaining to

pharyng/o	pharynx (throat)	**pharyng/o/**scope (făr-ĬN-gō-skōp): instrument for examining the pharynx *-scope:* instrument for examining
epiglott/o	epiglottis	**epiglott/**itis (ĕp-ĭ-glŏt-Ī-tĭs): inflammation of the epiglottis *-itis:* inflammation *Because the epiglottis seals the opening to the lungs, inflammation can lead to severe airway obstruction and death. Epiglottitis is treated as a medical emergency.*
laryng/o	larynx (voice box)	**laryng/o/**plegia (lă-rĭn-gō-PLĒ-jē-ă): paralysis of the (vocal cords and) larynx *-plegia:* paralysis
trache/o	trachea (windpipe)	**trache/o/**plasty (TRĀ-kē-ō-plăs-tē): surgical repair of the trachea *-plasty:* surgical repair *Tracheoplasty is performed to correct a narrow or stenotic trachea.*

Element	Meaning	Word Analysis
Lower Respiratory Tract		
bronchi/o	bronchus (plural, bronchi)	**bronchi**/ectasis (brŏng-kē-ĔK-tă-sĭs): dilation of the bronchi *-ectasis:* dilation, expansion *Bronchiectasis is associated with various lung conditions and is commonly accompanied by chronic infection.*
bronch/o		**bronch/o**/scope (BRŎNG-kō-skōp): instrument for examining the bronchus or bronchi *-scope:* instrument for examining *A bronchoscope is a flexible tube that is passed through the nose or mouth to enable inspection of the lungs and collection of tissue biopsies and secretions for analysis.*
bronchiol/o	bronchiole	**bronchiol**/itis (brŏng-kē-ō-LĪ-tĭs): inflammation of the bronchioles *-itis:* inflammation
alveol/o	alveolus; air sac	**alveol**/ar (ăl-VĒ-ō-lăr): pertaining to the alveoli *-ar:* pertaining to
pleur/o	pleura	**pleur/o**/centesis (ploo-rō-sĕn-TĒ-sĭs): surgical puncture of the pleural cavity; also called *thoracocentesis* or *thoracentesis* *-centesis:* surgical puncture
pneum/o	air; lung	**pneum**/ectomy (nūm-ĔK-tō-mē): excision of (all or part of) a lung *-ectomy:* excision
pneumon/o		**pneumon**/ia (nū-MŌ-nē-ă): condition of the lungs *-ia:* condition *The usual causes of pneumonia are infections due to bacteria, viruses, or other pathogenic organisms.*
pulmon/o	lung	**pulmon/o**/logist (pŭl-mŏ-NŎL-ŏ-jĭst): specialist in the study (and treatment) of lungs (and respiratory diseases) *-logist:* specialist in the study of
Other		
anthrac/o	coal, coal dust	**anthrac**/osis (ăn-thră-KŌ-sĭs): abnormal condition of coal dust (in the lungs); also called *black lung disease* *-osis:* abnormal condition; increase (used primarily with blood cells) *Anthracosis is a chronic occupational disease found in coal miners and those associated with the coal industry.*
atel/o	incomplete; imperfect	**atel**/ectasis (ăt-ĕ-LĔK-tă-sĭs): incomplete expansion of the lung; also called *airless lung* or *collapsed lung* *-ectasis:* dilation, expansion

(continued)

Element	Meaning	Word Analysis
coni/o	dust	pneum/o/**coni**/osis (nū-mō-kō-nē-Ō-sĭs): condition of dust in the lungs *pneum/o:* air; lung *-osis:* abnormal condition; increase (used primarily with blood cells) *Pneumoconiosis is usually caused by mineral dusts of occupational or environmental origin. Forms of pneumoconiosis include silicosis, asbestosis, and anthracosis.*
cyan/o	blue	**cyan**/osis (sī-ă-NŌ-sĭs): abnormal condition of blueness *-osis:* abnormal condition; increase (used primarily with blood cells) *Cold temperatures, heart failure, lung diseases, and smothering cause unusual blueness of the skin and mucous membranes due to the build-up of carbon dioxide in the blood.*
lob/o	lobe	**lob**/ectomy (lō-BĔK-tō-mē): excision of a lobe *-ectomy:* excision *Lobectomies are performed when a malignancy is confined to a single lobe of any lobed organ, such as the lungs, liver, and thyroid gland.*
orth/o	straight	**orth/o**/pnea (or-THŎP-nē-ă): breathing in a straight (or upright position) *-pnea:* breathing *Various lung disorders cause a patient to experience difficulty breathing in any position other than sitting or standing.*
ox/i	oxygen (O_2)	**ox/i**/meter (ŏk-SĬM-ě-těr): instrument used for measuring O_2 *-meter:* instrument for measuring *An oximeter is usually attached to the tip of a finger but may also be placed on a toe or ear lobe. It provides a measurement of O_2 saturation level of the blood.*
ox/o		hyp/**ox**/emia (hī-pŏks-Ē-mē-ă): deficiency of O_2 in blood *hyp-:* under, below, deficient *-emia:* blood condition
pector/o	chest	**pector**/algia (pĕk-tō-RĂL-jē-ă): pain in the chest; also called *thoracalgia* or *thoracodynia,* *-algia:* pain
steth/o		**steth/o**/scope (STĔTH-ō-skōp): instrument used for examining the chest *-scope:* instrument for examining *A stethoscope enables evaluation of sounds in the chest as well as the abdomen.*
thorac/o		**thorac/o**/pathy (thō-răk-ŎP-ă-thē): disease of the chest *-pathy:* disease
phren/o	diaphragm; mind	**phren/o**/spasm (FRĔN-ō-spăzm): involuntary contraction of the diaphragm *-spasm:* involuntary contraction, twitching
spir/o	breathe	**spir/o**/meter (spī-RŎM-ět-ěr): instrument for measuring breathing *-meter:* instrument for measuring *A spirometer measures how much air the lungs can hold (vital capacity) as well as how much and how quickly air can be exhaled.*

Element	Meaning	Word Analysis
Suffixes		
-capnia	carbon dioxide (CO_2)	hyper/**capnia** (hī-pĕr-KĂP-nē-ă): excessive CO_2 *hyper-:* excessive, above normal
-osmia	smell	an/**osmia** (ăn-ŎZ-mē-ă): without (the sense of) smell *an-:* without, not
-phonia	voice	dys/**phonia** (dĭs-FŌ-nē-ă): bad (impaired) voice (quality) *dys-:* bad; painful; difficult *Dysphonia includes hoarseness, voice fatigue, or decreased projection.*
-pnea	breathing	a/**pnea** (ăp-NĒ-ă): not breathing *a-:* without, not *Apnea is a temporary loss of breathing and includes sleep apnea, cardiac apnea, and apnea of the newborn.*
-ptysis	spitting	hem/o/**ptysis** (hē-MŎP-tĭ-sĭs): (coughing up or) spitting of blood *hem/o:* blood *Bloody sputum is usually a sign of a serious condition of the lungs.*
-thorax	chest	py/o/**thorax** (pī-ō-THŌ-răks): pus in the chest (cavity); also called *empyema* *py/o:* pus *Pyothorax is usually caused by a penetrating chest wound or spreading of infection from another part of the body.*
Prefixes		
brady-	slow	**brady**/pnea (brăd-ĭp-NĒ-ă): slow breathing *-pnea:* breathing
dys-	bad; painful; difficult	**dys**/pnea (dĭsp-NĒ-ă): difficult breathing *-pnea:* breathing *Dyspnea includes any discomfort or significant breathlessness.*
eu-	good, normal	**eu**/pnea (ūp-NĒ-ă): normal breathing *-pnea:* breathing *The normal range for a resting adult respiratory rate is 12 to 20 breaths/minute.*
tachy-	rapid	**tachy**/pnea (tăk-ĭp-NĒ- ă): rapid breathing *-pnea:* breathing

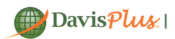

Visit the *Medical Terminology Systems* online resource center at Davis*Plus* for an audio exercise of the terms in this table. Other activities are also available to reinforce content.

It is time to review medical word elements by completing Learning Activities 7–1 and 7–2.

Pathology

Common signs and symptoms of many respiratory disorders include cough (dry or productive), chest pain, altered breathing patterns, shortness of breath (SOB), cyanosis, fever, and exercise intolerance. Many disorders of the respiratory system, including bronchitis and emphysema, begin as an acute problem but become chronic over time. Chronic respiratory diseases are usually difficult to treat. Their damaging effects are commonly irreversible.

For diagnosis, treatment, and management of respiratory disorders, the medical services of a specialist may be warranted. **Pulmonology** is the medical specialty concerned with disorders of the respiratory system. The physician who treats these disorders is called a **pulmonologist.**

Chronic Obstructive Pulmonary Disease

Chronic obstructive pulmonary disease (COPD) includes respiratory disorders that produce a chronic partial obstruction of the air passages. Because of its chronic nature, the disease usually progresses to limited airflow into and out of the lungs with increased shortness of breath (SOB) and difficulty breathing (dyspnea). COPD is insidious and is commonly first diagnosed after some lung capacity has already been lost. It is possible to have early stages of COPD without knowing it. (See Table 7-1.) The three major disorders of COPD included asthma, chronic bronchitis, and emphysema. (See Figure 7-3.)

Asthma

Asthma produces spasms in the bronchial passages **(bronchospasms)** that may be sudden and violent **(paroxysmal)** and lead to dyspnea. Asthma is commonly caused by exposure to allergens or irritants. Other causes include stress, cold, and exercise. During recovery, coughing episodes produce large amounts of mucus **(productive cough).** Over time, the epithelium of the bronchial passages thickens, breathing becomes more difficult, and flare-ups **(exacerbations)** occur more frequently. Treatment includes agents that loosen and break down mucus **(mucolytics)** and medications that expand the bronchi **(bronchodilators)** by relaxing their smooth muscles. Most cases of asthma can be treated effectively. However, when treatment does not reverse bronchospasm, a life-threatening condition called **status asthmaticus** can occur, requiring hospitalization.

Table 7-1	**Stages of COPD**	
The table below lists the levels of severity of COPD and describes their characteristics.		
Severity Level	**Description**	
At risk, mild	• Minor difficulty with airflow	
	• Possible presence of chronic cough with sputum production	
	• Patient possibly unaware of disease	
Moderate	• Apparent limitation in airflow	
	• Possible shortness of breath	
	• Patient possibly seeking medical intervention at this level	
Severe	• Inadequate airflow	
	• Increase in shortness of breath with activity	
	• Patient experiencing diminished quality of life	
Very severe	• Severe airflow limitations	
	• Significant impairment in quality of life	
	• Possible life-threatening exacerbations	
	• Possible development of complications, such as respiratory or heart failure	

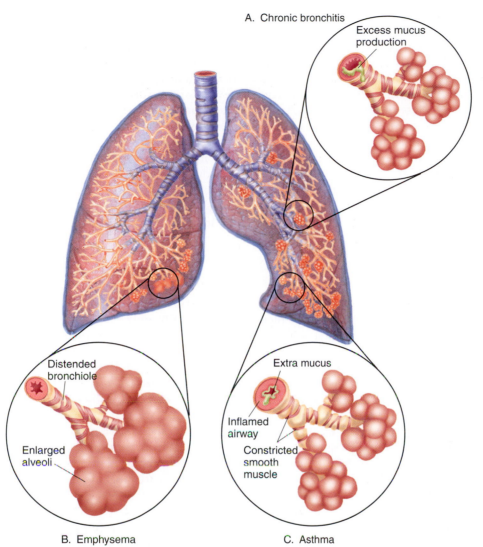

Figure 7-3 COPD. **(A)** Chronic bronchitis with inflamed airways and excessive mucus. **(B)** Emphysema with distended bronchioles and alveoli. **(C)** Asthma with narrowed bronchial tubes and swollen mucous membranes.

Chronic Bronchitis

Chronic bronchitis is an inflammation of the bronchi caused mainly by smoking and air pollution. However, other agents, such as viruses and bacteria, may also cause the disorder. Bronchitis is characterized by swelling of the mucosa and a heavy, productive cough that is commonly accompanied by chest pain. Patients usually seek medical help when they suffer exercise intolerance, wheezing, and shortness of breath (SOB). Bronchodilators and medications that aid in the removal of mucus **(expectorants)** help widen air passages. Steroids may be prescribed if the disease progresses or becomes chronic.

Emphysema

Emphysema is characterized by decreased elasticity of the alveoli. The alveoli expand (dilate) but are unable to contract to their original size. The air that remains trapped in the chest results in a characteristic "barrel-chested" appearance. This disease commonly occurs with another respiratory disorder, such as asthma, tuberculosis, or chronic bronchitis. It is also found in long-term heavy smokers. Most emphysema sufferers find it easier to breathe when sitting upright or standing erect **(orthopnea).** As the disease progresses, relief—even in the orthopneic position—is not possible. Treatment for emphysema is similar to that of chronic bronchitis.

Influenza

Influenza (flu) is an acute infectious respiratory viral disease. Three major viral types are of concern: type A, type B, and type C. Type A is of primary concern because it is associated with worldwide epidemics **(pandemics)** and its causative organism is highly infectious **(virulent).** Influenza type A epidemics occur about every 2 to 3 years. Type B is usually limited geographically and tends to be less severe than type A. Both viruses undergo antigenic changes; consequently, new vaccines must be developed in anticipation of outbreaks. Type C is a mild flu and is not associated with epidemics.

The onset of the flu is usually rapid. Symptoms include fever, chills, headache, generalized muscle pain **(myalgia),** and loss of appetite, but recovery occurs in about 7 to 10 days. The flu virus rarely causes death. If death occurs, it is usually the result of a secondary pneumonia caused by bacteria or viruses that invade the lungs. Children should not use aspirin for relief of symptoms caused by viruses because there appears to be a relationship between Reye syndrome and the use of aspirin by children ages 2 to 15.

Pleural Effusions

Any abnormal fluid in the pleural cavity, the space between the visceral and parietal pleura, is called a **pleural effusion.** Normally, the pleural cavity contains only a small amount of lubricating fluid. However, some disorders may cause excessive fluid to collect in the pleural cavity. Two initial techniques used to diagnose pleural effusion are auscultation and percussion. **Auscultation** is listening to sounds made by organs of the body using a stethoscope. **Percussion** is gentle tapping on the chest with the fingers and listening to the resultant sounds to determine the position, size, or consistency of the underlying structures. Chest x-ray (CXR) or magnetic resonance imaging (MRI) tends to confirm the diagnosis.

Effusions are classified as transudates and exudates. A **transudate** is a noninflammatory fluid that resembles serum but with slightly less protein. It results from an imbalance in venous-arterial pressure or a decrease of protein in blood. Both of these conditions allow serum to leak from the vascular system and collect in the pleural space. Common causes include heart failure and liver disorders. An **exudate** is usually high in protein and commonly contains blood and immune cells. Common causes include tumors, infections, and inflammation.

Various types of pleural effusions include serum **(hydrothorax),** pus **(empyema** or **pyothorax),** and blood **(hemothorax).** Although not considered a pleural effusion, air can enter the pleural space **(pneumothorax),** resulting in a partial or complete collapse of a lung. (See Figure 7-4.)

Treatment consists of correcting the underlying cause of the effusion. It commonly includes surgical puncture of the chest using a hollow-bore needle **(thoracocentesis, thoracentesis)** to remove excess fluid for diagnostic or therapeutic purposes. (See Figure 7-5.) Sometimes a physician will insert chest tubes to drain fluid or remove air in pneumothorax.

Tuberculosis

Tuberculosis (TB) is a communicable disease caused by the bacterium *Mycobacterium tuberculosis.* TB spreads by droplets of respiratory secretions **(droplet nuclei)** from an infected individual when he coughs, laughs, or sneezes. The waxy coat of the TB organism keeps it alive **(viable)** and infectious for 6 to 8 months outside the body. The waxy coat of this bacterium resists staining in the laboratory, but once stained it is difficult to remove even when an acid rinse is employed. Hence, TB is also known as the **acid-fast bacillus** (AFB).

Not everyone infected with TB bacteria becomes ill. As a result, two TB-related conditions exist: latent TB infection and active TB disease. With latent TB infection, the first time the TB organism enters the body **(primary tuberculosis)** the disease develops slowly. It eventually produces typical inflammatory nodules **(granulomas)** called **tubercles,** which encase the organism. These granulomas usually remain dormant for years and the patient is asymptomatic. The only evidence of the latent infection is a positive skin test for TB. In the dormant stage, the patient cannot transmit the disease to others.

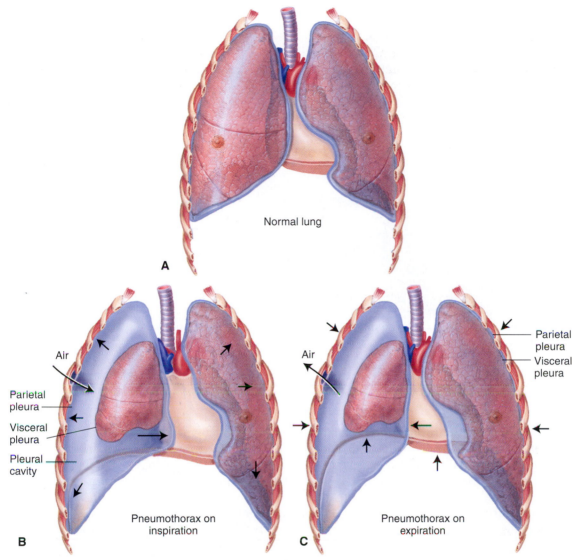

Figure 7-4 Pneumothorax. **(A)** Normal. **(B)** Open pneumothorax during inspiration. **(C)** Open pneumothorax during expiration.

When the immune system becomes impaired (**immunocompromised**) or when the patient is re-exposed to the bacterium, the active disease may develop and the patient becomes infectious to others. Sign and symptoms include hemoptysis, weakness, chills, fever, loss of appetite, and night sweats.

Although primarily a lung disease, TB can infect the bones, genital tract, meninges, and peritoneum. Some TB strains that infect AIDS patients have become resistant and do not respond to standard medications. Treatment may include using several antibiotics (**combination therapy**) at the same time.

Pneumonia

Pneumonia is any inflammatory disease of the lungs. It may be caused by bacteria, viruses, fungi, chemicals, or other agents that cause lung inflammation. In addition, some unrelated diseases cause various forms of pneumonia. For example, one type of pneumonia is associated with influenza and may be fatal. Other potentially fatal pneumonias may result from food or liquid inhalation (**aspiration pneumonias**). Some pneumonias affect only one lobe of the lung (**lobar pneumonia**), but

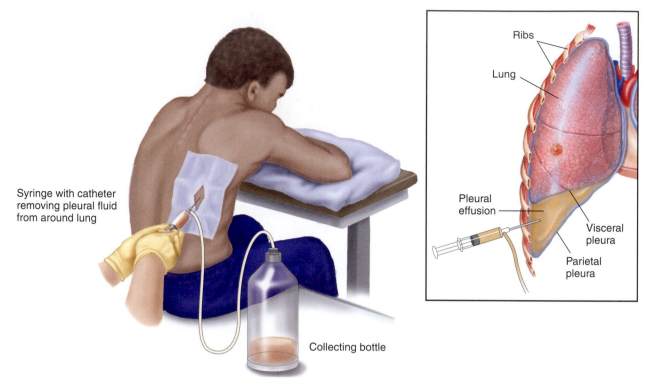

Syringe with catheter removing pleural fluid from around lung

Collecting bottle

Ribs

Lung

Pleural effusion

Visceral pleura

Parietal pleura

Figure 7-5 Thoracentesis.

some are more diffuse **(bronchopneumonia).** Chest pain, mucopurulent sputum, and spitting of blood **(hemoptysis)** are common signs and symptoms of the disease. If the air in the lungs is replaced by fluid and inflammatory debris, the lung tissue looses its spongy texture and becomes swollen and engorged **(consolidation).** Consolidation is primarily associated with bacterial pneumonias, not viral pneumonias.

Pneumocystis **pneumonia** (PCP) is a type of pneumonia closely associated with AIDS. Recent evidence suggests that it is caused by organisms that reside in or on most people **(normal flora)** but causes no harm as long as the individual remains healthy. When the immune system begins to fail, this organism becomes infectious **(opportunistic).** Diagnosis relies on examination of biopsied lung tissue or bronchial washings **(lavage).**

Cystic Fibrosis

Cystic fibrosis is a hereditary disorder of the exocrine glands that causes the body to secrete extremely thick **(viscous)** mucus. This thickened mucus clogs ducts of the pancreas and digestive tract. As a result, digestion is impaired and the patient may suffer from malnutrition. It also blocks ducts of the sweat glands, causing the skin to become highly "salty." In the lungs, mucus blocks airways and impedes natural disease-fighting mechanisms, causing repeated infections. Medications in the form of mists **(aerosols)** along with postural drainage provide relief.

An important diagnostic test called the **sweat test** measures the amount of salt excreted in sweat. When elevated, it indicates cystic fibrosis. Although the disease is fatal, improved methods of treatment have extended life expectancy, and patient survival is approximately 30 years.

Acute Respiratory Distress Syndrome

Acute respiratory distress syndrome (ARDS) is a condition in which the lungs no longer function effectively, threatening the life of the patient. It usually occurs as a result of very serious lung conditions, such as trauma, severe pneumonia, and other major infections that affect the entire body **(systemic infections)** or blood **(sepsis).** In ARDS, the alveoli fill with fluid **(edema)** caused by inflammation and then collapse, making oxygen exchange impossible. Mechanical ventilation is commonly required to save the life of the patient.

Hyaline membrane disease (HMD), also called **infant respiratory distress syndrome (IRDS),** is a form of respiratory distress syndrome. It is most commonly seen in preterm infants or infants born to diabetic mothers. It is caused by insufficient **surfactant,** a phospholipid substance that helps keep alveoli open. With insufficient surfactant, the alveoli collapse and breathing becomes labored. Clinical signs may include blueness **(cyanosis)** of the extremities. Flaring of the nostrils **(nares)** and central cyanosis are typically present. Other signs include rapid breathing **(tachypnea),** intercostal retraction, and a characteristic grunt audible during exhalation. Radiography shows a membrane that has a ground-glass appearance **(hyaline membrane),** bilateral decrease in volume, and alveolar consolidation. Although severe cases of HMD result in death, some forms of therapy are effective.

Oncology

Lung cancer, also called **bronchogenic carcinoma,** is a malignancy that arises from the epithelium of the bronchial tree. As masses form, they block air passages and alveoli. Within a short time they spread **(metastasize)** to other areas of the body usually lymph nodes, liver, bones, brain, and kidneys. Cigarette smoking causes most lung cancers. High levels of pollution, radiation and asbestos exposure may also increase risk.

Very few lung cancers are found in the early stages when the cure rate is high. Treatment of lung cancers include surgery, radiation, chemotherapy, or a combination of these methods depending on the type and stage of the tumor, and the general health of the patient. The prognosis for patients with cancer (CA) is generally poor.

Diseases and Conditions

This section introduces diseases and conditions of the respiratory system with their meanings and pronunciation. Word analyses for selected terms are also provided.

Term	Definition
acidosis ăs-ĭ-DŌ-sĭs *acid:* acid *-osis:* abnormal condition; increase (used primarily with blood cells)	Excessive acidity of body fluids *Respiratory acidosis is commonly associated with pulmonary insufficiency and the subsequent retention of carbon dioxide.*
anosmia ăn-ŎZ-mē-ă *an-:* without, not *-osmia:* smell	Absence of the sense of smell *Anosmia usually occurs as a temporary condition resulting from an upper respiratory infection or a condition that causes intranasal swelling.*

(continued)

Term	Definition
apnea ăp-NĒ-ă *a-:* without, not *-pnea:* breathing	Temporary loss of breathing *There are three types of apnea: obstructive (enlarged tonsils and adenoids), central (failure of the brain to transmit impulses for breathing), and mixed (combination of obstructive and central apnea).*
sleep	Sleeping disorder in which breathing stops repeatedly for more than 10 seconds, causing measurable blood deoxygenation (See Figure 7-6.) Enlarged tonsil causing obstructive sleep apnea — Uvula — Epiglottis — Trachea **A** Nasal mask (pillows) — Positive pressure provided by a fan **B** **Figure 7-6** Sleep apnea. **(A)** Airway obstruction caused by enlarged tonsils, which eventually leads to obstructive sleep apnea. **(B)** Continuous positive airway pressure (CPAP) machine used to treat sleep apnea.
asphyxia ăs-FĬK-sē-ă *a-:* without, not *-sphyxia:* pulse	Condition caused by insufficient intake of oxygen *Some common causes of asphyxia are drowning, electric shock, lodging of a foreign body in the respiratory tract, inhalation of toxic smoke, and poisoning.*
atelectasis ăt-ĕ-LĔK-tă-sĭs *atel:* incomplete; imperfect *-ectasis:* dilation, expansion	Collapsed or airless state of the lung, which may be acute or chronic and affects all or part of a lung *Atelectasis is a potential complication of some surgical procedures, especially those of the chest, because breathing is commonly shallow after surgery to avoid pain from the surgical incision. In fetal atelectasis, the lungs fail to expand normally at birth.*
Cheyne-Stokes respiration chān-STŌKS	Repeated breathing pattern characterized by fluctuation in the depth of respiration: first deeply, then shallow, then not at all *Cheyne-Stokes respirations are usually caused by diseases that affect the respiratory centers of the brain (such as heart failure and brain damage).*

Term	Definition
coryza kŏ-RĪ-ză	Acute inflammation of the membranes of the nose; also called *head cold* or *upper respiratory infection* (URI)
crackle KRĂK-ĕl	Abnormal respiratory sound heard on auscultation, caused by exudates, spasms, hyperplasia, or when air enters moisture-filled alveoli; also called *rale*
croup CROOP	Common childhood condition involving inflammation of the larynx, trachea, bronchial passages and, sometimes, lungs *Signs and symptoms of croup include a resonant, barking cough with suffocative, difficult breathing; laryngeal spasms; and, sometimes, the narrowing of the top of the air passages.*
deviated nasal septum DĒ-vē-āt-ĕd NĀ-zl SĔP-tŭm *nas:* nose *-al:* pertaining to	Displacement of cartilage dividing the nostrils that causes reduced airflow and, sometimes, nosebleed
epiglottitis ĕp-ĭ-glŏt-Ī-tĭs *epiglott:* epiglottis *-itis:* inflammation	Severe, life-threatening infection of the epiglottis and supraglottic structures that occurs most commonly in children between 2 and 12 years of age *Signs and symptoms of epiglottitis include fever, dysphagia, inspiratory stridor, and severe respiratory distress. Intubation or tracheostomy may be required to open the obstructed airway.*
epistaxis ĕp-ĭ-STĂK-sĭs	Nasal hemorrhage; also called *nosebleed*
finger clubbing KLŬB-ĭng	Enlargement of the terminal phalanges of the fingers and toes commonly associated with pulmonary disease
hypoxemia hī-pŏks-Ē-mē-ă *hyp-:* under, below, deficient *ox:* oxygen *-emia:* blood condition	Oxygen deficiency in arterial blood; usually a sign of respiratory impairment
hypoxia hī-PŎKS-ē-ă *hyp-:* under, below, deficient *-oxia:* oxygen	Oxygen deficiency in body tissues; usually a sign of respiratory impairment
pertussis pĕr-TŬS-ĭs	Acute, infectious disease characterized by a cough that has a "whoop" sound; also called *whooping cough* *Immunization of infants as part of the diphtheria-pertussis-tetanus (DPT) vaccination is effective in preventing pertussis.*
pleurisy PLOO-rĭs-ē *pleur:* pleura *-isy:* state of; condition	Inflammation of the pleural membrane characterized by a stabbing pain that is intensified by coughing or deep breathing; also called *pleuritis*

(continued)

Term	Definition
pneumoconiosis nū-mō-kō-nē-Ō-sĭs *pneum/o:* air; lung *coni:* dust *-osis:* abnormal condition; increase (used primarily with blood cells)	Disease caused by inhaling dust particles, including coal dust (anthracosis), stone dust (chalicosis), iron dust (siderosis), and asbestos particles (asbestosis)
pulmonary edema PŬL-mō-nĕ-rē ĕ-DĒ-mă *pulmon:* lung *-ary:* pertaining to	Accumulation of extravascular fluid in lung tissues and alveoli, most commonly caused by heart failure *Excessive fluid in the lungs induces coughing and dyspnea.*
pulmonary embolism PŬL-mō-nĕ-rē ĔM-bō-lĭzm *pulmon:* lung *-ary:* pertaining to *embol:* plug *-ism:* condition	Blockage in an artery of the lungs caused by a mass of undissolved matter (such as a blood clot, tissue, air bubbles, and bacteria) (See Figure 7-7.)

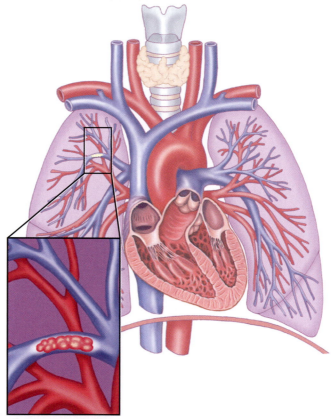

Pulmonary embolism

Figure 7-7 Pulmonary embolism. From Williams and Hopper: *Understanding Medical-Surgical Nursing,* 4th edition. FA Davis, Philadelphia, 2011, p 664, with permission.

Term	Definition
rhonchus RŎNG-kŭs	Abnormal breath sound heard on auscultation of an obstructed airway *A rhonchus is described as a course, rattling noise that resembles snoring, commonly suggesting secretions in the larger airways.*
stridor STRĪ-dor	High-pitched, harsh, adventitious breath sound caused by a spasm or swelling of the larynx or an obstruction in the upper airway *The presence of stridor requires immediate intervention.*
sudden infant death syndrome (SIDS)	Completely unexpected and unexplained death of an apparently normal, healthy infant, usually less than age 12 months; also called *crib death* *The rate of SIDS has decreased more than 30% since parents have been instructed to place babies on their backs for sleeping rather than on their stomachs.*
wheeze HWĔZ	Whistling or sighing sound heard on auscultation that results from narrowing of the lumen of the respiratory passageway *Wheezing is a sign of asthma, croup, hay fever, obstructive emphysema, and other obstructive respiratory conditions.*

It is time to review pathology, diseases, and conditions by completing Learning Activity 7-3.

Medical, Surgical, and Diagnostic Procedures

This section introduces medical, surgical and diagnostic procedures used to treat and diagnose respiratory disorders. Descriptions are provided as well as pronunciations and word analyses for selected terms.

Procedure	Description
Medical	
aerosol therapy ĂR-ō-sŏl THĔR-ă-pē	Lung treatment using various techniques to deliver medication in mist form directly to the lungs or air passageways *Techniques include nebulizers, metered-dose inhalers (MDIs), and dry powder inhalers (DPIs). Nebulizers change liquid medications into droplets to be inhaled through a mouthpiece. (See Figure 7-8.) MDIs deliver a specific amount when activated. Children and the elderly can use a spacer to synchronize inhalation with medication release. (See Figure 7-9.) A DPI is activated by a quick inhalation by the user.* **Figure 7-8** Nebulizer. **Figure 7-9** Metered-dose inhaler.
antral lavage ĂN-trăl lă-VĂZH	Washing or irrigating of the paranasal sinuses to remove mucopurulent material in an immunosuppressed patient or one with known sinusitis that has failed medical management

Procedure	Description
oximetry ŏk-SĬM-ĕ-trē *ox/i:* oxygen *-metry:* act of measuring	Noninvasive method of monitoring the percentage of hemoglobin (Hb) saturated with oxygen; also called *pulse oximetry* *In oximetry, a probe attached to the patient's finger or ear lobe links to a computer that displays the percentage of hemoglobin saturated with oxygen.*
polysomnography pŏl-ē-sŏm-NŎG-ră-fē *poly-:* many, much *somn/o:* sleep *-graphy:* process of recording	Test of sleep cycles and stages using continuous recordings of brain waves (EEGs), electrical activity of muscles, eye movement, respiratory rate, blood pressure, blood oxygen saturation, heart rhythm and, sometimes, direct observation of the person during sleep using a video camera (See Figure 7-10.) Face and scalp sensors measure eye movement and brain activity. Nose sensor measures air flow. Wires transmit data to a computer. Elastic belt sensors measure amount of effort to breathe. Finger sensor measures amount of oxygen in blood. **Figure 7-10** Polysomnography.
postural drainage PŎS-tū-răl	Method of positioning a patient so that gravity aids in the drainage of secretions from the bronchi and lobes of the lungs
pulmonary function tests (PFTs) PŬL-mō-nĕ-rē *pulmon:* lung *-ary:* pertaining to	Variety of tests used to evaluate respiratory function, the ability of the lungs to take in and expel air as well as perform gas exchange across the alveolocapillary membrane *Measurement of different portions of lung volume provides an indication of breathing impairments, as does measurement of the volume of air expelled during a rapid, vigorous exhalation.*

(continued)

Procedure	Description
spirometry spī-RŎM-ĕ-trē *spir/o:* breathe *-metry:* act of measuring	PFT that measures the breathing capacity of the lungs, including the time necessary for exhaling the total volume of inhaled air (See Figure 7-11.) *A spirometer produces a graphic record of spirometry results for placement in the patient's chart.* 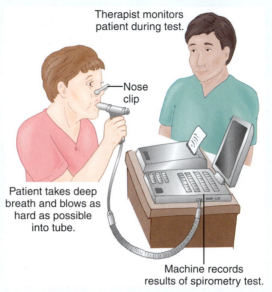 **Figure 7-11** Spirometry.

Surgical

Procedure	Description
endotracheal intubation ĕn-dŏ-TRĀ-kē-ăl ĭn-tū-BĀ-shŭn *endo-:* in, within *trache:* trachea *-al:* pertaining to	Procedure in which a plastic tube is inserted into the trachea to maintain an open airway *Endotracheal intubation is commonly performed before surgery when the patient is first placed under sedation or in emergency situations to facilitate ventilation if necessary. (See Figure 7-12.)* 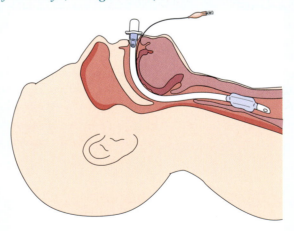 Placement of tube in airway **Figure 7-12** Endotracheal intubation. Williams and Hopper: *Understanding Medical-Surgical Nursing,* 4th edition. FA Davis, Philadelphia, 2011, p 617, with permission.

Procedure	Description
pleurectomy ploor-ĔK-tō-mē *pleur:* pleura *-ectomy:* excision, removal	Excision of part of the pleura, usually the parietal pleura *Pleurectomy is performed to reduce pain caused by a tumor mass or to prevent the recurrence of pleural effusion but is generally ineffective in the treatment of malignancy of the pleura.*
pneumectomy nūm-ĔK-tō-mē *pneum:* air; lung *-ectomy:* excision, removal	Excision of a lung or a portion of the lung, commonly for treatment of cancer (See Figure 7-13.)

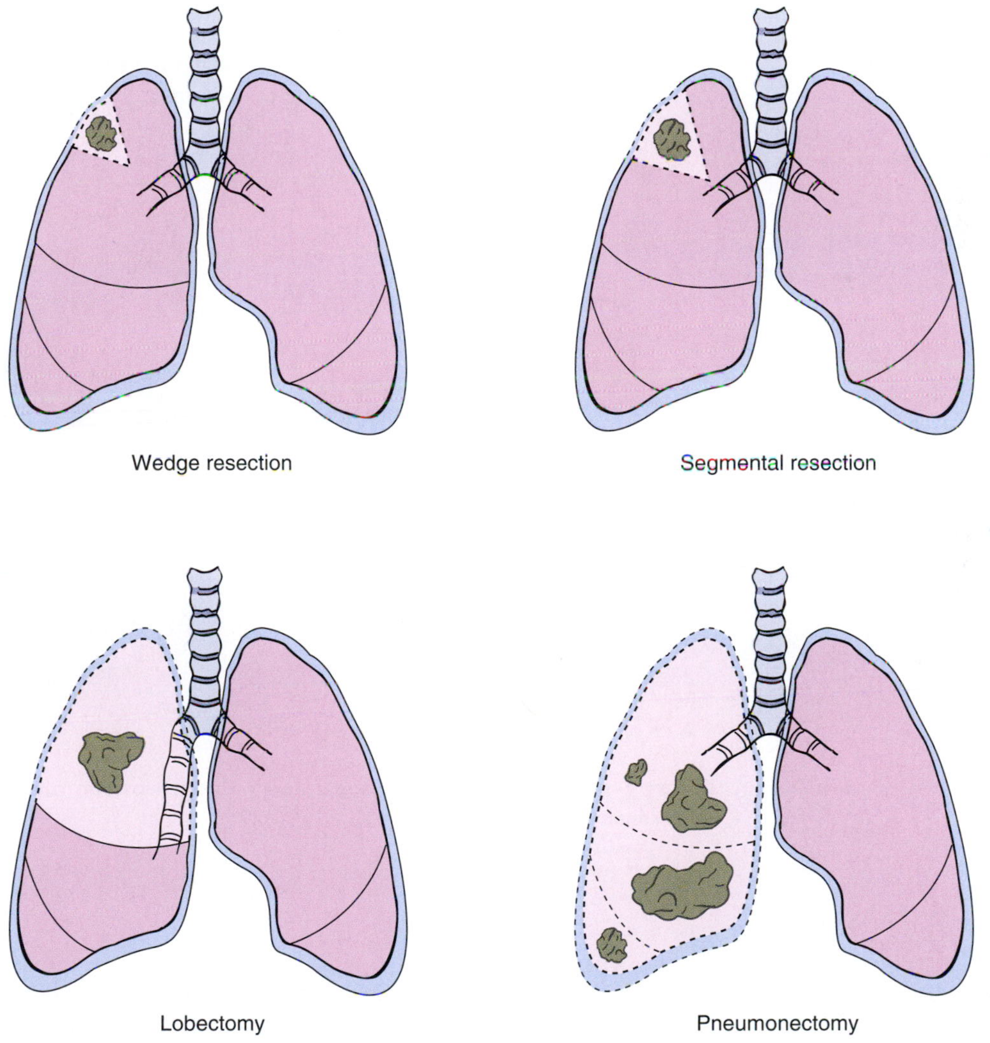

Wedge resection

Segmental resection

Lobectomy

Pneumonectomy

Figure 7-13 Types of pneumonectomies. Williams and Hopper: *Understanding Medical-Surgical Nursing,* 4th edition. FA Davis, Philadelphia, 2011, p 673, with permission.

(continued)

Procedure	Description
septoplasty sĕp-tō-PLĂS-tē *sept/o:* septum *–plasty:* surgical repair	Surgical repair of a deviated nasal septum usually performed when the septum is encroaching on the breathing passages or nasal structures *Common complications of a deviated septum include interference with breathing and a predisposition to sinus infections.*
thoracentesis thō-ră-sĕn-TĒ-sĭs	Surgical puncture and drainage of the pleural cavity; also called *pleurocentesis* or *thoracocentesis* *Thoracentesis as a diagnostic procedure helps determine the nature and cause of an effusion and, as a therapeutic procedure, relieves the discomfort caused by the effusion.*
tracheostomy trā-kē-ŎS-tō-mē *trache/o:* trachea *–stomy:* forming an opening (mouth)	Surgical procedure in which an opening is made in the neck and into the trachea into which a breathing tube may be inserted (See Figure 7-14.)

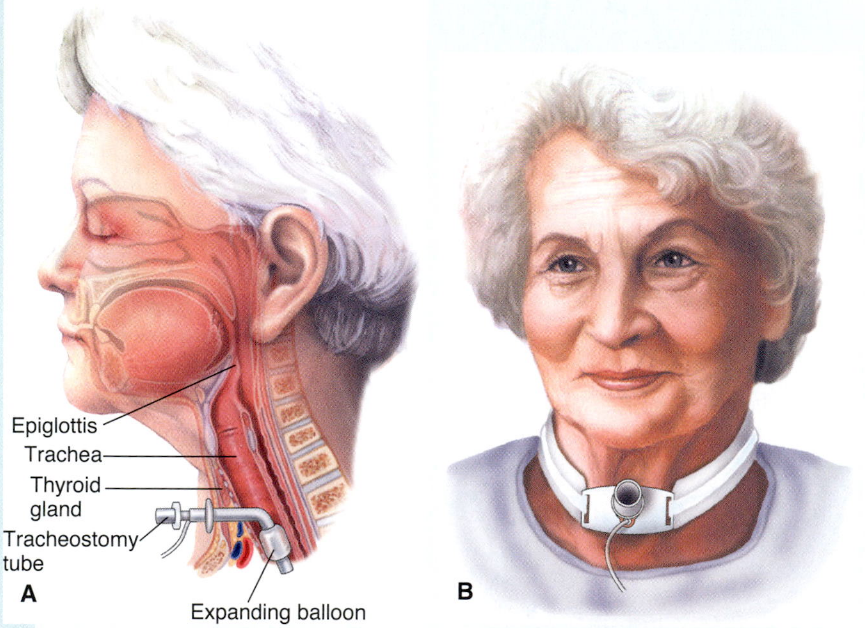

Epiglottis
Trachea
Thyroid gland
Tracheostomy tube
A
Expanding balloon
B

Figure 7-14 Tracheostomy. **(A)** Lateral view with tracheostomy tube in place. **(B)** Frontal view.

Diagnostic

Clinical

Mantoux test măn-TŪ	Intradermal test to determine tuberculin sensitivity based on a positive reaction where the area around the test site becomes red and swollen *A positive test suggests a past or present exposure to TB or past TB vaccination. However, the Mantoux test does not differentiate between active and inactive infection.*

Procedure	Description
Endoscopy	
bronchoscopy brŏng-KŎS-kō-pē *bronch/o:* bronchus *-scopy:* visual examination	Visual examination of the bronchi using an endoscope (flexible fiberoptic or rigid) inserted through the mouth and trachea for direct viewing of structures or for projection on a monitor (See Figure 7-15.) *Attachments on the bronchoscope can be used to suction mucus, remove foreign bodies, collect sputum, or perform biopsy.* **Figure 7-15** Bronchoscopy of the left bronchus.
laryngoscopy lăr-ĭn-GŎS-kō-pē *laryng/o:* larynx (voice box) *-scopy:* visual examination	Visual examination of the larynx to detect tumors, foreign bodies, nerve or structural injury, or other abnormalities
mediastinoscopy mē-dē-ăs-tĭ-NŎS-kō-pē *mediastin/o:* mediastinum *-scopy:* visual examination	Visual examination of the mediastinal structures, including the heart, trachea, esophagus, bronchus, thymus, and lymph nodes *The mediastinoscope is inserted through a small incision made above the sternum. The attached camera projects images on a monitor. Additional incisions may be made if nodes are removed or other diagnostic or therapeutic procedures are performed.*
Laboratory	
arterial blood gas (ABG) ăr-TĒ-rē-ăl *arteri/o:* artery *-al:* pertaining to	Test that measures dissolved oxygen and carbon dioxide in arterial blood *ABG analysis evaluates acid-base state and how well oxygen is being carried to body tissues.*

(continued)

Procedure	Description
sputum culture SPŪ-tŭm	Microbial test used to identify disease-causing organisms of the lower respiratory tract, especially those that cause pneumonias
sweat test	Measurement of the amount of salt (sodium chloride) in sweat *A sweat test is used almost exclusively in children to confirm cystic fibrosis.*
throat culture	Test used to identify pathogens, especially group A streptococci *Untreated streptococcal infections may lead to serious secondary complications, including kidney and heart disease.*
Imaging	
computed tomography pulmonary angiography (CTPA) kŏm-PŪ-tĕd tō-MŎG-ră-fē PŬL-mō-nĕr-ē ăn-jē-ŎG-ră-fē *tom/o:* to cut *-graphy:* process of recording *pulmon:* lung *-ary:* pertaining to *angi/o:* vessel (usually blood or lymph) *-graphy:* process of recording	Minimally invasive imaging that combines computed tomography scanning and angiography to produce images of the pulmonary arteries *This test is highly sensitive and specific for the presence of pulmonary emboli.*
ventilation-perfusion (V-Q) scan	Nuclear test scan that evaluates both airflow (ventilation) and blood flow (perfusion) in the lungs for evidence of a blood clot in the lungs; also called *V-Q lung scan*

Pharmacology

Several classes of drugs are prescribed to treat pulmonary disorders. These include antibiotics, which are used to treat respiratory infections, and bronchodilators, which are especially effective in treating COPD and exercise-induced asthma. (See Table 7-2.) Bronchodilators relax smooth muscles of the bronchi, thus increasing airflow. Some bronchodilators are delivered as a fine mist directly to the airways via aerosol delivery devices, including nebulizers and metered-dose inhalers (MDIs). Another method of delivering medications directly to the lungs is dry-powder inhalers (DPIs) that dispense medications in the form of a powder. Steroidal and nonsteroidal anti-inflammatory drugs are important in the control and management of many pulmonary disorders.

Table 7-2   Drugs Used to Treat Respiratory Disorders

This table lists common drug classifications used to treat respiratory disorders, their therapeutic actions, and selected generic and trade names.

Classification	Therapeutic Action	Generic and *Trade* Names
antibiotics ăn-tĭ-bī-ĂW-tĭks	Destroy or inhibit the growth of bacteria by disrupting their membranes or one or more of their metabolic processes	**azythromycin** ā-ZĬTH-rō-mī-sĭn *Zithromax* **erythromycin** ĕr-ĭth-rō-MĪ-sĭn *Ery-tab*

Table 7-2 **Drugs Used to Treat Respiratory Disorders—cont'd**

Classification	Therapeutic Action	Generic and *Trade* Names
antihistamines ăn-tĭ-HĬS-tă-mēnz	Block histamines from binding with histamine receptor sites in tissues *Histamines cause sneezing, runny nose, itchiness, and rashes.*	**fexofenadine** fĕk-sō-FĔN-ă-dēn *Allegra* **loratadine** lor-ĂH-tă-dēn *Claritin*
antitussives ăn-tĭ-TŬS-ĭvz	Relieve or suppress coughing by blocking the cough reflex in the medulla of the brain *Antitussives alleviate nonproductive dry coughs and should not be used with productive coughs.*	**hydrocodone** hī-drō-KŌ-dōn *Hycodan* **dextromethorphan** dĕk-strō-mĕth-OR-făn *Vicks Formula 44*
bronchodilators brŏng-kō-DĪ-lă-torz	Stimulate bronchial muscles to relax, thereby expanding air passages, resulting in increased air flow *Bronchodilators are used to treat chronic symptoms and prevent acute attacks in respiratory diseases, such as asthma and COPD, and may be delivered by an inhaler, orally, or intravenously.*	**albuterol** ăl-BŪ-tĕr-ŏl *Proventil, Ventolin* **salmeterol** săl-MĔT-ĕr-ŏl *Serevent*
corticosteroids kor-tĭ-kō-STĔR-oyds	Act on the immune system by blocking production of substances that trigger allergic and inflammatory actions *Corticosteroids are available as nasal sprays, in metered-dose-inhalers (inhaled steroids), and in oral forms (pills or syrups) to treat chronic lung conditions, such as asthma and COPD.*	**beclomethasone dipropionate** bĕ-klō-MĔTH-ă-sōn dī-PRŌ-pĕ-ō-nāt *Vanceril, Beclovent* **triamcinolone** trī-ăm-SĬN-ō-lōn *Azmacort*
decongestants dē-kŏn-JĔST-ănts	Constrict blood vessels of nasal passages and limit blood flow, which causes swollen tissues to shrink so that air can pass more freely through the passageways *Decongestants are commonly prescribed for allergies and colds and are usually combined with antihistamines in cold remedies. They can be administered orally or topically as nasal sprays and nasal drops.*	**oxymetazoline** ŏks-ē-mĕt-ĂZ-ō-lēn *Dristan* **pseudoephedrine** soo-dō-ĕ-FĔD-rĭn *Drixoral, Sudafed*
expectorants ĕk-SPĔK-tō-rănts	Liquefy respiratory secretions so that they are more easily dislodged during coughing episodes *Expectorants are prescribed for productive coughs.*	**guaifenesin** gwī-FĔN-ĕ-sĭn *Robitussin, Mucinex*

Abbreviations

This section introduces respiratory-related abbreviations and their meanings.

Abbreviation	Meaning	Abbreviation	Meaning
ABG	arterial blood gas(es)	MRI	magnetic resonance imaging
AFB	acid-fast bacillus (TB organism)	NMT	nebulized mist treatment
ARDS	acute respiratory distress syndrome	O_2	oxygen
CA	cancer	PA	posteroanterior; pernicious anemia
CO_2	carbon dioxide	Pco_2	partial pressure of carbon dioxide
COPD	chronic obstructive pulmonary disease	PCP	Pneumocystis carinii pneumonia; primary care physician
CPAP	continuous positive airway pressure	PFT	pulmonary function test
CPR	cardiopulmonary resuscitation	pH	degree of acidity or alkalinity
CT	computed tomography	PND	paroxysmal nocturnal dyspnea
CTPA	computed tomography pulmonary angiography	Po_2	partial pressure of oxygen
CXR	chest x-ray, chest radiograph	RD	respiratory distress
DPI	dry powder inhaler	RDS	respiratory distress syndrome
DPT	diphtheria, pertussis, tetanus	SIDS	sudden infant death syndrome
Hb, Hgb	hemoglobin	SOB	shortness of breath
HMD	hyaline membrane disease	T&A	tonsillectomy and adenoidectomy
IRDS	infant respiratory distress syndrome	TB	tuberculosis
MDI	metered-dose inhaler	URI	upper respiratory infection

It is time to review procedures, pharmacology, and abbreviations by completing Learning Activity 7-4.

LEARNING ACTIVITIES

The following activities provide review of the respiratory system terms introduced in this chapter. Complete each activity and review your answers to evaluate your understanding of the chapter.

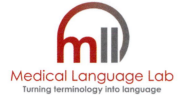

Visit the Medical Language Lab at the web site: medicallanguagelab.com. Use it to enhance your study and reinforcement of this chapter with the flash-card activity. We recommend you complete the flash-card activity before starting Learning Activities 7-1 and 7-2 below.

Learning Activity 7-1
Combining Forms, Suffixes, and Prefixes

Use the elements listed in the table to build medical words. You may use these elements more than once.

Combining Forms		Suffixes		Prefixes
bronch/o	rhin/o	-capnia	-osis	brady-
bronchi/o	sept/o	-centesis	-phonia	dys-
cyan/o	sinus/o	-ectasis	-plasty	eu-
laryng/o	tonsill/o	-ectomy	-plegia	hyper-
ox/i		-emia	-pnea	
pleur/o		-ia	-scope	
pneumon/o		-meter	-tomy	

1. surgical puncture of the pleura _____

2. instrument for examining the bronchus _____

3. excision of the tonsils _____

4. slow breathing _____

5. difficult voice _____

6. abnormal condition of blue(ness) _____

7. instrument to measure oxygen (saturation) _____

8. paralysis of the voice box _____

9. surgical repair of the septum _____

10. incision of the sinus _____

11. excessive carbon dioxide _____

12. good, normal breathing _____

13. expansion of a bronchi _____

14. surgical repair of the nose _____

15. condition of the lungs _____

 Check your answers in Appendix A. Review any material that you did not answer correctly.

Correct Answers _____ X 6.67 = _____ % Score

Learning Activity 7-2
Building Medical Words

Use *rhin/o* (nose) to build words that mean:

1. discharge from the nose _____
2. inflammation of (mucous membranes of the) nose _____

Use *laryng/o* (larynx [voice box]) to build words that mean:

3. visual examination of the larynx _____
4. inflammation of the larynx _____
5. stricture or narrowing of the larynx _____

Use *bronch/o* or *bronchi/o* (bronchus) to build words that mean:

6. dilation or expansion of the bronchus _____
7. disease of the bronchus _____
8. spasm of the bronchus _____

Use *pneumon/o* or *pneum/o* (air; lung) to build words that mean:

9. air in the chest (pleural space) _____
10. inflammation of the lungs _____

Use *pulmon/o* (lung) to build words that mean:

11. specialist in lung (diseases) _____
12. pertaining to the lung _____

Use *-pnea* (breathing) to build words that mean:

13. difficult breathing _____
14. slow breathing _____
15. rapid breathing _____
16. absence of breathing _____

Build surgical words that mean:

17. surgical repair of the nose _____
18. surgical puncture of the chest _____
19. removal of a lung _____
20. forming an opening (mouth) in the trachea _____

✓ *Check your answers in Appendix A. Review material that you did not answer correctly.*

Correct Answers _____ X 5 = _____ % Score

Learning Activity 7-3

Pathology, Diseases, and Conditions

Match the following terms with the definitions in the numbered list.

anosmia	deviated septum	hemoptysis	pneumoconiosis
apnea	emphysema	hypoxemia	pulmonary edema
atelectasis	empyema	hypoxia	surfactant
consolidation	epistaxis	pertussis	transudate
coryza	exudate	pleurisy	tubercles

1. collapsed or airless lung _____

2. pus in the pleural cavity _____

3. phospholipid that allows the lungs to expand with ease _____

4. deficiency of oxygen in the tissues _____

5. inflammatory fluid high in protein with blood and immune cells _____

6. absence or decrease in the sense of smell _____

7. deficiency of oxygen in the blood _____

8. granulomas associated with tuberculosis _____

9. temporary loss of breathing _____

10. disease characterized by a decrease in alveolar elasticity _____

11. spitting of blood _____

12. nosebleed; nasal hemorrhage _____

13. excessive fluid in the lungs that induces cough and dyspnea _____

14. noninflammatory fluid that resembles serum but with less protein _____

15. displacement of the cartilage dividing the nostrils _____

16. acute inflammation of the membranes of the nose; also called *head cold* _____

17. condition in which dust particles are found in the lungs _____

18. inflammation of the pleural membrane _____

19. loss of sponginess of lungs due to engorgement _____

20. whooping cough _____

Check your answers in Appendix A. Review material that you did not answer correctly.

Correct Answers _____ X 5 = _____ % Score

Learning Activity 7-4
Matching Procedures, Pharmacology, and Abbreviations

Match the following terms with the definitions in the numbered list.

ABGs	antral lavage	Mantoux test	rhinoplasty
aerosol therapy	CXR	oximetry	septoplasty
AFB	decongestant	pneumectomy	sputum culture
antihistamine	expectorant	polysomnography	sweat test
antitussive	laryngoscopy	pulmonary function tests	throat culture

1. microbial test used to identify disease-causing organisms of the lower respiratory tract _____

2. test of sleep cycles and stages _____

3. imaging procedure to evaluate the lungs _____

4. washing or irrigating sinuses _____

5. relieves sneezing, runny nose, itchiness, and rashes _____

6. relieves or suppresses coughing _____

7. used primarily in children to confirm cystic fibrosis _____

8. noninvasive test used to monitor the percentage of hemoglobin saturated with oxygen _____

9. TB organism _____

10. inhalation of medication directly into the respiratory system via a nebulizer _____

11. decreases mucous membrane swelling by constricting blood vessels _____

12. intradermal test to determine tuberculin sensitivity _____

13. laboratory tests to assess gases and pH of arterial blood _____

14. reduces the viscosity of sputum to facilitate productive coughing _____

15. used to identify pathogens, especially group A streptococci _____

16. multiple tests used to determine the ability of lungs and capillary membranes to exchange oxygen _____

17. visual examination of the voice box to detect tumors and other abnormalities _____

18. procedure to correct a deviated nasal septum _____

19. excision of the entire lung _____

20. reconstructive surgery of the nose, commonly for cosmetic purposes _____

✔ *Check your answers in Appendix A. Review any material that you did not answer correctly.*

Correct Answers _____ X 5 = _____ % Score

Learning Activity 7-5
Medical Scenarios

To construct chart notes, replace the italicized terms in each of the two scenarios with one of the medical terms listed below.

antitussive	dyspnea	septoplasty
cephalodynia	myalgia	sinusitis
coryza	pharyngitis	T&A
deviated nasal septum		

Billy P., a 2-year-old boy, was referred to the ENT Clinic by his pediatrician. His mother states that, while sleeping, Billy experiences (1) **difficult breathing**, starts gasping for air, and then wakes up crying. This is especially true when he has a (2) **head cold**. The examination of his nasal passages show a (3) **septum displaced to one side**, causing impaired air flow through the nostrils. His tonsils and adenoids are also enlarged, making breathing even more difficult. The physician schedules a (4) **surgical repair of the septum** and (5) **removal of the tonsils and adenoids**.

1. _____
2. _____
3. _____
4. _____
5. _____

Betty L. presents to the Student Health Services on campus. She complains of (6) **muscle pain** and (7) **headache**. Betty L. states that she was up the entire night with a dry hacking cough. Upon examination, the physician confirms that Betty has flu and stated that her headache was probably due to (8) **inflamed sinuses**. He further notes an (9) **inflammation of the throat** without evidence of strep infection. Betty L. is advised to drink clear fluids and take Tylenol, as needed, to reduce fever and general discomfort. The physician also prescribes Hycodan, a (10) **medication to control coughing**.

6. _____
7. _____
8. _____
9. _____
10. _____

✓ *Check your answers in Appendix A. Review any material that you did not answer correctly.*

Correct Answers _____ X 10 = _____ % Score

MEDICAL RECORD ACTIVITIES

The two medical records included in the following activities use common clinical scenarios to show how medical terminology is used to document patient care. Complete the terminology and analysis sections for each activity to help you recognize and understand terms related to the respiratory system.

Medical Record Activity 7-1

SOAP Note: Respiratory Evaluation

Terminology

Terms listed in the following table are taken from *SOAP Note: Respiratory Evaluation* that follows. Use a medical dictionary such as *Taber's Cyclopedic Medical Dictionary;* the appendices of *Systems,* 7th ed.; or other resources to define each term. Then review the pronunciations for each term and practice by reading the medical record aloud.

Term	Definition
anteriorly ăn-TĔR-ē-or-lē	
bilateral bī-LĂT-ĕr-ăl	
COPD	
exacerbation ĕks-ăs-ĕr-BĀ-shŭn	
heart failure	
Hx	
hypertension hī-pĕr-TĔN-shŭn	
interstitial ĭn-tĕr-STĬSH-ăl	
PE	
peripheral vascular disease pĕr-ĬF-ĕr-ăl VĂS-kū-lăr	

(continued)

Term	Definition
pleural PLOO-răl	
posteriorly pŏs-TĒR-ē-or-lē	
rhonchi RŎNG-kī	
SOB	
wheezes HWĒZ-ĕz	

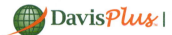 | Visit the *Medical Terminology Systems* online resource center at Davis*Plus* to practice pronunciation and reinforce the meanings of the terms in this medical report.

SOAP NOTE: RESPIRATORY EVALUATION

Emergency Department Record

Date: February 1, 20xx   Time Registered: 1345 hours
Patient: Flowers, Richard   Physician: Samara Batichara, MD
Chief Complaint: SOB

Medications: Vytorin 10/20 mg daily; Toprol-XL 50 mg daily; Azmacort 2 puffs three times a day; Proventil 2 puffs every six hours.

S:　This 49-year-old man with Hx of COPD is admitted because of exacerbation of SOB over the past few days. Patient was a heavy smoker and states that he quit smoking for a short while but now smokes 3-4 cigarettes a day. He has a Hx of difficult breathing, hypertension, COPD, and peripheral vascular disease. The patient underwent triple bypass surgery in 19xx.

O:　T: 98.9 F. BP: 180/90. Pulse: 80 and regular. R: 20 and shallow. PE indicates scattered bilateral wheezes and rhonchi heard anteriorly and posteriorly. When compared with a portable chest film taken 22 months earlier, the current study most likely indicates interstitial vascular congestion. Some superimposed inflammatory change cannot be excluded. There may also be some pleural reactive change.

A:　1. Acute exacerbation of chronic obstructive pulmonary disease.
　　　2. Heart failure.
　　　3. Hypertension.
　　　4. Peripheral vascular disease.

P:　Admit to hospital.

Samara Batichara, MD
Samara Batichara, MD

SB:icc

D: 2/1/20xx; T: 2/1/20xx

Analysis

Review the medical record *SOAP Note: Respiratory Evaluation* to answer the following questions.

1. What symptom caused the patient to seek medical help?

_____

2. What was the patient's previous history?

_____

3. What were the abnormal findings of the physical examination?

_____

4. What changes were noted from the previous film?

_____

5. What are the present assessments?

_____

6. What new diagnosis was made that did not appear in the previous medical history?

_____

Medical Record Activity 7-2
SOAP Note: Chronic Interstitial Lung Disease

Terminology

Terms listed in the following table are taken from *SOAP Note: Chronic Interstitial Lung Disease* that follows. Use a medical dictionary such as *Taber's Cyclopedic Medical Dictionary;* the appendices of *Systems*, 7th ed.; or other resources to define each term. Then review the pronunciations for each term and practice by reading the medical record aloud.

Term	Definition
ABG	
adenopathy ăd-ě-NŎP-ă-thē	
basilar crackles BĂS-ĭ-lăr KRĂK-ĕlz	
cardiomyopathy kăr-dē-ō-mī- ŎP-ă-thē	
chronic KRŎN-ĭk	
diuresis dī-ū-RĒ-sĭs	
dyspnea dĭsp-NĒ-ă	
fibrosis fī-BRŌ-sĭs	
interstitial ĭn-tĕr-STĬSH-ăl	
kyphosis kī-FŌ-sĭs	
Lasix LĀ-sĭks	
neuropathy nū-RŎP-ă-thē	
P_{CO_2}	
pedal edema PĔD-ăl ē-DĒ-mă	

(continued)

Term	Definition
pH	
Po$_2$	
pulmonary fibrosis PŬL-mō-nĕ-rē fĭ-BRŌ-sĭs	
renal insufficiency RĒ-năl ĭn-sŭ-FĬSH-ĕn-sē	
rhonchi RŎNG-kī	
silicosis sĭl-ĭ-KŌ-sĭs	
thyromegaly thī-rō-MĔG-ă-lē	

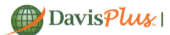 Visit the *Medical Terminology Systems* online resource center at Davis*Plus* to practice pronunciation and reinforce the meanings of the terms in this medical report.

SOAP NOTE: CHRONIC INTERSTITIAL LUNG DISEASE

O'Malley, Robert   09/01/20xx

SUBJECTIVE: Patient is an 84-year-old male with chief complaint of dyspnea with activity and pedal edema. He carries the dx cardiomyopathy, renal insufficiency, COPD, and pulmonary fibrosis. He also has peripheral neuropathy, which has improved with Elavil therapy.

OBJECTIVE: BP: 140/70. Pulse: 76. Neck is supple without thyromegaly or adenopathy. Mild kyphosis without scoliosis is present. Chest reveals basilar crackles without wheezing or rhonchi. Cardiac examination shows trace edema without clubbing or murmur. Abdomen is soft and nontender. ABGs on room air demonstrate a PO_2 of 55, PCO_2 of 45, and pH of 7.42.

ASSESSMENT: Chronic interstitial lung disease, likely a combination of pulmonary fibrosis and heart failure. We do believe he would benefit from further diuresis, which was implemented by Dr. Lu. Should there continue to be concerns about his volume status or lack of response to Lasix therapy, then he might benefit from right heart catheterization.

PLAN: Supplemental oxygen will be continued. We plan no change in his pulmonary medication at this time and will see him in return visit in 4 months. He has been told to contact us should he worsen in the interim.

Samara Batichara, MD
Samara Batichara, MD

SB:icc

Analysis

Review the medical record *SOAP Note: Chronic Interstitial Lung Disease* to answer the following questions.

1. When did the patient notice dyspnea?

_____

2. Other than the respiratory system, what other body systems are identified in the history of present illness?

_____

3. What were the findings regarding the neck?

_____

4. What was the finding regarding the chest?

_____

5. What appears to be the likely cause of the chronic interstitial lung disease?

_____

6. What did the cardiac examination reveal?

_____

CHAPTER

Cardiovascular System

8

Chapter Outline

Objectives

Upon completion of this chapter, you will be able to:

- Locate and describe the structures of the cardiovascular system.
- Describe the functional relationship between the cardiovascular system and other body systems.
- Pronounce, spell, and build words related to the cardiovascular system.
- Describe diseases, conditions, and procedures related to the cardiovascular system.
- Explain pharmacology related to the treatment of cardiovascular disorders.
- Demonstrate your knowledge of this chapter by completing the learning and medical record activities.

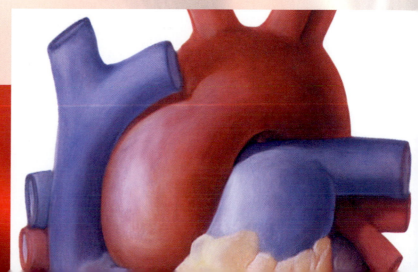

Anatomy and Physiology

The cardiovascular (CV) system is composed of the heart and blood vessels. The heart is a hollow, muscular organ lying in the mediastinum, the center of the thoracic cavity between the lungs. The pumping action of the heart propels blood that contains oxygen (O_2), nutrients, and other vital products from the heart to body cells through a vast network of blood vessels called **arteries.** Arteries branch into smaller vessels until they become microscopic vessels called **capillaries.** At the capillary level, an exchange of products occurs between body cells and blood. Capillaries merge to form larger blood vessels called **venules,** which then combine to form **veins,** the vessels that return blood to the heart to begin the cycle again. Millions of body cells rely on the cardiovascular system for their survival. When the CV system fails, life at the cellular level is not possible and, ultimately, death occurs.

Anatomy and Physiology Key Terms

This section lists important terms found in the anatomy and physiology section as well as their definitions and pronunciations.

Term	Definition
autonomic nervous system (ANS) aw-tō-NŎM-ĭk NĔR-vĕs	Portion of the nervous system that regulates involuntary actions, such as heart rate, digestion, and peristalsis
leaflet	Flat, leaf-shaped structure that comprises the valves of the heart and prevents backflow of blood
lumen LŪ-mĕn	Tubular space or channel within an organ or structure of the body; space within an artery, vein, intestine, or tube
regurgitation rē-gŭr-jĭ-TĀ-shŭn	Backflow or ejecting of contents through an opening
sphincter SFĬNGK-tĕr	Circular muscle found in a tubular structure or hollow organ that constricts or dilates to regulate passage of substances through its opening
vasoconstriction văs-ō-kŏn-STRĬK-shŭn	Narrowing of the lumen of a blood vessel that limits blood flow, usually as a result of diseases, medications, or physiological processes
vasodilation văs-ō-dī-LĀ-shŭn	Widening of the lumen of a blood vessel caused by the relaxing of the muscles of the vascular walls
viscosity vĭs-KŎS-ĭ-tē	State of being sticky or gummy *A solution that has high viscosity is relatively thick and flows slowly.*

Pronunciation Help Long Sound ā — rate ē — rebirth ī — isle ō — over ū — unite
Short Sound ă — alone ĕ — ever ĭ — it ŏ — not ŭ — cut

Vascular System

Three major types of vessels—(1) **artery,** (2) **capillary,** and (3) **vein**—carry blood throughout the body. (See Figure 8-1.) Each type of vessel differs in structure, depending on its function.

Arteries

Arteries carry blood from the heart to all cells of the body. Because blood is propelled thorough the arteries by the pumping action of the heart, the walls of the arteries must be strong and flexible enough to withstand the surge of blood that results from each contraction of the heart.

The walls of large arteries have three layers to provide toughness and elasticity. The (4) **tunica externa** is the outer coat, composed of connective tissue that provides strength and flexibility. The (5) **tunica media** is the middle layer, composed of smooth muscle. Depending on the needs of the body, this muscle can alter the size of the (7) lumen of the vessel. When it contracts, the tunica media causes **vasoconstriction**, resulting in decreased blood flow. When it relaxes, it causes

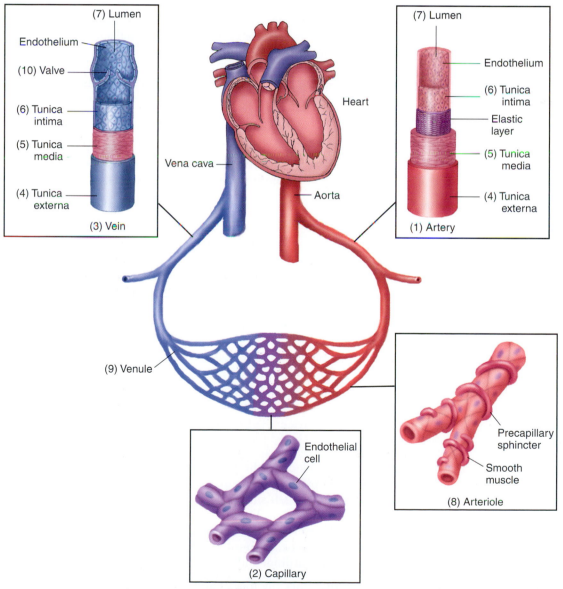

Figure 8-1 Vascular structures.

vasodilation, resulting in increased blood flow. The (6) **tunica intima** is the thin, inner lining of the lumen of the vessel, composed of endothelial cells that provide a smooth surface on the inside of the vessel.

The surge of blood felt in the arteries when blood is pumped from the heart is referred to as a **pulse**. Because of the pressure against arterial walls associated with the pumping action of the heart, a cut or severed artery may lead to profuse bleeding.

Arterial blood (except for that found in the pulmonary artery) contains a high concentration of O_2 **(oxygen)** and appears bright red in color. Oxygenated blood travels to smaller arteries called (8) **arterioles** and, finally, to the smallest vessels, the capillaries.

Capillaries

Capillaries are microscopic vessels that join the arterial system with the venous system. Although they seem like the most insignificant of the three vessel types owing to their microscopic size, they are actually the most important because of their function. Because capillary walls are composed of only a single layer of endothelial cells, they are very thin. This thinness enables the exchange of water, respiratory gases, macromolecules, metabolites, and wastes between the blood and the cells adjacent to the capillary bed. The vast number of capillaries branching from arterioles causes blood to flow very slowly, providing sufficient time for exchange of essential substances.

Blood flow through the capillary networks is slow and intermittent, rather than steady, and is regulated by the precapillary **sphincters**. When tissues require more blood, these sphincters open; when less blood is required, they close. Once the exchange of products is complete, blood enters the venous system for its return to the heart.

Veins

Veins return blood to the heart. They are formed from smaller vessels called (9) **venules** that develop from the union of capillaries. Because the extensive network of capillaries absorbs the propelling pressure exerted by the heart, veins use other methods to return blood to the heart, including:

• skeletal muscle contraction
• gravity
• respiratory activity
• valves.

The (10) **valves** are small structures within veins that prevent the backflow of blood. Valves are found mainly in the extremities and are especially important for returning blood from the legs to the heart because blood must travel a long distance against the force of gravity to reach the heart from the legs. Large veins, especially in the abdomen, contain smooth muscle that provides peristalsis and helps propel blood toward the heart.

Blood carried in veins (except for the blood in the pulmonary veins) contains a low concentration of O_2 with a corresponding high concentration of carbon dioxide (CO_2). This blood takes on a characteristic purple color, and is said to be deoxygenated. It continuously circulates from the heart to the lungs so that CO_2 can be exchanged for O_2.

Heart

The **heart** is a muscular pump that propels blood to the entire body through a closed vascular network. It allows a dual circulatory system: pulmonary circulation provided by the right side of the heart and systemic circulation provided by the left side of the heart. Pulmonary circulation delivers blood to the lungs where CO_2 is exchanged for O_2. Systemic circulation delivers blood to body tissues where O_2 is exchanged for CO_2, a waste product that will be expelled by the lungs. Both systemic and pulmonary circulatory activities occur simultaneously. (See Figure 8-2.)

The heart is found in a sac called the **pericardium** and is composed of three distinct tissue layers:

• **endocardium,** a serous membrane that lines the four chambers of the heart and its valves and is continuous with the endothelium of the arteries and veins
• **myocardium,** the muscular layer of the heart
• **epicardium,** the outermost layer of the heart.

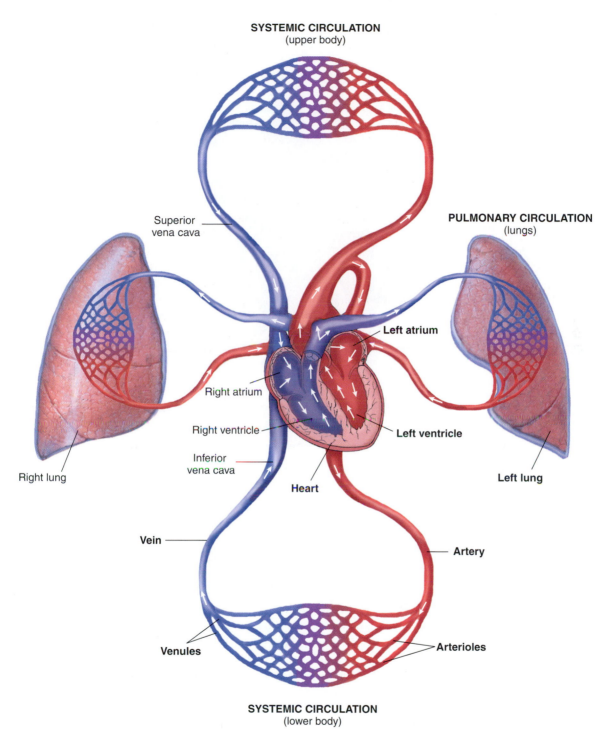

SYSTEMIC CIRCULATION
(upper body)

PULMONARY CIRCULATION
(lungs)

Superior
vena cava

Left atrium

Right atrium

Right ventricle

Left ventricle

Inferior
vena cava

Right lung

Left lung

Heart

Vein

Artery

Venules

Arterioles

SYSTEMIC CIRCULATION
(lower body)

Figure 8-2 Systemic and pulmonary circulation.

The heart is divided into four chambers. (See Figure 8-3.) The two upper chambers, the
(1) **right atrium (RA)** and (2) **left atrium (LA),** collect blood. The two lower chambers, the
(3) **right ventricle (RV)** and (4) **left ventricle (LV),** pump blood from the heart. The right
ventricle pumps blood to the lungs **(pulmonary circulation)** for oxygenation, and the left ventricle pumps oxygenated blood to the entire body **(systemic circulation).**

Deoxygenated blood from the body returns to the right atrium by way of two large
veins: the (5) **superior vena cava,** which collects and carries blood from the upper body, and

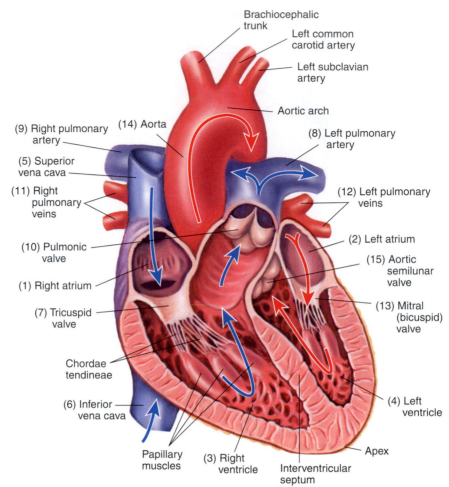

Brachiocephalic trunk
Left common carotid artery
Left subclavian artery
Aortic arch
(9) Right pulmonary artery
(14) Aorta
(8) Left pulmonary artery
(5) Superior vena cava
(12) Left pulmonary veins
(11) Right pulmonary veins
(2) Left atrium
(10) Pulmonic valve
(15) Aortic semilunar valve
(1) Right atrium
(7) Tricuspid valve
(13) Mitral (bicuspid) valve
Chordae tendineae
(4) Left ventricle
(6) Inferior vena cava
Apex
Papillary muscles
(3) Right ventricle
Interventricular septum

Figure 8-3 Internal structures of the heart, with red arrows designating oxygen-rich blood flow and blue arrows designating oxygen-poor blood flow.

the (6) **inferior vena cava,** which collects and carries blood from the lower body. From the right atrium, blood passes through the (7) **tricuspid valve,** consisting of three leaflets, to the right ventricle. When the heart contracts, blood leaves the right ventricle by way of the (8) **left pulmonary artery** and (9) **right pulmonary artery** and travels to the lungs. During contraction of the ventricle, the tricuspid valve closes to prevent a backflow of blood to the right atrium. The (10) **pulmonic valve (or pulmonary semilunar valve)** prevents regurgitation of blood into the right ventricle from the pulmonary artery. In the lungs the pulmonary artery branches into millions of capillaries, each lying close to an alveolus. Here, carbon dioxide in the blood is exchanged for oxygen that has been drawn into the lungs during inhalation.

Pulmonary capillaries unite to form four pulmonary veins—two (11) **right pulmonary veins** and two (12) **left pulmonary veins.** These vessels carry oxygenated blood back to the heart. They deposit blood in the left atrium. From there, blood passes to the left ventricle through the (13) **mitral (bicuspid) valve,** a structure consisting of two leaflets. Upon contraction of the ventricles, the oxygenated blood leaves the heart through the largest artery of the body, the (14) **aorta.** The aorta contains the (15) **aortic semilunar valve (aortic valve)** that permits blood to flow in only one direction—from the left ventricle to the aorta. The aorta branches into many smaller arteries that carry blood to all parts of the body.

It is important to understand that oxygen in the blood passing through the chambers of the heart cannot be used by the myocardium as a source of oxygen and nutrients. Instead, an arterial system composed of the coronary arteries branches from the aorta and provides the myocardium with its own blood supply. (See Figure 8-4.) The artery vascularizing the right side of the heart is the (1) **right coronary artery.** The artery vascularizing the left side of the heart is the (2) **left coronary**

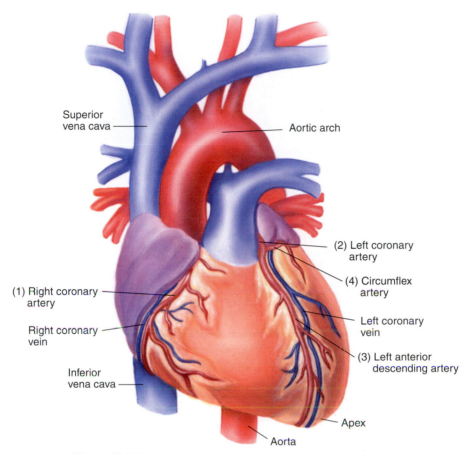

Superior vena cava

Aortic arch

(2) Left coronary artery

(4) Circumflex artery

(1) Right coronary artery

Left coronary vein

Right coronary vein

(3) Left anterior descending artery

Inferior vena cava

Apex

Aorta

Figure 8-4 Anterior view of the heart showing coronary arteries.

artery. The left coronary artery divides into two branches, the (3) **left anterior descending artery** and the (4) **circumflex artery.** If blood flow in the coronary arteries is diminished, damage to the heart muscle may result. When severe damage occurs, part of the heart muscle may die.

Conduction System of the Heart

Within the heart, specialized cardiac tissue known as **conduction tissue** has the sole function of initiating and spreading contraction impulses. (See Figure 8-5.) This tissue consists of four masses of highly specialized cells that possess characteristics of both nervous and cardiac tissue:

* sinoatrial (SA) node
* atrioventricular (AV) node
* bundle of His (AV bundle)
* Purkinje fibers.

The (1) **sinoatrial (SA) node** is located in the upper portion of the right atrium and possesses its own intrinsic rhythm. Without being stimulated by external nerves, it has the ability to initiate and propagate each heartbeat, thereby setting the basic pace for the cardiac rate. For this reason, the SA node is commonly known as the **pacemaker** of the heart. The cardiac rate may be altered by impulses from the **autonomic nervous system**. Such an arrangement allows outside influences to accelerate or decelerate heart rate. For example, the heart beats more quickly during physical exertion and more slowly during rest. Each electrical impulse discharged by the SA node is transmitted to the (2) **atrioventricular (AV) node,** causing the atria to contract. The AV node is located at the base of the right atrium. From this point, a tract of conduction fibers called the (3) **bundle of His (AV bundle),** composed of a right and left branch, relays the impulse to the (4) **Purkinje fibers.** These fibers extend up the ventricle walls. The Purkinje fibers transmit the impulse to the right and left ventricles, causing them to contract. Blood is now forced from the heart through the

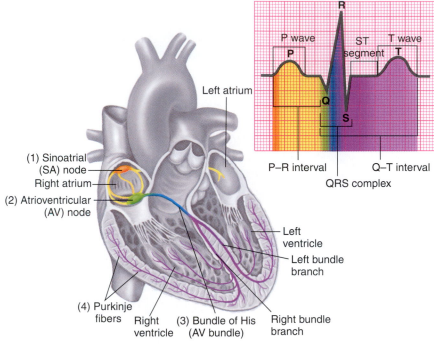

Figure 8-5 Conduction system.

pulmonary artery and aorta. Thus, the sequence of the four structures responsible for conduction of a contraction impulse is:

SA node → AV node → bundle of His → Purkinje fibers

Impulse transmission through the conduction system generates weak electrical impulses on the surface of the body. These impulses can be recorded on graph paper by an instrument called an **electrocardiograph.** The needle deflection of the electrocardiograph produces waves or peaks designated by the letters P, Q, R, S, and T, each of which is associated with a specific electrical event:

- The **P wave** is the depolarization (contraction) of the atria.
- The **QRS complex** is the depolarization (contraction) of the ventricles.
- The **T wave**, which appears a short time later, is the repolarization (recovery) of the ventricles.

Blood Pressure

Blood pressure (BP) is the force exerted by blood against the arterial walls during two phases of a heartbeat: the contraction phase **(systole)** when the blood is forced out of the heart, and the relaxation phase **(diastole)** when the ventricles are filling with blood. Systole produces the maximum force; diastole, the weakest. Blood pressure is measured with a **sphygmomanometer** and is recorded as two figures separated by a diagonal line. When recording a blood pressure reading, systolic pressure is listed first, followed by diastolic pressure. For instance, a blood pressure of *120/80 mm Hg* means a systolic pressure of 120 with a diastolic pressure of 80.

Several factors influence blood pressure:

- resistance of blood flow in blood vessels
- pumping action of the heart
- **viscosity**, or thickness, of blood
- elasticity of arteries
- quantity of blood in the vascular system.

Anatomy Review

To review the anatomy of the heart, label the illustration using the terms below.

aorta

aortic semilunar valve

inferior vena cava

left atrium

left pulmonary artery

left pulmonary veins

left ventricle

mitral (bicuspid) valve

pulmonic valve

right atrium

right pulmonary artery

right pulmonary veins

right ventricle

superior vena cava

tricuspid valve

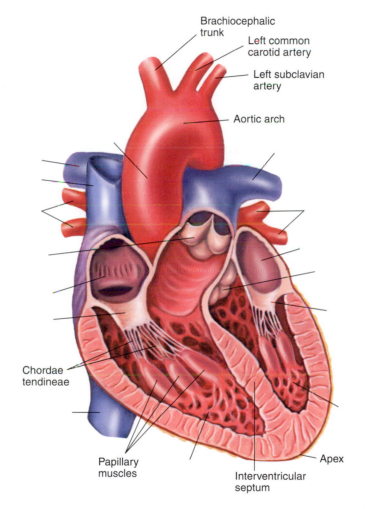

Brachiocephalic trunk

Left common carotid artery

Left subclavian artery

Aortic arch

Chordae tendineae

Papillary muscles

Apex

Interventricular septum

 Check your answers by referring to Figure 8–3 on page 212. Review material that you did not answer correctly.

CONNECTING BODY SYSTEMS—CARDIOVASCULAR SYSTEM

The main function of the cardiovascular (CV) system is to provide a network of vessels though which blood is pumped by the heart to all body cells. Specific functional relationships between the CV system and other body systems are discussed below.

Blood, Lymph, and Immune

- CV system transports the products of the immune system.

Digestive

- CV system delivers hormones that affect glandular activity of the digestive tract.
- Vessels of the CV system in the walls of the small intestine absorb nutrients.

Endocrine

- CV system delivers oxygen and nutrients to endocrine glands.
- CV system transports hormones from glands to target organs.

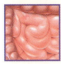

Female Reproductive

- CV system transports hormones that regulate the menstrual cycle.
- CV system influences the normal function of sex organs, especially erectile tissue.
- During pregnancy, vessels of the CV system in the placenta exchange nutrients and waste products.

Integumentary

- Blood vessels of the CV system in the skin regulate body temperature.
- CV system transports clotting factors to the skin to control bleeding.

Male Reproductive

- CV system transports reproductive hormones.
- CV system influences the normal function of sex organs, especially erectile tissue.

Musculoskeletal

- CV system removes heat and waste products generated by muscle contraction.
- CV system delivers oxygen for energy to sustain muscle contraction.
- CV system delivers calcium and nutrients and removes metabolic wastes from skeletal structures.
- CV system delivers hormones that regulate skeletal growth.

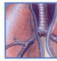

Nervous

- CV system carries electrolytes for transmission of electrical impulses.

Respiratory

- CV system transports oxygen and carbon dioxide between lungs and tissues.

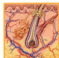

Urinary

- CV system delivers oxygen and nutrients.
- Blood pressure maintains kidney function.

Medical Word Elements

This section introduces combining forms, suffixes, and prefixes related to the cardiovascular system. Word analyses are also provided.

Element	Meaning	Word Analysis
Combining Forms		
aneurysm/o	widened blood vessel	**aneurysm/o/rrhaphy** (ăn-ū-rĭz-MŌR-ă-fē): suture of an aneurysm *-rrhaphy:* suture
angi/o	vessel (usually blood or lymph)	**angi/o/plasty** (ĂN-jē-ō-plăs-tē): surgical repair of a vessel *-plasty:* surgical repair *Angioplasty includes any endovascular procedure that reopens narrowed blood vessels and restores blood flow.*
vascul/o		**vascul/itis** (văs-kū-LĪ-tĭs): inflammation of (blood) vessels *-itis:* inflammation

Element	Meaning	Word Analysis
aort/o	aorta	**aort/o**/stenosis (ā-or-tō-stĕ-NŌ-sĭs): narrowing of the aorta -*stenosis:* narrowing, stricture
arteri/o	artery	**arteri/o**/rrhexis (ăr-tē-rē-ō-RĔK-sĭs): rupture of an artery -*rrhexis:* rupture
arteriol/o	arteriole	**arteriol**/itis (ăr-tēr-ē-ō-LĪ-tĭs): inflammation of an arteriole -*itis:* inflammation
atri/o	atrium	**atri/o**/megaly (ā-trē-ō-MĔG-ă-lē): enlargement of the atrium -*megaly:* enlargement
ather/o	fatty plaque	**ather**/oma (ăth-ĕr-Ō-mă): tumor of fatty plaque -*oma:* tumor *Atheromas are formed when fatty plaque builds up on the inner lining of arterial walls. As calcium and other minerals are absorbed by plaque, the vessel hardens.*
cardi/o	heart	**cardi/o**/megaly (kăr-dē-ō-MĔG-ă-lē): enlargement of the heart -*megaly:* enlargement
coron/o		**coron**/ary (KOR-ō-nă-rē): pertaining to the heart (vessels) -*ary:* pertaining to *The coronary arteries come down over the top of the heart like a crown.*
electr/o	electricity	**electr/o**/cardi/o/gram (ē-lĕk-trō-KĂR-dē-ō-grăm): record of the electrical (impulses) of the heart *cardi/o:* heart -*gram:* record, recording *An electrocardiogram is commonly used to diagnose abnormalities of the heart.*
embol/o	embolus (plug)	**embol**/ectomy (ĕm-bō-LĔK-tō-mē): removal of an embolus -*ectomy:* excision, removal *An embolectomy is the removal of a clot or other foreign material from a blood vessel.*
hemangi/o	blood vessel	**hemangi**/oma (hē-măn-jē-Ō-mă): tumor of blood vessels -*oma:* tumor *Infantile hemangiomas are also called* birthmarks. *They are not considered malignant and usually disappear over time.*
my/o	muscle	**my/o**/cardi/al (mī-ō-KĂR-dē-ăl): pertaining to heart muscle *cardi:* heart -*al:* pertaining to
phleb/o	vein	**phleb**/ectasis (flĕ-BĔK-tă-sĭs): expansion of a vein -*ectasis:* dilation, expansion
ven/o	vein	**ven/o**/stasis (vē-nō-STĀ-sĭs): standing still of (blood in) a vein; also called *phlebostasis* -*stasis:* standing still

(continued)

Element	Meaning	Word Analysis

scler/o	hardening; sclera (white of eye)	arteri/o/**scler**/osis (ăr-tē-rē-ō-sklĕ-RŌ-sĭs): abnormal condition of hardening of the artery
		  arteri/o: artery
		  -osis: abnormal condition; increase (used primarily with blood cells)
		The most common cause of arteriosclerosis is the presence of an atheroma in the vessel. Other common causes include smoking, diabetes, high blood pressure, obesity, and familial tendency.

sept/o	septum	**sept/o**/stomy (sĕp-TŎS-tō-mē): forming an opening in a septum *-stomy:* forming an opening (mouth) *Septostomy is a temporary procedure performed to increase systemic oxygenation in infants with congenital heart defects until corrective surgery can be performed.*
sphygm/o	pulse	**sphygm**/oid (SFĬG-moyd): resembling a pulse *-oid:* resembling
sten/o	narrowing, stricture	**sten/o**/tic (stĕ-NŎT-ĭk): pertaining to a narrowing or stricture *-tic:* pertaining to
thromb/o	blood clot	**thromb/o**/lysis (thrŏm-BŎL-ĭ-sĭs): destruction of a blood clot *-lysis:* separation; destruction; loosening *In thrombolysis, enzymes that destroy blood clots are infused into the occluded vessel.*
valv/o	valve	**valv/o**/tomy (văl-VŎT-ō-mē): incision of a valve *-tomy:* incision
valvul/o		**valvul/o**/plasty (VĂL-vū-lō-plăs-tē): surgical repair of a valve *-plasty:* surgical repair
vas/o	vessel; vas deferens; duct	**vas/o**/graphy (văs-ŎG-ră-fē): process of recording (an image of) a vessel *-graphy:* process of recording
ventricul/o	ventricle (of the heart or brain)	**ventricul**/ar (vĕn-TRĬK-ū-lăr): pertaining to a ventricle (chamber of the heart or brain) *-ar:* pertaining to
Suffixes		
-cardia	heart condition	tachy/**cardia** (tăk-ē-KĂR-dē-ă): rapid heart (beat) *tachy-:* rapid
-gram	record, writing	arteri/o/**gram** (ăr-TĒ-rē-ō-grăm): record of an artery *arteri/o:* artery *An arteriogram is used to visualize almost any artery, including those of the heart, head, kidneys, lungs, and other organs.*

-graph	instrument for recording	electr/o/cardi/o/**graph** (ē-lĕk-trō-KĂR-dē-ō-grăf): instrument for recording electrical (activity) of the heart
		  electr/o: electricity
		  cardi/o: heart

Element	Meaning	Word Analysis
-graphy	process of recording	angi/o/**graphy** (ăn-jē-ŎG-ră-fē): process of recording (an image of) a vessel *angi/o:* vessel (usually blood or lymph) ***Angiography is commonly used to identify atherosclerosis and diagnose heart and peripheral vascular disease.***
-stenosis	narrowing, stricture	aort/o/**stenosis** (ā-or-tō-stě-NŌ-sĭs): narrowing of the aorta *aort/o:* aorta

Prefixes		
brady-	slow	**brady/**cardia (brăd-ē-KĂR-dē-ă): slow heart (beat) *-cardia:* heart condition
endo-	in, within	**endo/**vascul/ar (ĕn-dō-VĂS-kū-lăr): pertaining to (the area) within a vessel *vascul:* vessel (usually blood or lymph) *-ar:* pertaining to
extra-	outside	**extra/**vascul/ar (ĕks-tră-VĂS-kū-lăr): pertaining to (the area) outside a vessel *vascul:* vessel (usually blood or lymph) *-ar:* pertaining to
peri-	around	**peri/**cardi/al (pĕr-ĭ-KĂR-dē-ăl): pertaining to (the area) around the heart *cardi:* heart *-al:* pertaining to
trans-	across	**trans/**sept/al (trăns-SĔP-tăl): across the septum *sept:* septum *-al:* pertaining to

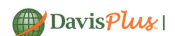 Visit the *Medical Terminology Systems* online resource center at Davis*Plus* for an audio exercise of the terms in this table. Other activities are also available to reinforce content.

 It is time to review medical word elements by completing Learning Activities 8–1 and 8–2.

Pathology

Many cardiac disorders, especially coronary artery disease, and valvular disorders are associated with a genetic predisposition. Thus, a complete history as well as a physical examination is essential in the diagnosis of cardiovascular disease. Although some of the most serious cardiovascular diseases have few signs and symptoms, when they occur they may include chest pain **(angina),** palpitations, breathing difficulties **(dyspnea),** cardiac irregularities **(arrhythmias),** and loss of consciousness **(syncope).** The location, duration, pattern of radiation, and severity of pain are important qualities in differentiating the various forms of cardiovascular disease. Because of the general nature of the signs and symptoms of cardiovascular disorders, invasive and noninvasive tests are usually required to confirm or rule out a suspected disease.

For diagnosis, treatment, and management of cardiovascular disorders, the medical services of a specialist may be warranted. **Cardiology** is the medical specialty concerned with disorders of the cardiovascular system. The physician who treats these disorders is called a **cardiologist.**

Arteriosclerosis

Arteriosclerosis is a progressive degenerative disease of arterial walls that causes them to become thickened and brittle. It is commonly caused by a buildup of a plaquelike substance composed of cholesterol, lipids, and cellular debris, called an *atheroma*, on the interior arterial wall. Over time, the atheroma hardens **(atherosclerosis)** and increases in size, causing the lumen of the artery to narrow. Atherosclerosis is the most common form of arteriosclerosis. In some instances, blood hemorrhages into the plaque and forms a clot called a thrombus. If the thrombus dislodges and travels though the vascular system, it is called an embolus **(plural, emboli).** Arterial emboli that completely block circulation cause localized tissue death, a condition called an **infarct.** A partial blocking of circulation causes localized tissue anemia, a condition called **ischemia.**

Major risk factors for developing arteriosclerosis include an elevated level of fatty substances in the blood **(hyperlipidemia),** age, family history, smoking, hypertension, and diabetes. Arteries commonly affected by arteriosclerosis include the coronary, carotid, cerebral, and femoral arteries and the aorta.

Treatment for arteriosclerosis varies depending on the location and symptoms. In one method, occluding material and plaque are removed from the innermost layer of the artery **(endarterectomy).** In this procedure, the surgeon opens the site and removes the plaque, thereby resuming normal blood flow. Physicians commonly use endarterectomy to treat carotid artery disease, peripheral artery disease, and diseases of the renal artery and aortic arch. (See Figure 8-6.)

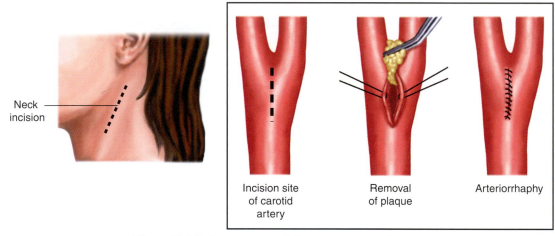

Neck incision

Incision site of carotid artery

Removal of plaque

Arteriorrhaphy

Figure 8-6 Endarterectomy of the common carotid artery.

Coronary Artery Disease

In order for the heart to function effectively, the myocardium must receive an adequate and uninterrupted supply of blood from the coronary arteries. Any disease that interferes with the ability of the coronary arteries to supply blood to the myocardium is called **coronary artery disease (CAD).** Arteriosclerosis is the major cause of CAD. The seriousness of the disease is dependant on the amount of occluding material blocking the coronary vessels. With a partial occlusion, the myocardium experiences ischemia. When the occlusion is total or almost total, the affected area experiences a myocardial infarction. (See Figure 8-7.) The clinical signs and symptoms of myocardial infarction (MI) typically include intense, suffocating pain, especially in the chest **(angina);** profuse sweating **(diaphoresis);** paleness **(pallor);** and labored breathing **(dyspnea).** Arrhythmia with an abnormally rapid heart rate **(tachycardia)** or an abnormally slow heart rate **(bradycardia)** may also accompany an MI.

As the heart muscle undergoes necrotic changes, it releases several highly specific cardiac enzymes. Their rapid elevation at predictable times following MI helps differentiate MI from pericarditis, abdominal aortic aneurysm (AAA), and acute pulmonary embolism.

When angina cannot be controlled with medication, surgical intervention may be necessary. Two types of angioplasty are commonly used to treat CAD, percutaneous transluminal coronary angioplasty (PTCA) and coronary artery bypass graft (CABG). In PTCA, a deflated balloon passes through a small incision in the skin and into the diseased blood vessel. When the balloon inflates, it presses the occluding material against the lumen walls to force open the channel. After

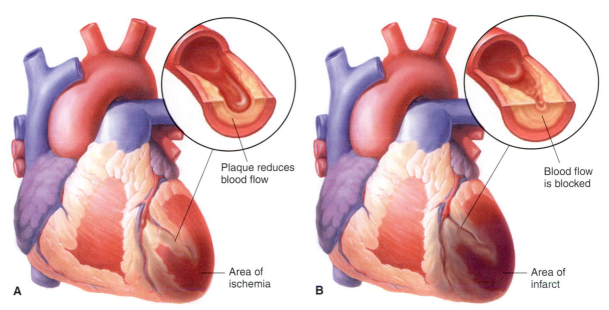

Plaque reduces
blood flow

Area of
ischemia

A

Blood flow
is blocked

Area of
infarct

B

Figure 8-7 Coronary artery occlusions. **(A)** Partial occlusion showing area of ischemia. **(B)** Complete occlusion showing a myocardial infarction.

the procedure, the physician deflates and removes the balloon. Sometimes, the physician will place a hollow, thin mesh tube called a **stent** on the balloon and position it against the artery wall. It remains in place after the balloon is deflated and the catheter removed to keep the artery open.

The more invasive procedure, CABG, involves rerouting blood around the occluded area using a vessel graft that bypasses the obstruction. One end of the graft vessel is sutured to the aorta and the other end is sutured to the coronary artery below the blocked area. This graft reestablishes blood flow to the heart muscle.

Endocarditis

Endocarditis is an inflammation of the inner lining of the heart and its valves. It may be noninfective in nature, caused by thrombi formation, or infective, caused by various microorganisms. Although the infecting organism can be viral or fungal, the usual culprit is a bacterium. Congenital valvular defects, scarlet fever, rheumatic fever, calcified bicuspid or aortic valves, mitral valve prolapse, and prosthetic valves are predisposing factors for developing endocarditis. Bacteria traveling in the bloodstream **(bacteremia)** may lodge in the weakened heart tissue and form small masses, called **vegetations,** composed of fibrin and platelets. Vegetations usually collect on the leaflets of the valves and their cords, causing a backflow of blood **(regurgitation)** or scarring. Vegetations may embolize and travel to the brain, lungs, kidneys, or spleen. Scarring of the valves may cause them to narrow **(stenosis)** or not close properly **(insufficiency).** (See Figure 8-8.) Although medications may prove helpful, if heart failure develops as a result of damaged heart valves, surgery may be the only treatment option. Whenever possible, the original valve is repaired. When the damage is extensive, a mechanical or bioprosthetic valve (replacement valve made of human or animal tissue) may be used.

Patients who are susceptible to endocarditis are given antibiotic treatment to protect against infection before invasive procedures **(prophylactic treatment).** Because many bacteria normally found in the mouth are also responsible for endocarditis, prophylactic treatment is essential for tooth removal, root canal procedures, and even routine cleaning in susceptible individuals.

Varicose Veins

Varicose veins are enlarged, engorged, twisted, superficial veins. They develop when the valves of the veins do not function properly **(incompetent)** and fail to prevent the backflow of blood.

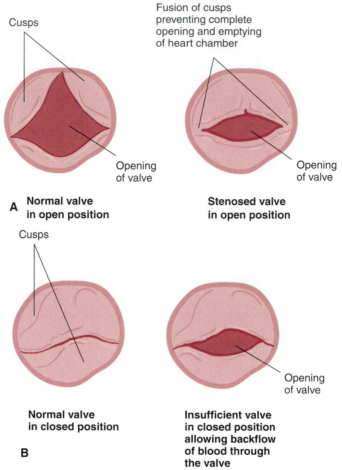

Figure 8-8 Openings of stenosed and insufficient valves compared with a normal valve. **(A)** Normal valve and a stenosed valve in open position. **(B)** Normal valve and an insufficient valve in closed position. From *Williams and Hopper: Understanding Medical-Surgical Nursing,* 4th ed. FA Davis, Philadelphia, 2011, p 430, with permission.

(See Figure 8-9.) Blood accumulates and the vein becomes engorged and distended. Excess fluid eventually seeps from the vein, causing **edema.** Varicose veins may develop in almost any part of the body, including the esophagus **(varices)** and rectum **(hemorrhoids),** but occur most commonly in the greater and lesser saphenous veins of the lower legs. Types of varicose veins include reticular veins, which appear as small blue veins seen through the skin, and "spider" veins **(telangiectases),** which look like short, fine lines, starburst clusters, or weblike mazes.

Varicose veins of the legs are not typically painful but may be unsightly in appearance. However, if open lesions, pain or vein inflammation **(phlebitis)** is present, treatment includes laser ablation, microphlebectomies, sclerotherapy and, occasionally, ligation and stripping for heavily damaged or diseased veins. The same methods are used as an elective procedure to improve the appearance of the legs. Treatment of mild cases of varicose veins includes use of elastic stockings and rest periods, during which the legs are elevated.

Oncology

Although rare, the most common primary tumor of the heart is composed of mucous connective tissue **(myxoma);** however, these tumors tend to be benign. Although some myxomas originate in the endocardium of the heart chambers, most arise in the left atrium. Occasionally, they impede mitral valve function and cause a decrease in exercise tolerance, dyspnea, fluid in the lungs

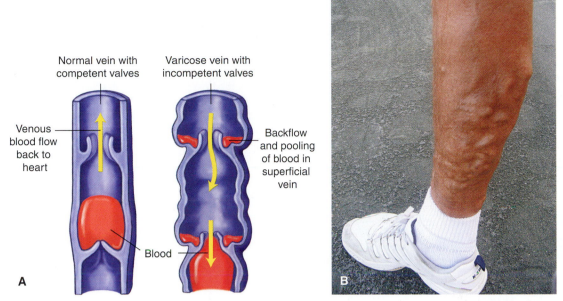

Figure 8-9 Healthy and unhealthy veins and valves. **(A)** Valve function in competent and incompetent valves. **(B)** Varicose veins.

(pulmonary edema), and systemic problems, including joint pain **(arthralgia),** malaise, and anemia. These tumors are usually identified and located by two-dimensional echocardiography. When present, they should be excised surgically.

Most malignant tumors of the heart are the result of a malignancy originating in another area of the body **(primary tumor)** that has spread **(metastasized)** to the heart. The most common type originates in a darkly pigmented mole or tumor **(malignant melanoma)** of the skin. Other primary sites of malignancy that metastasize to the heart are bone marrow and lymphatic tissue. Treatment of the metastatic tumor of the heart involves treating the primary tumor.

Diseases and Conditions

This section introduces diseases and conditions of the cardiovascular system with their meanings and pronunciations. Word analyses for selected terms are also provided.

Term	Definition
aneurysm ĂN-ū-rĭzm	Localized abnormal dilation of a vessel, usually an artery (See Figure 8-10.)

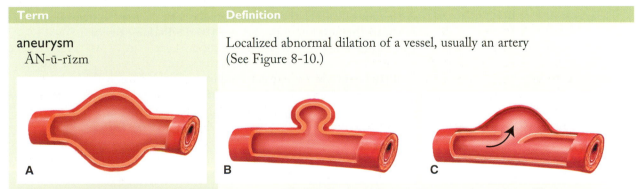

Figure 8-10 Types of aneurysms. **(A)** Fusiform, with dilation of the entire circumference of the artery. **(B)** Saccular, with dilation of one side of the artery. **(C)** Dissecting, in which a tear in the inner layer causes a cavity to form between the layers of the artery that fills with blood and expands with each heartbeat.

(continued)

Term	Definition
angina ĂN-jĭ-nă *angin:* choking pain *-a:* noun ending	Mild to severe suffocating pain that typically occurs in the chest and is caused by an inadequate blood flow to the myocardium; also called *angina pectoris* *Anginal pain can radiate down the left arm into the shoulder, neck, jaw, or back. (See Figure 8-11.) Women may experience anginal pain with different symptoms than those thought of as typical, including fatigue, nausea, and breathlessness. These atypical symptoms may be cardiac related and may require treatment.*

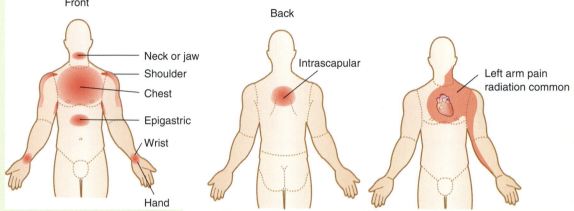

Figure 8-11 Common locations of anginal pain, which may vary in combination and intensity. From Williams and Hopper: *Understanding Medical-Surgical Nursing,* 4th ed. FA Davis, Philadelphia, 2011, p 464, with permission.

Term	Definition
arrhythmia ă-RĬTH-mē-ă	Irregularity in the rate or rhythm of the heart; also called *dysrhythmia*
bradycardia brăd-ē-KĂR-dē-ă *brady-:* slow *-cardia:* heart condition	Arrhythmia in which the heart beats abnormally slowly, usually fewer than 60 beats per minute in a resting adult
fibrillation fĭ-brĭl-Ā-shŭn	Arrhythmia in which there is an abnormally rapid, uncoordinated quivering of the myocardium that can affect the atria or the ventricles
heart block	Arrhythmia in which there is interference with the normal transmission of electric impulses from the SA node to the Purkinje fibers (See Figure 8-5.)
tachycardia tăk-ē-KĂR-dē-ă *tachy-:* rapid *-cardia:* heart condition	Arrhythmia in which there is a fast but regular rhythm, with the heart possibly beating up to 200 beats/minute *Patients with tachycardia may experience palpitations.*

Term	Definition
arteriosclerosis ăr-tē-rē-ō-sklĕ-RŌ-sĭs *arteri/o:* fatty plaque *-sclerosis:* abnormal condition of hardening	Hardening and narrowing of an artery along with the loss of its elasticity
atherosclerosis ăth-ĕr-ō-sklĕ-RŌ-sĭs *ather/o:* fatty plaque *-sclerosis:* abnormal condition of hardening	Form of arteriosclerosis characterized by the deposit of plaques containing cholesterol and lipids that narrows the lumen in the arteries
carotid artery disease kă-RŎT-ĭd	Narrowing of the carotid arteries, usually caused by atherosclerosis; may eventually lead to thrombus formation and stroke *Carotid artery disease can cause such symptoms as weakness on one side of the body, blurred vision, confusion, and memory loss. (See Figure 8-12.)*

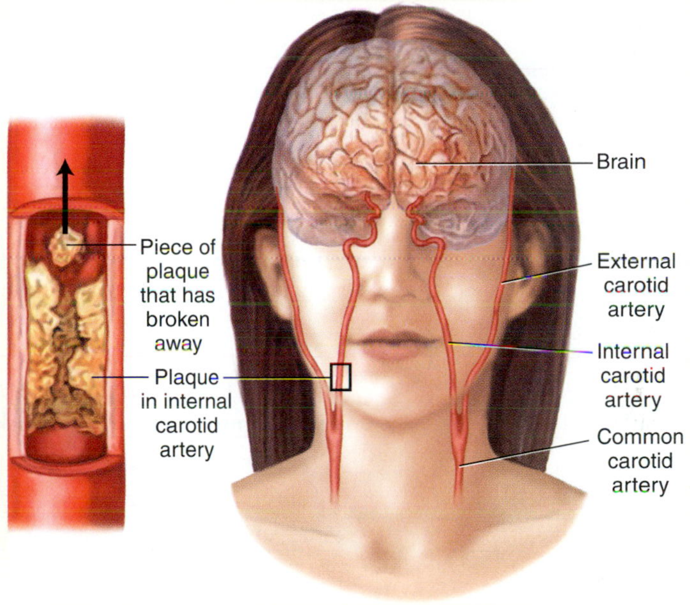

Figure 8-12 Atherosclerosis of the internal carotid artery.

Term	Definition
bruit BRWĒ	Soft blowing sound heard on auscultation, associated valvular action or with the movement of blood as it passes an obstruction or both; also called *murmur*
cardiomyopathy kăr-dē-ō-mī-ŎP-ă-thē *cardi/o:* heart *my/o:* muscle *-pathy:* disease	Disease or weakening of heart muscle that diminishes cardiac function *Causes of cardiomyopathy include viral or bacterial infections, metabolic disorders, or general systemic disease.*
coarctation kō-ărk-TĀ-shŭn	Narrowing of a vessel, especially the aorta

(continued)

Term	Definition
embolism ĔM-bō-lĭzm *embol:* embolus (plug) *-ism:* condition	Condition in which a mass (commonly a blood clot) becomes lodged in a blood vessel, obstructing blood flow
hyperlipidemia hī-pĕr-lĭp-ĭ-DĒ-mē-ă *hyper-:* excessive, above normal *lipid:* fat *-emia:* blood condition	Excessive amounts of lipids (cholesterol, phospholipids, and triglycerides) in the blood *Hyperlipidemia is associated with an increased risk of atherosclerosis.*
hypertension (HTN) hī-pĕr-TĔN-shŭn *hyper-:* excessive, above normal *-tension:* to stretch	Elevated blood pressure persistently higher than 140/90 mm Hg (See Table 8-1.)
hypotension hī-pō-TĔN-shŭn *hypo-:* under, below, deficient *-tension:* to stretch	Low blood pressure persistently lower than 90/60 mm Hg
infarction ĭn-FĂRK-shŭn	Localized tissue necrosis due to the cessation of blood supply
ischemia ĭs-KĒ-mē-ă	Local, temporary deficiency of blood supply to an organ or tissue due to circulatory obstruction
mitral valve prolapse (MVP) MĪ-trăl, PRŌ-lăps	Structural defect in which the mitral (bicuspid) valve leaflets prolapse into the left atrium during ventricular contraction (systole), resulting in incomplete closure and backflow of blood *Common signs and symptoms of MVP include a characteristic murmur heard on auscultation, and palpitations of the heart. Because of the possibility of valve infection, prophylactic treatment with antibiotics is advised before undergoing invasive procedures, such as dental work.*
palpitation păl-pĭ-TĀ-shŭn	Sensation of an irregular heartbeat, commonly described as pounding, racing, skipping a beat, or flutter
phlebitis flĕ-BĪ-tĭs *phleb:* vein *-itis:* inflammation	Inflammation of a deep or superficial vein of the arms or legs (more commonly the legs) *Thrombophlebitis, a more serious condition, is vein inflammation caused by the development of thrombi within the veins.*
syncope SĬN-kō-pē	Partial or complete loss of consciousness that is usually caused by a decreased supply of blood to the brain; also called *fainting*
thrombosis thrŏm-BŌ-sĭs *thromb:* blood clot *-osis:* abnormal condition; increase (used primarily with blood cells)	Abnormal condition in which a blood clot develops in a vessel and obstructs it at the site of its formation

Term	Definition
deep vein thrombosis (DVT) thrŏm-BŌ-sĭs *thromb:* blood clot *-osis:* abnormal condition; increase (used primarily with blood cells)	Blood clot that forms in the deep veins of the body, especially those in the legs or thighs; also called *deep venous thrombosis* (See Figure 8-13.) *In DVT, blood clots may break away from the vein wall and travel in the body, especially to the lungs.*

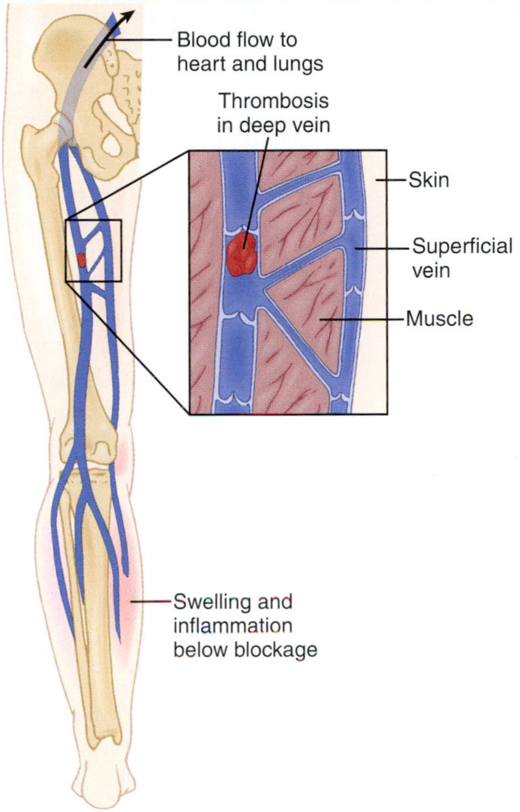

Figure 8-13 Deep vein thrombosis.

Table 8-1	**Hypertensive Blood Pressure Levels**		
Category	**Systolic**	**Diastolic**	
Normal	Less than 120 mm Hg	Less than 80 mm Hg	
Prehypertension (HTN)*	120 to 139 mm Hg	80 to 89 mm Hg	
Stage 1 HTN	140 to 159 mm Hg	90 to 99 mm Hg	
Stage 2 HTN	160 mm Hg or higher	100 mm Hg or higher	

*A blood pressure of 130/80 mm Hg or higher is considered hypertension in persons with diabetes and chronic kidney disease.

It is time to review pathology, diseases, and conditions by completing Learning Activity 8-3.

Medical, Surgical, and Diagnostic Procedures

This section introduces medical, surgical, and diagnostic procedures used to treat and diagnose cardiovascular disorders. Descriptions are provided as well as pronunciations and word analyses for selected terms.

Procedure	Description
Medical Procedures	
defibrillation dē-fĭb-rĭ-LĀ-shŭn	Electrical shock delivered randomly during the cardiac cycle to treat emergency life-threatening arrhythmias (See Figure 8-14.) *Defibrillation is performed when the patient does not have a pulse. Brief discharges of electricity are applied across the chest with a defibrillator to restore the normal heart rhythm.*
cardioversion KĂR-dē-ō-vĕr-zhŭn *cardi/o:* heart *-version:* turning	Defibrillation technique using low energy shocks to treat an arrhythmia (atrial fibrillation, atrial flutter, or ventricular tachycardia), and is usually synchronized with the large R waves of the ECG complex (see Figure 8-5) to restore normal heart rhythm *Cardioversion is used to treat arrhythmias that cannot be treated with antiarrhythmic drugs. This procedure is not typically performed in an emergency situation but in a hospital as an outpatient procedure.* **Figure 8-14** Placement of defibrillator pads on the chest. From Williams and Hopper: *Understanding Medical-Surgical Nursing,* 4th ed. FA Davis, Philadelphia, 2011, p 516, with permission.
sclerotherapy sklĕr-ō-THĔR-ă-pē *scler/o:* hardening; sclera (white of the eye) *-therapy:* treatment	Injection of a chemical irritant (sclerosing agent) into a vein to produce inflammation and fibrosis that destroys the lumen of the vein *Sclerotherapy is commonly performed to treat varicose veins and, sometimes, telangiectasias.*

Procedure	Description
thrombolysis thrŏm-BŎL-ĭ-sĭs *thromb/o:* blood clot *-lysis:* separation; destruction; loosening	Destruction of a blood clot using anticlotting agents called *clot-busters*, such as tissue plasminogen activator *Prompt thrombolysis can restore blood flow to tissue before irreversible damage occurs. However, many thrombolytic agents also pose a risk of hemorrhage.*

Surgical Procedures

Procedure	Description
angioplasty ĂN-jē-ō-plăs-tē *angi/o:* vessel (usually blood or lymph) *-plasty:* surgical repair	Any endovascular procedure that reopens narrowed blood vessels and restores forward blood flow *Most often angioplasties are performed on coronary, carotid, or peripheral arteries occluded by atherosclerosis.*
percutaneous transluminal coronary angioplasty (PTCA) pĕr-kū-TĀ-nē-ŭs trăns-LŪ-mĭ-năl KOR-ō-nă-rē ĂN-jē-ō-plăs-tē *per-:* through *cutane:* skin *-ous:* pertaining to	Angioplasty of the coronary arteries in which a balloon catheter is inserted through the skin into the right femoral artery and threaded to the site of the stenosis to enlarge the lumen of the artery and restore forward blood flow (See Figure 8-15.) *The inflated balloon dilates the narrowed vessel to restore forward blood flow. Then the balloon is deflated and the catheter is removed. Angioplasty can be done with or without the placement of a stent.*

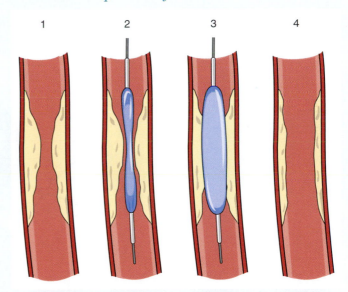

Figure 8-15 Angioplasty that opens an area of arterial blockage with a catheter that has an inflatable balloon. From Williams and Hopper: *Understanding Medical-Surgical Nursing,* 4th ed. FA Davis, Philadelphia, 2011, p 472, with permission.

(continued)

Procedure	Description
biopsy BĪ-ŏp-sē *bi:* life *-opsy:* view of	Removal of a small piece of tissue for diagnostic purposes
arterial ăr-TĒ-rē-ăl *arteri:* artery *-al:* pertaining to	Removal of a segment of an arterial vessel wall to confirm inflammation of the wall or arteritis, a type of vasculitis
catheter ablation KĂTH-ĕ-tĕr ăb-LĀ-shŭn	Treatment for cardiac arrhythmias; usually performed under fluoroscopic guidance *A special machine delivers energy through the catheter to tiny areas of the heart muscle that cause the abnormal heart rhythm. This energy removes the pathway of the abnormal rhythm.*
commissurotomy kŏm-ĭ-shūr-ŎT-ō-mē	Surgical separation of the leaflets of the mitral valve, which have fused together at their points of contact (commissures). *Many candidates for commissurotomy are now treated with balloon mitral valvuloplasty.*
coronary artery bypass graft (CABG) KOR-ō-nă-rē ĂR-tĕr-ē *coron:* heart *-ary:* pertaining to	Placement of a vessel graft from another part of the body to bypass the blocked part of a coronary artery and restore blood supply to the heart muscle (See Figure 8-16) **Figure 8-16** Coronary artery bypass graft (CABG) in which a blood vessel from the leg is used to reroute blood around a segment of the coronary artery that is narrowed by atherosclerosis. From Williams and Hopper: *Understanding Medical-Surgical Nursing,* 4th ed. FA Davis, Philadelphia, 2011, p 475, with permission.
embolectomy ĕm-bō-LĔK-tō-mē *embol:* plug *-ectomy:* excision, removal	Removal of an embolus *An embolus is any mass moving through the vascular channels, including air or a clump of bacteria or tissue. However, most emboli are blood clots.*

Procedure	Description
endarterectomy end-ăr-tĕr-ĔK-tō-mē *end-:* in, within *arter:* artery *-ectomy:* excision, removal	Removal of fatty plaque from the interior of an occluded vessel using a specially designed catheter fitted with a cutting or grinding device *Carotid endarterectomy is used to prevent stroke by correcting stenosis (narrowing) in the carotid arteries.*
automatic implantable cardioverter-defibrillator (AICD) insertion KĂR-dē-ō-vĕr-tĕr– dē-FĬB-rĭ-lā-tor	Implantation of a battery-powered device that monitors and automatically corrects ventricular tachycardia or fibrillation by sending electrical impulses to the heart in patients who are at risk of sudden cardiac death; also called *implantable cardioverter-defibrillator (ICD)* (See Figure 8-17.) *In ventricular fibrillation, the heart quivers rather than beats, and blood is not pumped to the brain. Unless treatment is received within 5 to 10 minutes, ventricular fibrillation causes death.* Electrodes inserted into cephalic vein leading to the heart AICD implanted under the skin Electrodes in heart Right atrium Right ventricle Lead delivering electrical shock Electrical charge **Figure 8-17** Automatic implantable cardioverter-defibrillator (AICD).
laser ablation LĀ-zĕr ăb-LĀ-shŭn	Procedure used to remove or treat varicose veins *In laser ablation, the laser's heat coagulates blood inside the vessel, causing it to collapse and seal. Later, the vessels dissolve within the body, becoming less visible, or disappear altogether.*
open heart surgery	Surgical procedure performed on or within the exposed heart, usually with the assistance of a heart–lung machine *During the operation, the heart–lung machine takes over circulation to allow surgery on the resting (nonbeating) heart. Types of open heart surgery include CABG, valve replacement, and heart transplant.*

(continued)

Procedure	Description
stent placement STĔNT	Placement of a mesh tube inserted into a natural passage or conduit in the body to prevent or counteract a disease-induced, localized flow constriction (See Figure 8-18.) *Stent placement may also refer to a tube used to temporarily hold such a natural conduit open to allow access for surgery.* **Figure 8-18** Insertion of a coronary artery stent. **(A)** Balloon catheter delivering the stent to the location of occlusion. **(B)** Inflation of the balloon, expanding the stent and compressing the occlusion. **(C)** Deflation and removal of the balloon, leaving the stent in the artery. From Williams and Hopper: *Understanding Medical-Surgical Nursing,* 4th ed. FA Davis, Philadelphia, 2011, p 472, with permission.
valvotomy văl-VŎT-ō-mē *valv/o:* valve *-tomy:* incision	Incision of a valve to increase the size of the opening; used in treating mitral stenosis

Procedure	Description
Diagnostic Procedures	
Clinical	
cardiac catheterization (CC) KĂR-dē-ăk kăth-ĕ-tĕr-ĭ-ZĀ-shŭn *cardi:* heart *-ac:* pertaining to	Passage of a catheter into the heart through a vein or artery to provide a comprehensive evaluation of the heart (See Figure 8-19.) *CC gathers information about the heart, including blood supply through the coronary arteries and blood flow and pressure through the heart's chambers, and enables blood sample collection and x-rays of the heart.*
electrophysiology study (EPS) ē-lĕk-trō-fĭz-ē-ŎL-ō-jē	Procedure used to determine the cause of life-threatening cardiac arrhythmias by mapping the heart's conduction system in a patient with an arrhythmia *While an EKG is performed, a specialized cardiac catheter sends out electrical impulses within the heart to stimulate rhythm disturbances; the response of the heart can be studied to pinpoint where the arrhythmia originates in the heart.*

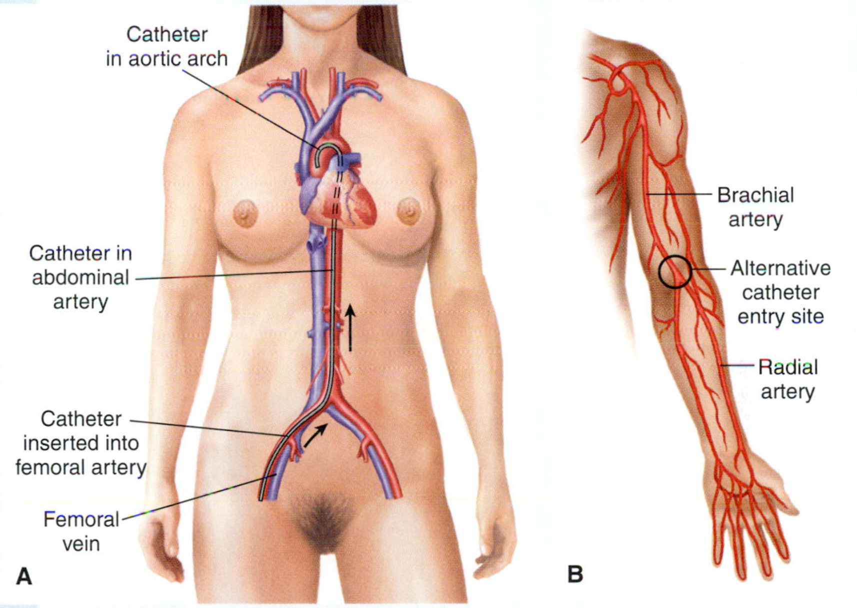

Figure 8-19 Cardiac catheterization. **(A)** Catheter insertion into a femoral vein or artery. **(B)** Catheter insertion into a brachial or radial artery.

(continued)

Procedure	Description
electrocardiography (ECG, EKG) ē-lĕk-trō-kăr-dē-ŎG-ră-fē *electr/o:* electricity *cardi/o:* heart *-graphy:* process of recording	Procedure that graphically records the spread of electrical excitation to different parts of the heart using small metal electrodes applied to the chest, arms, and legs *ECGs help diagnose abnormal heart rhythms and myocardial damage.*
Holter monitor test HŎL-tĕr	ECG taken with a small, portable recording system capable of storing up to 48 hours of ECG tracings; also called *event monitor test* (See Figure 8-20.) *Holter monitoring is particularly useful in obtaining a cardiac arrhythmia record that would be missed during an ECG of only a few minutes' duration.*
stress test	ECG taken under controlled exercise stress conditions (bicycle or treadmill) *A stress test may show abnormal ECG tracings that do not appear during an ECG taken when the patient is resting.*

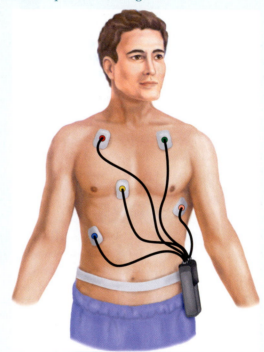

Figure 8-20 Holter monitor.

Laboratory

Procedure	Description
cardiac enzyme studies KĂR-dē-ăk ĔN-zīm *cardi:* heart *-ac:* pertaining to	Blood test that measures the presence and amount of cardiac enzymes in the blood, including troponin T, troponin I, and creatine kinase (CK-MB) *Cardiac enzymes are released into the bloodstream when heart muscle becomes damaged. Their presence and when they are first detected in a blood specimen help differentiate a myocardial infarction from other disorders that have similar signs and symptoms.*
lipid panel LĬP-ĭd	Series of blood tests (total cholesterol, high-density lipoprotein, low-density lipoprotein, and triglycerides) used to assess risk factors of ischemic heart disease

Procedure	Description
Imaging	
angiography ăn-jē-ŎG-ră-fē *angi/o:* vessel (usually blood or lymph) *-graphy:* process of recording	Radiographic image (angiogram) of the inside of a blood vessel after injection of a contrast medium; also called *arteriography* *Angiography is used to diagnose cardiovascular disease, especially blockages, narrowed areas, and aneurysms.*
aortography ā-or-TŎG-ră-fē *aort/o:* aorta *-graphy:* process of recording	Angiography of the aorta and its branches after injection of a contrast medium *Aortography is used to diagnose aortic insufficiency.*
coronary KOR-ō-nă-rē *coron:* heart *-ary:* pertaining to	Angiography that is used to determine the degree of stenosis or obstruction of the arteries that supply blood to the heart *In coronary angiography, the contrast medium is administered through a catheter inserted into the femoral artery and threaded to the aorta. This procedure is usually done along with cardiac catheterization.*
magnetic resonance imaging (MRI) măg-NĔT-ĭk RĔZ-ĕn-ăns ĬM-ĭj-ĭng	Noninvasive technique that uses radio waves and a strong magnetic field rather than an x-ray beam to produce highly detailed, multiplanar, cross-sectional views of soft tissues
cardiac KĂR-dē-ăk *cardi:* heart *-ac:* pertaining to	Specialized MRI that provides information on both static and moving images of the heart, including blood flow and velocity
magnetic resonance angiography (MRA) măg-NĔT-ĭk RĔZ-ĕn-ăns ăn-jē-ŎG-ră-fē *angi/o:* vessel (usually blood or lymph *-graphy:* process of recording	Type of MRI scan that uses a magnetic field and radio waves to provide detailed images of blood vessels *Unlike angiography, MRA detects blood flow, the condition of blood vessel walls, and blockages without using a contrast medium.*
multiple-gated acquisition (MUGA) scan	Nuclear procedure that uses radioactive tracers to detect how well the heart walls move as they contract and calculates the ejection fraction rate (amount of blood the ventricle can pump out in one contraction) *The ejection fraction rate is the most accurate predictor of overall heart function. The gamma camera is coordinated (gated) with the patient's ECG.*
single-photon emission computed tomography (SPECT) tō-MŎG-ră-fē *tom/o:* to cut *-graphy:* process of recording	MUGA scan of the heart in which the gamma camera moves in a circle around the patient to create individual images as "slices" of the heart (tomography)

(continued)

Procedure	Description
nuclear perfusion study pĕr-FŪ-zhŭn	Test used in conjunction with a stress test to detect the presence of coronary artery disease (CAD) that is causing partial obstruction of the coronary arteries; also called *thallium scan* or *cardiolite scan* *This test involves administration of a radioisotope and compares a resting image and one taken at the height of exercise. An area not receiving sufficient blood flow, called a* cold spot, *shows decreased uptake of the isotope.*
ultrasonography (US) ŭl-trǎ-sŏn-ŎG-rǎ-fē *ultra-:* excess, beyond *son/o:* sound *-graphy:* process of recording	High-frequency sound waves (ultrasound) are directed at soft tissue and reflected as "echoes" to produce an image on a monitor of an internal body structure; also called ultrasound, sonography, and echo *US is a noninvasive procedure that does not require a contrast medium. It is used to detect diseases and abnormalities in the cardiovascular system.*
Doppler DŎP-lĕr	Ultrasonography used to assess blood flow through blood vessels and the heart *Carotid Doppler ultrasound uses reflected sound waves to create detailed images of the inside of the carotid arteries in the neck to check for blood flow problems caused by blood clots or plaque on the walls of the arteries. The test can also detect tears in the carotid artery, which can interfere with blood flow. (See Figure 8-21.)*

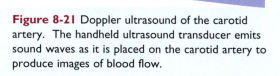

Figure 8-21 Doppler ultrasound of the carotid artery. The handheld ultrasound transducer emits sound waves as it is placed on the carotid artery to produce images of blood flow.

Procedure	Description

echocardiography (ECHO)
   ĕk-ō-kăr-dē-ŎG-rǎ-fē
   echo-: repeated sound
   cardi/o: heart
   -graphy: process of recording
	Ultrasonography that is used to visualize internal cardiac structures, produce images of the heart, and assess cardiac output
	Echocardiography involves placement of a transducer on the chest to direct ultra-high-frequency sound waves toward cardiac structures. Reflected echoes are then converted to electrical impulses and displayed on a screen.

venography
vē-NŎG-rǎ-fē
   ven/o: vein
   -graphy: process of recording
	Radiography of a vein after injection of a contrast medium to detect incomplete filling of a vein, indicating an obstruction
	Venography is used primarily to locate blood clots in veins of the leg.

Pharmacology

A healthy, functional cardiovascular system ensures adequate blood circulation and efficient delivery of oxygen and nutrients to all parts of the body. When any part of the cardiovascular system malfunctions or becomes diseased, drug therapy plays an integral role in establishing and maintaining perfusion and homeostasis.

Medications treat a variety of cardiovascular conditions, including angina pectoris, myocardial infarction, heart failure (HF), arrhythmias, hypertension, hyperlipidemia, and vascular disorders. (See Table 8-2.) Many cardiovascular drugs treat multiple problems simultaneously.

Table 8-2	Drugs Used to Treat Cardiovascular Disorders	
This table lists common drug classifications used to treat cardiovascular disorders, their therapeutic actions, and selected generic and trade names.		
Classification	**Therapeutic Action**	**Generic and *Trade* Names**
angiotensin-converting enzyme (ACE) inhibitors ăn-jē-ō-TĚN-sĭn ĚN-zīm ĭn-HĬB-ĭ-tŏrs	Lower blood pressure by inhibiting the conversion of angiotensin I (an inactive enzyme) to angiotensin II (a potent vasoconstrictor) *ACE inhibitors treat hypertension alone or with other agents and aid in the management of heart failure.*	**benazepril** bĕn-Ā-ză-prĭl *Lotensin* **captopril** KĂP-tō-prĭl *Capoten*
antiarrhythmics ăn-tē-ă-RĬTH-mĭks	Prevent, alleviate, or correct cardiac arrhythmias (dysrhythmias) by stabilizing the electrical conduction of the heart *Antiarrhythmics are used to treat atrial and ventricular dysrhythmias.*	**flecainide** flĕ-KĀ-nīd *Tambocor* **digoxin** dī-JŎX-ĭn *Lanoxin*
beta-blockers BĀ-tă	Block the effect of adrenaline, which slows nerve pulses through the heart, causing a decrease in heart rate *Beta-blockers are prescribed for hypertension, angina, and arrhythmias (dysrhythmias).*	**atenolol** ă-TĚN-ō-lŏl *Tenormin* **metoprolol** mĕ-TŌ-prō-lŏl *Lopressor, Toprol-XL*
calcium channel blockers KĂL-sē-ŭm	Block movement of calcium (required for blood vessel contraction) into myocardial cells and arterial walls, causing heart rate and blood pressure to decrease *Calcium channel blockers are used to treat angina pectoris, hypertension, arrhythmias, and heart failure.*	**amlodipine** ăm-LŌ-dĭ-pēn *Norvasc* **diltiazem** dĭl-TĪ-ă-zĕm *Cardizem CD* **nifedipine** nī-FĚD-ĭ-pēn *Adalat CC, Procardia*
diuretics dī-ū-RĚT-ĭks	Act on kidneys to increase excretion of water and sodium *Diuretics reduce fluid buildup in the body, including fluid in the lungs, a common symptom of heart failure. Diuretics are also used to treat hypertension.*	**furosemide** fū-RŌ-sĕ-mīd *Lasix* **bumetanide** bū-MĚT-ă-nīd *Bumex*

(continued)

Table 8-2	Drugs Used to Treat Cardiovascular Disorders—cont'd	
Classification	**Therapeutic Action**	**Generic and *Trade* Names**
nitrates NĪ-trāts	Dilate blood vessels of the heart, causing an increase in the amount of oxygen delivered to the myocardium, and widen blood vessels of the body, allowing more blood flow to the heart *Nitrates can be administered in several ways: sublingually as a spray or tablet, orally as a tablet, transdermally as a patch, topically as an ointment, or intravenously in an emergency setting.*	**nitroglycerin** nī-trō-GLĬS-ĕr-ĭn *Nitrolingual, Nitrogard, Nitrostat* **bumetanide** bu-MĔT-ă-nīd *Bumex*
statins STĂ-tĭnz	Lower cholesterol in the blood and reduce its production in the liver by blocking the enzyme that produces it *Combination of Vytorin, a statin drug, with a cholesterol absorption inhibitor not only lowers cholesterol in the blood and reduces its production in the liver, but also decreases absorption of dietary cholesterol from the intestine. Hypercholesterolemia is a major factor in development of heart disease.*	**atorvastatin** ăh-tor-vă-STĂ-tĭn *Lipitor* **simvastatin** SĬM-vă-stă-tĭn *Zocor* **simvastatin and ezetimibe** SĬM-vă-stă-tĭn, ĕ-ZĔ-tĭ-mīb *Vytorin*
vasodilators văs-ō-DĪ-l ā-torz	Reduce blood pressure by relaxing the smooth muscle in blood vessels, particularly in the large arteries, arterioles, and large veins, which decreases vascular resistance *Vasodilators are used to treat hypertension, heart failure, and angina.*	**hydralazine** hī-DRĂL-ă-zēn *Apresoline* **nitroprusside** nī-trō-PRŬS-īd *Nitropress*

Abbreviations

This section introduces cardiovascular-related abbreviations and their meanings.

Abbreviation	Meaning	Abbreviation	Meaning
AAA	abdominal aortic aneurysm	EPS	electrophysiology studies
ACE	angiotensin-converting enzyme (inhibitor)	HDL	high-density lipoprotein
AFib	atrial fibrillation	HF	heart failure
AICD	automatic implantable cardioverter-defibrillator	HTN	hypertension
AS	aortic stenosis	ICD	implantable cardioverter-defibrillator
ASHD	arteriosclerotic heart disease	LA	left atrium
AV	atrioventricular; arteriovenous	LDL	low-density lipoprotein
BP, B/P	blood pressure	LV	left ventricle
CA	cancer; cardiac arrest; chronological age	MI	myocardial infarction
CABG	coronary artery bypass graft	MRA	magnetic resonance angiogram, magnetic resonance angiography
CAD	coronary artery disease	MRI	magnetic resonance imaging
CC	cardiac catheterization	MUGA scan	multiple-gated acquisition scan
CHD	coronary heart disease	MVP	mitral valve prolapse
Chol	cholesterol	O_2	oxygen
CK	creatine kinase (cardiac enzyme); conductive keratoplasty	NSR	normal sinus rhythm
CO_2	carbon dioxide	PTCA	percutaneous transluminal coronary angioplasty
CPR	cardiopulmonary resuscitation	RA	right atrium
DVT	deep vein thrombosis, deep venous thrombosis	RV	residual volume; right ventricle
ECG, EKG	electrocardiogram, electrocardiography	SA, S-A	sinoatrial
ECHO	echocardiogram, echocardiography; echoencephalogram, echoencephalography	US	ultrasound

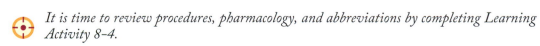 *It is time to review procedures, pharmacology, and abbreviations by completing Learning Activity 8–4.*

LEARNING ACTIVITIES

The following activities provide review of the cardiovascular system terms introduced in this chapter. Complete each activity and review your answers to evaluate your understanding of the chapter.

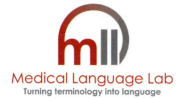

Medical Language Lab
Turning terminology into language

Visit the Medical Language Lab at the web site: medicallanguagelab.com. Use it to enhance your study and reinforcement of this chapter with the flash-card activity. We recommend you complete the flash-card activity before starting Learning Activities 8-1 and 8-2.

Learning Activity 8-1

Combining Forms, Suffixes, and Prefixes

Use the elements listed in the table to build medical words. You may use the elements more than once.

Combining Forms		Suffixes		Prefixes
aneurysm/o	scler/o	-ar	-megaly	a-
aort/o	thromb/o	-dynia	-oma	brady-
arteri/o	valvul/o	-ectasis	-osis	endo-
ather/o	vascul/o	-ectomy	-plasty	tachy-
cardi/o		-gram	-rrhexis	
phleb/o		-ia	-therapy	
rrhythm/o		-lysis		

1. enlargement of the heart _____
2. tumor composed of fatty plaque _____
3. rupture of an artery _____
4. pertaining to within a vessel _____
5. condition of a rapid heart (rate) _____
6. dilation or expansion of a vein _____
7. record of the aorta _____
8. surgical repair of a valve _____
9. abnormal condition of hardening _____
10. treatment that hardens (a varicose vein) _____
11. destruction of a blood clot _____
12. condition (of the heart being) without a rhythm _____
13. condition of a slow heart (rate) _____
14. pain in the heart _____
15. excision of an aneurysm _____

✓ *Check your answers in Appendix A. Review any material that you did not answer correctly.*

Correct Answers _____ X 6.67 = _____ % Score

Learning Activity 8-2
Building Medical Words

Use *ather/o* (fatty plaque) to build words that mean:

1. tumor of fatty plaque _____
2. abnormal condition of fatty plaque hardening _____

Use *phleb/o* (vein) to build words that mean:

3. inflammation of a vein (wall) _____
4. abnormal condition of a blood clot in a vein _____

Use *ven/o* (vein) to build words that mean:

5. pertaining to a vein _____
6. spasm of a vein _____

Use *cardi/o* (heart) to build words that mean:

7. specialist in the study of the heart _____
8. rupture of the heart _____
9. poisonous to the heart _____
10. enlargement of the heart _____

Use *angi/o* (vessel) to build words that mean:

11. softening of a vessel (wall) _____
12. tumor of a vessel _____

Use *thromb/o* (blood clot) to build words that mean:

13. beginning or formation of a blood clot _____
14. abnormal condition of a blood clot _____

Use *aort/o* (heart) to build words that mean:

15. abnormal condition of narrowing or stricture of the aorta _____
16. process of recording the aorta _____

Build surgical words that mean:

17. puncture of the heart _____
18. suture of an artery _____
19. removal of an embolus _____
20. separation, destruction, or loosening of a blood clot _____

Check your answers in Appendix A. Review material that you did not answer correctly.

Correct Answers _____ X 5 = _____ % Score

Learning Activity 8-3

Pathology, Diseases, and Conditions

Match the following terms with the definitions in the numbered list.

aneurysm	bradycardia	embolism	insufficiency	stenosis
angina	bruit	hyperlipidemia	ischemia	tachycardia
arrhythmia	coarctation	hypertension	palpitation	thrombosis
arteriosclerosis	diaphoresis	infarction	regurgitation	varices

1. area of tissue that undergoes necrosis _____

2. pain, usually in the chest, that is associated with lack of oxygen to the myocardium _____

3. failure of a valve to close completely _____

4. abnormally rapid heart rate _____

5. varicose veins of the esophagus _____

6. soft, blowing sound heard on auscultation; murmur _____

7. abnormally slow heart rate _____

8. awareness of an irregular heartbeat _____

9. abnormal condition in which a blood clot develops in a blood vessel _____

10. localized abnormal dilation of a vessel _____

11. condition in which a mass (usually blood clot) blocks a blood vessel _____

12. inability of the heart to maintain a normal sinus rhythm _____

13. backflow of blood due to valve failure _____

14. profuse sweating _____

15. disorder commonly caused by the buildup of fatty plaque on an artery wall _____

16. persistent elevated blood pressure _____

17. excessive amounts of lipids in the blood _____

18. narrowing of a vessel, especially the aorta _____

19. deficiency of blood supply due to circulatory obstruction _____

20. narrowing of a valve _____

Check your answers in Appendix A. Review any material that you did not answer correctly.

Correct Answers _____ X 5 = _____ % Score

Learning Activity 8-4

Procedures, Pharmacology, and Abbreviations

Match the following terms with the definitions in the numbered list.

angioplasty	commissurotomy	Holter monitor test	statins
biopsy	diuretics	ICD insertion	stent placement
CABG	Doppler	nitrates	stress test
cardiac enzyme studies	echocardiography	PTCA	thrombolysis
catheter ablation	endarterectomy	sclerotherapy	valvotomy

1. 24-hour ECG tracing taken with a small, portable recording system _____

2. US diagnostic test used to visualize internal cardiac structures _____

3. incision to increase the size of the opening of the mitral valve _____

4. agents used to treat angina _____

5. drugs that have powerful lipid-lowering properties _____

6. increase urine output; used to treat edema, hypertension, and heart failure _____

7. provides levels of troponin T, troponin I, and creatinine kinase in the blood _____

8. ultrasound procedure that measures blood flow through the heart and vessels _____

9. ECG taken under controlled exercise stress conditions _____

10. treatment of cardiac arrhythmias in which energy is transmitted through a catheter to remove the pathway of an abnormal heart rhythm _____

11. surgical separation of the leaflets of the mitral valve _____

12. removal of a small segment of tissue for diagnostic purposes _____

13. implanting of a device that corrects ventricular tachycardia or fibrillation _____

14. insertion of a device that holds open tubular structures _____

15. procedure that alters a vessel through surgery or dilation _____

16. treatment of a varicose vein using a chemical irritant _____

17. surgery that creates a bypass around a blocked segment of a coronary artery _____

18. removal of occluding material from the interior of an artery _____

19. dilation of an occluded vessel using a balloon catheter passed through the skin _____

20. destruction of a blood clot _____

 Check your answers in Appendix A. Review any material that you did not answer correctly.

Correct Answers _____ X 5 = _____ % Score

Learning Activity 8-5
Medical Scenarios

To construct chart notes, replace the italicized terms in each of the two scenarios with one of the medical terms listed below.

angina pectoris	edema	myocardial infarction
angioplasty	hypertension	palpitations
catheter	ischemia	stent
diaphoresis		

Mr. J. presented to the emergency room with complaints of (1) *chest pains*, (2) *profuse sweating*, and (3) *an awareness of his heart skipping beats*. He takes medication for (4) *persistent high blood pressure*. He also takes diuretics to promote urine excretion and to control fluid retention that is causing (5) *puffiness* in his ankles and legs.

1. _____
2. _____
3. _____
4. _____
5. _____

Mrs. R. has a family history of coronary artery disease. Her 60-year-old uncle died of a (6) *heart attack* two years ago. Last year, her father was diagnosed with an occlusion of the coronary artery. He was also diagnosed with (7) *decreased blood flow* of the coronary vessels. He was admitted to the hospital for a (8) *surgical repair of the vessel*. During this surgery, the surgeon threaded a (9) *tube* with a deflated balloon into the blocked vessel and used it to press the fatty plaque against the arterial walls. The surgeon then inserted an (10) *expandable mesh tube* to keep the artery open after surgery.

6. _____
7. _____
8. _____
9. _____
10. _____

Check your answers in Appendix A. Review any material that you did not answer correctly.

Correct Answers _____ X 10 = _____ % Score

MEDICAL RECORD ACTIVITIES

The two medical records included in the following activities use common clinical scenarios to show how medical terminology is used to document patient care. Complete the terminology and analysis sections for each activity to help you recognize and understand terms related to the cardiovascular system.

Medical Record Activity 8-1
Chart Note: Acute Myocardial Infarction

Terminology

Terms listed in the following table are taken from *Chart Note: Acute Myocardial Infarction* that follows. Use a medical dictionary such as *Taber's Cyclopedic Medical Dictionary;* the appendices of *Systems,* 7th ed.; or other resources to define each term. Then review the pronunciations for each term and practice by reading the medical record aloud.

Term	Definition
acute	
cardiac enzymes KĂR-dē-ăk ĔN-zīmz	
CCU	
ECG	
heparin HĔP-ă-rĭn	
infarction ĭn-FĂRK-shŭn	
inferior	
ischemia ĭs-KĒ-mē-ă	
lateral LĂT-ĕr-ăl	
MI	
myocardial mī-ō-KĂR-dē-ăl	

(continued)

Term	Definition
partial thromboplastin time thrŏm-bō-PLĂS-tĭn	
streptokinase strĕp-tō-KĪ-nās	
substernal sŭb-STĔR-năl	

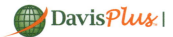 **DavisPlus** | Visit the *Medical Terminology Systems* online resource center at Davis*Plus*. Use it to practice pronunciation and reinforce the meanings of the terms in this medical report.

CHART NOTE: ACUTE MYOCARDIAL INFARCTION

Gately, Mary   **March 15, 20xx**

PRESENT ILLNESS: Patient is a 68-year-old woman hospitalized for acute anterior myocardial infarction. She has a history of sudden onset of chest pain. Approximately 2 hours before hospitalization, she had severe substernal pain with radiation to the back. ECG showed evidence of abnormalities. She was given streptokinase and treated with heparin at 800 units per hour. She will be evaluated with a partial thromboplastin time and cardiac enzymes in the morning.

PAST HISTORY: Patient was seen in 20xx, with a history of an inferior MI in 19xx, but she was stable and underwent a treadmill test. Test results showed no ischemia and she had no chest pain. Her records confirmed an MI with enzyme elevation and evidence of a previous inferior MI.

IMPRESSION: Acute lateral anterior myocardial infarction and a previous healed inferior myocardial infarction.

PLAN: At this time the patient is stable, is in the CCU, and will be given appropriate follow-up and supportive care.

Juan Perez, MD
Juan Perez, MD

D: 03-15-20xx
T: 03-15-20xx

bg

Analysis

Review the medical record *Chart Note: Acute Myocardial Infarction* to answer the following questions.

1. How long had the patient experienced chest pain before she was seen in the hospital?

_____

2. Did the patient have a previous history of chest pain?

_____

3. Initially, what medications were administered to stabilize the patient?

_____

4. What two laboratory tests will be used to evaluate the patient?

_____

5. During the current admission, what part of the heart was damaged?

_____

6. Was the location of damage to the heart for this admission the same as for the initial MI?

_____

Operative Report: Right Temporal Artery Biopsy

Terminology

Terms listed in the following table are taken from *Operative Report: Right Temporal Artery Biopsy* that follows. Use a medical dictionary such as *Taber's Cyclopedic Medical Dictionary;* the appendices of *Systems,* 7th ed.; or other resources to define each term. Then review the pronunciations for each term and practice by reading the medical record aloud.

Term	Definition
arteritis ăr-tĕ-RĪ-tĭs	
Betadine BĂ-tă-dīn	
biopsy BĪ-ŏp-sē	
dissected dī-SĔKT-ĕd	
distally DĬS-tă-lē	
incised ĭn-SĪZD	
IV	
ligated LĪ-gā-tĕd	
palpable PĂL-pă-b'l	
preauricular prē-aw-RĬK-ū-lăr	
proximally PRŎK-sĭ-mă-lē	
superficial fascia soo-pĕr-FĬSH-ăl FĂSH-ē-ă	
supine sū-PĪN	

Term	Definition
temporal TĔM-por-ăl	
Xylocaine ZĪ-lō-kăn	

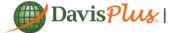 | Visit the *Medical Terminology Systems* online resource center at Davis*Plus*. Use it to practice pronunciation and reinforce the meanings of the terms in this medical report.

OPERATIVE REPORT: RIGHT TEMPORAL ARTERY BIOPSY

General Hospital

1511 Ninth Avenue ■■ Sun City, USA 12345 ■■ (555) 802-1887

OPERATIVE REPORT

Date: May 14, 20xx   Physician: Dante Riox, MD
Patient: Gonzolez, Roberto   Room: 703

PREOPERATIVE DIAGNOSIS: Rule out right temporal arteritis.

POSTOPERATIVE DIAGNOSIS: Rule out right temporal arteritis.

PROCEDURE: Right temporal artery biopsy.

SPECIMEN: 1.5-cm segment of right temporal artery.

ESTIMATED BLOOD LOSS: Nil.

COMPLICATIONS: None.

TIME UNDER SEDATION: 25 minutes.

PROCEDURE AND FINDINGS: Informed consent was obtained. Patient was taken to the surgical suite and placed in the supine position. IV sedation was administered. Patient was turned to his left side and the preauricular area was prepped for surgery using Betadine. Having been draped in sterile fashion, 1% Xylocaine was infiltrated along the palpable temporal artery and a vertical incision was made. Dissection was carried down through the subcutaneous tissue and superficial fascia, which was incised. The temporal artery was located and dissected proximally and distally. Then the artery was ligated with 6-0 Vicryl proximally and distally and a large segment of approximately 1.5 cm was removed. The specimen was sent to the pathology laboratory and then the superficial fascia was closed with interrupted stitches of 6-0 Vicryl and the skin was closed with interrupted stitches of 6-0 Prolene. A sterile dressing was applied. Patient tolerated the procedure well and was transferred to the postanesthesia care unit in stable condition.

Dante Riox, MD
Dante Riox, MD

dr:bg

D: 5-14-20xx; T: 5-14-20xx

Analysis

Review the medical record *Operative Report: Right Temporal Artery Biopsy* to answer the following questions.

1. Why was the right temporal artery biopsied?

_____

2. In what position was the patient placed?

_____

3. What was the incision area?

_____

4. How was the temporal artery located for administration of Xylocaine?

_____

5. How was the dissection carried out?

_____

6. What was the size of the specimen?

_____

Blood, Lymph, and Immune Systems

CHAPTER

9

Chapter Outline

Objectives

Upon completion of this chapter, you will be able to:

- Identify and describe the components of blood.
- Locate and identify the structures associated with the lymph system.
- List the cells associated with the acquired immune response and describe their function.
- Describe the functional relationships among the blood, lymph, and immune systems and other body systems.
- Pronounce, spell, and build words related to the blood, lymph, and immune systems.
- Describe diseases, conditions, and procedures related to the blood, lymph, and immune systems.
- Explain pharmacology related to the treatment of blood, lymph, and immune disorders.
- Demonstrate your knowledge of this chapter by completing the learning and medical record activities.

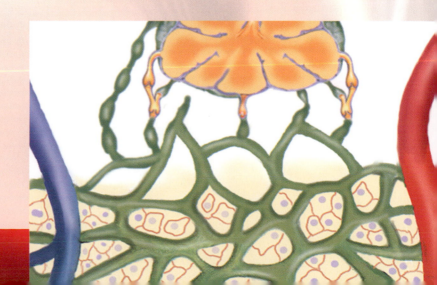

Anatomy and Physiology

The blood, lymph, and immune systems share common cells, structures, and functions. Blood is a body tissue composed of cells suspended in a liquid medium called plasma. Two important blood cells, monocytes and lymphocytes, provide protection to the body against invasion by disease-causing organisms and other harmful substances. As such, these two blood cells are considered part of the immune system. As blood circulates through capillaries, a small quantity of plasma exits the vascular system and enters interstitial spaces. Plasma, now in the form of interstitial fluid, exchanges its beneficial products for cellular waste found in the surrounding tissues. After the exchange of products, some interstitial fluid enters an extensive network of lymph vessels as lymph and becomes part of the lymph system. Lymph vessels return lymph to the vascular system for reintegration into blood as plasma. Although blood, lymph, and immune systems are discussed separately, their functions and structures overlap.

Anatomy and Physiology Key Terms

This section introduces important blood, lymph, and immune system terms and their definitions. Word analyses for selected terms are also provided.

Term	Definition
antibody (Ab) ĂN-tĭ-bŏd-ē	Protective protein produced by B lymphocytes in response to the presence of a foreign substance called an *antigen* *Antibodies are also known as **immunoglobulins (Igs)**.*
antigen ĂN-tĭ-jĕn	Substance, recognized as harmful to the host, that stimulates formation of antibodies in an immunocompetent individual
bile pigment BĪL	Substance derived from the breakdown of hemoglobin and excreted by the liver *Interference with the excretion of bile may lead to jaundice.*
cytokine SĪ-tō-kīn	Chemical substance produced by certain cells that initiates, inhibits, increases, or decreases activity in other cells *Cytokines are important chemical communicators in the immune response, regulating many activities associated with immunity and inflammation.*
immunocompetent ĭm-ū-nō-KŎM-pĕ-tĕnt	Ability to develop an immune response or recognize antigens and respond to them
natural killer (NK) cells	Specialized lymphocytes that kill abnormal cells by releasing chemicals that destroy the cell membrane, causing its intercellular fluids to leak out *NK cells destroy virally infected cells and tumor cells.*

Pronunciation Help	Long Sound	ā — rate	ē — rebirth	ī — isle	ō — over	ū — unite
	Short Sound	ă — alone	ĕ — ever	ĭ — it	ŏ — not	ŭ — cut

Blood

Although blood makes up only about 8% of all body tissues, it is essential to life. Blood is connective tissue composed of a liquid medium called **plasma** in which solid components are suspended. The solid components of blood include:

- red blood cells **(erythrocytes)**
- white blood cells **(leukocytes)**
- platelets **(thrombocytes).** (See Figure 9-1.)

Blood cells have a finite life span; the body must continually replace them. The body produces millions of them every second to replace those that are destroyed or worn out. In adults, blood cells are formed in the bone marrow of the skull, ribs, sternum, vertebrae, pelvis, and ends of the long bones of the arms and legs. The stem cells in the bone marrow give rise to embryonic **(blastic)** forms of all blood cell types. In the embryonic stages, monocytes and lymphocytes migrate to the lymph system for maturation and specialization. All other embryonic cells remain in the bone marrow to complete their development. Once blood cells mature, they enter the circulatory system. The development of blood cells to their mature form is called **hematopoiesis** or **hemopoiesis.** (See Figure 9-2.)

Red Blood Cells

Red blood cells (RBCs), or **erythrocytes,** transport oxygen (O_2) and carbon dioxide (CO_2). They are the most numerous of the circulating blood cells. During red cell development **(erythropoiesis),** RBCs decrease in size and, just before reaching maturity, extrude their nuclei. They also develop a specialized iron-containing compound called **hemoglobin (Hb, Hgb)** that gives them their red color. Hemoglobin carries oxygen to body tissues and exchanges it for carbon dioxide. When mature, RBCs are shaped like biconcave disks.

RBCs live about 120 days and then rupture, releasing hemoglobin and cell fragments. Hemoglobin breaks down into an iron compound called **hemosiderin** and several bile pigments. Most hemosiderin returns to the bone marrow and is reused in a different form to manufacture new blood cells. The liver eventually excretes bile pigments.

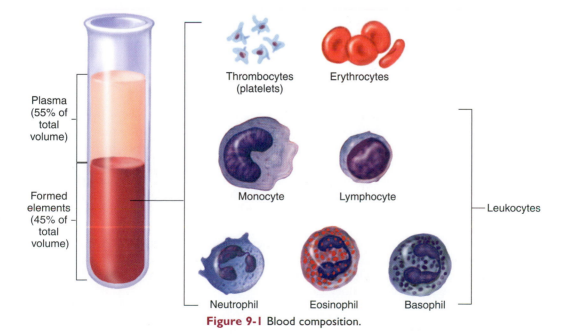

Figure 9-1 Blood composition.

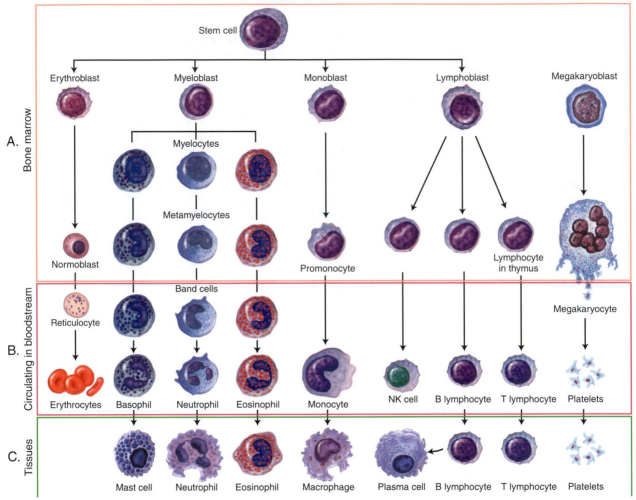

Figure 9-2 Hematopoiesis. **(A)** Bone marrow, where blood cells originate from a highly undifferentiated stem cell and develop into blastic (embryonic) blood cells. **(B)** Bloodstream, which blood cells enter once they are mature. **(C)** Tissues, which leukocytes enter for defense and protection after eventually leaving the bloodstream.

White Blood Cells

White blood cells (WBCs), or **leukocytes,** protect the body against invasion by pathogens and foreign substances, remove debris from injured tissue, and aid in the healing process. Leukocytes are crucial to the body's defense against disease. Unlike RBCs that remain in the bloodstream, WBCs migrate through endothelial walls of capillaries and venules, and enter tissue spaces by a process called **diapedesis.** (See Figure 9-3.) Leukocytes are classified as either **granulocytes** or **agranulocytes** depending on whether their cytoplasm contains or lacks visible granules.

Granulocytes

The different types of granulocytes are named for their staining properties when a blood smear is prepared for microscopic examination. The stain used in its preparation is composed of several dyes, including a red acidic dye called **eosin** and an **alkaline** (basic) dye that stains a dark purple color. There are three types of granulocytes:

• **Neutrophils** contain granules that stain a pale lilac color. They do not show a marked affinity for either an acid dye (red) or alkaline (basic) dye (dark purple), hence they are called **neutrophils.** They are also known as **polymorphonuclear leukocytes (PMNs)** or **polys** because their nuclei are segmented. Neutrophils are phagocytic cells and are responsible for ingesting and destroying bacteria and other foreign particles. They are the most numerous

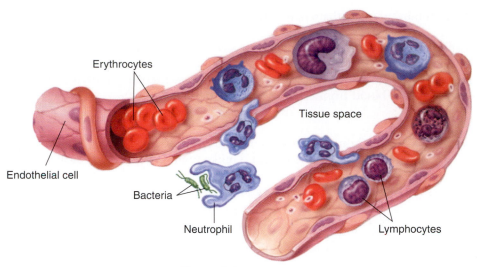

Figure 9-3 Diapedesis.

circulating leukocyte. Neutrophils are the first cells to appear at a site of injury or infection to initiate phagocytosis of foreign material. (See Figure 9-4.) Their importance in body protection cannot be underestimated. A person with a serious deficiency of this blood cell type is highly vulnerable to infection, despite protective attempts by other body defenses.

• **Eosinophils** contain granules that stain red because of their affinity for the red acid dye eosin. Their main function is detoxification. They are especially numerous during allergic reactions and animal parasite infestations.

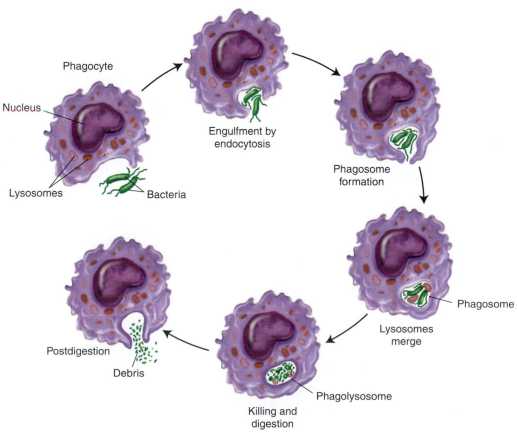

Figure 9-4 Phagocytosis.

• **Basophils** contain granules that stain dark purple because of their affinity for the purple alkaline (basic) dye. Their main function is to release **histamines** and **heparin** at sites of injury. Histamines initiate the inflammatory process by increasing blood flow. As more blood flows to the damaged area, it carries with it additional nutrients, immune substances, and immune cells that help in damage containment and tissue repair. Heparin, an anticoagulant, acts to prevent blood from clotting at the injury site.

Agranulocytes

Agranulocytes arise in the bone marrow from stem cells but mature in lymph tissues. They play an integral part in the specific immune system. Unlike granulocytes that typically have lobed nuclei, agranulocytes have nuclei that do not form lobes. Thus, they are commonly called **mononuclear leukocytes (MNLs).** There are two types of mononuclear leukocytes:

• **Monocytes** are mildly phagocytic when found within blood vessels. However, they remain in the vascular channels only a short time. When they exit, they transform into **macrophages,** avid phagocytes capable of ingesting pathogens, dead cells, and other debris found at sites of inflammation.
• **Lymphocytes** include **B cells**, **T cells**, and **natural killer (NK) cells**. B cells and T cells provide a highly specific body defense called acquired immunity. In acquired immunity, lymphocytes learn to recognize and destroy potential threats to the well-being of the individual. NK cells provide a generalized defense and respond whenever a potentially dangerous or abnormal cell is encountered. They "kill" by releasing potent chemicals that rupture the cell membrane of abnormal cells. NK cells are highly effective against cancer cells and cells harboring pathogens. They have the ability to kill over and over again before they die. (See Table 9-1.)

Platelets

Platelets, also called **thrombocytes,** are the smallest formed elements found in blood. They are not true cells but merely cell fragments. Platelets initiate blood clotting when they encounter damaged vessel walls that have been injured or traumatized. Control of bleeding **(hemostasis)** is not a single reaction but a complex series of interdependent reactions. Initially, platelets become sticky and aggregate at the injury site to form a barrier to control blood loss. Clotting factors in platelets and injured tissue release **thromboplastin,** a substance that initiates clot formation. In the final step of coagulation, **fibrinogen** (a soluble blood protein) becomes insoluble and forms

Table 9-1	**Protective Actions of White Blood Cells**

This chart lists the two main categories of white blood cells along with their cellular components and their protective actions.

Cell Type	Protective Action
Granulocytes	
Neutrophils	Phagocytosis
Eosinophils	Allergy, animal parasites
Basophils	Inflammation mediators, anticoagulant properties
Agranulocytes	
Monocytes (macrophages)	Phagocytosis
Lymphocytes	
• B cells	Adaptive immunity (humoral)
• T cells	Adaptive immunity (cellular)
• Natural killer cells	Destruction without specificity

fibrin strands that act as a net, entrapping blood cells. This jellylike mass of blood cells and fibrin is called a **thrombus** or **blood clot.**

Plasma

Plasma is the liquid portion of blood in which blood cells are suspended. When blood cells are removed, plasma appears as a thin, almost colorless fluid. It is composed of about 92% water and contains such products as **plasma proteins** (albumins, globulins, and fibrinogen), gases, nutrients, salts, hormones, and waste materials. A small amount of plasma continuously leaks from capillaries to bathe the surrounding cells in their products and remove waste material making cellular communication possible throughout the body. Blood serum is a product of blood plasma. If fibrinogen and clotting elements are removed from plasma, the resulting fluid is called *serum.*

Blood Types

Human blood is divided into four types, A, B, AB, and O, based on the presence or absence of specific **antigens** on the surface of RBCs. (See Figure 9-5.) In each of these four blood types, the plasma does not contain the **antibody** against the antigen that is present on the RBCs. Rather, the plasma contains the opposite antibodies. Thus, type A blood contains A antigen on the surface of the RBC and the plasma contains B antibody in the plasma. (See Table 9-2.)

In addition to antigens of the four blood types, there are numerous other antigens that may be present on RBCs. Blood types are medically important in transfusions, transplants, and maternal–fetal incompatibilities. Although **hematologists** have identified more than 300 different blood antigens, most of these are not of medical concern.

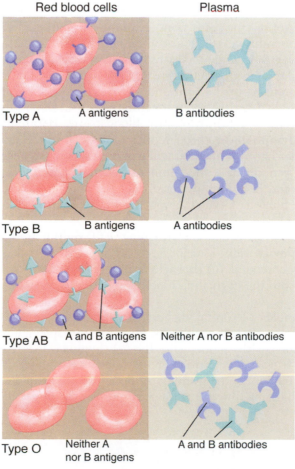

Red blood cells   Plasma

Type A   A antigens   B antibodies

Type B   B antigens   A antibodies

Type AB   A and B antigens   Neither A nor B antibodies

Type O   Neither A nor B antigens   A and B antibodies

Figure 9-5 ABO blood types. From Venes, ed.: *Tabers' Cyclopedic Medical Dictionary,* 21st ed. FA Davis, Philadelphia, 2009, p 787, with permission.

Table 9-2	ABO System		

The table below lists the four blood types along with their respective antigens and antibodies and the percentage of the population that have each type.

Blood Type	Antigen (RBCs)	Antibody (plasma)	% Population
A	A	anti-B	41
B	B	anti-A	10
AB	A and B	Neither anti-A nor anti-B	4
O	neither A nor B	anti-A and anti-B	45

Lymph System

The lymph system consists of a fluid called **lymph** (in which lymphocytes and monocytes are suspended), a network of transporting vessels called **lymph vessels,** and a multiplicity of other structures, including nodes, spleen, thymus, and tonsils. Functions of the lymph system include:

- maintaining fluid balance of the body by draining interstitial fluid from tissue spaces and returning it to the blood
- transporting lipids away from the digestive organs for use by body tissues
- filtering and removing unwanted or infectious products in lymph nodes.

Lymph vessels begin as closed-ended capillaries in tissue spaces and terminate at the right lymphatic duct and the thoracic duct in the chest cavity. (See Figure 9-6.) As whole blood circulates, a small amount of plasma seeps from (1) **blood capillaries.** This fluid, now called **interstitial** or **tissue fluid,** resembles plasma but contains slightly less protein. Interstitial fluid carries needed products to tissue cells while removing their wastes. As interstitial fluid moves through tissues, it collects cellular debris, bacteria, and particulate matter. Upon completing these functions, interstitial fluid returns to the surrounding venules to become plasma or enters closed-ended microscopic vessels called (2) **lymph capillaries** to become lymph. Lymph passes into larger and larger vessels on its return trip to the bloodstream. Before it reaches its final destination, it first enters (3) **lymph nodes** through afferent vessels. In the node, macrophages phagocytize bacteria and other harmful material while T cells and B cells exert their protective influence. When a local infection exists, the number of bacteria entering a node is so great and the destruction by T cells and B cells so powerful that the node commonly enlarges and becomes tender. Once lymph is filtered, it exits the node by way of efferent vessels to continue its return to the circulatory system.

Lymph vessels from the right chest and arm join the (4) **right lymphatic duct.** This duct drains into the (5) **right subclavian vein,** a major vessel in the cardiovascular system. Lymph from all other areas of the body enters the (6) **thoracic duct** and drains into the (7) **left subclavian vein.** Lymph is redeposited into the circulating blood and becomes plasma. This cycle continually repeats itself.

The (8) **spleen** resembles a lymph node because it acts as a filter by removing cellular debris, bacteria, parasites, and other infectious agents. However, the spleen also destroys old RBCs and serves as a repository for healthy blood cells. The (9) **thymus** is located in the upper part of the chest **(mediastinum).** It partially controls the immune system by transforming certain lymphocytes into T cells to function in the immune system. The (10) **tonsils** are masses of lymphatic tissue located in the pharynx. They act as filters to protect the upper respiratory structures from invasion by pathogens.

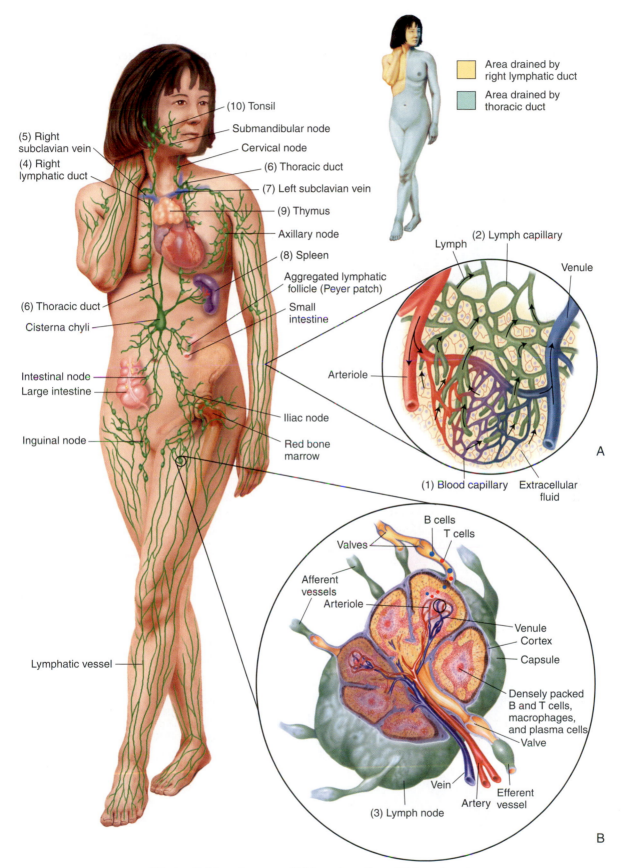

(10) Tonsil

Submandibular node

Cervical node

(5) Right subclavian vein

(4) Right lymphatic duct

(6) Thoracic duct

(7) Left subclavian vein

(9) Thymus

Axillary node

(8) Spleen

Aggregated lymphatic follicle (Peyer patch)

Small intestine

(6) Thoracic duct

Cisterna chyli

Intestinal node

Large intestine

Inguinal node

Iliac node

Red bone marrow

Lymphatic vessel

Area drained by right lymphatic duct

Area drained by thoracic duct

Lymph

(2) Lymph capillary

Venule

Arteriole

(1) Blood capillary

Extracellular fluid

A

B cells

T cells

Valves

Afferent vessels

Arteriole

Venule

Cortex

Capsule

Densely packed B and T cells, macrophages, and plasma cells

Valve

Vein

Artery

Efferent vessel

(3) Lymph node

B

Figure 9-6 Lymph system. **(A)** Lymph capillary. **(B)** Lymph node.

Anatomy Review

To review the anatomy of the lymph system, label the following illustration using the terms listed below.

blood capillary   *right lymphatic duct*   *thoracic duct*

left subclavian vein   *right subclavian vein*   *thymus*

lymph capillary   *spleen*   *tonsil*

lymph node

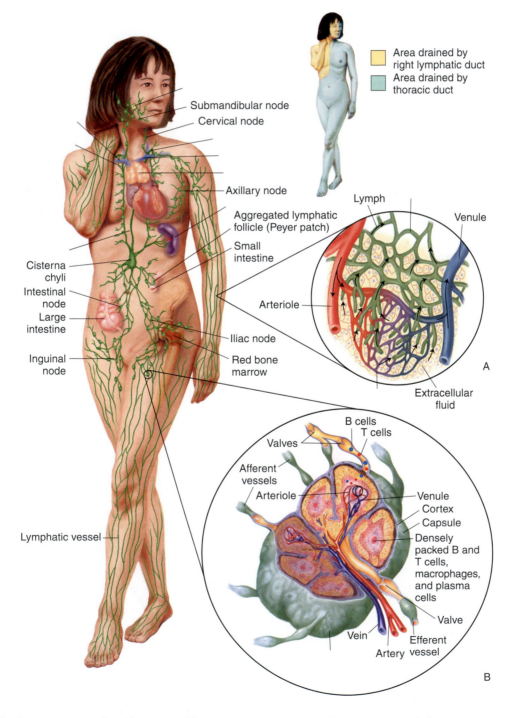

Submandibular node

Cervical node

Axillary node

Aggregated lymphatic
follicle (Peyer patch)

Small
intestine

Cisterna
chyli

Intestinal
node

Large
intestine

Inguinal
node

Iliac node

Red bone
marrow

Lymphatic vessel

Area drained by
right lymphatic duct

Area drained by
thoracic duct

Lymph

Venule

Arteriole

Extracellular
fluid

A

B cells

T cells

Valves

Afferent
vessels

Arteriole

Venule

Cortex

Capsule

Densely
packed B and
T cells,
macrophages,
and plasma
cells

Valve

Vein

Efferent
vessel

Artery

B

*Check your answers by referring to Figure 9-6 on page 261. Review material that you
did not answer correctly.*

Immune System

Although exposed to a vast number of harmful substances, most people suffer relatively few diseases throughout their lifetime. Numerous body defenses called **resistance** work together to protect against disease. Resistance includes first-line barriers that keep pathogens from entering the body. It includes skin and mucous membranes, tears, saliva and gastric secretions. The second-line barriers protect the body once pathogens have gained entry. These protective barriers include phagocytic cells and inflammation. Because these forms of resistance are present at birth, they are said to be **innate.**

The last and most complicated type of body resistance is called **acquired immunity** and develops only after birth in an **immunocompetent** individual. This type of immunity is a lifelong monitoring system that remains vigilant to disease causing microbes and other potentially dangerous substances. Once encountered, the adaptive immune system reacts with incredible efficiency and speed to destroy microbes or neutralize their toxic effects. The white blood cells chiefly responsible for the adaptive immune response are monocytes and lymphocytes.

Monocytes

After a brief stay in the vascular system, monocytes enter tissue spaces and become highly phagocytic **macrophages.** In this form, they consume large numbers of pathogens, including bacteria and viruses. After macrophages engulf a pathogen, they process it in such a way that the highly specific antigenic properties of the pathogen are placed on the cell surface of the macrophage. Thus, the macrophage becomes an **antigen-presenting cell (APC).** The APC awaits an encounter with a lymphocyte capable of responding to (matching) that specific antigen. When this occurs, the acquired immune system begins the operations required for the systematic destruction of the antigen.

Lymphocytes

Two types of **lymphocytes,** B cells and T cells, are the active cells of the adaptive immune response. B cells are formed and mature in the bone marrow and then migrate to the lymph system. They are responsible for humoral immunity. T cells are formed in the bone marrow but migrate to the thymus where the mature before entering the lymph system. T cells are responsible for cellular immunity.

Humoral Immunity

Humoral immunity is the component of the specific immune system that protects primarily against extracellular antigens, such as bacteria and viruses that have not yet entered a cell. Upon an encounter with its matching antigen, B cells produce a clone of cells called **plasma cells** that produce highly specific proteins called **antibodies.** Antibodies travel in plasma, tissue fluid, and lymph. If an antibody encounters its matching antigen, it attaches to it and forms an **antigen–antibody complex.** Once this complex forms, the antigen is inactivated, neutralized, or tagged for destruction. After all antigens have been eliminated, memory B cells migrate to lymph tissue and remain available for immediate recall if that same antigen is encountered again.

Cellular Immunity

Cellular immunity is the component of the specific immune system that protects primarily against intracellular antigens, such as viruses and cancer cells. The four types of T cells include the cytotoxic T cell, helper T cell, suppressor T cell, and memory T cell. The **cytotoxic T cell** is the cell that actually destroys the invading antigen. It determines the antigen's specific weakness and uses this weakness as a point of attack to destroy it. The **helper T cell** is essential to the proper functioning of both humoral and cellular immunity. It uses chemical messengers called **cytokines** to activate, direct, and regulate the activity of most of the other components of the immune system, especially B cells. If the number of helper T cells is deficient, the immune system essentially shuts down and the patient becomes a victim of even the most harmless organisms. The **suppressor T cell** monitors the progression of infection. When infection resolves, the suppressor T cell "shuts down" the immune response. Finally, like the humoral response, the cellular response also produces memory cells. These **memory T cells** find their way to the lymph system and remain there long after the encounter with the antigen, ready for combat if the antigen reappears. (See Table 9-3.)

The memory component is unique to the acquired immune response. Memory B and T cells are able to "recall" how they previously disposed of a particular antigen and are able to repeat the process. The repeat performance is immediate, powerful, and sustained. Disposing of the antigen during the second and all subsequent exposures is extremely rapid and much more effective than it was during the first exposure.

Table 9-3	Lymphocytes and Immune Response

The chart below lists the lymphocytes involved in humoral and cellular immunity along with their functions and sites of origin and maturation.

Lymphocyte	Function	Origin	Maturation
Humoral immunity			
B lymphocytes		Bone marrow	Bone marrow
• Plasma cells	• Antibody formation for destruction of extracellular antigens		
• Memory cells	• Active immunity		
Cellular immunity			
T lymphocytes		Bone marrow	Thymus, immune system
• Cytotoxic T cell	• Destruction of infected cells and cancer cells		
• Helper T cell	• Assistance for B cells, cytotoxic T cells, and other components of the immune system		
• Suppressor T cell	• Suppression (shutting down) of humoral and cellular response when infection resolves		
• Memory T cell	• Active immunity		

CONNECTING BODY SYSTEMS—BLOOD, LYMPH, AND IMMUNE SYSTEMS

The main functions of the blood, lymph, and immune systems are to provide a way to transport and exchange products throughout the body and protect and repair cells that are damaged by disease or trauma. Specific functional relationships between the blood, lymph, and immune systems and other body systems are summarized below.

Cardiovascular
- Blood delivers oxygen needed for contraction of the heart.
- Lymph system returns interstitial fluid to the vascular system to maintain blood volume.
- Immune system protects against infections.

Digestive
- Blood transports products of digestion to nourish body cells.
- Immune system provides surveillance mechanisms to detect and destroy cancer cells in the digestive tract.
- An innate component of the immune system, the acidic environment of the stomach helps control pathogens of the digestive tract.

CONNECTING BODY SYSTEMS—BLOOD, LYMPH, AND IMMUNE SYSTEMS—cont'd

Endocrine
- Blood and lymph systems transport hormones to target organs.
- Immune system protects against infection in endocrine glands.

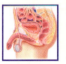

Female Reproductive
- Blood, lymph, and immune systems transport nourishing and defensive products across the placental barrier for the developing fetus.
- Immune system provides specific defense against pathogens that enter the body through the reproductive tract.
- Immune system supplies antibodies for breast milk that protect the baby until its immune system is established.

Integumentary
- Blood provides leukocytes, especially neutrophils, to the integumentary system when breaches or injury occurs in the skin.
- Lymph system supplies antibodies to the dermis for defense against pathogens.
- Blood found in the skin, the largest organ of the body, helps maintain temperature homeostasis.

Male Reproductive
- Immune system provides surveillance against cancer cells.
- Blood delivers hormones and other essential products for male fertility.
- Lymph maintains fluid balance in the male organs of reproduction.

Musculoskeletal
- Blood removes lactic acid that accumulates in muscles during strenuous exercise.
- Blood transports calcium to bones for strength and healing.
- Lymph system maintains interstitial fluid balance in muscle tissue.
- Immune system aids in repair of muscle tissue following trauma.

Nervous
- Immune system responds to nervous stimuli in order to identify injury or infection sites and initiate tissue defense and repair.
- Plasma and lymph provide the medium in which nervous stimuli cross from one neuron to another.
- Lymph system removes excess interstitial fluid from tissues surrounding nerves.

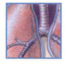

Respiratory
- Red blood cells transport respiratory gases to and from the lungs.
- Tonsils harbor immune cells to combat pathogens that enter through the nose and mouth.

Urinary
- Blood transports waste products, especially urea, to the kidneys for removal via the production of urine.
- Blood in peritubular capillaries reabsorbs essential products that have been filtered by the nephron.

Medical Word Elements

This section introduces combining forms, suffixes, and prefixes related to the blood, lymph, and immune systems. Word analyses are also provided.

Element	Meaning	Word Analysis
Combining Forms		
aden/o	gland	**aden/**oid (ĂD-ĕ-noyd): resembling a gland *–oid*: resembling
agglutin/o	clumping, gluing	**agglutin/**ation (ă-gloo-tĭ-NĀ-shŭn): process of clumping *–ation*: process (of)
bas/o	base (alkaline, opposite of acid)	**bas/o/**phil (BĀ-sō-fĭl): attraction to base (alkaline dyes) *–phil*: attraction for *The granules of the basophil appear dark blue when stained with a dye used in hematology.*

(continued)

Element	Meaning	Word Analysis
blast/o	embryonic cell	erythr/o/**blast**/osis (ĕ-rĭth-rō-blăs-TŌ-sĭs): abnormal increase of embryonic red (cells) *erythr/o:* red *-osis:* abnormal condition; increase (used primarily with blood cells) *Erythroblastosis fetalis is a potentially fatal disease of newborns occurring when a blood incompatibility exists between the mother and fetus.*
chrom/o	color	hypo/**chrom**/ic (hī-pō-KRŌM-ĭk): under (decrease in) color *hypo-:* under, below *-ic:* pertaining to *Hypochromic cells are erythrocytes that contain inadequate hemoglobin. These cells are commonly associated with iron-deficiency anemia.*
eosin/o	dawn (rose-colored)	**eosin/o**/phil (ē-ō-SĬN-ō-fĭl): attraction for rose colored (dye) *-phil:* attraction for *The granules of an eosinophil appear rose-colored when stained with eosin, a dye used in hematology.*
erythr/o	red	**erythr/o**/cyte (ĕ-RĬTH-rō-sīt): red cell *-cyte:* cell *An erythrocyte is a red blood cell.*
granul/o	granule	**granul/o**/cyte (GRĂN-ū-lō-sīt): cell (containing) granules *-cyte:* cell
hem/o	blood	**hem/o**/phobia (hē-mō-FŌ-bē-ă): fear of blood *-phobia:* fear *People who suffer from hemophobia commonly faint at the sight of blood.*
hemat/o		**hemat**/oma (hē-mă-TŌ-mă): blood tumor *-oma:* tumor *A hematoma is a mass of extravasated, usually clotted blood caused by a break or leak in a blood vessel. It may be found in any organ, tissue, or space within the body.*
immun/o	immune, immunity, safe	**immun/o**/logy (ĭm-ū-NŎL-ō-jē): study of immunity *-logy:* study of *Immunology includes the study of autoimmune diseases, hypersensitivities, and immune deficiencies.*
kary/o	nucleus	**kary/o**/lysis (kăr-ē-ŎL-ĭ-sĭs): destruction of the nucleus *-lysis:* separation; destruction; loosening *Karyolysis results in cell death.*
nucle/o	nucleus	mono/**nucle**/ar (mŏn-ō-NŪ-klē-ăr): pertaining to a single nucleus *mono-:* one *-ar:* pertaining to
leuk/o	white	**leuk**/emia (loo-KĒ-mē-ă): white blood condition *-emia:* blood condition *Leukemia causes a profoundly elevated white blood cell count and a very low red blood cell count.*

Element	Meaning	Word Analysis
lymphaden/o	lymph gland (node)	**lymphaden/o/**pathy (lĭm-făd-ĕ-NŎP-ă-thē): disease of lymph nodes *-pathy:* disease *Lymphadenopathy is characterized by changes in the size, consistency, or number of lymph nodes.*
lymph/o	lymph	**lymph/**oid (LĬM-foyd): resembling lymph *-oid:* resembling
lymphangi/o	lymph vessel	**lymphangi/**oma (lĭm-făn-jē-Ō-mă): tumor (composed of) lymph vessels *-oma:* tumor
morph/o	form, shape, structure	**morph/o/**logy (mor-FŎL-ō-jē): study of form, shape, and structure *-logy:* study of
myel/o	bone marrow; spinal cord	**myel/o/**gen/ic (mī-ĕ-lō-JĔN-ĭk): relating to the origin in bone marrow *gen:* forming, producing, origin *-ic:* pertaining to *Granulocytes are formed in the bone marrow and are, thus, considered myelogenic.*
neutr/o	neutral, neither	**neutr/o/**phil/ic (nū-trō-FĬL-ĭk): pertaining to an attraction for neutral dyes *-phil:* attraction for *-ic:* pertaining to, relating to *A neutrophil is a leukocyte whose granules stain easily with neutral dyes.*
phag/o	swallowing, eating	**phag/o/**cyte (FĂG-ō-sīt): cell that eats (foreign material) *-cyte:* cell *The neutrophil is phagocytic and protects the body by consuming foreign substances that may cause disease or injury.*
plas/o	formation, growth	a/**plas/**tic (ā-PLĂS-tĭk): pertaining to a failure to form *a-:* without, not *-tic:* pertaining to *Aplastic anemia is a failure of the bone marrow to produce adequate blood cells.*
poikil/o	varied, irregular	**poikil/o/**cyte (POY-kĭl-ō-sīt): cell that is irregular or varied (in shape) *-cyte:* cell
reticul/o	net, mesh	**reticul/o/**cyte (rĕ-TĬK-ū-lō-sīt): cell (that contains a) net or meshwork *-cyte:* cell *A reticulocyte is an immature erythrocyte that contains strands of nuclear material. This material appears as a tiny net when observed microscopically.*
ser/o	serum	**ser/o/**logy (sē-RŎL-ō-jē): study of serum *-logy:* study of *Serology includes the study of antigens and antibodies in serum as well as sources other than serum, including plasma, saliva, and urine.*

(continued)

Element	Meaning	Word Analysis
sider/o	iron	**sider/o**/penia (sĭd-ĕr-ō-PĒ-nē-ă): deficiency of iron *-penia:* decrease, deficiency *Sideropenia usually results from inadequate iron uptake or from hemorrhage.*
splen/o	spleen	**splen/o**/rrhagia (splē-nō-RĀ-jē-ă): bursting forth of the spleen *-rrhagia:* bursting forth *Splenorrhagia is a hemorrhage from a ruptured spleen.*
thromb/o	blood clot	**thromb**/osis (thrŏm-BŌ-sĭs): abnormal condition of a blood clot *-osis:* abnormal condition; increase (used primarily with blood cells) *Thrombosis is the formation of blood clots in the blood vessels.*
thym/o	thymus gland	**thym/o**/pathy (thī-MŎP-ă-thē): disease of the thymus gland *-pathy:* disease
xen/o	foreign, strange	**xen/o**/graft (ZĔN-ō-grăft): foreign transplantation, also called heterograft *-graft:* transplantation *A xenograft is a cross-species transplant, such as a pig heart valve to a human recipient. A xenograft is used as a temporary measure when there is insufficient tissue available from the patient or other human donors.*

Suffixes		
-blast	embryonic cell	erythr/o/**blast** (ĕ-RĬTH-rō-blăst): embryonic red cell *erythr/o:* red
-emia	blood condition	an/**emia** (ă-NĒ-mē-ă): without blood *an-:* without, not *Anemia is any condition characterized by a reduction in the number of red blood cells or a deficiency in their hemoglobin.*
-globin	protein	hem/o/**globin** (HĒ-mō-glō-bĭn): blood protein *hem/o:* blood *Hemoglobin is an iron-containing protein found in RBCs that transports oxygen and gives blood its red color.*
-graft	transplantation	auto/**graft** (AW-tō-grăft): self transplantation *auto-:* self, own *An autograft is a surgical transplantation of tissue from one location of the body to another in the same individual.*
-osis	abnormal condition; increase (used primarily with blood cells)	leuk/o/cyt/**osis** (loo-kō-sī-TŌ-sĭs): abnormal increase in white (blood) cells *leuk/o:* white *cyt:* cell
-penia	decrease, deficiency	erythr/o/**penia** (ĕ-rĭth-rō-PĒ-nē-ă): abnormal decrease in red (blood) cells *erythr/o:* red

Element	Meaning	Word Analysis
-phil	attraction for	neutr/o/**phil** (NŪ-trō-fĭl): attraction for a neutral (dye) *neutr/o:* neutral, neither *Neutrophils are the most numerous type of leukocyte. They provide phagocytic protection for the body.*
-phoresis	carrying, transmission	electr/o/**phoresis** (ē-lĕk-trō-fō-RĒ-sĭs): carrying an electric (charge) *electr/o:* electricity *Electrophoresis is a laboratory technique used to separate proteins based on their electrical charge, size, and shape. It is commonly used in deoxyribonucleic acid (DNA) testing.*
-phylaxis	protection	ana/**phylaxis** (ăn-ă-fĭ-LĂK-sĭs): against protection *ana-:* against, up, back *Anaphylaxis is an exaggerated, life-threatening hypersensitivity reaction to a previously encountered antigen. It is treated as a medical emergency.*
-poiesis	formation, production	hem/o/**poiesis** (hē-mō-poy-Ē-sĭs): formation of blood *hem/o:* blood
-stasis	standing still	hem/o/**stasis** (hē-mō-STĀ-sĭs): standing still of blood *hem/o:* blood *Hemostasis is the control or arrest of bleeding, commonly using chemical agents.*
Prefixes		
a-	without, not	**a**/morph/ic (ā-MOR-fĭk): without a (definite) form *morph:* form, shape, structure *ic:* pertaining to
allo-	other, differing from the normal	**allo**/graft (ĂL-ō-grăft): transplantation from another; also called homograft *-graft:* transplantation *An allograft is a transplant between two individuals who are not identical twins but are genetically compatible.*
aniso-	unequal, dissimilar	**aniso**/cyt/osis (ăn-ī-sō-sĭ-TŌ-sĭs): abnormal increase in cells that are unequal *cyt:* cell *-osis:* abnormal condition; increase (used primarily with blood cells) *Anisocytosis generally refers to red blood cells that vary in size from normal (normocytic) to abnormally large (macrocytic) or abnormally small (microcytic).*
iso-	same, equal	**iso**/chrom/ic (ī-sō-KRŌM-ĭk): pertaining to the same color *chrom:* color *ic:* pertaining to
macro-	large	**macro**/cyte (MĂK-rō-sīt): large (red) cell *-cyte:* cell
micro-	small	**micro**/cyte (MĪ-krō-sīt): small (red) cell *-cyte:* cell

(continued)

Element	Meaning	Word Analysis
mono-	one	**mono**/nucle/osis (mŏn-ō-nū-klē-Ō-sĭs): abnormal increase of mononuclear (cells) *nucle:* nucleus *-osis:* abnormal condition; increase (used primarily with blood cells) *In infectious mononucleosis, there is an increase in monocytes and lymphocytes.*
poly-	many, much	**poly**/morph/ic (pŏl-ē-MOR-fĭk): pertaining to many forms or shapes *morph:* form, shape, structure *-ic:* pertaining to

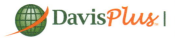

Visit the *Medical Terminology Systems* online resource center at DavisPlus for an audio exercise of the terms in this table. Other activities are also available to reinforce content.

It is time to review medical word elements by completing Learning Activities 9-1 and 9-2.

Pathology

Anemias, leukemias, and coagulation disorders typically share common signs and symptoms that generally include paleness, weakness, shortness of breath, and heart palpitations. Lymphatic disorders are commonly associated with edema and lymphadenopathy. In these disorders, tissues are swollen with enlarged, tender nodes. Immune disorders include abnormally heightened immune responses to antigens (allergies, hypersensitivities), abnormally depressed responses (immunodeficiencies and cancers) and autoimmune diseases where the body fails to recognize its own tissue and mounts a response that results in its destruction. Many immunological disorders are manifested in other body systems. For example, asthma and hay fever are immunological disorders that affect the respiratory system; atopic dermatitis and eczema are immunological disorders that affect the integumentary system. Some of the most devastating diseases, such as rheumatoid arthritis (RA) and AIDS, are caused by disordered immunity.

For diagnosis, treatment, and management of diseases that affect blood and blood-forming organs, the medical services of a specialist may be warranted. **Hematology** is the branch of medicine that studies blood cells, blood-clotting mechanisms, bone marrow, and lymph nodes. The physician who specializes in this branch of medicine is called a **hematologist. Allergy and immunology** is the branch of medicine involving disorders of the immune system, including asthma and anaphylaxis, adverse reactions to drugs, autoimmune diseases, organ transplantations, and malignancies of the immune system. Physicians who specialize in this combined branch of medicine are called **allergists and immunologists.**

Anemias

Anemia is a deficiency of erythrocytes or hemoglobin in the blood. It is not a disease but a symptom of other illnesses. The most common type of anemia is iron-deficiency anemia, which is caused by lack of iron that is required for hemoglobin production. Other causes of anemias include excessive blood loss **(hemorrhagic anemia),** excessive blood-cell destruction **(hemolytic anemia),** decreased blood formation within bone marrow **(aplastic anemia),** and faulty hemoglobin production. The faulty hemoglobin molecule causes the RBCs to assume a bizarre shape, commonly resembling a crescent, or sickle, when oxygen levels are low. The RBCs then have difficulty passing through the small capillaries. (See Figure 9-7.) The sickle cells are fragile and easily break apart **(hemolyze).** Tissue distal to the blockage undergoes ischemia, resulting in severe pain called a **sickle cell crisis** that can last from several hours to several days. Sickle cell anemia affects only those who have inherited the trait from both parents. If the trait is inherited from only one parent,

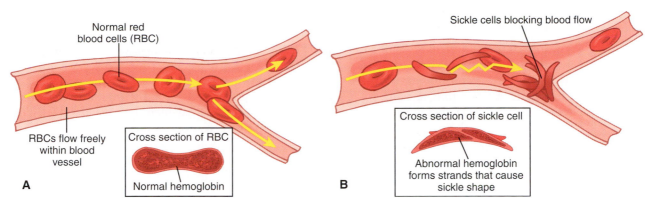

Figure 9-7 Sickle cell anemia. **(A)** Normal RBCs passing easily through capillaries. **(B)** Sickle cells becoming trapped and obstructing normal blood flow.

the offspring will be a carrier but will not have the disorder. Treatment is designed to control or limit the number of crises. Folic acid is commonly recommended and some medications are proving to be helpful in controlling the disease.

Signs and symptoms associated with most anemias include difficulty breathing **(dyspnea),** weakness, rapid heartbeat **(tachycardia),** paleness **(pallor),** low blood pressure **(hypotension),** and, commonly, a slight fever. (See Table 9-4.)

Table 9-4	**Common Anemias**	
This table lists various types of anemia along with descriptions and causes for each.		
Type of Anemia	**Description**	**Causes**
Aplastic (hypoplastic)	Serious form of anemia associated with bone marrow failure and resulting in erythropenia, leukopenia, and thrombocytopenia	Commonly caused by some autoimmune disorders, chemotherapy, radiation therapy, and exposure to certain cytotoxic agents
Folic-acid deficiency anemia	Inability to produce sufficient red blood cells (RBCs) due to the lack of folic acid, a B vitamin essential for erythropoiesis	Caused by insufficient folic acid intake due to poor diet, impaired absorption, prolonged drug therapy, or increased requirements (pregnancy or rapid growth as seen in children)
Hemolytic	Destruction of RBCs, commonly resulting in jaundice	Associated with some inherited immune and blood (sickle cell anemia) disorders, medications, and incompatible transfusions
Iron-deficiency anemia	Lack of sufficient iron in RBCs	Caused by a greater demand for stored iron than can be supplied, usually as a result of inadequate dietary iron intake or malabsorption of iron
Pernicious anemia	Chronic, progressive anemia found mostly in people older than age 50 due to lack of sufficient vitamin B_{12} needed for blood cell development	Commonly the result of insufficient intrinsic factor in the stomach, which is essential for absorption of vitamin B_{12}
Sickle cell anemia	Inherited anemia that causes RBCs to become crescent- or sickle-shaped when oxygen levels are low	Caused by a defect in the gene responsible for hemoglobin synthesis

Acquired Immune Deficiency Syndrome (AIDS)

Acquired immune deficiency syndrome (AIDS) is an infectious disease caused by the human immunodeficiency virus **(HIV),** which slowly destroys the immune system. The immune system becomes so weak **(immunocompromised)** that, in the final stage of the disease, the patient falls victim to infections that usually do not affect healthy individuals **(opportunistic infections).** Symptoms of AIDS begin to appear gradually, and include swollen lymph glands **(lymphadenopathy),** malaise, fever, night sweats, and weight loss. **Kaposi sarcoma,** a neoplastic disorder, and *Pneumocystis* pneumonia (PCP) are two diseases closely associated with AIDS and are considered AIDS-defining diseases.

Transmission of HIV occurs primarily through body fluids—mostly blood, semen, and vaginal secretions. The virus attacks the most important cell in the immune system, the helper T cell. Once infected with HIV, the helper T cell becomes a "mini-factory" for the replication of the virus. More important, the virus destroys the helper T cell, which impairs the effective functioning of the humoral and cellular arms of the immune system, ultimately causing the patient's death.

Although there is no cure for HIV, treatments are available that can slow the development of the virus and the progression of the disease. These medications have serious adverse effects; however, once the decision for medical management is made, the patient should continue treatment. Failure to do so causes the virus to become highly resistant to current treatment options.

Allergy

An **allergy** is an acquired abnormal immune response. It requires initial exposure **(sensitization)** to an allergen **(antigen).** Subsequent exposures to the allergen produce increasing allergic reactions that cause a broad range of inflammatory changes. Common signs and symptoms include hives **(urticaria),** eczema, allergic rhinitis, asthma and, in the extreme, **anaphylactic shock,** a life-threatening condition.

The offending allergens are identified by allergy-sensitivity tests. In one such test, small scratches are made on the patient's back and a liquid suspension of the allergen is introduced into the scratch. If antibodies to the allergen are present, the scratch becomes red, swollen, and hardened **(indurated).**

An immunotherapy treatment **(allergy shots)** desensitize the patient and reduces the reaction of the patient to the offending allergen. This treatment involves repeated injections of highly diluted solutions containing the allergen. The initial concentration of the solution is too weak to cause symptoms. Additional exposure to higher concentrations promotes tolerance of the allergen.

Autoimmune Disease

Autoimmunity is the failure of the body to distinguish accurately between "self" and "nonself." In this abnormal response, the immune system attacks the antigens found on its own cells to such an extent that tissue injury results. Types of autoimmune disorders range from those that affect only a single organ to those that affect many organs and tissues **(multisystemic).**

Myasthenia gravis is a chronic, progressive autoimmune neuromuscular disease that affects the voluntary muscles of the body, causing sporadic weakness. The muscles most frequently affected are the limbs, eyes, and those affecting speech and swallowing. This disease is caused by circulating antibodies that block receptors at the neuromuscular junction. There is no cure, but treatment can help relieve signs and symptoms such as weakness of arm or leg muscles. Other autoimmune diseases include **rheumatoid arthritis (RA)** and **systemic lupus erythematosus (SLE).**

Treatment of myasthenia gravis consists of attempting to reach a balance between suppressing the immune response to avoid tissue damage, while still maintaining the immune mechanism sufficiently to protect against disease. Most autoimmune diseases have periods of flare-up **(exacerbations)** and latency **(remissions).** Autoimmune diseases are usually chronic, requiring lifelong care and monitoring, even when the person may look or feel well. Currently, few autoimmune diseases can be cured; however, with treatment, those afflicted can live relatively normal lives.

Edema

Edema is an abnormal accumulation of fluids in the intercellular spaces of the body. A major cause of edema is a decrease in the blood protein level **(hypoproteinemia),** especially albumin, which controls the amount of plasma leaving the vascular channels. Other causes of edema include poor lymph drainage commonly associated with surgery, high sodium intake, increased capillary permeability, and heart failure.

Edema limited to a specific area **(localized)** may be relieved by elevation of that body part and application of cold packs. Systemic edema may be treated with medications that promote urination **(diuretics).**

Closely associated with edema is a condition called **ascites,** in which fluid collects within the peritoneal or pleural cavity. The chief causes of ascites are interference in venous return in cardiac disease, obstruction of lymphatic flow, disturbances in electrolyte balance, and liver disease.

Hemophilia

Hemophilia, also called **bleeder's disease,** is a hereditary disorder in which the blood-clotting mechanism is impaired. There are two main types of hemophilia: **hemophilia A,** a deficiency in clotting factor VIII, and **hemophilia B,** a deficiency in clotting factor IX. The degree of deficiency varies from mild to severe. The disease is sex-linked and found most commonly in men. Women are carriers of the trait but generally do not have symptoms of the disease.

Mild symptoms include nosebleeds, easy bruising, and bleeding from the gums. Severe symptoms produce areas of blood seepage **(hematomas)** deep within muscles. If blood enters joints **(hemarthrosis),** it is associated with pain and, possibly, permanent deformity. Uncontrolled bleeding in the body may lead to shock and death. Treatment consists of intravenous administration of the deficient factor. The amount of factor replaced depends on the seriousness of the hemorrhage and the amount of blood lost.

Infectious Mononucleosis

Infectious mononucleosis is one of the acute infections caused by the Epstein-Barr virus (EBV). It is usually found in young adults and tends to appear in early spring and fall. Saliva and respiratory secretions have been implicated as significant infectious agents, hence the name "kissing disease." Sore throat, fever, and enlarged cervical lymph nodes characterize this disease. Other signs and symptoms include gum infection **(gingivitis),** headache, tiredness, loss of appetite **(anorexia),** and general malaise. In most cases, the disease resolves spontaneously and without complications. In some cases, however, the liver and spleen enlarge **(hepatomegaly** and **splenomegaly).** Less common clinical findings include hemolytic anemia with jaundice and thrombocytopenia. Recovery usually ensures a lasting immunity.

Oncology

Oncological disorders associated with the blood, lymph, and immune systems include leukemia, Hodgkin disease, and Kaposi sarcoma.

Leukemia

Leukemia is an oncological disorder of the blood-forming organs, characterized by an overgrowth **(proliferation)** of blood cells. With this condition, malignant cells replace healthy bone marrow cells. The disease is generally categorized by the type of leukocyte population affected: granulocytic **(myelogenous)** or lymphocytic.

The various types of leukemia may be further classified as **chronic** or **acute.** In the acute form, there is a sudden onset of the disease and the cells are highly embryonic **(blastic)** with few mature forms. In the acute form, severe anemia, infections, and bleeding disorders appear early in the disease. This form of leukemia is life-threatening. In the chronic form, signs and symptoms are slow to develop. Although there is a proliferation of blastic cells in chronic forms of leukemia, there are usually enough mature cells to carry on the functions of the various cell types. As the chronic form progresses, signs and symptoms develop.

Although the causes of leukemia are unknown, viruses, environmental conditions, high-dose radiation, and genetic factors have been implicated. Bone marrow aspiration and bone marrow biopsy are used to diagnose leukemia. Treatment includes chemotherapy, radiation, biological therapy, bone marrow transplant, or a combination of these modalities. Left untreated, leukemias are fatal.

Hodgkin Disease

Hodgkin disease, also called **Hodgkin lymphoma,** is a malignant disease of the lymph system, primarily the lymph nodes. Although malignancy usually remains only in neighboring nodes, it may spread to the spleen, GI tract, liver, or bone marrow.

Hodgkin disease usually begins with a painless enlargement of lymph nodes, typically on one side of the neck, chest, or underarm. Other symptoms include severe itching **(pruritus),** weight loss, progressive anemia, and fever. If nodes in the neck become excessively large, they may press on the trachea, causing difficulty breathing **(dyspnea),** or on the esophagus, causing difficulty swallowing **(dysphagia).**

Radiation and chemotherapy are important methods of controlling the disease. Newer methods of treatment include bone marrow transplants. Treatment is highly effective.

Kaposi Sarcoma

Kaposi sarcoma is a malignancy of connective tissue, including bone, fat, muscle, and fibrous tissue. It is closely associated with AIDS and is commonly fatal because the tumors readily metastasize to other organs. The lesions emerge as purplish brown macules and develop into plaques and nodules. The lesions initially appear over the lower extremities and tend to spread symmetrically over the upper body, particularly the face and oral mucosa. Treatment for AIDS-related Kaposi sarcoma is usually palliative, relieving the pain and discomfort that accompany the lesions, but there is little evidence that it prolongs life.

Diseases and Conditions

This section introduces diseases and conditions of the blood, lymph, and immune systems with their meanings and pronunciations. Word analyses for selected terms are also provided.

Term	Definition
disseminated intravascular coagulation (DIC) ĭn-tră-VĂS-kū-lăr kō-ăg-ū-LĀ-shŭn *intra-:* in, within *vascul:* vessel, (usually blood or lymph) *-ar:* pertaining to	Abnormal activation of the proteins involved in blood coagulation, causing small blood clots to form in vessels and cutting off the supply of oxygen to distal tissues *Eventually, clotting proteins are exhausted, leading to profuse bleeding, even with the slightest trauma. (See Figure 9-8.)* **Figure 9-8** Extensive hemorrhage into the skin in disseminated intravascular coagulation (DIC), with an area outlined in pen to assess if the hemorrhage is spreading. From Harmening: *Clinical Hematology and Fundamentals of Hemostasis,* 3rd ed. FA Davis, Philadelphia, 1997, p 520, with permission.
graft rejection GRĂFT	Process in which a recipient's immune system attacks a transplanted organ or tissue *The transplanted organ or tissue may fail to function when this process occurs.*
graft-versus-host disease (GVHD) GRĂFT	Complication that occurs following a stem cell or bone marrow transplant in which the transplant produces antibodies against recipient's organs that can be severe enough to cause death
hematoma hēm-ă-TŌ-mă *hemat:* blood *-oma:* tumor	Localized accumulation of blood, usually clotted, in an organ, space, or tissue due to a break in or severing of a blood vessel
hemoglobinopathy hē-mō-glō-bĭ-NŎP-ă-thē *hem/o:* blood *globin/o:* protein *-pathy:* disease	Any disorder caused by abnormalities in the hemoglobin molecule *One of the most common hemoglobinopathies is sickle cell anemia.*
lymphadenopathy lĭm-făd-ĕ-NŎP-ă-thē *lymph:* lymph *aden/o:* gland *-pathy:* disease	Any disease of the lymph nodes *In localized lymphadenopathy, only one area of the body is affected. In systemic lymphadenopathy, two or more noncontiguous areas of the body are affected.*

(continued)

Term	Definition

lymphedema
lĭmf-ĕ-DĒ-mă
  lymph: lymph
  -edema: swelling
	Swelling, primarily in a single arm or leg, due to an accumulation of lymph within tissues caused by obstruction or disease in the lymph vessels
	The most common causes of lymphedema are surgery, radiation therapy, and infection of the lymph vessels.

multiple myeloma
mī-ĕ-LŌ-mă
  myel: bone marrow; spinal cord
  -oma: tumor
	Malignant tumor of plasma cells (cells that help the body fight infection by producing antibodies) in the bone marrow
	In multiple myeloma, malignant plasma cells spread throughout bone marrow and invade the harder outer portion of the bone, causing soft spots of holes in the bone. The goal of treatment is to relieve symptoms, avoid complications, and prolong life.

sepsis SĔP-sĭs	Presence of bacteria or their toxins in the blood; also called septicemia or blood poisoning *Usual causes of sepsis are peritonitis, urinary tract infections, meningitis, cellulitis, and bacterial pneumonias.*
systemic lupus erythematosus (SLE) sĭs-TĔM-ĭk LŪ-pŭs ĕr-ĭ-thē-mă-TŌ-sŭs	Widespread autoimmune disease that may affect the skin, brain, kidneys, and joints and causes chronic inflammation; also called discoid lupus if symptoms are limited to the skin *A typical "butterfly rash" appears over the nose and cheeks in about 50% of people afflicted with SLE and tends to get worse in direct sunlight. (See Figure 9-9.)*

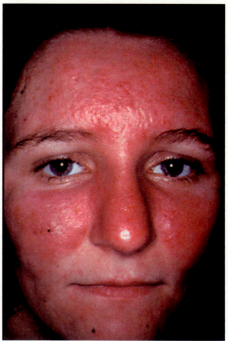

Figure 9-9 Red papules and plaques of systemic lupus erythematosus (SLE) in butterfly pattern on the face. From Goldsmith and Tharp: *Adult and Pediatric Dermatology: A Color Guide to Diagnosis and Treatment.* FA Davis, Philadelphia, 1997, p 230, with permission.

Term	Definition
thrombocythemia thrŏm-bō-sī-THĒ-mē-ă	Overproduction of platelets, leading to thrombosis or bleeding disorders due to platelet malformations
thrombocytopenia thrŏm-bō-sī-tō-PĒ-nē-ă *thromb/o:* blood clot *cyt/o:* cell *-penia:* decrease, deficiency	Abnormal decrease in platelets caused by low production of platelets in the bone marrow or increased destruction of platelets in the blood vessels (intravascular), spleen (extravascular), or liver (extravascular) *A common sign of thrombocytopenia is the development of pinpoint hemorrhages called petechiae that appear primarily on the lower leg. (See Figure 9–10.)*

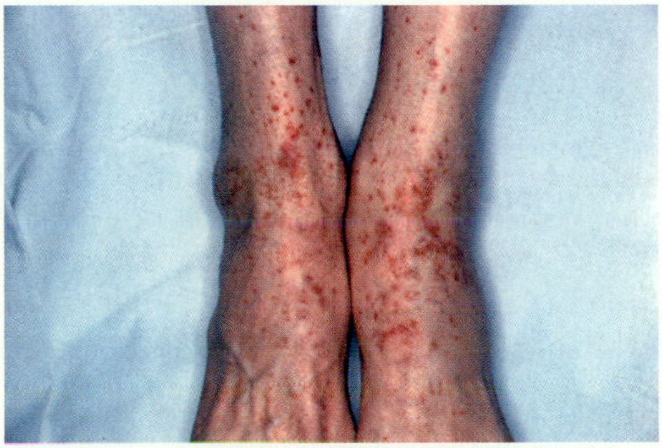

Figure 9-10 Petechiae on the skin from thrombocytopenia.
From Goldsmith and Tharp: *Adult and Pediatric Dermatology: A Color Guide to Diagnosis and Treatment.* FA Davis, Philadelphia, 1997, p 61, with permission.

Term	Definition
von Willebrand disease WĬL-ĕ-brănd	Bleeding disorder caused by a deficiency of von Willebrand factor, a "sticky" protein that lines blood vessels and reacts with platelets to form a plug that leads to clot formation

 It is time to review pathology, diseases, and conditions by completing Learning Activity 9–3.

Medical, Surgical, and Diagnostic Procedures

This section introduces medical, surgical, and diagnostic procedures used to treat and diagnose blood, lymph, and immune system disorders. Descriptions are provided as well as pronunciations and word analyses for selected terms.

Procedure	Description
Medical	
immunotherapy ĭm-ū-nō-THĔR-ă-pē *immun/o:* immune, immunity, safe *-therapy:* treatment	Any form of treatment that alters, enhances, stimulates or restores the body's natural immune mechanisms to treat disease
allergy injections ĂL-ĕr-jē	Injection with increasing strengths of the offending antigen given over a period of months or years to increase tolerance to an antigen responsible for severe allergies
biological bī-ō-LŎJ-ĭk-ăl	Use of immune system stimulators to enhance the immune response in the treatment of certain forms of cancer, rheumatoid arthritis, and Crohn disease; also called *biologic therapy* or *biotherapy*
Surgical	
bone marrow aspiration BŌN MĂR-ō ăs-pĭ-RĀ-shŭn	Removal of a small sample of bone marrow using a thin aspirating needle (usually from the pelvis) for microscopic examination (See Figure 9-11.) *Bone marrow aspiration identifies blood disorders or determines if infection has spread to the bone marrow.* **Figure 9-11** Bone marrow aspiration.
bone marrow transplant BŌN MĂR-ō TRĂNS-plănt	Infusion of healthy bone marrow stem cells after the diseased bone marrow is destroyed by chemotherapy and/or radiation therapy; used to treat leukemia, aplastic anemia, and certain cancers *The infusion is administered either to the same person or to another person.*
autologous aw-TŎL-ō-gŭs	Infusion of the patient's own bone marrow or stem cells after a course of chemotherapy and/or radiation therapy
homologous hō-MŎL-ō-gŭs	Infusion of bone marrow or stem cells from a compatible donor after a course of chemotherapy and/or radiation; also called *allogenic transplant*

Procedure	Description
lymphadenectomy lĭm-făd-ĕ-NĔK-tō-mē *lymph:* lymph *aden:* gland *-ectomy:* excision	Removal of lymph nodes, especially in surgical procedures undertaken to remove malignant tissue *A limited or modified lymphadenectomy removes only some of the lymph nodes in the area around a tumor; a total or radical lymphadenectomy removes all of the lymph nodes in the area.*
sentinel node excision SĔNT-ĭ-nĕl NŌD	Removal of the first node (sentinel node) that receives drainage from cancer-containing areas and the one most likely to contain malignant cells *If the sentinel node does not contain malignant cells, there may be no need to remove regional lymph nodes during cancer surgery. (See Figure 9–12.)* **Figure 9-12** Sentinel node, the first to receive drainage from a tumor site.
transfusion	Infusion of blood or blood products from one person (donor) to another person (recipient) *Transfusion is usually preformed as a life-saving maneuver when there is serious blood loss or for treatment of severe anemias.*

Diagnostic	
Laboratory	
antinuclear antibody (ANA)	Test to identify antibodies that attack the nucleus of the individual's own body cells (auto-antibodies) *Presence of ANAs indicates the potential for autoimmunity and directs the physician to explore possible autoimmune diseases.*
blood culture	Test to determine the presence of pathogens in the bloodstream *Sepsis, the most serious form of bacteremia, is life-threatening and usually the result of an overwhelming infection in another area of the body.*
complete blood count (CBC)	Series of tests that includes hemoglobin; hematocrit; red and white blood cell counts, platelet count; and differential (diff) count; also called *hemogram* *CBC is a broad screening test for anemias, coagulation disorders, and infections.*

(continued)

Procedure	Description
monospot	Nonspecific rapid serological test for the presence of the heterophile antibody, which develops several days after infection by Epstein-Barr virus, the organism that caused infectious mononucleosis
partial thromboplastin time (PTT) thrŏm-bō-PLĂS-tĭn	Test that measures the length of time it takes blood to clot to screen for deficiencies of some clotting factors; also called *activated partial thromboplastin time (APTT)* *PTT is a valuable tool in preoperative screening for bleeding tendencies.*
prothrombin time (PT) prō-THRŎM-bĭn	Test that measures the time it takes for prothrombin to form a clot; also called *pro time* *PT is commonly used to manage patients receiving the anticoagulant warfarin (Coumadin) and is also used to evaluate liver function.*
Shilling test	Test used to diagnose pernicious anemia by determining if the body properly absorbs vitamin B$_{12}$ through the digestive tract *Pernicious anemia is caused by the failure of the body to absorb vitamin B$_{12}$ due to lack of intrinsic factor, a glycoprotein required for its absorption.*
Imaging	
bone marrow magnetic resonance imaging (MRI)	Highly sensitive imaging procedure that detects lesions and changes in bone tissue and bone marrow, especially in multiple myeloma

lymphangiography
lĭm-făn-jē-ŎG-ră-fē
  lymph: lymph
  angi/o: vessel
  -graphy: process of recording
	Visualization of lymphatic channels and lymph nodes using a contrast medium to determine blockages or other pathologies of the lymph system
	
	Because lymph nodes filter and trap cancer cells, this test is commonly used to determine lymph flow in areas that contain malignancy.

lymphoscintigraphy lĭm-fō-sĭn-TĬGră-fē	Introduction of a radioactive tracer into the lymph channels to determine lymph flow, identify obstructions, and locate the sentinel node *Lymphoscintigraphy is also used to biopsy the lymph node, assess the stage of cancer, and determine a plan of treatment.*

Pharmacology

Various drugs are prescribed to treat blood, lymph, and immune systems disorders. (See Table 9-5.) These drugs act directly on individual components of each system. For example, anticoagulants are used to prevent clot formation but are ineffective in destroying formed clots. Instead, thrombolytics are used to dissolve clots that obstruct coronary, cerebral, or pulmonary arteries and, conversely, hemostatics are used to prevent or control hemorrhage. In addition, chemotherapy and radiation are commonly used to treat diseases of the blood and immune system. For example, antineoplastics prevent cellular replication to halt the spread of cancer in the body; antivirals prevent viral replication within cells and have been effective in slowing the progression of HIV and AIDS.

Table 9-5 — **Drugs Used to Treat Blood, Lymph, and Immune Disorders**

This table lists common drug classifications used to treat blood, lymph, and immune disorders, their therapeutic actions, and selected generic and trade names.

Classification	Therapeutic Action	Generic and *Trade* Names
anticoagulants ăn-tĭ-kō-ĂG-ū-lănts	Prevent blood clot formation by inhibiting the synthesis or inactivating one or more clotting factors *Anticoagulants prevent deep vein thrombosis (DVT) and postoperative clot formation and decrease the risk of Stroke.*	**heparin** HĔP-ă-rĭn *heparin sodium* **warfarin** WĂR-făr-ĭn *Coumadin*
antifibrinolytics ăn-tĭ-fī-brĭ-nō-LĬT-ĭks	Neutralize fibrinolytic chemicals in the mucous membranes of the mouth, nose, and urinary tract to prevent the breakdown of blood clots *Antifibrinolytics are used to treat serious bleeding following certain surgeries and dental procedures, especially in patients with such medical problems as hemophilia.*	**aminocaproic acid** ă-mē-nō-kă-PRŌ-ĭk ĂS-ĭd *Amicar*
antimicrobials ăn-tĭ-mī-KRŌ-bē-ălz	Destroy bacteria, fungi, and protozoa, depending on the particular drug, generally by interfering with the functions of their cell membrane or their reproductive cycle *HIV patients are commonly treated prophylactically with antimicrobials to prevent development of Pneumocystis pneumonia (PCP).*	**trimethoprim, sulfamethoxazole** trĭ-MĔTH-ō-prĭm, sŭl-fă-mĕth-ŎK-să-zōl *Bactrim, Septra* **metronidazole** mĕ-trō-NĬ-dă-zōl *Flagyl*
antivirals ăn-tĭ-VĪ-rălz	Prevent replication of viruses within host cells *Antivirals are used in treatment of HIV infection and AIDS.*	**nelfinavir** nĕl-FĬN-ă-vēr *Viracept* **lamivudine/zidovudine** lă-MĬV-ū-dēn, zī-DŌ-vū-dēn *Combivir*
fat-soluble vitamins SŌL-ū-bl	Prevent and treat bleeding disorders resulting from a lack of prothrombin, which is commonly caused by vitamin K deficiency	**phytonadione** fī-tō-nă-DĪ-ōn *Vitamin K1 Mephyton*
thrombolytics thrŏm-bō-LĬT-ĭks	Dissolve blood clots by destroying their fibrin strands *Thrombolytics are used to break apart, or lyse, thrombi, especially those that obstruct coronary, pulmonary, and cerebral arteries.*	**alteplase** ĂL-tĕ-plās *Activase, t-PA* **streptokinase** strĕp-tō-KĪ-nās *Streptase*

Abbreviations

This section introduces blood, lymph, and immune system abbreviations and their meanings.

Abbreviation	Meaning	Abbreviation	Meaning
AB, Ab, ab	antibody, abortion	eos	eosinophil (type of white blood cell)
A, B, AB, O	blood types in ABO blood group	Hb, Hgb	hemoglobin
AIDS	acquired immune deficiency syndrome	HIV	human immunodeficiency virus
ALL	acute lymphocytic leukemia	Igs	immunoglobulins
AML	acute myelogenous leukemia	MNL	mononuclear leukocytes
ANA	antinuclear antibody		
APC	antigen-presenting cell	NK cell	natural killer cell
APTT	activated partial thromboplastin time	PCP	*Pneumocystis* pneumonia; primary care physician
BMT	bone marrow transplant	PMN	polymorphonuclear
CBC	complete blood count	PMNL, poly	polymorphonuclear leukocyte
CLL	chronic lymphocytic leukemia	PT	prothrombin time, physical therapy
CML	chronic myelogenous leukemia	PTT	partial thromboplastin time
DIC	disseminated intravascular coagulation	RA	right atrium; rheumatoid arthritis
diff	differential count (white blood cells)	RBC, rbc	red blood cell
DVT	deep vein thrombosis; deep venous thrombosis	segs	segmented neutrophils
EBV	Epstein-Barr virus	SLE	systemic lupus erythematosus
GVHD	graft-versus-host disease	WBC, wbc	white blood cell

It is time to review procedures, pharmacology, and abbreviations by completing Learning Activity 9-4.

LEARNING ACTIVITIES

The following activities provide review of the blood, lymph, and immune system terms introduced in this chapter. Complete each activity and review your answers to evaluate your understanding of the chapter.

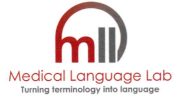

Medical Language Lab
Turning terminology into language

Visit the Medical Language Lab at the web site: medicallanguagelab.com. Use it to enhance your study and reinforcement of this chapter with the flash-card activity. We recommend you complete the flash-card activity before starting Learning Activities 9-1 and 9-2 below.

Learning Activity 9-1
Combining Forms, Suffixes, and Prefixes

Use the elements listed in the table to build medical words. You may use elements more than once.

Combining Forms		Suffixes		Prefixes
aden/o	leukocyt/o	-blast	-oma	a-
chrom/o	lymphangi/o	-ectomy	-osis	aniso-
cyt/o	morph/o	-ic	-penia	iso-
electr/o	phag/o	-itis	-phoresis	macro-
embol/o	splen/o	-lysis	-poiesis	
erythr/o	thromb/o	-megaly		
hem/o	thym/o	-oid		

1. inflammation of a lymph vessel _____
2. decrease of leukocytes _____
3. enlargement of the spleen _____
4. abnormal condition of clots _____
5. excision of an embolus _____
6. tumor of the thymus _____
7. pertaining to the same color _____
8. abnormal condition of unequal cell (sizes) _____
9. pertaining to a large eating (cell) _____
10. embryonic red (cell) _____
11. destruction of blood _____
12. carrying an electric (charge) _____
13. resembling a gland _____
14. pertaining to without a shape _____
15. formation (production) of white blood cells _____

 Check your answers in Appendix A. Review any material that you did not answer correctly.

Correct Answers _____ X 6.67 = _____ % Score

Learning Activity 9-2
Building Medical Words

Use *-osis* (abnormal condition; increase [used primarily with blood cells]) to build words that mean:

1. abnormal increase in erythrocytes _____
2. abnormal increase in leukocytes _____
3. abnormal increase in lymphocytes _____
4. abnormal increase in reticulocytes _____

Use *-penia* (deficiency, decrease) to build words that mean:

5. decrease in leukocytes _____
6. decrease in erythrocytes _____
7. decrease in thrombocytes _____
8. decrease in lymphocytes _____

Use *-poiesis* (formation, production) to build words that mean:

9. production of blood _____
10. production of white cells _____
11. production of thrombocytes _____

Use *immun/o* (immune, immunity, safe) to build words that mean:

12. specialist in the study of immunity _____
13. study of immunity _____

Use *splen/o* (spleen) to build words that mean:

14. herniation of the spleen _____
15. destruction of the spleen _____

Build surgical words that mean:

16. excision of the spleen _____
17. removal of the thymus _____
18. destruction of the thymus _____
19. incision of the spleen _____
20. fixation of (a displaced) spleen _____

✔ *Check your answers in Appendix A. Review any material that you did not answer correctly.*

Correct Answers _____ X 5 = _____ % Score

Learning Activity 9-3

Pathology, Diseases, and Conditions

Match the following terms with the definitions in the numbered list.

anaphylaxis	hematoma	lymphadenopathy	sepsis
aplastic	hemoglobinopathy	mononucleosis	sickle cell
edema	hemolytic	multiple myeloma	splenomegaly
erythropenia	Hodgkin disease	myelogenous	thrombocythemia
graft rejection	Kaposi sarcoma	opportunistic	thrombocytopenia

1. disorder in the development of hemoglobin _____

2. abnormal accumulation of fluid in tissues _____

3. disease of a lymph node _____

4. anemia associated with bone marrow failure _____

5. life-threatening allergic response _____

6. denotes an infection that affects only those who are immunocompromised _____

7. malignant disease of the lymph nodes _____

8. enlargement of the spleen _____

9. decrease in RBCs _____

10. malignancy of plasma cells in the bone marrow _____

11. infectious disorder caused by the Epstein-Barr virus _____

12. presence of bacteria or their toxins in blood _____

13. leukemia that affects granulocytes _____

14. malignancy associated with HIV _____

15. hereditary anemia found mostly in the those of African descent _____

16. decrease of platelets in the circulatory system _____

17. anemia caused by destruction of erythrocytes _____

18. excessive number of platelets in circulation _____

19. area of blood seepage into tissues due to a ruptured blood vessel _____

20. destruction of a transplanted organ or tissue by the recipient's immune system _____

 Check your answers in Appendix A. Review any material that you did not answer correctly.

Correct Answers _____ X 5 = _____ % Score

Learning Activity 9-4

Procedures, Pharmacology, and Abbreviations

Match the following terms with the definitions in the numbered list.

ANA	homologous	RBC
anticoagulants	lymphadenectomy	Shilling
antimicrobials	lymphangiography	thrombolytics
autologous	lymphoscintigraphy	transfusion
biological	monospot	WBC

1. immunotherapy that uses stimulators to enhance the immune system _____

2. procedure that uses a contrast dye to determine blockages of the lymph vessels _____

3. serologic test for infectious mononucleosis _____

4. used to prevent blood clot formation _____

5. leukocyte _____

6. procedure that describes a transplantation from a compatible donor _____

7. test that identifies antibodies that attack an individual's own cells _____

8. procedure that uses a radioactive tracer to identify the location of the sentinel node _____

9. laboratory test to diagnose pernicious anemia _____

10. excision of lymph nodes _____

11. procedure that describes a transplantation using the recipient's own stem cells _____

12. destroy bacteria, fungi, and protozoa _____

13. erythrocyte _____

14. used to dissolve blood clots _____

15. lifesaving procedure to replenish blood loss or for treatment of severe anemia _____

✅ *Check your answers in Appendix A. Review any material that you did not answer correctly.*

Correct Answers _____ X 6.67 = _____ % Score

Learning Activity 9-5
Medical Scenarios

To construct chart notes, replace the italicized terms in each of the two scenarios with one of the medical terms listed below.

arthralgia	*hematologist*	*leukocytosis*
ecchymoses	*hemophilia*	*lymphadenopathy*
erythropenia	*hemostasis*	*splenomegaly*
hemarthrosis		

Mr. X., a 53-year-old male, presents with complaints of feeling "poorly" and not sleeping well for the past three months. Upon examination, the physician notes that Mr. X's gums are red and swollen. Also, there is evidence of (1) ***disease in the glands*** under the patient's left arm and on the back of his neck. Upon palpation, the physician also notes an (2) ***enlarged spleen***. The patient's CBC shows an (3) ***abnormal increase of leukocytes*** and a moderate (4) ***decrease of erythrocytes***. The patient is referred to Dr. Jordan, a (5) ***specialist in blood diseases***.

1. _____
2. _____
3. _____
4. _____
5. _____

Mr. J. states that his father and uncle have (6) ***bleeder's disease***. The patient also states that he often develops (7) ***large bruises*** under his skin even with a minimal "bump or scrape." Today he presents with swelling and (8) ***pain in his joints***, especially the knees. His present complaints are likely due to (9) ***abnormal bleeding into the joint*** cavity. The physician prescribes an infusion of Mr. J's deficient clotting factor to (10) ***stop the bleeding***.

6. _____
7. _____
8. _____
9. _____
10. _____

✓ *Check your answers in Appendix A. Review any material that you did not answer correctly.*

Correct Answers _____ X 10 = _____ % Score

MEDICAL RECORD ACTIVITIES

The two medical records included in the following activities use common clinical scenarios to show how medical terminology is used to document patient care. Complete the terminology and analysis sections for each activity to help you recognize and understand terms related to the blood, lymph, and immune systems.

Medical Record Activity 9-1

Discharge Summary: Sickle Cell Crisis

Terminology

Terms listed in the following table are taken from *Discharge Summary: Sickle Cell Crisis* that follows. Use a medical dictionary such as *Taber's Cyclopedic Medical Dictionary;* the appendices of *Systems,* 7th ed.; or other resources to define each term. Then review the pronunciations for each term and practice by reading the medical record aloud.

Term	Definition
ambulating ĂM-bū-lāt-ĭng	
analgesia ăn-ăl-JĒ-zē-ă	
anemia ă-NĒ-mē-ă	
crisis KRĪ-sĭs	
CT	
hemoglobin HĒ-mō-glō-bĭn	
ileus ĬL-ē-ŭs	
infarction ĭn-FĂRK-shŭn	
morphine MOR-fēn	
sickle cell SĬK-ăl SĚL	

Term	Definition
splenectomy splē-NĔK-tō-mē	
Vicodin VĪ-kō-dĭn	

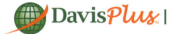 | Visit the *Medical Terminology Systems* online resource center at Davis*Plus* to practice pronunciation and reinforce the meanings of the terms in this medical report.

DISCHARGE SUMMARY: SICKLE CELL CRISIS

General Hospital

1511 Ninth Avenue ■■ Sun City, USA 12345 ■■ (555) 802-1887

DISCHARGE SUMMARY

ADMISSION DATE: June 21, 20xx   **DISCHARGE DATE:** June 23, 20xx

ADMITTING AND DISCHARGE DIAGNOSES:
1. Sickle cell crisis.
2. Abdominal pain.

PROCEDURES: Two units of packed red blood cells and CT scan of the abdomen.

REASON FOR ADMISSION: This is a 46-year-old African American man who reports a history of sickle cell anemia, which results in abdominal cramping when he is in crisis. His hemoglobin was 6 upon admission. He says his baseline runs 7 to 8. The patient states that he has not had a splenectomy. He describes the pain as midabdominal and cramplike. He denied any chills, fevers, or sweats.

HOSPITAL COURSE BY PROBLEM:
Problem 1. Sickle cell crisis. Patient was admitted to a medical-surgical bed, and placed on oxygen and IV fluids. He received morphine for analgesia as well as Vicodin. At discharge, his abdominal pain had resolved; however, he reported weakness. He was kept for an additional day for observation.

Problem 2. CT scan was performed on the belly and showed evidence of ileus in the small bowel with somewhat dilated small-bowel loops and also an abnormal enhancement pattern in the kidney. The patient has had no nausea or vomiting. He is moving his bowels without any difficulty. He is ambulating. He even goes outside to smoke cigarettes, which he has been advised not to do. Certainly, we should obtain some information on his renal function and have his regular doctor assess this problem.

DISCHARGE INSTRUCTIONS: Patient advised to stop smoking and to see his regular doctor for follow-up on renal function.

Michael R. Saadi, MD
Michael R. Saadi, MD

MRS:dp

D: 6-23-20xx
T: 6-23-20xx

Patient: Evans, Joshua   Physician: Michael R. Saadi, MD
Room #: 609 P   Patient ID#: 532657

Analysis

Review the medical record *Discharge Summary: Sickle Cell Crisis* to answer the following questions.

1. What blood product was administered to the patient?

_____

2. Why was this blood product given to the patient?

_____

3. Why was a CT scan performed on the patient?

_____

4. What were the three findings of the CT scan?

_____

5. Why should the patient see his regular doctor?

_____

Discharge Summary: PCP and HIV

Terminology

Terms listed in the following table are taken from *Discharge Summary: PCP and HIV* that follows. Use a medical dictionary such as *Taber's Cyclopedic Medical Dictionary;* the appendices of *Systems,* 7th ed.; or other resources to define each term. Then review the pronunciations for each term and practice by reading the medical record aloud.

Term	Definition
alveolar lavage ăl-VĒ-ō-lăr lă-VĂZH	
Bactrim BĂK-trĭm	
bronchoscopy brŏng-KŎS-kō-pē	
diffuse dĭ-FŪS	
HIV	
human immunodeficiency virus ĭm-ū-nō-dē-FĬSH-ĕn-sē	
infiltrate ĬN-fĭl-trāt	
Kaposi sarcoma KĂP-ō-sē săr-KŌ-mă	
leukoencephalopathy loo-kō-ĕn-sĕf-ă-LŎP-ă-thē	
multifocal mŭl-tĭ-FŌ-kăl	
PCP	
PMN	

Term	Definition
Pneumocystis pneumonia nū-mō-SĬS-tĭs nū-MŌ-nē-ă	
thrush THRŬSH	
vaginal candidiasis VĂJ-ĭn-ăl kăn-dĭ-DĪ-ă-sĭs	

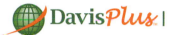

Visit the *Medical Terminology Systems* online resource center at Davis*Plus* to practice pronunciation and reinforce the meanings of the terms in this medical report.

DISCHARGE SUMMARY: PCP AND HIV

General Hospital

1511 Ninth Avenue ■■ Sun City, USA 12345 ■■ (544) 802-1887

DISCHARGE SUMMARY

Age: 31

ADMISSION DATE: March 5, 20xx   **DISCHARGE DATE:** March 6, 20xx

ADMITTING AND DISCHARGE DIAGNOSES:
Pneumocystis pneumonia.
Human immunodeficiency virus infection.
Wasting.

SOCIAL HISTORY: Patient's husband is deceased from AIDS 1 year ago with progressive multifocal leukoencephalopathy and Kaposi sarcoma. She denies any history of intravenous drug use, transfusion, and identifies three lifetime sexual partners.

PAST MEDICAL HISTORY: Patient's past medical history is significant for HIV and several episodes of diarrhea, sinusitis, thrush, and vaginal candidiasis. She gave a history of a 10-pound weight loss. The chest x-ray showed diffuse lower lobe infiltrates, and she was diagnosed with presumptive *Pneumocystis* pneumonia and placed on Bactrim. She was admitted for a bronchoscopy with alveolar lavage to confirm the diagnosis.

PROCEDURE: The antiretroviral treatment was reinitiated, and she was counseled as to the need to strictly adhere to her therapeutic regimen.

DISCHARGE INSTRUCTIONS: Complete medication regimen. Patient discharged to the care of Dr. Amid Shaheen.

Michael R. Saadi, MD
Michael R. Saadi, MD

MRS:dp

D: 3-06-20xx
T: 3-06-20xx

Patient: Smart, Joann   Physician: Michael R. Saadi, MD
Room #: 540   Patient ID#: 532850

Analysis

Review the medical record *Discharge Summary: PCP and HIV* to answer the following questions.

1. How do you think the patient acquired the HIV infection?

_____

2. What were the two diagnoses of the husband?

_____

3. What four disorders in the medical history are significant for HIV?

_____

4. What was the x-ray finding?

_____

5. What two procedures are going to be performed to confirm the diagnosis of *pneumocystis* pneumonia?

_____

Musculoskeletal System

Chapter Outline

Objectives

Upon completion of this chapter, you will be able to:

- Locate and describe the structures of the musculoskeletal system.
- Describe the functional relationship between the musculoskeletal systems and other body systems.
- Pronounce, spell, and build words related to the musculoskeletal system.
- Describe pathological conditions, diagnostic and therapeutic procedures, and other terms related to the musculoskeletal system.
- Explain pharmacology related to the treatment of musculoskeletal disorders.
- Demonstrate your knowledge of this chapter by completing the learning and medical record activities.

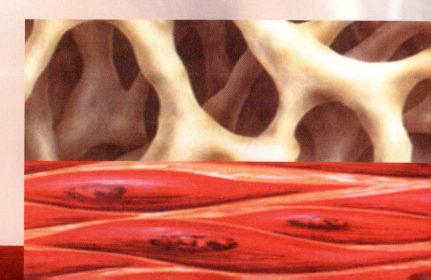

Anatomy and Physiology

The musculoskeletal system includes muscles, bones, joints, and related structures, such as the tendons and connective tissue that function in support and movement of body parts and organs. (See Figure 10-1.)

Anatomy and Physiology Key Terms

This section introduces important terms along with their definitions and pronunciations. Word analyses are also provided.

Term	Definition
appendage ă-PĔN-dĭj	Any body part attached to a main structure *Examples of appendages include the arms and legs.*
articulation ăr-tĭk-ū-LĀ-shŭn	Place of union between two or more bones; also called *joint*
cancellous KĂN-sĕl-ŭs	Latticelike arrangement of bony plates occurring at the ends of long bones
cruciate ligaments KROO-shē-āt *cruci:* cross *-ate:* having the form of; possessing	Ligaments that cross each other, forming an X within the notch between the femoral condyles *Along with other structures, the cruciate ligaments help secure and stabilize the knee.*
hematopoiesis hĕm-ă-tō-poy-Ē-sĭs *hemat/o:* blood *-poiesis:* formation, production	Production and development of blood cells, normally in the bone marrow

Pronunciation Help	Long Sound	ā — rate	ē — rebirth	ī — isle	ō — over	ū — unite
	Short Sound	ă — alone	ĕ — ever	ĭ — it	ŏ — not	ŭ — cut

Muscles

Muscle tissue is composed of contractile cells, or **fibers,** that provide movement of an organ or body part. Muscles contribute to posture, produce body heat, and act as a protective covering for internal organs. Muscles make up the bulk of the body. They have the ability to be excited by a stimulus, contract, relax, and return to their original size and shape. Whether muscles are attached to bones or to internal organs and blood vessels, their primary responsibility is movement. (See Table 10-1.) Apparent motions provided by muscles include walking and talking. Less apparent motions include the passage and elimination of food through the digestive system, propulsion of blood through the arteries, and contraction of the bladder to eliminate urine.

There are three types of muscle tissue in the body:

- **Skeletal muscles,** also called **voluntary** or **striated muscles,** are muscles whose action is under voluntary control. Some examples of voluntary muscles are muscles that move the eyeballs, tongue, and bones.
- **Cardiac muscle** is found only in the heart. It is unique for its branched interconnections, and makes up most of the wall of the heart. Cardiac muscle shares similarities with both

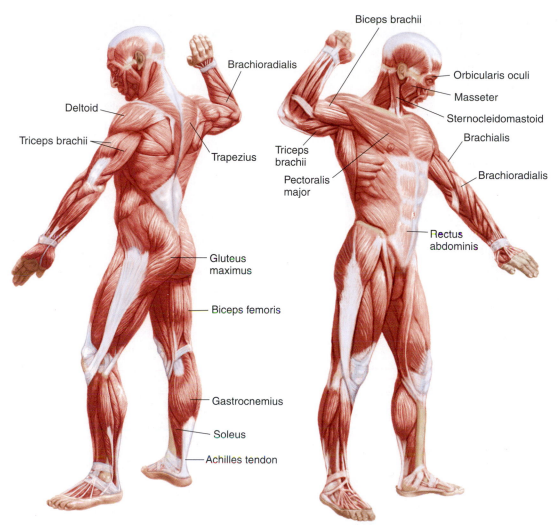

Figure 10-1 Selected muscles of the body.

skeletal and smooth muscles. Like skeletal muscle, it is striated, but it produces rhythmic involuntary contractions like smooth muscle.

- **Smooth muscles,** also called **involuntary** or **visceral muscles,** are muscles whose actions are involuntary. They are found principally in the visceral organs, walls of arteries and respiratory passages, and urinary and reproductive ducts. The contraction of smooth muscle is controlled by the autonomic (involuntary) nervous system.

Attachments

Muscles attach to bones by fleshy or fibrous attachments. In **fleshy attachments,** muscle fibers arise directly from bone. Although these fibers distribute force over wide areas, they are weaker than a fibrous attachment. In **fibrous attachments,** the connective tissue converges at the end of the muscle to become continuous and indistinguishable from the periosteum. When the fibrous attachment spans a large area of a bone, the attachment is called an **aponeurosis.** Such attachments are found in the lumbar region of the back. In some instances, this connective tissue penetrates the bone itself. When connective tissue fibers form a cord or strap, it is referred to as a **tendon.** This arrangement localizes a great deal of force in a small area of bone. **Ligaments** are flexible bands of fibrous tissue that are highly adapted for resisting strains and are one of the principal mechanical factors that hold bones close together in a synovial joint. An example are the **cruciate ligaments** of the knee that help to prevent anterior–posterior displacement of the articular surfaces and to secure articulating bones when we stand.

Table 10-1	Body Movements Produced by Muscle Action	

This table lists body movements and the resulting muscle action. With the exception of rotation, these movements are in pairs of opposing functions.

Motion	Action
Adduction	Moves closer to the midline
Abduction	Moves away from the midline

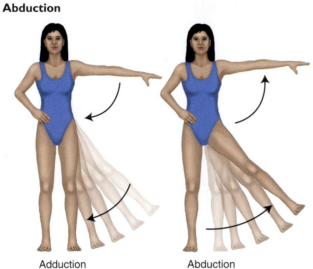

Adduction   Abduction

Motion	Action
Flexion	Decreases the angle of a joint
Extension	Increases the angle of a joint

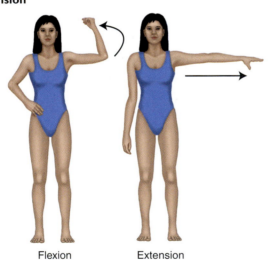

Flexion   Extension

Table 10-1	**Body Movements Produced by Muscle Action—cont'd**

Motion	Action
Rotation	Moves a bone around its own axis

Rotation

Pronation	Turns the palm down
Supination	Turns the palm up

Pronation   Supination

Inversion	Moves the sole of the foot inward
Eversion	Moves the sole of the foot outward

Eversion   Inversion

Dorsiflexion	Elevates the foot
Plantar flexion	Lowers the foot (points the toes)

Dorsiflexion

Plantar flexion

Anatomy Review: Musculoskeletal System

To review the anatomy of the muscular system, label the illustration using the terms below.

Achilles tendon   *gastrocnemius*   *rectus abdominus*

biceps brachii   *gluteus maximus*   *soleus*

biceps femoris   *masseter*   *sternocleidomastoid*

brachioradialis   *orbicularis oculi*   *trapezius*

deltoid   *pectoralis major*

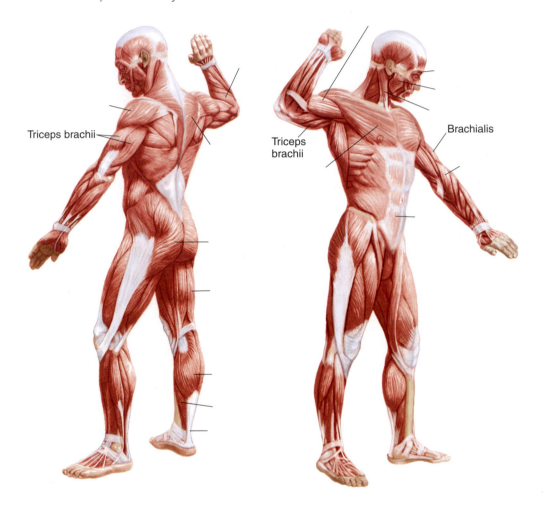

Triceps brachii

Triceps brachii

Brachialis

 Check your answers by referring to Figure 10-1 on page 299. Review material that you did not answer correctly.

Bones

Bones provide the framework of the body, protect internal organs, store calcium and other minerals, and produce blood cells within bone marrow (**hematopoiesis**). Together with soft tissue, most vital organs are enclosed and protected by bones. For example, bones of the skull protect the brain; the rib cage protects the heart and lungs. In addition to support and protection, the skeletal system carries out a number of other important functions. Movement is possible because bones provide points of attachment for muscles, tendons, and ligaments. As muscles contract, tendons and ligaments pull on bones and cause skeletal movement. Bone marrow, found within the larger bones, is responsible for hematopoiesis, continuously producing millions of blood cells to replace those that have been destroyed. Bones serve as a storehouse for minerals, particularly phosphorus and calcium. When the body experiences a need for a certain mineral, such as calcium during pregnancy, and a sufficient dietary supply is not available, calcium is withdrawn from the bones.

Bone Types

There are four principal types of bone:

- **Short bones** are somewhat cube-shaped. They consist of a core of spongy bone, also known as **cancellous** bone, enclosed in a thin surface layer of compact bone. Examples of short bones include the bones of the ankles, wrists, and toes.
- **Irregular bones** include the bones that cannot be classified as short or long because of their complex shapes. Examples of irregular bones include vertebrae and the bones of the middle ear.
- **Flat bones** are exactly what their name suggests. They provide broad surfaces for muscular attachment or protection for internal organs. Examples of flat bones include bones of the skull, shoulder blades, and sternum.
- **Long bones** are found in the **appendages** (extremities) of the body, such as the legs, arms, and fingers. (See Figure 10-2.) There are three main parts of a long bone:
  - The (1) **diaphysis** is the shaft, or long, main portion of a bone. It consists of (2) **compact bone** that forms a cylinder and surrounds a central canal called the (3) **medullary cavity.** The medullary cavity, also called **marrow cavity,** contains fatty yellow marrow in adults and consists primarily of fat cells and a few scattered blood cells.
  - The (4) **distal epiphysis** and (5) **proximal epiphysis** (plural, **epiphyses**) are the two ends of the bones. Both ends have a somewhat bulbous shape to provide space for muscle and ligament attachments near the joints. The epiphyses are covered with (6) **articular cartilage,** a type of elastic connective tissue that provides a smooth surface for movement of joints. It also reduces friction and absorbs shock at the freely movable joints. In addition, the epiphyses are made up largely of a porous chamber of (7) **spongy bone** surrounded by a layer of compact bone. Within spongy bone is red bone marrow, which is richly supplied with blood and consists of immature and mature blood cells in various stages of development.
  - The (8) **periosteum,** a dense, white, fibrous membrane, covers the remaining surface of the bone. It contains numerous blood and lymph vessels and nerves. In growing bones, the inner layer contains the bone-forming cells known as **osteoblasts.** Because blood vessels and osteoblasts are located here, the periosteum provides a means for bone repair and general bone nutrition. Bones that lose periosteum through injury or disease usually scale or die. The periosteum also serves as a point of attachment for muscles, ligaments, and tendons.

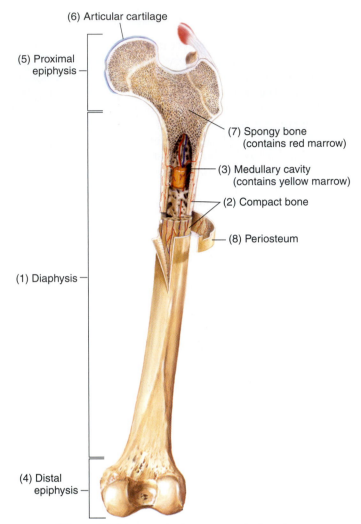

(6) Articular cartilage

(5) Proximal epiphysis

(7) Spongy bone (contains red marrow)

(3) Medullary cavity (contains yellow marrow)

(2) Compact bone

(8) Periosteum

(1) Diaphysis

(4) Distal epiphysis

Figure 10-2 Longitudinal structure of a long bone.

Surface Features of Bones

Surfaces of bones are rarely smooth but consist of projections, depressions, and openings that provide sites for muscle and ligament attachment. They also provide pathways and openings for blood vessels, nerves, and ducts. Various types of projections are evident in bones, some of which serve as points of **articulation**. Surfaces of bones may be rounded, sharp, or narrow or contain ridges. (See Table 10-2.)

Divisions of the Skeletal System

The skeletal system of a human adult consists of 206 individual bones. Here, we will discuss the major bones of the skeletal system. For anatomical purposes, the human skeleton is divided into the axial skeleton and appendicular skeleton. (See Figure 10-3.)

Axial Skeleton

The axial skeleton is divided into three major regions: skull, rib cage, and vertebral column. It contributes to the formation of body cavities and provides protection for internal organs, such as

---

Table 10-2   **Surface Features of Bones**

This table lists the most common types of bone projections, depressions, and openings along with the bones involved, descriptions, and examples for each. Becoming familiar with these terms will help you identify parts of individual bones described in medical reports related to orthopedics.

Surface Type	Bone Marking	Description	Example
Projections			
• Nonarticulating surfaces	• Trochanter	• Very large, irregularly shaped process found only on the femur	• Greater trochanter of the femur
• Sites of muscle and ligament attachment	• Tubercle	• Small, rounded process	• Tubercle of the femur
	• Tuberosity	• Large, rounded process	• Tuberosity of the humerus
Articulating Surfaces			
• Projections that form joints	• Condyle	• Rounded, articulating knob	• Condyle of the humerus
	• Head	• Prominent, rounded, articulating end of a bone	• Head of the femur
Depressions and Openings			
• Sites for blood vessel, nerve, and duct passage	• Foramen	• Rounded opening through a bone to accommodate blood vessels and nerves	• Foramen of the skull through which cranial nerves pass
	• Fissure	• Narrow, slitlike opening	• Fissure of the sphenoid bone
	• Meatus	• Opening or passage into a bone	• External auditory meatus of the temporal bone
	• Sinus	• Cavity or hollow space in a bone	• Cavity of the frontal sinus containing a duct that carries secretions to the upper part of the nasal cavity

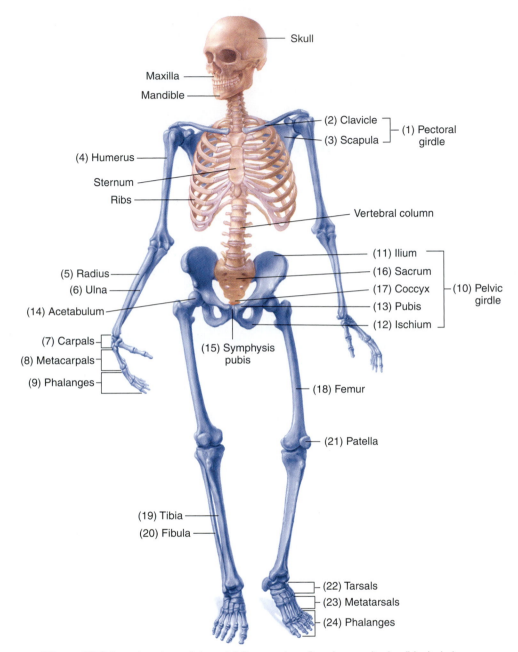

Skull

Maxilla

Mandible

(2) Clavicle ⌉
(3) Scapula ⌋ ⊢ (1) Pectoral girdle

(4) Humerus

Sternum

Ribs

Vertebral column

(11) Ilium ⌉
(16) Sacrum
(5) Radius
(17) Coccyx ⊢ (10) Pelvic girdle
(6) Ulna
(13) Pubis
(14) Acetabulum
(12) Ischium ⌋

(7) Carpals
(15) Symphysis pubis
(8) Metacarpals

(9) Phalanges

(18) Femur

(21) Patella

(19) Tibia
(20) Fibula

(22) Tarsals
(23) Metatarsals
(24) Phalanges

Figure 10-3 Anterior view of the axial (bone-colored) and appendicular (blue) skeleton.

the brain, spinal cord, and organs enclosed in the thorax. The axial skeleton is distinguished with bone color in Figure 10-3.

Skull

The bony structure of the skull consists of cranial bones and facial bones. (See Figure 10-4.) With the exception of one facial bone, all other bones of the skull are joined together by sutures. Sutures are the lines of junction between two bones, especially of the skull, and are usually immovable.

Cranial Bones

Eight bones, collectively known as the **cranium (skull),** enclose and protect the brain and the organs of hearing and equilibrium. Cranial bones are connected to muscles to provide head movements, chewing motions, and facial expressions.

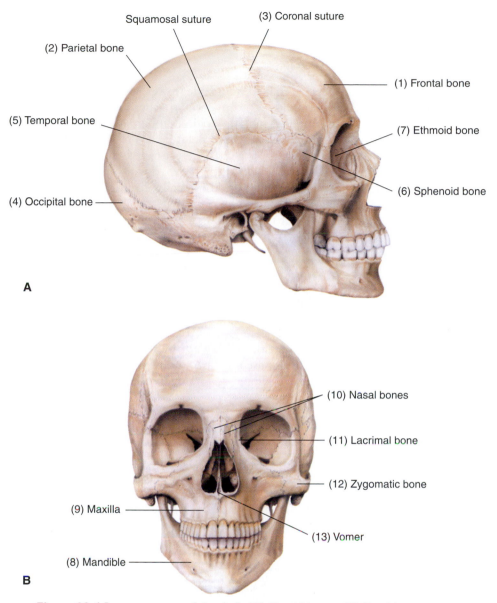

Squamosal suture

(3) Coronal suture

(2) Parietal bone

(1) Frontal bone

(5) Temporal bone

(7) Ethmoid bone

(6) Sphenoid bone

(4) Occipital bone

A

(10) Nasal bones

(11) Lacrimal bone

(12) Zygomatic bone

(9) Maxilla

(13) Vomer

(8) Mandible

B

Figure 10-4 Bony structures of the skull. **(A)** Cranial bones. **(B)** Facial bones.

An infant's skull contains an unossified membrane, or **soft spot** (incomplete bone formation), called a **fontanel** that lies between the cranial bones. The pulse of blood vessels can be felt under the skin in that area. The chief function of the fontanels is to allow the bones to move as the fetus passes through the birth canal during the delivery process. With age, the fontanels begin to fuse together and become immobile in early childhood.

The (1) **frontal bone** forms the anterior portion of the skull **(forehead)** and the roof of the bony cavities that contain the eyeballs. One (2) **parietal bone** is situated on each side of the skull just behind the frontal bone. Together they form the upper sides and roof of the cranium. Each parietal bone meets the frontal bone along the (3) **coronal suture.** A single (4) **occipital bone** forms the back and base of the skull. It contains an opening in its base through which the spinal cord passes. Two (5) **temporal bone(s),** one on each side of the skull, form part of the lower cranium. Each temporal bone has a complicated shape that contains various cavities and recesses associated with the internal ear, the essential part of the organ of hearing. The temporal bone projects downward to form the **mastoid process,** which provides a point of attachment for several neck muscles. The (6) **sphenoid bone,** located at the middle part of the base of the skull, forms a central wedge that joins with all other cranial bones, holding them together. A very light and spongy bone, the (7) **ethmoid bone,** forms most of the bony area between the nasal cavity and parts of the orbits of the eyes.

Facial Bones

All facial bones, with the exception of the (8) **mandible** (lower jaw bone), are joined together by sutures and are immovable. Movement of the mandible is needed for speaking and chewing **(mastication).** The (9) **maxillae** (singular, **maxilla**), paired upper jawbones, are fused in the midline by a suture. They form the upper jaw and **hard palate** (roof of the mouth). If the maxillary bones do not fuse properly before birth, a congenital defect called **cleft palate** results. The maxillae and mandible contain sockets for the roots of the teeth. Two thin, nearly rectangular bones, the (10) **nasal bones,** lie side-by-side and are fused medially, forming the shape and the bridge of the nose. Two paired (11) **lacrimal bones** are located at the corner of each eye. These thin, small bones unite to form the groove for the lacrimal sac and canals through which the tear ducts pass into the nasal cavity. The paired (12) **zygomatic bones** are located on the side of the face below the eyes and form the higher portion of the cheeks below and to the sides of the eyes. The zygomatic bone is commonly referred to as the **cheekbone.** The (13) **vomer** is a single, thin bone that forms the lower part of the nasal septum.

Other important structures, the **paranasal sinuses,** are cavities located within the cranial and facial bones. As their name implies, the frontal, ethmoidal, sphenoidal, and maxillary sinuses are named after the bones in which they are located. (See Figure 10-5.) The paranasal sinuses open into the nasal cavities and are lined with the **ciliary epithelium,** which is continuous with the mucosa of the nasal cavities. When sinuses are unable to drain properly, a feeling of being "stuffed up" ensues. This commonly occurs during upper respiratory infections (URIs) or with allergies.

Thorax

The term *thorax* refers to the entire chest. The internal organs of the thorax include the heart and lungs, which are enclosed and protected by the "rib cage," also known as the **thoracic cage.** The thoracic cage consists of 12 pairs of ribs, all attached to the spine. (See Figure 10-6.) The first seven pairs, the (1) **true ribs,** are attached directly to the (2) **sternum** by a strip of (3) **costal cartilage.** The costal cartilage of the next five pairs of ribs is not fastened directly to the sternum, so these ribs are known as (4) **false ribs.** The last two pairs of false ribs are not joined, even indirectly,

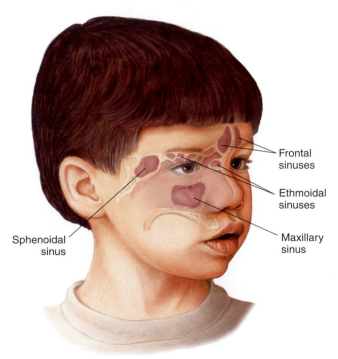

Frontal sinuses

Ethmoidal sinuses

Maxillary sinus

Sphenoidal sinus

Figure 10-5 Paranasal sinuses.

to the sternum but attach posteriorly to the thoracic vertebrae. These last two pairs of false ribs are known as (5) **floating ribs.**

Vertebral Column

The vertebral column of the adult is composed of 26 bones called **vertebrae** (singular, **vertebra**). The vertebral column supports the body and provides a protective bony canal for the spinal cord. A healthy, normal spine has four curves that help make it resilient and maintain balance. The cervical and lumbar regions curve forward, whereas the thoracic and sacral regions curve backward. Abnormal curves may be due to a congenital defect, poor posture, or bone disease. (See Figure 10-7.)

The vertebral column consists of five regions of bones, each deriving its name from its location within the spinal column. The seven (1) **cervical vertebrae** form the skeletal framework of the neck. The first cervical vertebra, the (2) **atlas,** supports the skull. The second cervical vertebra, the (3) **axis,** makes possible the rotation of the skull on the neck. Under the seventh cervical vertebra are 12 (4) **thoracic vertebrae,** which support the chest and serve as a point of articulation for the ribs. The next five vertebrae, the (5) **lumbar vertebrae,** are situated in the lower back area and carry most of the weight of the torso. Below this area are five sacral vertebrae, which are fused into a single bone in the adult and are referred to as the (6) **sacrum.** The tail of the vertebral column consists of four or five fragmented fused vertebrae referred to as the (7) **coccyx.**

Vertebrae are separated by flat, round structures, the (8) **intervertebral disks,** which are composed of a fibrocartilaginous substance with a gelatinous mass in the center **(nucleus pulposus).**

Appendicular Skeleton

The appendicular skeleton consists of bones of the upper and lower limbs and their girdles, which attach the limbs to the axial skeleton. The appendicular skeleton is distinguished with a blue color in Figure 10-3. The difference between the axial and appendicular skeletons is that the axial skeleton protects internal organs and provides central support for the body; the appendicular skeleton enables the body to move. The ability to walk, run, or catch a ball is possible because of the movable joints of the limbs that make up the appendicular skeleton.

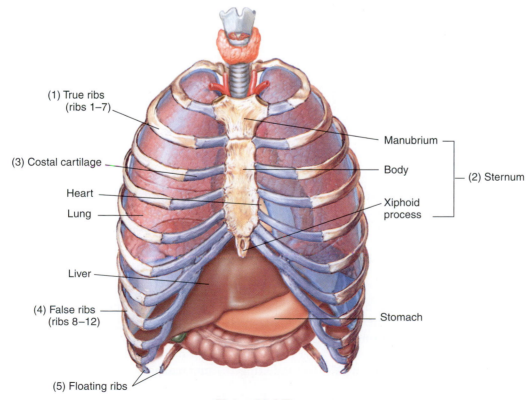

(1) True ribs (ribs 1–7)

(3) Costal cartilage

Heart

Lung

Liver

(4) False ribs (ribs 8–12)

(5) Floating ribs

Manubrium

Body

(2) Sternum

Xiphoid process

Stomach

Figure 10-6 Thorax.

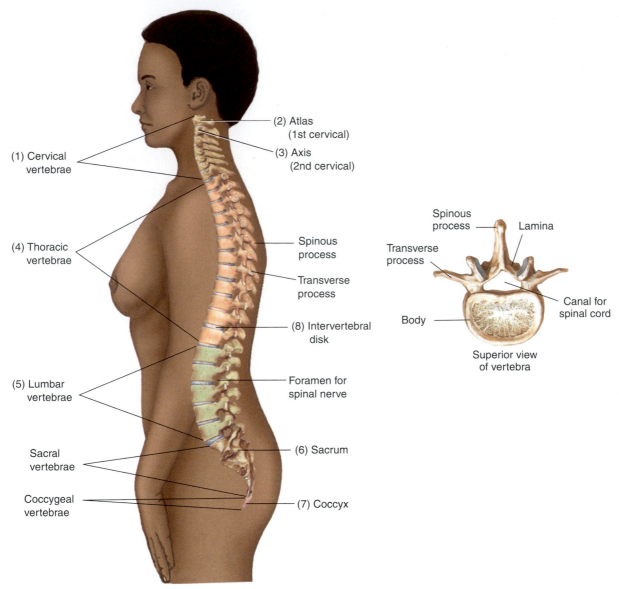

(1) Cervical vertebrae

(2) Atlas (1st cervical)

(3) Axis (2nd cervical)

(4) Thoracic vertebrae

Spinous process

Transverse process

(8) Intervertebral disk

(5) Lumbar vertebrae

Foramen for spinal nerve

Sacral vertebrae

(6) Sacrum

Coccygeal vertebrae

(7) Coccyx

Spinous process

Lamina

Transverse process

Canal for spinal cord

Body

Superior view of vertebra

Figure 10-7 Lateral view of the vertebral column.

Pectoral Girdle

The (1) **pectoral (shoulder) girdle** consists of two bones, the anterior (2) **clavicle** (collar bone) and the posterior (3) **scapula** (triangular shoulder blade). The primary function of the pectoral girdle is to attach the bones of the upper limbs to the axial skeleton and provide attachments for muscles that aid upper limb movements. The paired pectoral structures and their associated muscles form the shoulders of the body.

Upper Limbs

The skeletal framework of each upper limb includes the arm, forearm, and hand. Anatomically speaking, the arm is only that part of the upper limb between the shoulder and elbow. Each appendage consists of a (4) **humerus** (upper arm bone), which articulates with the (5) **radius** and (6) **ulna** at the elbow. The radius and ulna form the skeleton of the forearm. The bones of each hand include eight (7) **carpals** (wrist); five radiating (8) **metacarpals** (palm); and ten radiating (9) **phalanges** (fingers).

Pelvic Girdle

The (10) **pelvic (hip) girdle** is a basin-shaped structure that attaches the lower limbs to the axial skeleton. Along with its associated ligaments, it supports the trunk of the body and provides protection for the visceral organs of the pelvis (lower organs of digestion and urinary and reproductive structures).

Male and female **pelves** (singular, **pelvis**) differ considerably in size and shape but share the same basic structures. Generally, the bones of males are larger and heavier and possess larger surface markings than those of females of comparable age and physical stature. Some of the differences are attributable to the function of the female pelvis during childbearing. The female pelvis is shallower than the male pelvis but wider in all directions. The female pelvis not only supports the enlarged uterus as the fetus matures, but also provides a large opening to allow the infant to pass through during birth. Regardless of these differences, the female and male pelves are both divided into the (11) **ilium,** (12) **ischium,** and (13) **pubis.** These three bones are fused together in the adult to form a single bone called the **innominate (hip) bone.** The ilium travels inferiorly to form part of the (14) **acetabulum** (the deep socket of the hip joint) and medially to join the pubis. The bladder is located behind the (15) **symphysis pubis;** the rectum is in the curve of the (16) **sacrum** and (17) **coccyx.** In the female, the uterus, fallopian tubes, ovaries, and vagina are located between the bladder and the rectum.

Lower Limbs

The lower limbs support the complete weight of the erect body and are subjected to exceptional stresses, especially in running or jumping. To accommodate for these types of forces, the lower limb bones are stronger and thicker than comparable bones of the upper limbs. The difference between the upper and lower limb bones is that the lighter bones of the upper limbs are adapted for mobility and flexibility; the massive bones of the lower limbs are specialized for stability and weight bearing.

There are three parts of each lower limb: the thigh, the leg, and the foot. The thigh consists of a single bone called the (18) **femur.** It is the largest, longest, and strongest bone in the body. The leg is formed by two parallel bones: the (19) **tibia** and the (20) **fibula.** A small triangular bone, the (21) **patella,** or kneecap, is located anterior to the knee joint. The seven (22) **tarsals** (ankle bones) resemble metacarpals (wrist bones) in structure. Last, the bones of each foot include the (23) **metatarsals,** which consists of five small long bones numbered 1 to 5 and beginning with the great toe on the medial side of the foot, and the much smaller (24) **phalanges** (toes).

Joints or Articulations

To allow for body movements, bones must have points where they meet **(articulate).** These articulating points form joints that have various degrees of mobility. Some are freely movable **(diarthroses),** others are only slightly movable **(amphiarthroses),** and the remaining are immovable **(synarthroses).** All three types are necessary for smooth, coordinated body movements.

Joints that allow movement are called **synovial joints.** The ends of the bones that comprise these joints are encased in a sleevelike extension of the periosteum called the **joint capsule.** This capsule binds the articulating bones to each other. In most synovial joints, the capsule is strengthened by ligaments that lash the bones together, providing additional strength to the joint capsule. A membrane called the **synovial membrane** surrounds the inside of the capsule. It secretes a lubricating fluid **(synovial fluid)** within the entire joint capsule. The ends of each of the bones are covered with a smooth layer of cartilage that serves as a cushion.

Anatomy Review: Long Bone

To review the anatomy of a typical long bone, label the following illustration of the femur using the terms below.

articular cartilage   *distal epiphysis*   *proximal epiphysis*

compact bone   *medullary cavity*   *spongy bone*

diaphysis   *periosteum*

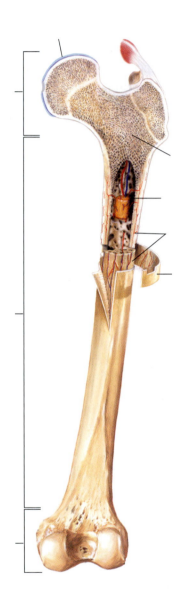

 Check your answers by referring to Figure 10–2 on page 304. Review material that you did not answer correctly.

Anatomy Review: Skeletal Structures

To review the skeletal structures, label the following illustration using the terms below.

acetabulum	*humerus*	*pelvic girdle*	*sternum*
carpals	*ilium*	*phalanges*	*symphysis pubis*
clavicle	*ischium*	*pubis*	*tarsals*
coccyx	*metatarsals*	*radius*	*tibia*
femur	*metacarpals*	*sacrum*	*ulna*
fibula	*pectoral girdle*	*scapula*	

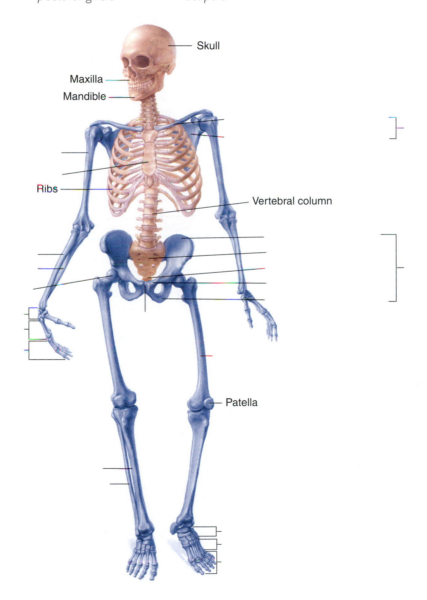

Skull

Maxilla

Mandible

Ribs

Vertebral column

Patella

 Check your answers by referring to Figure 10–3 on page 306. Review material that you did not answer correctly.

CONNECTING BODY SYSTEMS—MUSCULOSKELETAL SYSTEM

The main function of the musculoskeletal system is to provide support, protection, and movement of body parts. Specific functional relationships between the musculoskeletal system and other body systems are summarized below.

Blood, Lymph, and Immune
• Muscle action pumps lymph through lymphatic vessels.
• Bone marrow provides a place for cells of the immune system to develop.

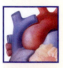

Cardiovascular
• Bone helps regulate blood calcium levels, which are important to heart function.

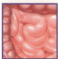

Digestive
• Muscles play an important role in swallowing and propelling food through the digestive tract.
• Muscles of the stomach mechanically break down food to prepare it for chemical digestion.

Endocrine
• Exercising skeletal muscles stimulates release of hormones to increase blood flow.

Female Reproductive
• Muscles are important in sexual activity and during delivery of the fetus.
• Bones provide a source of calcium during pregnancy and lactation if dietary intake is lacking or insufficient.
• Pelvis helps support the enlarged uterus during pregnancy.

Integumentary
• Involuntary muscle contractions (shivering) help regulate body temperature.

Male Reproductive
• Muscles play an important role in sexual activity.

Nervous
• Bones protect the brain and spinal cord.

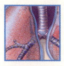

Respiratory
• Muscles elevate ribs and contract the diaphragm to assist in the breathing process.

Urinary
• Bones work in conjunction with the kidneys to help regulate blood calcium levels.
• Skeletal muscles help control urine elimination.

Medical Word Elements

This section introduces combining forms, suffixes, and prefixes related to the musculoskeletal system. Word analyses are also provided.

Element	Meaning	Word Analysis
Combining Forms		
Skeletal System		
General		
ankyl/o	stiffness; bent, crooked	**ankyl**/osis (ăng-kĭ-LŌ-sĭs): abnormal condition of stiffness *-osis:* abnormal condition; increase (used primarily with blood cells) *Ankylosis results in immobility and stiffness of a joint. It may be the result of trauma, surgery, or disease and most commonly occurs in rheumatoid arthritis.*
arthr/o	joint	**arthr**/itis (ăr-THRĪ-tĭs): inflammation of a joint *-itis:* inflammation
kyph/o	humpback	**kyph**/osis (kī-FŌ-sĭs): abnormal condition of a humpback posture *-osis:* abnormal condition; increase (used primarily with blood cells)
lamin/o	lamina (part of vertebral arch)	**lamin**/ectomy (lăm-ĭ-NĔK-tō-mē): excision of the lamina *-ectomy:* excision, removal *Laminectomy is usually performed to relieve compression of the spinal cord or to remove a lesion or herniated disk.*
lord/o	curve, swayback	**lord**/osis (lor-DŌ-sĭs): abnormal condition of a swayback posture *-osis:* abnormal condition; increase (used primarily with blood cells)
myel/o	bone marrow; spinal cord	**myel/o**/cyte (MĪ-ĕl-ō-sīt): bone marrow cell *-cyte:* cell

orth/o	straight	**orth/o**/ped/ist (or-thō-PĒ-dĭst): specialist in treatment of musculoskeletal disorders
		   ped: foot; child
		   -ist: specialist
		 Initially, an orthopedist corrected deformities and straightened children's bones. In today's medical practice, however, the orthopedist treats musculoskeletal disorders and associated structures in persons of all ages.

oste/o	bone	**oste**/oma (ŏs-tē-Ō-mă): tumor composed of bone *-oma:* tumor *Osteomas are benign bony tumors.*
ped/o	foot; child	**ped/o**/graph (PĔD-ō-grăf): instrument for recording the foot *-graph:* instrument for recording *A pedograph is an instrument for recording an imprint of the foot and studying the gait (manner of walking).*
ped/i		**ped/i**/cure* (PĔD-ĭ-kūr): care of feet

*The *i* in *ped/i/cure* is an exception to the rule of using the connecting vowel *o.*

(continued)

Element	Meaning	Word Analysis
scoli/o	crooked, bent	**scoli/**osis (skō-lē-Ō-sĭs): abnormal bending of the spine *-osis:* abnormal condition; increase (used primarily with blood cells)
thorac/o	chest	**thorac/o/**dynia (thō-răk-ō-DĬN-ē-ă): pain in the chest *-dynia:* pain
Specific Bones		
acromi/o	acromion (projection of the scapula)	**acromi/**al (ăk-RŌ-mē-ăl): pertaining to the acromion *-al:* pertaining to
brachi/o	arm	**brachi/**algia (brā-kē-ĂL-jē-ă): pain in the arm *-algia:* pain
calcane/o	calcaneum (heel bone)	**calcane/o/**dynia (kăl-kā-nē-ō-DĬN-ē-ă): pain in the heel *-dynia:* pain
carp/o	carpus (wrist bone)	**carp/o/**ptosis (kăr-pŏp-TŌ-sĭs): downward displacement of the wrist; also called *wrist drop* *-ptosis:* prolapse, downward displacement
cephal/o	head	**cephal/**ad (SĔF-ă-lăd): toward the head *-ad:* toward
cervic/o	neck; cervix uteri (neck of the uterus)	**cervic/o/**dynia (sĕr-vĭ-kō-DĬN-ē-ă): pain in the neck; also called cervical neuralgia *-dynia:* pain
clavicul/o	clavicle (collar bone)	**clavicul/**ar (klă-VĬK-ū-lăr): pertaining to the clavicle *-ar:* pertaining to
cost/o	ribs	**cost/**ectomy (kŏs-TĔK-tō-mē): excision of a rib *-ectomy:* excision, removal
crani/o	cranium (skull)	**crani/o/**tomy (krā-nē-ŎT-ō-mē): incision of the cranium *-tomy:* incision
dactyl/o	fingers; toes	**dactyl/**itis (dăk-tĭl-Ī-tĭs): inflammation of fingers or toes *-itis:* inflammation
femor/o	femur (thigh bone)	**femor/**al (FĔM-or-ăl): pertaining to the femur *-al:* pertaining to
fibul/o	fibula (smaller bone of the lower leg)	**fibul/o/**calcane/al (fĭb-ū-lō-kăl-KĀ-nē-ăl): pertaining to the fibula and calcaneus *calcane:* calcaneum (heel bone) *-al:* pertaining to

Element	Meaning	Word Analysis
humer/o	humerus (upper arm bone)	**humer/o**/scapul/ar (hū-měr-ō-SKĂP-ū-lăr): relating to the humerus and scapula *scapul:* scapula (shoulder blade) *-ar:* pertaining to
ili/o	ilium (lateral, flaring portion of the hip bone)	**ili/o**/pelv/ic (ĭl-ē-ō-PĔL-vĭk): pertaining to the iliac area of the pelvis *pelv:* pelvis *-ic:* pertaining to
ischi/o	ischium (lower portion of the hip bone)	**ischi/o**/dynia (ĭs-kē-ō-DĬN-ē-ă): pain in the ischium *-dynia:* pain
lumb/o	loins (lower back)	**lumb/o**/dynia (lŭm-bō-DĬN-ē-ă): pain in the lumbar region of the back; also called *lumbago* *-dynia:* pain
metacarp/o	metacarpus (hand bones)	**metacarp**/ectomy (mět-ă-kăr-PĔK-tō-mē): excision of metacarpal bone(s) *-ectomy:* excision, removal
metatars/o	metatarsus (foot bones)	**metatars**/algia (mět-ă-tăr-SĂL-jē-ă): pain in the metatarsus *-algia:* pain *Metatarsalgia emanates from the heads of the metatarsus and worsens with weight bearing or palpation.*
patell/o	patella (kneecap)	**patell**/ectomy (păt-ě-LĔK-tō-mē): removal of the patella *-ectomy:* excision, removal
pelv/i	pelvis	**pelv/i**/metry** (pěl-VĬM-ět-rē): act of measuring the pelvis *-metry:* act of measuring *Pelvimetry is routinely performed in obstetrical management.*
phalang/o	phalanges (bones of the fingers and toes)	**phalang**/ectomy (făl-ăn-JĔK-tō-mē): excision of phalanges *-ectomy:* excision, removal
pod/o	foot	**pod**/iatry (pō-DĪ-ă-trē): treatment of the feet *-iatry:* medicine, treatment
pub/o	pelvis bone (anterior part of the pelvic bone)	**pub/o**/coccyg/eal (pū-bō-kŏk-SĬJ-ē-ăl): pertaining to the pubis and the coccyx *coccyg:* coccyx (tailbone) *-eal:* pertaining to
radi/o	radiation, x-ray; radius (lower arm bone on the thumb side)	**radi**/al (RĀ-dē-ăl): pertaining to the radius *-al:* pertaining to

**The *i* in *pelv/i/metry* is an exception to the rule of using the connecting vowel o.

(continued)

Element	Meaning	Word Analysis
spondyl/o	vertebrae (backbone)	**spondyl/**itis (spŏn-dĭl-Ī-tĭs): inflammation of the vertebrae *-itis:* inflammation *The combining form* spondyl/o *is used to describe diseases and conditions.*

vertebr/o		inter/**vertebr/**al (ĭn-tĕr-VĔRT-ĕ-brĕl): relating to the area between two vertebrae
		  inter-: between
		  -al: pertaining to
		The combining form vertebr/o *is used to indicate anatomical terms.*

stern/o	sternum (breastbone)	**stern/**ad (STĔR-năd): toward the sternum *-ad:* toward

tibi/o	tibia (larger bone of the lower leg)	**tibi/o/**femor/al (tĭb-ē-ō-FĔM-or-ăl) pertaining to the tibia and femur
		  femor: femur
		  -al: pertaining to

Muscular System		
leiomy/o	smooth muscle (visceral)	**leiomy/**oma (lī-ō-mī-Ō-mă): tumor of smooth muscle *-oma:* tumor
muscul/o	muscle	**muscul/**ar (MŬS-kū-lăr): pertaining to muscles *-ar:* pertaining to
my/o		**my/**oma (mī-Ō-mă): tumor of muscle (tissue) *-oma:* tumor
rhabd/o	rod-shaped (striated)	**rhabd/**oid (RĂB-doyd): resembling a rod *-oid:* resembling
rhabdomy/o	rod-shaped (striated) muscle	**rhabdomy/**oma (răb-dō-mī-Ō-mă): tumor composed of striated muscular tissue *-oma:* tumor
Related Structures		
chondr/o	cartilage	**chondr/**itis (kŏn-DRĪ-tĭs): inflammation of cartilage *-itis:* inflammation
fasci/o	band, fascia (fibrous membrane supporting and separating muscles)	**fasci/o/**plasty (FĂSH-ē-ō-plăs-tē): surgical repair of a fascia *-plasty:* surgical repair

Element	Meaning	Word Analysis
fibr/o	fiber, fibrous tissue	**fibr**/oma (fī-BRŌ-mă): tumor of fibrous tissue –*oma:* tumor
synov/o	synovial membrane, synovial fluid	**synov**/ectomy (sĭn-ō-VĔK-tō-mē): removal of a synovial membrane –*ectomy:* excision, removal
ten/o	tendon	**ten/o**/desis (tĕn-ŌD-ĕ-sĭs): surgical binding or fixation of a tendon –*desis:* binding, fixation (of a bone or joint)
tend/o		**tend/o**/plasty (TĔN-dō-plăs-tē): surgical repair of a tendon –*plasty:* surgical repair
tendin/o		**tendin**/itis (tĕn-dĭn-Ī-tĭs): inflammation of a tendon –*itis:* inflammation

Suffixes		
-asthenia	weakness, debility	my/**asthenia** (mī-ăs-THĒ-nē-ă): weakness of muscle (and abnormal fatigue) *my:* muscle
-blast	embryonic cell	my/o/**blast** (MĪ-ō-blăst): embryonic cell that develops into muscle *my/o:* muscle
-clasia	to break; surgical fracture	oste/o/**clasia** (ŏs-tē-ō-KLĀ-zē-ă): surgical fracture of a bone *oste/o:* bone *Osteoclasia is the intentional fracture of a bone to correct a deformity and is also called* **osteoclasis**.
-clast	to break; surgical fracture	oste/o/**clast** (ŎS-tē-ō-klăst): (multinucleated cell that) breaks down bone *oste/o:* bone *An osteoclast destroys the matrix of bone. Osteoblasts and osteoclasts work together to maintain a constant bone size in adults. An osteoclast also refers to an instrument used to surgically fracture a bone (osteoclasis).*
-desis	binding, fixation (of a bone or joint)	arthr/o/**desis** (ăr-thrō-DĒ-sĭs): binding together of a joint *arthr/o:* joint
-malacia	softening	chondr/o/**malacia** (kŏn-drō-măl-Ā-shē-ă): softening of cartilage *chondr/o:* cartilage *Chondromalacia is a softening of the articular cartilage, usually involving the patella.*
-physis	growth	epi/**physis** (ĕ-PĬF-ĭ-sĭs): growth upon (the end of a long bone) *epi-:* above, upon *The epiphyses are the enlarged proximal and distal ends of a long bone.*

(continued)

Element	Meaning	Word Analysis
-porosis	porous	oste/o/**porosis** (ŏs-tē-ō-pŏ-RŌ-sĭs): porous bone *oste/o:* bone *Osteoporosis is a disorder characterized by loss of bone density. It may cause pain, especially in the lower back; pathological fractures; loss of stature; and hairline fractures.*
-sarcoma	malignant tumor of connective tissue	chondr/o/**sarcoma** (kŏn-drō-săr-KŌ-mă): malignant tumor from cartilage (cells) *Although bone cancer is rare, chondrosarcoma is the second most common type of bone cancer after osteosarcoma. The tumors typically develop in the pelvis, legs, or shoulders of adults over 40.*
-scopy	visual examination	arthr/o/**scopy** (ăr-THRŎS-kō-pē): visual examination of a joint *arthr/o:* joint *Arthroscopy is an endoscopic examination of the interior of a joint. It is performed by inserting small surgical instruments to remove and repair damaged tissue, such as cartilage fragments or torn ligaments.*
Prefixes		
a-	without, not	**a**/trophy (ĂT-rō-fē): without nourishment *-trophy:* development, nourishment *Atrophy is a wasting or decrease in size or physiological activity of a part of the body because of disease or other influences.*
dys-	bad; painful; difficult	**dys**/trophy (DĬS-trō-fē): disorder caused by defective nutrition or metabolism *-trophy:* development, nourishment
sub-	under, below	**sub**/patell/ar (sŭb-pă-TĔL-ăr): pertaining to below the patella *patell:* patella (kneecap) *-ar:* pertaining to
supra-	above; excessive; superior	**supra**/cost/al (soo-pră-KŎS-tăl): pertaining to above the ribs *cost:* ribs *-al:* pertaining to
syn-	union, together, joined	**syn**/dactyl/ism (sĭn-DĂK-tĭl-ĭzm): condition of joined fingers or toes *dactyl:* fingers, toes *-ism:* condition *Syndactylism is a fusion of two or more fingers or toes.*

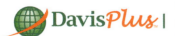

Visit the *Medical Terminology Systems* online resource center at Davis*Plus* for an audio exercise of the terms in this table. Other activities are also available to reinforce content.

 It is time to review medical word elements by completing Learning Activities 10-1 and 10-2.

Pathology

Joints are especially vulnerable to constant wear and tear. Repeated motion, disease, trauma, and aging affect joints as well as muscles and tendons. Overall, disorders of the musculoskeletal system are more likely to be caused by injury than disease. Other disorders of structure and bone strength—such as osteoporosis, which occurs primarily in elderly women—affect the health of the musculoskeletal system.

For diagnosis, treatment, and management of musculoskeletal disorders, the medical services of a specialist may be warranted. **Orthopedics** is the branch of medicine concerned with prevention, diagnosis, care, and treatment of musculoskeletal disorders. The physician who specializes in the diagnoses and treatment of musculoskeletal disorders is known as an **orthopedist.** These physicians use medical, physical, and surgical methods to restore function that has been lost as a result of musculoskeletal injury or disease. Another physician who specializes in treating joint disease is the **rheumatologist.** Still another physician, a **Doctor of Osteopathy (DO),** maintains that good health requires proper alignment of bones, muscles, ligaments, and nerves. Like the medical doctor, osteopathic physicians combine manipulative procedures with state-of-the-art methods of medical treatment, including prescribing drugs and performing surgeries. Also, the osteopathic physician has the same rights, privileges, and responsibilities as the Doctor of Medicine (MD).

Bone Disorders

Disorders involving the bones include fractures, infections, osteoporosis, and spinal curvatures.

Fractures

A broken bone is called a **fracture.** The different types of fractures are classified by extent of damage. (See Figure 10-8.) A (1) **closed (simple) fracture** is one in which the bone is broken but no external wound exists. An (2) **open (compound)** fracture involves a broken bone and an external wound that leads to the site of fracture. Fragments of bone commonly protrude through the skin. A (3) **complicated fracture** is one in which a broken bone has injured an internal organ, such as when a broken rib pierces a lung. In a (4) **comminuted fracture,** the bone has broken or splintered into pieces. An (5) **impacted fracture** occurs when the bone is broken and one end is wedged into the interior of another bone. An (6) **incomplete fracture** occurs when the line of fracture does not completely transverse the entire bone. A (7) **greenstick fracture** is when the broken bone does not extend through the entire thickness of the bone; that is, one side of the bone is broken and one side of the bone is bent. It occurs most often in children as part of the bone is still composed of flexible cartilage. The term greenstick refers to new branches on a tree that bend rather than break. A greenstick fracture is also known as an **incomplete fracture.** A (8) **Colles fracture,** a break at the lower end of the radius, occurs just above the wrist. It causes displacement of the hand and usually occurs as a result of flexing a hand to cushion a fall. A **hairline fracture** is a minor fracture in which all portions of the bone are in perfect alignment. The fracture is seen on radiographic examination as a very thin hairline between the two segments but not extending entirely through the bone. **Pathological (spontaneous) fractures** are usually caused by a disease process such as a neoplasm or osteoporosis.

Unlike other repairs of the body, bones sometimes require months to heal. Several factors influence the rate at which fractures heal. Some fractures need to be immobilized to ensure that bones unite soundly in their proper position. In most cases, this is achieved with bandages, casts, traction, or a fixation device. Certain fractures, particularly those with bone fragments, require surgery to reposition and fix bones securely, so that surrounding tissues heal. In addition to promoting healing, immobilization prevents further injury and reduces pain.

Some bones have a natural tendency to heal more rapidly than others. For instance, the long bones of the arms usually mend twice as fast as those of the legs. Age also plays an important role in bone fracture healing rate; older patients require more time for healing. In addition, an adequate blood supply to the injured area and the nutritive state of the individual are crucial to the healing process.

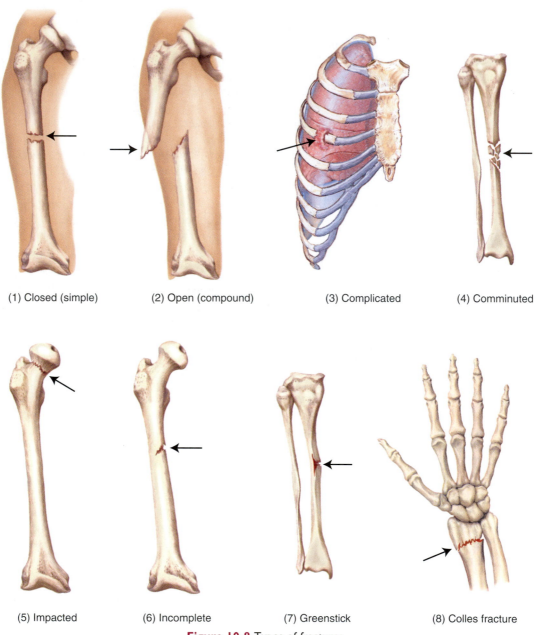

(1) Closed (simple)   (2) Open (compound)   (3) Complicated   (4) Comminuted

(5) Impacted   (6) Incomplete   (7) Greenstick   (8) Colles fracture

Figure 10-8 Types of fractures.

Infections

Bone infection, also known as **osteomyelitis,** is an infective process that encompasses all bone **(osseous)** components, including the bone marrow. When bone infection is chronic, it can lead to bone sclerosis and deformity. The most common causes of osteomyelitis are bacterial in origin. (See Figure 10-9.) Bacteria may gain entry into bone in several ways. They may spread to a bone from infected tissue lying adjacent to bone such as muscles, tendons, or ulcerated skin lying over the bone. Bacteria may travel in the bloodstream **(bacteremia)** from elsewhere in the body (lungs, urinary structures, and so forth) and eventually establish an infection in a bone. A bone infection can also start after bone surgery, especially if the surgery is performed after an injury or if metal plates are inserted in the bone.

Once bone, is infected, leukocytes are attracted to the area and release enzymes that lyse the bone causing an abscess with pus formation. Pus spreads into the bone's blood vessels, impairing their flow, and areas of devitalized infected bone, known as *sequestra* form the basis of a chronic

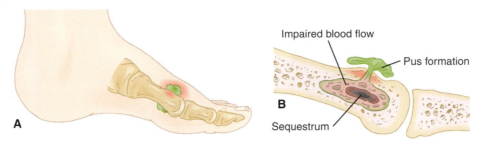

Figure 10-9 Osteomyelitis. **(A)** Bone infection in the toe. **(B)** Blocked blood flow in the area of infection, with **sequestrum** (bone death) and pus formation at infection site.

infection. Often, the body will try to create new bone around the area of necrosis. It becomes difficult for the immune system and antibiotics to penetrate the sequestra and they continue forming pus and other necrotic substances.

The goal of treatment is to eliminate the infection and reduce damage to the bone and surrounding tissues. Multiple antibiotics are simultaneously administered intravenously **(IV)** rather than by mouth **(orally)**. Surgery may be needed to remove **sequestrum (sequestrectomy)** when antibiotic treatment fails. If there are metal plates near the infection, they may need to be removed. With early treatment, prognosis for acute osteomyelitis is good; prognosis for the chronic form of the disease is poor.

Paget disease, also known as **osteitis deformans,** is a chronic inflammation of bones, resulting in thickening and softening of bones. It can occur in any bone but most commonly affects the long bones of the legs, the lower spine, the pelvis, and the skull. This disease is found in persons over age 40. Although a variety of causes have been proposed, a slow virus (not yet isolated) is currently thought to be the most likely cause.

Osteoporosis

Osteoporosis is a common metabolic bone disorder in the elderly, particularly in postmenopausal women and especially women older than age 60. It usually begins as a decrease in bone mineral density **(osteopenia)** and becomes progressively worse. Osteoporosis is characterized by decreased bone density that occurs when the rate of bone resorption (loss of substance) exceeds the rate of bone formation. Among the many causes of osteoporosis are disturbances of protein metabolism, protein deficiency, disuse of bones due to prolonged periods of immobilization, estrogen deficiencies associated with menopause, a diet lacking vitamins or calcium, and long-term administration of high doses of corticosteroids.

Patients with osteoporosis commonly complain of bone pain, typically in the back, which may be caused by repeated microscopic fractures. Thin areas of porous bone are also evident. Deformity associated with osteoporosis is usually the result of pathological fractures.

Spinal Curvatures

Any persistent, abnormal deviation of the vertebral column from its normal position may cause an abnormal spinal curvature. Three common deviations are **scoliosis, kyphosis,** and **lordosis.** (See Figure 10-10.)

An abnormal lateral curvature of the spine, either to the right or left, is called **scoliosis.** Some rotation of a portion of the vertebral column may also occur. **Scoliosis,** or **C-shaped curvature of the spine,** may be congenital, caused by chronic poor posture during childhood while the vertebrae are still growing, or the result of one leg being longer than the other. Treatment depends on the severity of the curvature and may vary from exercises, physical therapy, and back braces to surgical intervention. Untreated scoliosis may result in pulmonary insufficiency (curvature may decrease lung capacity), back pain, sciatica, disk disease, or even degenerative arthritis.

An abnormal curvature of the upper portion of the spine is called **kyphosis,** more commonly known as **humpback** or **hunchback.** Rheumatoid arthritis, rickets, poor posture, or chronic respiratory diseases may cause kyphosis. Treatment consists of spine-stretching exercises, sleeping with a board under the mattress, and wearing a brace to straighten the kyphotic curve; surgery is rarely required.

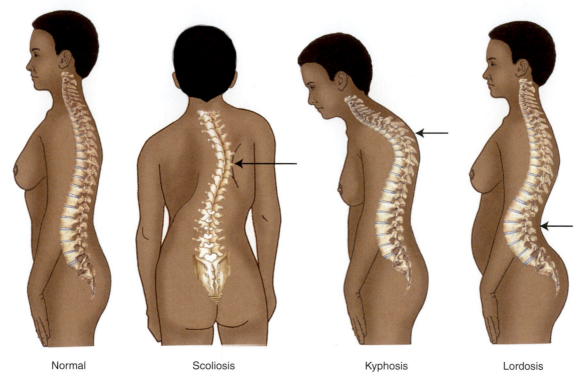

| Normal | Scoliosis | Kyphosis | Lordosis |

Figure 10-10 Spinal curvatures.

An abnormal, inward curvature of a portion of the lower portion of the spine is called **lordosis,** more commonly known as **swayback.** It may be caused by increased weight of the abdominal contents, resulting from obesity or excessive weight gain during pregnancy. Kyphosis and lordosis also occur in combination with scoliosis.

Joint Disorders

Arthritis, a general term for many joint diseases, is an inflammation of a joint usually accompanied by pain, swelling and, commonly, changes in structure. Because of their location and constant use, joints are prone to stress injuries and inflammation. The main types of arthritis include rheumatoid arthritis, osteoarthritis, and gouty arthritis, or gout.

Rheumatoid arthritis (RA), a systemic disease characterized by inflammatory changes in joints and their related structures, results in crippling deformities. (See Figure 10-11.) This form of arthritis is believed to be caused by an autoimmune reaction of joint tissue. It occurs most commonly in women between ages 23 and 35 but can affect people of any age group. Intensified aggravations **(exacerbations)** of this disease are commonly associated with periods of increased physical or emotional stress. In addition to joint changes, muscles, bones, and skin adjacent to the affected joint atrophy. There is no specific cure, but nonsteroidal anti-inflammatory drugs (NSAIDs), physical therapy, and orthopedic measures are used in treatment of less severe cases.

Osteoarthritis, also known as **degenerative joint disease (DJD)**, is by far the most common form of arthritis. It is a progressive, degenerative disease that occurs when the protective cartilage at the end of the bones wear down. A variety of causes, such as aging, hereditary, metabolic, and injury from trauma or disease may initiate processes leading to loss of cartilage. In osteoarthritis, there may also be development of new bone growth (**bone spur**, or **osteophyte**) at articular surfaces.

Osteoarthritis can occur in any joint, but usually it affects the hands, knees, hips, or spine. It results from normal wear and tear on the joints and is most common in the elderly. Almost everyone has some symptoms by age 70, but these symptoms may be minor. However, there is a higher risk of DJD in overweight individuals of all ages and of younger athletes. Playing sports that involve direct impact on the joint (such as tennis or football), twisting (such as basketball or soccer), or throwing also increases the risk of arthritis. In osteoarthritis, there is a tendency for the smallest joints at the ends of the fingers to be affected by spur formation that leads to the

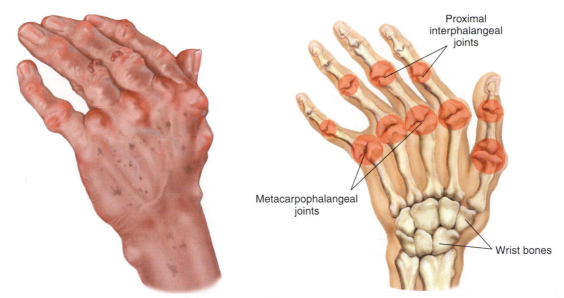

Figure 10-11 Rheumatoid arthritis.

classic bony enlargement referred to as **Heberden nodes.** Degenerative changes in the spinal vertebrae and the joints of the pelvis can lead to abnormal curvature and local pain. Pain and stiffness in the joints are the most common symptoms. The pain is often worse after exercise and when putting weight or pressure on the joint. Over time, the joints become stiffer and harder to move. There may also be a rubbing, grating, or crackling sound **(crepitation)** when there is movement in the joint. Nevertheless, some persons are asymptomatic, even though x-rays show the changes of osteoarthritis.

Gout, also called **gout arthritis,** is a metabolic disease caused by the accumulation of uric acid crystals in the blood. These crystals may become deposited in joints and soft tissue near joints, causing painful swelling and inflammation. Although the joint chiefly affected is the big toe, any joint may be involved. Sometimes, renal calculi **(nephroliths)** form because of uric acid crystals collecting in the kidney.

Muscle Disorders

Disorders involving the muscles include muscular dystrophy and myasthenia gravis.

Muscular Dystrophy

Muscular dystrophy, a genetic disease, is characterized by gradual **atrophy** and weakening of muscle tissue. There are several types of muscular dystrophy. The most common type, **Duchenne dystrophy,** affects children; boys more commonly than girls. It is transmitted as a sex-linked disease passed from mother to son. As muscular dystrophy progresses, the loss of muscle function affects not only skeletal muscle but also cardiac muscle. At present, there is no cure for this disease, and most children with muscular dystrophy die before age 30.

Myasthenia Gravis

Myasthenia gravis (MG), a neuromuscular disorder, causes fluctuating weakness of certain skeletal muscle groups (of the eyes, face and, sometimes, limbs). It is characterized by destruction of the receptors in the synaptic region that respond to acetylcholine, a substance that transmits nerve impulses **(neurotransmitter).** As the disease progresses, the muscle becomes increasingly weak and may eventually cease to function altogether. Women tend to be affected more often than men. Initial symptoms include a weakness of the eye muscles and difficulty swallowing **(dysphagia).** Later, the individual has difficulty chewing and talking. Eventually, the muscles of the limbs may become involved. Myasthenia gravis can be controlled, and medical management is the usual form of treatment.

Oncology

Two major types of malignancies that affect bone are those that arise directly from bone or bone tissue, called **primary bone cancer,** and those that arise in another region of the body and spread **(metastasize)** to bone, called **secondary bone cancer.** Primary bone cancers are rare, but secondary bone cancers are quite prevalent. They are usually caused by malignant cells that have metastasized to the bone from the lungs, breast, or prostate.

Malignancies that originate from bone, fat, muscle, cartilage, bone marrow, and cells of the lymphatic system are called **sarcomas.** Three major types of sarcomas are fibrosarcoma, osteosarcoma, and Ewing sarcoma. **Fibrosarcoma** develops in cartilage and generally affects the pelvis, upper legs, and shoulders. Patients with fibrosarcoma are usually between ages 50 and 60. **Osteosarcoma** develops from bone tissue and generally affects the knees, upper arms, and upper legs. Patients with osteosarcoma are usually between ages 20 and 25. **Ewing sarcoma** develops from primitive nerve cells in bone marrow. It usually affects the shaft of long bones but may occur in the pelvis or other bones of the arms or legs. This disease usually affects boys between ages 10 and 20.

Signs and symptoms of sarcoma include swelling and tenderness, with a tendency toward fractures in the affected area. Magnetic resonance imaging (MRI), bone scan, and computed tomography (CT) scan are diagnostic tests that assist in identifying bone malignancies. All malignancies, including Ewing sarcoma, are staged and graded to determine the extent and degree of malignancy. This staging helps the physician determine an appropriate treatment modality. Generally, combination therapy is used, including chemotherapy for management of metastasis and radiation when the tumor is radiosensitive. In some cases, amputation is required.

Diseases and Conditions

This section introduces diseases and conditions of the musculoskeletal system with their meanings and pronunciations. Word analyses for selected terms are also provided.

Term	Definition
ankylosis ăng-kĭ-LŌ-sĭs *ankyl:* stiffness, bent, crooked *-osis:* abnormal condition, increase (used primarily with blood cells)	Stiffening and immobility of a joint as a result of disease, trauma, surgery, or abnormal bone fusion
bunion (hallux valgus) BŬN-yŭn (HĂL-ŭks VĂL-gŭs)	Deformity characterized by lateral deviation of the great toe as it turns in toward the second toe (angulation), which may cause the tissues surrounding the joint to become swollen and tender (See Figure 10-12.) *The term is used to refer to the pathological bump on the side of the great toe joint.* A B **Figure 10-12** Bunion. **(A)** Preoperative. **(B)** Postoperative.

Term	Definition
carpal tunnel syndrome (CTS) KĂR-păl	Painful condition resulting from compression of the median nerve within the carpal tunnel (wrist canal through which the flexor tendons and the median nerve pass)
claudication klăw-dĭ-KĀ-shŭn	Lameness, limping
contracture kŏn-TRĂK-chūr	Fibrosis of connective tissue in the skin, fascia, muscle, or joint capsule that prevents normal mobility of the related tissue or joint
crepitation krĕp-ĭ-TĀ-shŭn	Dry, grating sound or sensation caused by bone ends rubbing together, indicating a fracture or joint destruction
exacerbation ĕks-ăs-ĕr-BĀ-shŭn	Increase in severity of a disease or any of its symptoms; also called *flare*
ganglion cyst GĂNG-lē-ŏn SĬST	Fluid-filled tumor that most commonly develops along the tendons or joint of the wrists or hands, but may also appear in the feet (See Figure 10-13.) *In most instances, ganglion cysts cause no pain and require no treatment. They commonly go away on their own. Reasons for treatment are cosmetic or when the cyst causes pain or interference with joint movement. Treatment involves removing the fluid or excising the cyst.*

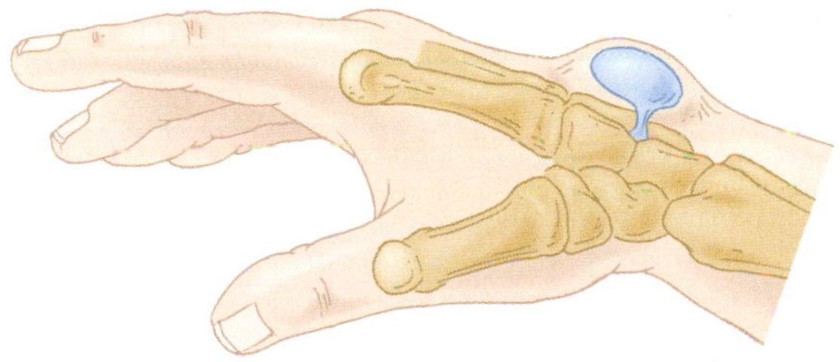

Figure 10-13 Ganglion cyst of the wrist.

Term	Definition
hemarthrosis hĕm-ăr-THRŌ-sĭs *hem:* blood *arthr:* joint *-osis:* abnormal condition; increase (used primarily with blood cells)	Effusion of blood into a joint cavity

(continued)

Term	Definition
herniated disk HĔR-nē-āt-ĕd	Rupture of a vertebral disk's center (nucleus pulposus) through its outer edge and back toward the spinal canal with pressure on the adjacent spinal nerve that results in pain, numbness, or weakness in one or both legs (See Figure 10-14.) *Herniated disk occurs most commonly in the lower spine and is referred to as herniation of an intervertebral disk, herniated nucleus pulposus (HNP), ruptured disk, prolapsed disk, or slipped disk.* **Figure 10-14** Herniated disk.
hypotonia hī-pō-TŌ-nē-ă *hypo-:* under, below, deficient *ton:* tension *-ia:* condition	Loss of muscular tone or a diminished resistance to passive stretching
multiple myeloma mī-ĕ-LŌ-mă *myel:* bone marrow; spinal cord *-oma:* tumor	Malignant tumor of plasma cells (cells that help the body fight infection by producing antibodies) in the bone marrow *In multiple myeloma, malignant plasma cells spread throughout bone marrow and invade the harder outer portion of the bone, causing soft spots of holes in the bone. The goal of treatment is to relieve symptoms, avoid complications, and prolong life.*
phantom limb FĂN-tŭm	Perceived sensation, following amputation of a limb, that the limb still exists *The sensation that pain exists in the removed part is known as phantom limb pain.*
rickets RĬK-ĕts	Form of osteomalacia in children caused by vitamin D deficiency; also called *rachitis*
sequestrum sē-KWĔS-trŭm *sequestr:* separation *-um:* structure, thing	Fragment of necrosed bone that has become separated from surrounding tissue

Term	Definition
spondylolisthesis spŏn-dĭ-lō-lĭs-THĒ-sĭs *spondyl/o:* vertebrae (backbone) *-listhesis:* slipping	Any slipping (subluxation) of a vertebra from its normal position in relationship to the one beneath it
spondylosis spŏn-dĭ-LŌ-sĭs *spondyl:* vertebrae (backbone) *-osis:* abnormal condition; increase (used primarily with blood cells)	Degeneration of the cervical, thoracic, and lumbar vertebrae and related tissues *Spondylosis may cause pressure on nerve roots with subsequent pain or paresthesia in the extremities.*
sprain SPRĀN	Tearing of ligament tissue that may be slight, moderate, or complete *A complete tear of a major ligament is especially painful and disabling. Ligamentous tissue does not heal well because of poor blood supply. Treatment usually consists of surgical reconstruction of the severed ligament.*
strain STRĀN	Muscular trauma caused by violent contraction or an excessive forcible stretch
subluxation sŭb-lŭk-SĀ-shŭn	Partial or incomplete dislocation
talipes equinovarus TĂL-ĭ-pēz ē-kwī-nō-VĀ-rŭs	Congenital deformity of one or both feet in which the foot is pulled downward and laterally to the side; also called *clubfoot* (See Figure 10-15.) *In talipes, the heel never rests on the ground. Treatment consists of applying casts to progressively straighten the foot and surgical correction for severe cases.*

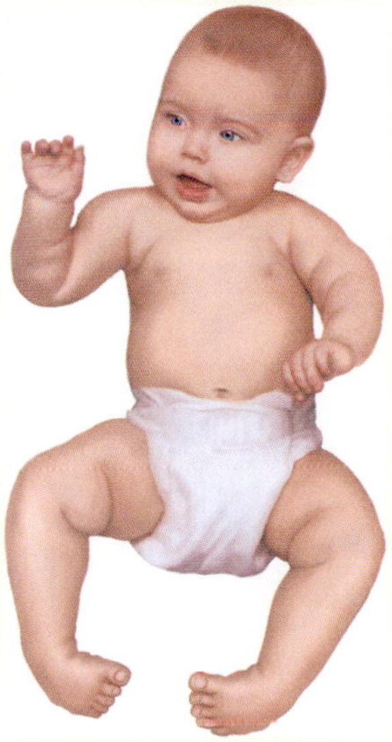

Figure 10-15 Talipes equinovarus.

⊕   *It is time to review pathology, diseases, and conditions by completing Learning Activity 10–3.*

Medical, Surgical, and Diagnostic Procedures

This section introduces medical, surgical, and diagnostic procedures used to treat and diagnose musculoskeletal disorders. Descriptions are provided as well as pronunciations and word analyses for selected terms.

Procedure	Description
Medical	
electromyography (EMG) ē-lĕk-trō-mī-ŎG-ră-fē *electr/o:* electric *my/o:* muscle *-graphy:* process of recording	Use of electrical stimulation to diagnose the health of muscles and the nerve cells that control them (motor neurons) *Motor neurons transmit electrical signals that cause muscles to contract. An EMG translates these signals into graphs, sounds, or numerical values that a specialist interprets.*
reduction	Procedure that restores a bone to its normal position *Following reduction, the bone is immobilized to maintain proper alignment during the healing process.*
closed	Reduction in which fractured bones are realigned by manipulation rather than surgery.
open	Reduction in which fractured bones are placed in their proper position during surgery *In open reduction of a complicated fracture, an incision is made at the fracture site and the fracture is reduced. Placing fracture fragments in their correct anatomical position commonly requires internal fixation devices, such as nails, screws, and plates.*
bone immobilization	Procedures used to restrict movement, stabilize and protect a fracture, and facilitate the healing process
casting	Bone immobilization by application of a solid, stiff dressing formed with plaster of Paris or similar material
splinting	Bone immobilization by application of an orthopedic device to the injured body part *A splint is constructed from wood, metal, or plaster of Paris and may be moveable or immovable.*
traction	Bone immobilization by application of weights and pulleys to align or immobilize a fracture

Procedure	Description
Surgical	
amputation ăm-pŭ-TĀ-shŭn	Partial or complete removal of an extremity due to trauma or a circulatory disease *After the extremity is removed, the surgeon cuts a shaped flap from muscle and cutaneous tissue to cover the end of the bone and provide cushion and support for a prosthesis. The most common reason for limb loss is peripheral vascular disease caused by a blood flow blockage from cigarette smoking, physical inactivity, or uncontrolled diabetes mellitus.*

arthrocentesis
ăr-thrō-sĕn-TĒ-sĭs
  arthr/o: joint
  -centesis: surgical puncture
	Puncture of a joint space using a needle to remove accumulated fluid

arthroclasia
ăr-thrō-KLĀ-zē-ă
  arthr/o: joint
  -clasia: to break; surgical fracture
	Surgical breaking of an ankylosed joint to provide movement

arthroscopy
ăr-THRŎS-kō-pē
  arthr/o: joint
  -scopy: visual examination
	Visual examination of the interior of a joint and its structures using a thin, flexible fiberoptic scope called an arthroscope that contains a magnifying lens, fiberoptic light, and miniature camera that projects images on a monitor (See Figure 10-16.)
	
	Instruments are introduced into the joint space through a small incision in order to carry out diagnostic and treatment procedures. Arthroscopy is also performed to correct defects, excise tumors, and obtain biopsies.

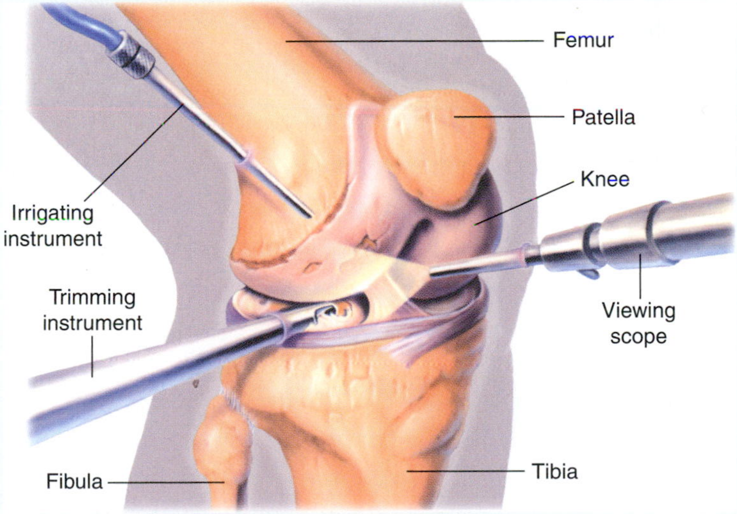

Figure 10-16 Arthroscopy.

(continued)

Procedure	Description
bone grafting BŌN GRĂFT-ĭng	Implantation or transplantation of bone tissue from another part of the body or from another person to serve as replacement for damaged or missing bone tissue
bursectomy bĕr-SĔK-tō-mē	Excision of bursa (padlike sac or cavity found in connective tissue, usually in the vicinity of joints)
laminectomy lăm-ĭ-NĔK-tō-mē *lamin:* lamina (part of vertebral arch) *-ectomy:* excision, removal	Excision of the posterior arch of a vertebra *Laminectomy is most commonly performed to relieve the symptoms of a ruptured (slipped) intervertebral disk.*
prosthesis fitting prŏs-THĒ-sĭs	Replacement of a missing part by an artificial substitute, such as an artificial extremity
revision surgery	Surgery repeated to correct problems of a previously unsuccessful surgery or to replace a worn-out prosthesis *Revision surgery is usually more complicated than the original surgery.*
bone	Revision surgery to correct misalignment of bones, broken prostheses, and bone fractures occurring around the prostheses
sequestrectomy sē-kwĕs-TRĔK-tō-mē *sequestr:* separation *-ectomy:* excision, removal	Excision of a sequestrum (segment of necrosed bone)
synovectomy sĭn-ō-VĔK-tō-mē *synov:* synovial membrane, synovial fluid *-ectomy:* excision, removal	Excision of a synovial membrane

Procedure	Description
total hip replacement (THR)	Surgical procedure to replace a hip joint damaged by a degenerative disease, commonly arthritis (See Figure 10-17.) *In THR, the femoral head and the acetabulum are replaced with a metal ball and stem (prosthesis). The acetabulum is coated with plastic to avoid metal-to-metal contact on articulating surfaces; the stem is anchored into the central core of the femur to achieve a secure fit.*

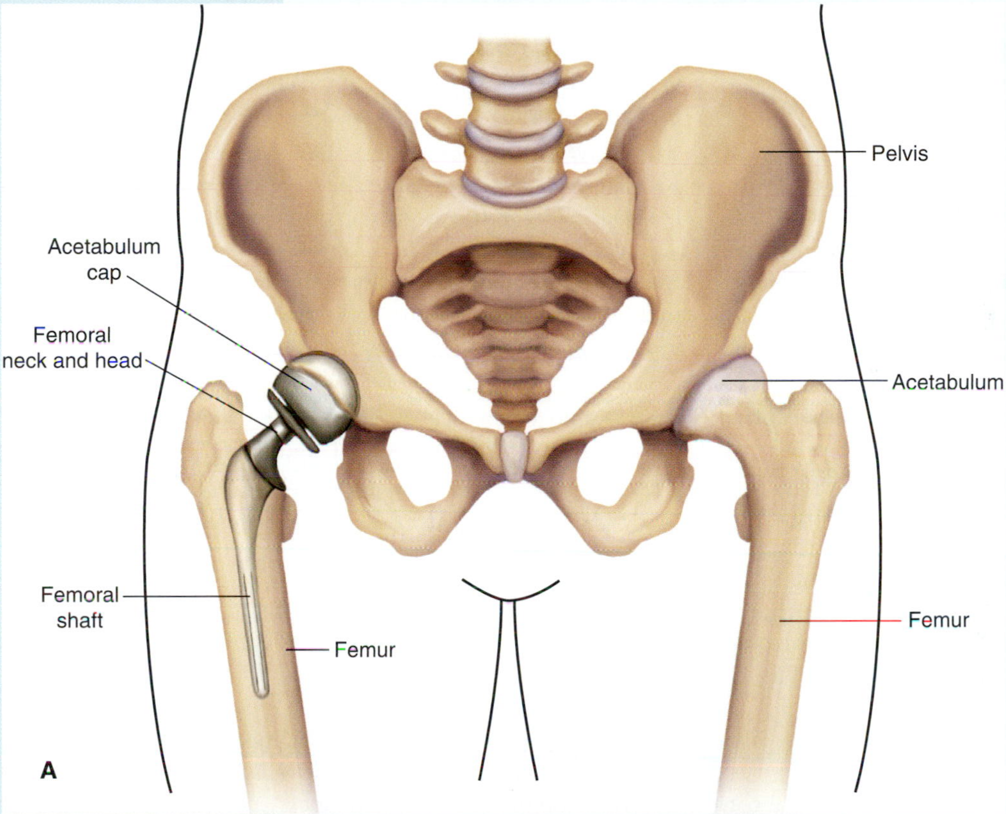

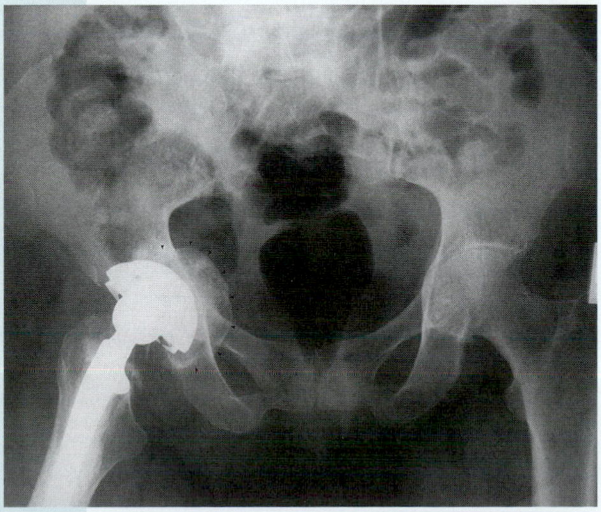

Figure 10-17 Total hip replacement. **(A)** Right total hip replacement. **(B)** Radiograph showing total hip replacement of an arthritic hip. From McKinnis: *Fundamentals of Musculoskeletal Imaging,* 2nd ed. FA Davis, Philadelphia, 2005, p 314, with permission.

(continued)

Procedure	Description
Diagnostic	
Imaging	

arthrography
ăr-THRŎG-ră-fē
   arthr/o: joint
   -graphy: process of recording
	Series of radiographs taken after injection of contrast material into a joint cavity, especially the knee or shoulder, to outline the contour of the joint

bone density test **(bone densitometry)**	Noninvasive procedure that uses low-energy x-ray absorption to measure bone mineral density (BMD) and usually measures bones of the spine, hip, and forearm; also called *dual-energy x-ray absorptiometry (DEXA)* *The x-rays measure how many grams of calcium and other bone minerals are packed into a segment of bone. The higher the mineral content, the denser is the bone. Areas of decreased density indicate osteopenia and osteoporosis.*
discography dĭs-KŎG-ră-fē	Radiological examination of the intervertebral disk structures with injection of a contrast medium *Discography is used to diagnose suspected cases of herniated disk.*

lumbosacral spinal radiography
LŬM-bō-sā-krăl
SPĪ-năl rā-dē-ŎG-ră-fē
   lumb/o: loins (lower back)
   sacr: sacrum
   -al: pertaining to, relating to
   radi/o: radiation, x-ray, radius
   (lower arm bone on thumb side)
   -graphy: process of recording
	Radiography of the five lumbar vertebrae and the fused sacral vertebrae, including anteroposterior, lateral, and oblique views of the lower spine
	
	The most common indication for lumbosacral (LS) spinal radiography is lower back pain. It is used to identify or differentiate traumatic fractures, spondylosis, spondylolisthesis, and metastatic tumor.

myelography
mī-ĕ-LŎG-ră-fē
   myel/o: bone marrow, spinal cord
   -graphy: process of recording
	Radiography of the spinal cord after injection of a contrast medium to identify and study spinal distortions caused by tumors, cysts, herniated intervertebral disks, or other lesions

scintigraphy sĭn-TĬG-ră-fē	Nuclear medicine procedure that visualizes various tissues and organs after administration of a radionuclide *After absorption of the radioactive substance, a scanner detects the radioactive tracer and makes a photographic recording (scintigram) of radionuclide distribution using a gamma camera to detect areas of uptake, called* hot spots.
bone	Scintigraphy in which the radionuclide is injected intravenously and taken up into the bone *Bone scintigraphy is used to detect bone disorders, especially arthritis, fractures, osteomyelitis, bone cancers, or areas of bony metastases. Areas of increased uptake (hot spots) are abnormal and may be infection or cancer.*

Pharmacology

Unlike other medications that treat specific diseases, most pharmacological agents for musculoskeletal disorders are used to treat symptoms. (See Table 10-3.) Acute musculoskeletal conditions, such as strains, sprains, and "pulled" muscles, are treated with analgesics and anti-inflammatory drugs. Nonsteroidal anti-inflammatory drugs (NSAIDs), salicylates, muscle relaxants, opioid analgesics, or narcotics are commonly used to treat pain by anesthetizing (numbing) the area or decreasing the inflammation. NSAIDs and salicylates are also used to treat arthritis, in addition to gold salts. Calcium supplements are used to treat hypocalcemia.

Table 10-3	Drugs Used to Treat Musculoskeletal Disorders	

This table lists common drug classifications used to treat musculoskeletal disorders, their therapeutic actions, and selected generic and trade names.

Classification	Therapeutic Action	Generic and *Trade* Names
calcium supplements KĂL-sē-ŭm	Treat and prevent hypocalcemia *Over-the-counter calcium supplements are numerous and are contained in many antacids as a secondary therapeutic effect. They are used to prevent osteoporosis when normal diet is lacking adequate amounts of calcium.*	**calcium carbonate** KĂL-sē-ŭm KĂR-bŏn-āt *Calci-Mix, Tums* **calcium citrate** KĂL-sē-ŭm SĬT-rāt *Cal-Citrate 250, Citracal*
gold salts	Treat rheumatoid arthritis by inhibiting activity within the immune system *Gold salts contain actual gold in capsules or in solution for injection. This agent prevents further disease progression but cannot reverse past damage.*	**auranofin** aw-RĂN-ŏ-fĭn *Ridaura* **aurothioglucose** aw-rō-thī-ō-GLOO-kōs *Solganal*
nonsteroidal anti-inflammatory drugs (NSAIDs) nŏn-STĒR-oyd-ăl ăn-tē-ĭn-FLĂM-ă-tō-rē	Decrease pain and suppress inflammation *NSAIDs are used to treat acute musculoskeletal conditions, such as sprains and strains, and inflammatory disorders, including rheumatoid arthritis, osteoarthritis, bursitis, gout, and tendinitis.*	**ibuprofen** ī-bū-PRŌ-fĕn *Advil, Motrin* **naproxen** nă-PRŎK-sĕn *Aleve, Naprosyn*
salicylates săl-ĬS-ĭl-ātz	Relieve mild to moderate pain and reduce inflammation *Salicylates have anti-inflammatory abilities and alleviate pain. Aspirin (acetylsalicylic acid) is the oldest drug in this classification that is used to treat arthritis.*	**aspirin** ĂS-pĕr-ĭn *Acuprin, Aspergum, Bayer Aspirin* **magnesium salicylate** măg-NĒ-zē-ŭm să-LĬS-ĭ-lāt *Magan, Mobidin*
muscle relaxants	Relieve muscle spasms and stiffness *Muscle relaxants are also prescribed for muscle spasms due to multiple sclerosis, spinal cord injury, cerebral palsy, and stroke.*	**cyclobenzaprine** sī-klō-BĔN-ză-prēn *Flexeril* **methocarbamol and aspirin** mĕth-ō-KĂR-bă-mōl *Robaxin*

Abbreviations

This section introduces musculoskeletal-related abbreviations and their meanings.

Abbreviation	Meaning	Abbreviation	Meaning
ACL	anterior cruciate ligament	LS	lumbosacral spine
BE	barium enema; below the elbow	MG	myasthenia gravis
C1, C2, and so on	first cervical vertebra, second cervical vertebra, and so on	MRI	magnetic resonance imaging
Ca	calcium; cancer	MS	musculoskeletal; multiple sclerosis; mental status; mitral stenosis
CDH	congenital dislocation of the hip	NSAIDs	nonsteroidal anti-inflammatory drugs
CTS	carpal tunnel syndrome	ORTH, ortho	orthopedics
DEXA, DXA	dual-energy x-ray absorptiometry	P	phosphorus; pulse
DJD	degenerative joint disease	PCL	posterior cruciate ligament
DO	Doctor of Osteophathy	RA	rheumatoid arthritis; right atrium
EMG	electromyography	RF	rheumatoid factor; radio frequency
Fx	fracture	ROM	range of motion
HD	hemodialysis; hip disarticulation; hearing distance	SD	shoulder disarticulation
HNP	herniated nucleus pulposus (herniated disk)	THA	total hip arthroplasty
HP	hemipelvectomy	THR	total hip replacement
IM	intramuscular; infectious mononucleosis	TKA	total knee arthroplasty
IS	intracostal space	TKR	total knee replacement
IV	intravenous	TRAM	transverse rectus abdominis muscle
L1, L2, and so on	first lumbar vertebra, second lumbar vertebra, and so on		

It is time to review procedures, pharmacology, and abbreviations by completing Learning Activity 10–5.

LEARNING ACTIVITIES

The following activities provide review of the musculoskeletal system terms introduced in this chapter. Complete each activity and review your answers to evaluate your understanding of the chapter.

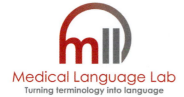

Medical Language Lab
Turning terminology into language

Visit the Medical Language Lab at the web site: medicallanguagelab.com. Use it to enhance your study and reinforcement of this chapter with the flash-card activity. We recommend you complete the flash-card activity before starting Learning Activities 10-1 and 10-2 below.

Learning Activity 10-1

Combining Forms, Suffixes, and Prefixes

Use the elements listed in the table to build medical words. You may use elements more than once.

Combining Forms		Suffixes		Prefixes
ankyl/o	leiomy/o	-al	-oma	dys-
arthr/o	oste/o	-ar	-osis	infra-
chondr/o	patell/o	-clasia	-plasty	syn-
cost/o	synov/o	-desis	-tome	
crani/o	ten/o	-ism	-trophy	
dactyl/o		-itis		
fasci/o		-malacia		

1. binding, fixation of a tendon _____

2. tumor of smooth muscle _____

3. inflammation of the synovial membrane _____

4. pertaining to the patella (knee cap) _____

5. poor, painful development _____

6. pertaining to under, below the ribs _____

7. abnormal condition of (being) bent or crooked _____

8. softening the cranium _____

9. instrument to incise a bone _____

10. inflammation of a joint _____

11. condition of joined fingers or toes _____

12. surgical fracture of a bone _____

13. instrument to incise the cranium _____

14. tumor of cartilage _____

15. surgical repair of fascia _____

 Check your answers in Appendix A. Review any material that you did not answer correctly.

Correct Answers _____ X 6.67 = _____ % Score

Learning Activity 10-2
Building Medical Words

Use *oste/o* (bone) to build words that mean:

1. bone cells _____
2. pain in bones _____
3. disease of bones and joints _____
4. beginning or formation of bones _____

Use *cervic/o* (neck) to build words that mean:

5. pertaining to the neck _____
6. pertaining to the neck and arm _____
7. pertaining to the neck and face _____

Use *myel/o* (bone marrow; spinal cord) to build words that mean:

8. tumor of bone marrow _____
9. sarcoma of bone marrow (cells) _____
10. bone marrow cell _____
11. resembling bone marrow _____

Use *stern/o* (sternum) to build words that mean:

12. pertaining to above the sternum _____
13. resembling the breastbone _____

Use *arthr/o* (joint) or *chondr/o* (cartilage) to build words that mean:

14. embryonic cell that forms cartilage _____
15. inflammation of a joint _____
16. inflammation of bones and joints _____

Use *pelv/i* (pelvis) to build a word that means:

17. instrument for measuring the pelvis _____

Use *my/o* (muscle) to build words that mean:

18. twitching of a muscle _____
19. any disease of muscle _____
20. rupture of a muscle _____

Build surgical words that mean:

21. excision of one or more of the phalanges (bones of a finger or toe) _____

22. incision of the thorax (chest wall) _____

23. excision of a vertebra _____

24. binding of a joint _____

25. repair of muscle (tissue) _____

Check your answers in Appendix A. Review material that you did not answer correctly.

Correct Answers _____ X 4 = _____ % Score

Learning Activity 10-3
Pathology, Diseases, and Conditions

Match the following terms with the definitions in the numbered list.

ankylosis	ganglion cyst	necrosis	spondylitis
bunion	gout	osteoporosis	spondylolisthesis
carpal tunnel	greenstick fracture	phantom limb	subluxation
chondrosarcoma	hypotonia	pyogenic	talipes
claudication	kyphosis	rickets	
comminuted fracture	muscular dystrophy	scoliosis	
Ewing	myasthenia gravis	sequestrum	

1. incomplete or partial dislocation _____

2. softening of the bones caused by vitamin D deficiency _____

3. slipped vertebrae _____

4. limping _____

5. disease causing degeneration of muscles _____

6. congenital deformity of the foot, which is twisted out of shape or position _____

7. part of necrosed bone that has become separated from surrounding tissue _____

8. neuromuscular disorder characterized by weakness manifested in ocular muscles _____

9. painful condition caused by compression of the median nerve within the wrist canal _____

10. joint capsule tumor, commonly found in the wrist _____

11. loss of muscular tonicity; diminished resistance of muscles to passive stretching _____

12. type of sarcoma that attacks the shafts rather than the ends of long bones _____

13. bone that is partially bent and partially broken; occurs in children _____

14. exaggeration of the thoracic curve of the vertebral column; humpback _____

15. disease caused by a decrease in bone density; occurs in the elderly _____

16. deviation of the spine to the right or left _____

17. cartilaginous sarcoma _____

18. describes a bone that has splintered into pieces _____

19. inflammation of the vertebrae _____

20. accumulation of uric acid, usually in the big toe _____

21. lateral deviation of the great toe as it turns in toward the second toe (angulation), which may cause the surrounding joint to become swollen _____

22. formation of pus _____

23. death of cells, tissues, or organs _____

24. stiffening and immobility of a joint _____

25. perceived sensation, following amputation, that the limb still exists _____

Check your answers in Appendix A. Review material that you did not answer correctly.

Correct Answers _____ X 4 = _____ % Score

Procedures, Pharmacology, and Abbreviations

Match the following terms with the definitions in the numbered list.

ACL	*closed reduction*	*myelography*
amputation	*CTS*	*open reduction*
arthrodesis	*gold salts*	*relaxants*
arthrography	*HNP*	*salicylates*
arthroscopy	*laminectomy*	*sequestrectomy*

1. images of the spinal cord after injection of a contrast medium _____
2. surgery to place fractured bones in normal position _____
3. used to treat rheumatoid arthritis by inhibiting activity with the immune system _____
4. painful disorder of the wrist due to compression of the median nerve _____
5. excision of the posterior arch of a vertebra _____
6. joint radiographs preceded by injection of a radiopaque substance or air into the joint cavity _____
7. surgical binding or immobilizing of a joint _____
8. partial or complete removal of a limb _____
9. herniated nucleus pulposus _____
10. relieve mild to moderate pain and reduce inflammation _____
11. visual examination of a joint's interior, especially the knee _____
12. excising a segment of necrosed bone _____
13. anterior cruciate ligament _____
14. relieve muscle spasms and stiffness _____
15. manipulative treatment of bone fractures by placing the bones in normal position without incision _____

Check your answers in Appendix A. Review material that you did not answer correctly.

Correct Answers _____ X 6.67 = _____ % Score

Learning Activity 10-5
Medical Scenarios

To construct chart notes, replace the italicized terms in each of the two scenarios with one of the medical terms listed below.

clavicle	*open fracture*	*pathological fractures*
comminuted	*orthopedist*	*spondylalgia*
femur	*osteopenia*	
kyphosis	*osteoporosis*	

Mr. L., a 30-year-old male, was brought to the ER following a head-on car collision. X-rays revealed a minor (1) ***splintered*** fracture of the right (2) ***collar bone***. The more serious injury was a (3) ***broken bone protruding through the skin surface*** with laceration of the surrounding soft tissue of the right thigh. Mr. L. was immediately prepped for a surgical reduction of the right (4) ***thigh bone***. Dr. Michaels, the (5) ***specialist in treating bone disorders***, will undertake management of this patient.

1. _____
2. _____
3. _____
4. _____
5. _____

Mrs. P.'s previous surgical history shows an appendectomy at age 10 and a hysterectomy with the removal of the ovaries and fallopian tubes at 35. She has a history of (6) ***a decrease in bone minerals***. She is stooped over with a prominent (7) ***hump back*** and complains of (8) ***pain in the vertebrae***. The results of her DEXA scan show (9) ***porous bones***. She is at risk for (10) ***bone fractures related to disease***.

6. _____
7. _____
8. _____
9. _____
10. _____

✓ *Check your answers in Appendix A. Review material that you did not answer correctly.*

Correct Answers _____ X 10 = _____ % Score

MEDICAL RECORD ACTIVITIES

The two medical records included in the following activities use common clinical scenarios to show how medical terminology is used to document patient care. Complete the terminology and analysis sections for each activity to help you recognize and understand terms related to the musculoskeletal system.

Medical Record Activity 10-1
Operative Report: Right Knee Arthroscopy and Medial Meniscectomy

Terminology

Terms listed in the following table are taken from *Operative Report: Right Knee Arthroscopy and Medial Meniscectomy* that follows. Use a medical dictionary such as *Taber's Cyclopedic Medical Dictionary;* the appendices of *Systems,* 7th ed.; or other resources to define each term. Then review the pronunciations for each term and practice by reading the medical record aloud.

Term	Definition
ACL	
arthroscopy ăr-THRŎS-kō-pē	
effusions ĕ-FŪ-zhŭnz	
intracondylar ĭn-tră-KŎN-dĭ-lăr	
Lachman test	
McMurray sign test	
meniscectomy měn-ĭ-SĔK-tō-mē	
MRI	
PCL	
synovitis sĭn-ō-VĪ-tĭs	

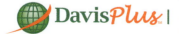 | Visit the *Medical Terminology Systems* online resource center at Davis*Plus.* Use it to practice pronunciation and reinforce the meanings of the terms in this medical report.

OPERATIVE REPORT: RIGHT KNEE ARTHROSCOPY AND MEDIAL MENISCECTOMY

General Hospital

1511 Ninth Avenue ■■ Sun City, USA 12345 ■■ (555) 802-1887

OPERATIVE REPORT

Date: August 14, 20xx   Physician: Robert L. Mead, MD
Patient: Jay, Elizabeth   Patient ID#: 20798

PREOPERATIVE DIAGNOSIS: Tear, medial meniscus, right knee.

POSTOPERATIVE DIAGNOSIS: Tear, medial meniscus, right knee.

CLINICAL HISTORY: This 42-year-old woman has jogged for the past 10 years, an average of 25 miles each week. She has persistent posteromedial right knee pain with occasional effusions. The patient has MRI-documented medial meniscal tear.

PROCEDURE: Right knee arthroscopy and medial meniscectomy.

ANESTHESIA: General.

COMPLICATIONS: None.

OPERATIVE SUMMARY: Examination of the knee under anesthesia showed a full range of motion, no effusion, no instability, and negative Lachman and negative McMurray sign tests. Arthroscopic evaluation showed a normal patellofemoral groove and normal intracondylar notch with normal ACL and PCL, some anterior synovitis, and a normal lateral meniscus and lateral compartment to the knee. The medial compartment of the knee showed an inferior surface, posterior and mid-medial meniscal tear that was flipped up on top of itself. This was resected, and then the remaining meniscus contoured back to a stable rim. A sterile dressing was applied.

Patient was taken to the postanesthesia care unit in stable condition.

Robert L. Mead, MD
Robert L. Mead, MD

rlm:bg

D: 8-14-20xx
T: 8-14-20xx

Analysis

Review the medical record *Operative Report: Right Knee Arthroscopy and Medial Meniscectomy* to answer the following questions.

1. Describe the meniscus and identify its location.

   _____

   _____

2. What is the probable cause of the tear in the patient's meniscus?

   _____

   _____

3. What does normal ACL and PCL refer to in the report?

   _____

   _____

4. Explain the McMurray sign test.

   _____

   _____

5. Because Lachman and McMurray tests were negative (normal), why was the surgery performed?

   _____

   _____

Radiographic Consultation: Tibial Diaphysis Nuclear Scan

Terminology

Terms listed in the following table are taken from *Radiographic Consultation: Tibial Diaphysis Nuclear Scan* that follows. Use a medical dictionary such as *Taber's Cyclopedic Medical Dictionary*; the appendices of *Systems*, 7th ed.; or other resources to define each term. Then review the pronunciations for each term and practice by reading the medical record aloud.

Term	Definition
buttressing BŬ-trĕs-ĭng	
cortical KOR-tĭ-kăl	
diaphysis dī-ĂF-ĭ-sĭs	
endosteal ĕn-DŎS-tē-ăl	
focal FŌ-kăl	
fusiform FŪ-zĭ-form	
NSAIDs	
nuclear scan NŪ-klē-ăr	
periosteal pĕr-ē-ŎS-tē-ăl	
resorption rē-SORP-shŭn	
tibial TĬB-ē-ăl	

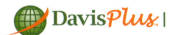

Visit the *Medical Terminology Systems* online resource center at Davis*Plus*. Use it to practice pronunciation and reinforce the meanings of the terms in this medical report.

RADIOGRAPHIC CONSULTATION:
TIBIAL DIAPHYSIS NUCLEAR SCAN

Physician Center

2422 Rodeo Drive ■■ **Sun City, USA 12345** ■■ **(555)333-2427**

September 3, 20xx

Grant Hammuda, MD
1115 Forest Ave
Sun City, USA 12345

Dear Doctor Hammuda:

We are pleased to provide the following in response to your request for consultation.

This is an 18-year-old male cross-country runner. He complains of pain of more than 1 month's duration, with persistent symptoms over middle one-third of left tibia with resting. He finds no relief with NSAIDs.

FINDINGS: Nuclear scan reveals the following: There is focal increased blood flow, blood pool, and delayed radiotracer accumulation within the left mid posterior tibial diaphysis. The delayed spot planar images demonstrate focal fusiform uptake involving 50% to 75% of the tibial diaphysis width.

It is our opinion that with continued excessive, repetitive stress, the rate of resorption will exceed the rate of bone replacement. This will lead to weakened cortical bone with buttressing by periosteal and endosteal new bone deposition. If resorption continues to exceed replacement, a stress fracture will occur.

Please let me know if I can be of any further assistance.

Sincerely yours,

Adrian Jones, MD
Adrian Jones, MD

aj:bg

Analysis

Review the medical record *Radiographic Consultation: Tibial Diaphysis Nuclear Scan* to answer the following questions.

1. Where was the pain located?

_____

_____

2. What medication was the patient taking for pain, and did it provide relief?

_____

_____

3. How was the blood flow to the affected area described by the radiologist?

_____

_____

4. How was the radiotracer accumulation described?

_____

_____

5. What will be the probable outcome with continued excessive repetitive stress?

_____

_____

6. What will happen if resorption continues to exceed replacement?

_____

_____

Urinary System

Chapter Outline

Objectives

Upon completion of this chapter, you will be able to:

- Locate and describe urinary structures.
- Describe the functional relationship between the urinary system and other body systems.
- Pronounce, spell, and build words related to the urinary system.
- Describe diseases, conditions, and procedures related to the urinary system.
- Explain pharmacology related to the treatment of urinary disorders.
- Demonstrate your knowledge of this chapter by completing the learning and medical record activities.

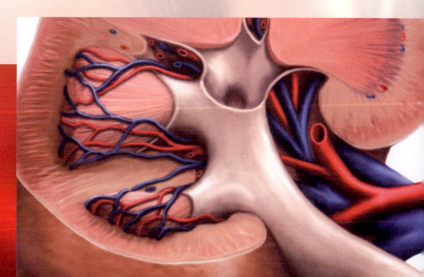

Anatomy and Physiology

The urinary system consists of two kidneys, two ureters, the urinary bladder, and the urethra. However, the kidneys carry out the major work of the urinary system, while the other structures are mainly passageways and storage areas. The primary function of the urinary system is regulation of the extracellular fluids of the body (primarily plasma and tissue fluid). The kidneys accomplish this function through the formation of urine. Urine passes out of the kidneys via the ureters to the urinary bladder, where it is temporarily stored before it is excreted from the body through the urethra.

Anatomy and Physiology Key Terms

This section introduces important urinary system terms along with their definitions and pronunciations. Word analyses are provided for selected terms.

Term	Definition
electrolyte ē-LĚK-trō-līt	Mineral salt (sodium, potassium, or calcium) that carries an electrical charge when in solution
filtrate FĬL-trāt	Fluid that passes from the blood through the capillary walls of the glomeruli into Bowman capsule *Filtrate is similar to plasma but with less protein. Urine is formed from filtrate.*
nitrogenous waste nī-TRŎJ-ĕn-ŭs	Product of protein metabolism that include urea, uric acid, creatine, creatinine, and ammonia
peristaltic wave pĕr-ĭ-STĂL-tĭk	Sequence of rhythmic contraction of smooth muscles of a hollow organ to force material forward and prevent backflow
peritoneum pĕr-ĭ-tō-NĒ-ŭm	Serous membrane that lines the abdominopelvic cavity and covers most of the organs within the cavity
pH	Symbol that expresses the alkalinity or acidity of a solution *A solution with a pH of 7.0 is neutral; greater than 7.0 is alkaline; less than 7.0 is acidic.*
plasma PLĂZ-mă	Liquid portion of blood that is filtered by the nephrons to remove dissolved wastes

Pronunciation Help	Long Sound	ā — rate	ē — rebirth	ī — isle	ō — over	ū — unite
	Short Sound	ă — alone	ĕ — ever	ĭ — it	ŏ — not	ŭ — cut

Macroscopic Structures

The harmful products excreted by the urinary system include **nitrogenous wastes** and excess **electrolytes.** Nitrogenous products are toxic, and must be continuously eliminated form the body or death can occur within a few days. The proper balance of **electrolytes** is vital for proper functioning of the muscles, heart, and nerves. Along with regulating the composition of extracellular fluids, the kidneys also secrete the hormone **erythropoietin.** This hormone acts on bone marrow to stimulate production of red blood cells when blood oxygen levels are low. The macroscopic structures that make up the urinary system include two kidneys, two ureters, a bladder, and a urethra. (See Figure 11-1.)

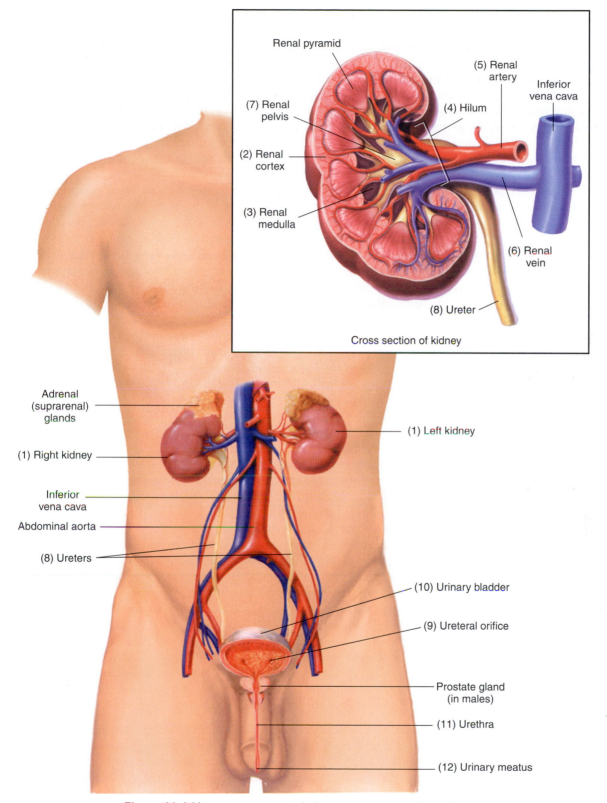

Figure 11-1 Urinary structures, including a cross-section of the kidney.

The (1) **left and right kidneys,** each about the size of a fist, are located in the abdominal cavity slightly above the waistline. Because they lie outside of the peritoneum, their location is said to be **retroperitoneal**. A concave medial border gives the kidney its beanlike shape. In the frontal section, two distinct areas are visible: an outer area, the (2) **renal cortex,** and a middle area, the (3) **renal medulla.** These structures contain portions of the microscopic filtering units of the kidney called **nephrons.** Near the medial border is the (4) **hilum** (also called **hilus**), an opening through which the (5) **renal artery** enters and the (6) **renal vein** exits the kidney. The renal artery carries blood that contains waste products to the nephrons for filtering. After waste products are removed, blood leaves the kidney by way of the renal vein. The process of urine formation helps maintain the normal composition, volume, and pH of blood and tissue fluid.

Waste material, now in the form of urine, passes to a hollow chamber, the (7) **renal pelvis.** This cavity is formed where the (8) **ureter** merges with the kidney. Each ureter is a slender tube about 10" to 12" long. They carry urine in peristaltic waves to the bladder. These waves keep urine flowing to the bladder, rather than regurgitating back into the kidney when bladder pressure is high during urination. Urine enters the bladder at the (9) **ureteral orifice.** The (10) **urinary bladder,** an expandable hollow organ, acts as a temporary reservoir for urine. The bladder has small folds called **rugae** that expand as the bladder fills. A triangular area at the base of the bladder called the **trigone** is delineated by the openings of the ureters and the urethra.

The base of the trigone forms the (11) **urethra,** a tube that discharges urine from the bladder. The length of the urethra is approximately 1.5" in women and about 7" to 8" in men. In the male, the urethra passes through the prostate gland and the penis. During urination **(micturition),** urine is expelled from the body through the urethral opening, the (12) **urinary meatus.**

Microscopic Structures

Microscopic examination of kidney tissue reveals the presence of approximately 1 million nephrons. These microscopic structures are responsible for maintaining homeostasis by continually adjusting and regulating the contents of blood plasma. Substances removed by nephrons are nitrogenous wastes, the end products of protein metabolism, excess electrolytes, and many other products that exceed the amount tolerated by the body.

Each nephron includes a renal corpuscle and a renal tubule. (See Figure 11-2.) The **renal corpuscle** is composed of a tuft of capillaries called the (1) **glomerulus** and a modified, enlarged extension of the renal tubule known as (2) **Bowman capsule** that encapsulates the glomerulus. A larger (3) **afferent arteriole** carries blood to the glomerulus, and a smaller (4) **efferent arteriole** carries blood from the glomerulus. The difference in the size of these vessels provides the needed pressure to force blood plasma into Bowman capsule. Once this happens, the fluid is no longer plasma but is called filtrate. The efferent arteriole passes behind the renal corpuscle to form the (5) **peritubular capillaries,** a network of capillaries that surround the renal tubule. The renal tubule consists of four sections: the (6) **proximal convoluted tubule,** followed by the narrow (7) **loop of Henle,** then the larger (8) **distal tubule,** and, finally, the (9) **collecting tubule.** The collecting tubule transports newly formed urine to the renal pelvis for excretion by the kidneys.

The nephron performs three physiological functions as it produces urine:

1. **Filtration** occurs in the renal corpuscle, where plasma containing water, electrolytes, sugar, and other small molecules is forced from the blood within the glomerulus into Bowman capsule to form filtrate. Filtrate resembles plasma except that the amount of protein in filtrate is less than that found in blood.

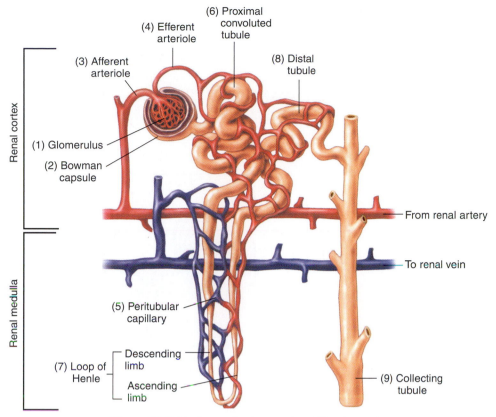

Figure 11-2 Nephron with its associated blood vessels.

2. **Reabsorption** begins as filtrate travels through the long, twisted pathway of the tubule. Most of the water and some of the electrolytes and amino acids are returned to the peritubular capillaries and reenter the circulating blood.
3. **Secretion** is the final stage of urine formation. Substances are actively secreted from the blood in the peritubular capillaries into the filtrate in the renal tubules. Waste products, such as ammonia, uric acid, and metabolic products of medications, are secreted into the filtrate to be eliminated in the urine. Urine leaves the collecting tubule and enters the renal pelvis. From here it passes to the bladder until urination takes place.

Anatomy Review: Urinary Structures

Label the following illustration using the terms listed below.

hilum	*renal medulla*	*right kidney*	*urethra*
left kidney	*renal pelvis*	*ureteral orifice*	*urinary bladder*
renal artery	*renal vein*	*ureters*	*urinary meatus*
renal cortex			

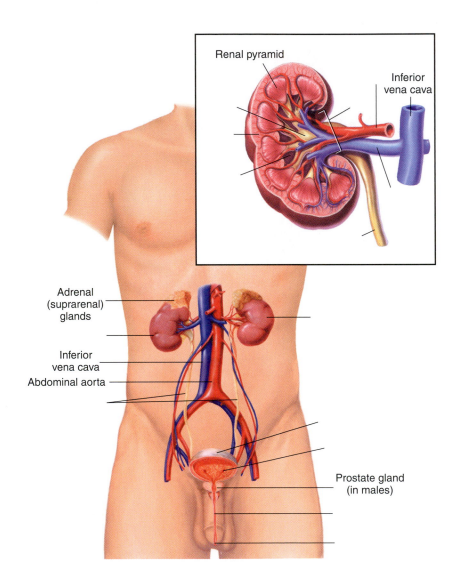

 Check your answers by referring to Figure 11–1 on page 351. Review material that you did not answer correctly.

Anatomy Review: Nephron

Label the following illustration using the terms listed below.

afferent arteriole   *distal tubule*   *loop of Henle*

Bowman capsule   *efferent arteriole*   *peritubular capillary*

collecting tubule   *glomerulus*   *proximal convoluted tubule*

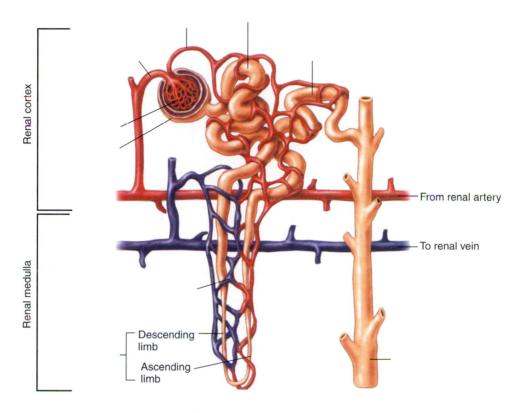

 Check your answers by referring to Figure 11–2 on page 353. Review material that you did not answer correctly.

CONNECTING BODY SYSTEMS—URINARY SYSTEM

The main function of the urinary system is to regulate extracellular fluids of the body. Specific functional relationships between the urinary system and other body systems are summarized below.

Blood, Lymph, and Immune
- Urinary system filters plasm, thereby regulating composition, quantity, and quality of blood plasma and lymph.
- Urinary system retains needed products and integrates them back into plasma as it removes products that are excessive or toxic to the body.

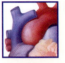

Cardiovascular
- Urinary system helps regulate essential electrolytes needed for contraction of the heart.

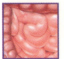

Digestive
- Urinary system aids in removing glucose from the blood when excessive amounts are consumed.
- Urinary system removes excessive fluids absorbed from the gastrointestinal (GI) tract.

Endocrine
- Urinary system regulates electrolyte and fluid balance, which is essential for hormone transport in the blood.
- Urinary system produces erythropoietin, a hormone synthesized mainly in the kidneys to stimulate bone marrow production of blood cells.

Female Reproductive
- Urinary system aids in removing waste products produced by the fetus in the pregnant woman.

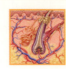

Integumentary
- Urinary system compensates for extracellular fluid loss due to hyperhidrosis by regulating fluid loss during urine production.
- Urinary system adjusts electrolytes, especially potassium and sodium, in response to their loss through sweating.

Male Reproductive
- Urinary system shares the urethra with the male reproductive system for delivery of semen to the female.

Musculoskeletal
- Urinary system works in conjunction with bone tissue to maintain a constant calcium level.

Nervous
- Urinary system regulates sodium, potassium, and calcium, which are the electrolytes responsible for the transmission of nervous stimuli.

Respiratory
- Urinary system assists the lungs in regulating acid–base balance of the body.

Medical Word Elements

This section introduces combining forms, suffixes, and prefixes related to the urinary system. Word analyses are also provided.

Element	Meaning	Word Analysis
Combining Forms		
albumin/o	albumin, protein	**albumin**/oid (ăl-BŪ-mĭ-noyd): resembling albumin *-oid:* resembling
azot/o	nitrogenous compounds	**azot**/emia (ăz-ō-TĒ-mē-ă): nitrogenous compounds in the blood *-emia:* blood condition *Nitrogenous products, especially urea, are toxic. If they are not removed from the body, death will result.*

Element	Meaning	Word Analysis
bacteri/o	bacteria (singular, bacterium)	**bacteri**/uria (băk-tē-rē-Ū-rē-ă): bacteria in urine *-uria:* urine
cyst/o	bladder	**cyst/o**/scope (SĬST-ō-skōp): instrument for examining the bladder *-scope:* instrument for examining
vesic/o		**vesic/o**/cele (VĔS-ĭ-kō-sēl): hernia of the bladder; also called *cystocele* *-cele:* hernia, swelling *With a vesicocele, the bladder herniates into the vaginal wall, which may lead to incomplete emptying of the bladder.*
glomerul/o	glomerulus	**glomerul/o**/pathy (glō-měr-ū-LŎP-ă-thē): disease of the glomerulus *-pathy:* disease
kal/i*	potassium (an electrolyte)	hypo/**kal**/emia (hī-pō-kă-LĒ-mē-ă): abnormally low concentration of potassium in the blood *hypo-:* under, below *-emia:* blood condition *Hypokalemia may result from excessive urination, which depletes potassium from the body.*
keton/o	ketone bodies (acids and acetones)	**keton**/uria (kē-tō-NŪ-rē-ă): presence of ketone bodies in the urine *-uria:* urine *Ketonuria is commonly found in diabetes mellitus, starvation, and excessive dieting.*
lith/o	stone, calculus	**lith/o**/tripsy (LĬTH-ō-trĭp-sē): crushing of a stone *-tripsy:* crushing *The most common method of lithotripsy is extracorporeal shock-wave lithotripsy (ESWL). Percutaneous nephrolithotomy or ureteroscopic stone removal are alternatives to lithotripsy when stones are large or lithotripsy is not recommended.*
meat/o	opening, meatus	**meat/o**/tomy (mē-ă-TŎT-ō-mē): incision of the urinary meatus *-tomy:* incision *A meatotomy is performed to relieve stenosis of the urethra by enlarging the urethral opening, which may be inhibiting the proper passage of urine or semen.*
nephr/o	kidney	**nephr/o**/pexy (NĔF-rō-pĕks-ē): fixation of kidney *-pexy:* fixation (of an organ)
ren/o		**ren**/al (RĒ-năl): pertaining to the kidney *-al:* pertaining to
noct/o	night	**noct**/uria (nok-TŪ-rē-ă): excessive and frequent urination after going to bed *-uria:* urine *Nocturia is associated with prostate disease, urinary tract infection, and uncontrolled diabetes.*

*The *i* in *kal/i* is an exception to the rule of using the connecting vowel *o*.

(continued)

Element	Meaning	Word Analysis
olig/o	scanty	**olig**/uria (ŏl-ĭg-Ū-rē-ă): scanty (decreased production) urine *-uria:* urine *Oliguria is usually caused by fluid and electrolyte imbalances, renal lesions, or urinary tract obstruction.*
py/o	pus	**py/o**/rrhea (pī-ō-RĒ-ă): flow or discharge of pus *-rrhea:* discharge, flow
pyel/o	renal pelvis	**pyel/o**/plasty (PĪ-ĕ-lō-plăs-tē): surgical repair of the renal pelvis *-plasty:* surgical repair
ur/o	urine, urinary tract	**ur/o**/lith (Ū-rō-lĭth): stone in the urinary tract *-lith:* stone, calculus
ureter/o	ureter	**ureter**/ectasis (ū-rē-tĕr-ĔK-tă-sĭs): dilation of the ureter *-ectasis:* dilation, expansion
urethr/o	urethra	**urethr/o**/stenosis (ū-rē-thrō-stĕn-Ō-sĭs): narrowing or stricture of the urethra *-stenosis:* narrowing, stricture

Suffixes		
-genesis	forming, producing, origin	lith/o/**genesis** (lĭth-ō-JĔN-ĕ-sĭs): forming or producing stones *lith/o:* stone, calculus
-iasis	abnormal condition (produced by something specified)	lith/**iasis** (lĭth-Ī-ă-sĭs): abnormal condition of stones or calculi *lith/o:* stone, calculus
-uria	urine	poly/**uria** (pŏl-ē-Ū-rē-ă): much (excretion of) urine *poly-:* many, much ***Polyuria is generally considered the excretion of over 2.5 L per 24 hours.***

Prefixes		
dia-	through, across	**dia**/lysis (dī-ĂL-ĭ-sĭs): separation across *-lysis:* separation; destruction; loosening *Renal dialysis is a procedure that uses a membrane to separate and selectively remove waste products from blood when kidneys are unable to complete this function.*

retro-	backward, behind	**retro**/peritone/al (rĕt-rō-pĕr-ĭ-tō-NĒ-ăl): pertaining to (the area) behind the peritoneum
		   peritone: peritoneum
		   -al: pertaining to

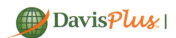 **|** Visit the *Medical Terminology Systems* online resource center at Davis*Plus* for an audio exercise of the terms in this table. Other activities are also available to reinforce content.

 It is time to review medical word elements by completing Learning Activities 11-1 and 11-2.

Pathology

Causes of urinary system disorders include congenital anomalies, infectious diseases, trauma, or conditions that secondarily involve the urinary structures. Frequently, asymptomatic urinary diseases are first diagnosed when a routine urinalysis identifies abnormalities. Forms of glomerulonephritis and chronic urinary tract infection are two such disorders. Symptoms specific to urinary disorders include changes in urination pattern, output, or dysuria. Endoscopic tests, radiological evaluations, and laboratory tests that evaluate renal function are typically used to diagnose disorders of the urinary system.

For diagnosis, treatment, and management of urinary disorders, the medical services of a specialist may be warranted. **Urology** is the branch of medicine concerned with urinary disorders and diseases of the male reproductive system. The physician who specializes in diagnosis and treatment of genitourinary disorders is known as a **urologist.** However, the branch of medicine concerned specifically with diseases of the kidney, electrolyte imbalance, renal transplantation, and dialysis therapy is known as **nephrology.** Physicians who practice in this specialty are called **nephrologists.**

Pyelonephritis

Pyelonephritis, also called **kidney infection** or **nephritis,** is an inflammation of the kidney and renal pelvis. It is the most common form of kidney disease that may affect one or both kidneys. The infection may lead to destruction or scarring of renal tissue, impairing kidney function. The disease is often a result of an ascending infection from the bladder. It is more common in women than in men due in part to the anatomic difference between men and women. The onset of the disease is usually acute, with symptoms that may include painful urination **(dysuria),** pain in the kidneys **(nephralgia),** fatigue, urinary urgency and frequency, chills, fever, nausea, and vomiting. Results of a urinalysis usually reveals bacteria in the urine **(bacteriuria),** pus in the urine **(pyuria),** and when lesions are present, blood in the urine **(hematuria).** Antibiotic therapy, appropriate to the infecting organism, is the treatment of choice.

Glomerulonephritis

Glomerulonephritis is an inflammation of the glomerular membrane in the nephrons, causing it to become "leaky" **(permeable).** Red blood cells and protein, which normally remain in the blood, pass through the inflamed glomerulus and enter the tubule. Retention of water and salts follows, resulting in injury to the glomeruli. Urinalysis reveals blood in the urine **(hematuria),** and protein in the urine **(proteinuria).** Signs and symptoms include high blood pressure **(hypertension),** edema, and impaired renal function. One of the most common causes of glomerular inflammation is a reaction to the toxins given off by pathogenic bacteria, especially streptococci that have recently infected another part of the body, usually the throat. Most patients with acute glomerulonephritis associated with a streptococcal infection recover with no lasting kidney damage.

Nephrolithiasis

Stones **(calculi)** may form in any part of the urinary tract **(urolithiasis),** but most arise in the kidney, a condition called **nephrolithiasis.** (See Figure 11-3.) They commonly form when dissolved urine salts begin to solidify. If they increase in size, they obstruct urinary structures. When they lodge in the ureters, a condition called **ureterolithiasis,** they cause an intense throbbing pain known as **colic.** Because urine is hindered from passing into the bladder, it flows backward **(refluxes)** into the renal pelvis, causing it to dilate.

In one method of treatment called **extracorporeal shock-wave lithotripsy,** calculi are pulverized using concentrated ultrasound waves, called **shock waves,** directed at the stones from a machine outside the body. (See Figure 11-4.) For excessively large stones or patients who have contraindications to ESWL, an alternative treatment is **percutaneous nephrolithotomy (PCNL).** In this procedure, a surgeon makes a small incision in the skin, and forms an opening

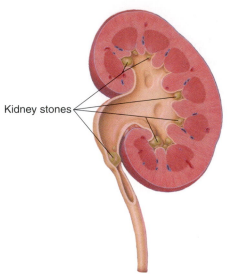

Figure 11-3 Kidney stones in the calices and ureter.

in the kidney. The surgeon then inserts a nephroscope into the kidney to locate and remove the stone. If the stone is large, the surgeon uses an ultrasonic or electrohydraulic probe to break it into smaller fragments, which are then more easily removed. The surgeon may also insert a nephrostomy tube, which remains in place during the healing process. For stones that have descended into the ureters, it may be possible to remove them using a specialized ureteroscope fitted with a small basket. The surgeon passes the ureteroscope through the urethra and bladder and into the ureter and collects the stone in the basket. For larger stones, it may be necessary to break them into smaller pieces using an endoscope fitted with a laser beam before removing the fragments. This procedure is called **ureteroscopic stone removal,** and no incision is required.

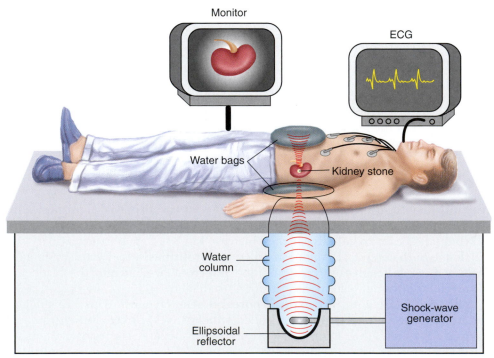

Figure 11-4 Extracorporeal shock-wave lithotripsy.

Acute Tubular Necrosis

In **acute tubular necrosis (ATN),** the tubular portion of the nephron is injured by a decrease in blood supply **(ischemic ATN)** or after the ingestion of toxic chemicals **(nephrotoxic ATN).** Ischemia may occur because of circulatory collapse, severe hypotension, hemorrhage, dehydration, or other disorders that affect blood supply. ATN does not produce specific signs and symptoms, and diagnosis relies on a positive history of risk factors. General signs and symptoms of ATN include scanty urine production **(oliguria),** fluid retention, mental apathy, nausea, vomiting, and increased blood levels of calcium **(hypercalcemia).** When tubular damage is not severe, the disorder is usually reversible.

Oncology

The fourth most common cancer in men and the eighth most common cancer in women is bladder cancer. This malignancy usually arises from the lining of the bladder. The two most common types in the United States are transitional cell carcinoma and adenocarcinoma. Transitional cells line the bladder and the inside of the ureters and urethra. These cells are able to expand when the bladder is full and contract when it is empty. The less common type, adenocarcinomas, arise from mucus-secreting glands in the bladder. Signs and symptoms include hematuria, frequency, dysuria, and abdominal or back pain. Diagnostic tests include cystoscopy with biopsy of suspicious lesions as well as urine cytology, in which a urine sample is checked for malignant cells.

Treatment depends on the type, stage, and grade of the malignancy. Early stages confined to the bladder lining respond to transurethral resection of bladder tumor (TURBT), in which malignant tissue is destroyed with an electric current or high-energy lasers with devices passed through the urethra. More advanced cancers are treated with more aggressive surgeries, including removal of the bladder **(cystectomy).** Surgery may be combined with biological therapy **(immunotherapy),** which stimulates the immune system to attack cancer cells, and chemotherapy, commonly delivered into the vein **(intravenous)** or directly into the bladder **(intravesical).** Finally, radiation therapy provides another modality in treating bladder cancer. This method uses high-energy beams directed at the malignancy from a machine outside of the body **(teletherapy)** or through "seeds" planted within the tumor **(brachytherapy).** Bladder cancer is commonly found early, and treatment is usually effective.

Diseases and Conditions

This section introduces diseases and conditions of the urinary system along with their meanings and pronunciation. Word analyses for selected terms are also provided.

Term	Definition
anuria ăn-Ū-rē-ă *an-:* without, not *uria:* urine	Absence of urine production or output *Anuria may be obstructive, in which there is blockage proximal to the bladder, or unobstructive, which is caused by severe damage to the nephrons of the kidneys.*
bladder neck obstruction (BNO)	Blockage at the base of the bladder that reduces or prevents urine from passing into the urethra *BNO can be caused by benign prostatic hyperplasia, bladder stones, bladder tumors, or tumors in the pelvic cavity.*

(continued)

Term	Definition
cystocele SĬS-tō-sēl *cyst/o:* bladder *-cele:* hernia, swelling	Prolapsing or downward displacement of the bladder due to weakening of the supporting tissues between a woman's bladder and vagina (See Figure 11-5.) *Cystocele is commonly the result of vaginal childbirth, frequent straining with constipation, or lifting of heavy objects.* Cystocele **Figure 11-5** Cystocele.
dysuria dĭs-Ū-rē-ă *dys-:* bad; painful; difficult *uria:* urine	Painful or difficult urination, commonly described as a "burning sensation" while urinating *Dysuria is a symptom of numerous conditions but, most commonly, urinary tract infection (UTI).*
end-stage renal disease (ESRD) RĒ-năl *ren:* kidney *-al:* pertaining to	Any type of kidney disease in which there is little or no remaining kidney function, requiring the patient to undergo dialysis or kidney transplant for survival *The two most common causes of ESRD are diabetes and hypertension.*
enuresis ĕn-ū-RĒ-sĭs *en-:* in, within *ur:* urine *-esis:* condition	Involuntary discharge of urine; also called *incontinence* *Enuresis that occurs during the night is called* nocturnal enuresis; *during the day,* diurnal enuresis.
fistula FĬS-tū-lă	Abnormal passage from a hollow organ to the surface or from one organ to another *The most common type of urinary fistula is vesicovaginal fistula, in which a passage forms between the bladder and vagina. Its causes include previous pelvic surgery such as hysterectomy, difficult and prolonged labor, or reduced blood supply to the area.*

Term	Definition
hydronephrosis hī-drō-nĕf-RŌ-sĭs *hydr/o:* water *nephr:* kidney *-osis:* abnormal condition; increase (used primarily with blood cells)	Abnormal dilation of the renal pelvis and the calyces of one or both kidneys due to pressure from accumulated urine that cannot flow past an obstruction in the urinary tract *The causes of hydronephrosis are enlargement of the prostate, urethral strictures, and calculi that lodge in the ureter. When dilation affects the ureter, it is called* hydroureter. *(See Figure 11-6.)*

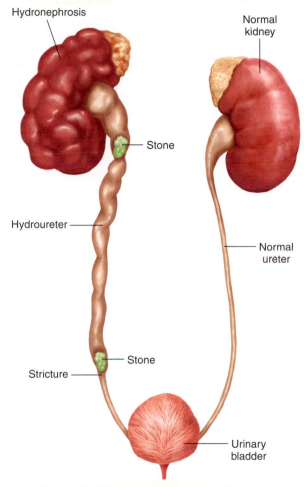

Figure 11-6 Hydronephrosis and hydroureter.

interstitial cystitis (IC) ĭn-tĕr-STĬSH-ăl sĭs-TĪ-tĭs *cyst:* bladder *-itis:* inflammation	Chronic inflammation of the bladder wall that is not caused by bacterial infection and is not responsive to conventional antibiotic therapy; also called *painful bladder syndrome*
nephrotic syndrome nĕ-FRŎT-ĭk *nephr/o:* kidney *-tic:* pertaining to	Loss of large amounts of plasma protein, usually albumin, through urine due to an increased permeability of the glomerular membrane *Hypoproteinemia, edema, and hyperlipidemia are commonly associated with nephrotic syndrome.*

(continued)

Term	Definition
neurogenic bladder nū-rō-JĔN-ĭk *neur/o:* nerve *gen:* forming, producing, origin *-ic:* pertaining to	Impairment of bladder control due to brain or nerve conduction *Nerve damage due to trauma or disease are common causes of neurogenic bladder.*
polycystic kidney disease (PKD) pŏl-ē-SĬS-tĭk *poly:* many, much *cyst:* bladder *-ic:* pertaining to	Inherited disease in which sacs of fluid called *cysts* develop in the kidneys *If cysts increase in number or size or if they become infected, kidney failure may result. Dialysis or kidney transplant may be necessary for renal failure caused by PKD.*
urgency ŬR-jĕn-sē	Sensation of the need to void immediately *Urinary urgency commonly occurs in UTI.*
vesicoureteral reflux (VUR) vĕs-ĭ-kō-ū-RĒ-tĕr-ăl *vesic/o:* bladder *ureter:* ureter *-al:* pertaining to	Disorder caused by the failure of urine to pass through the ureters to the bladder, usually due to impairment of the valve between the ureter and bladder or obstruction in the ureter *VUR may result in hydronephrosis if the obstruction is in the proximal portion of the ureter or hydroureter and hydronephrosis if the obstruction is in the distal portion of the ureter.*
Wilms tumor VĬLMZ	Rapidly developing malignant neoplasm of the kidney that usually occurs in children *Diagnosis of Wilms tumor is established by an excretory urogram (EU) with tomography. The tumor is well encapsulated in the early stage but may metastasize to other sites, such as lymph nodes and lungs, at later stages.*

 It is time to review pathology, diseases, and conditions by completing Learning Activity 11-3.

Medical, Surgical, and Diagnostic Procedures

This section introduces medical, surgical, and diagnostic procedures used to diagnose and treat urinary disorders. Descriptions are provided as well as pronunciations and word analyses for selected terms.

Procedure	Description
Medical	
dialysis dī-ĂL-ĭ-sĭs *dia-:* through, across *-lysis:* separation; destruction; loosening	Mechanical filtering process used to cleanse the blood of toxic substances, such as nitrogenous wastes, when kidneys fail to function properly. *Nitrogenous waste products are collected in a solution called dialysate, which is discarded at the end of the procedure. There are two primary methods of dialysis: hemodialysis and peritoneal dialysis.*
hemodialysis hē-mō-dī-ĂL-ĭ-sĭs *hem/o:* blood *dia:* through, across *-lysis:* separation; destruction; loosening	Type of dialysis in which an artificial kidney machine receives waste-filled blood, filters the blood, and returns the dialyzed (clean) blood to the patient's bloodstream. (See Figure 11-7.)

Procedure	Description

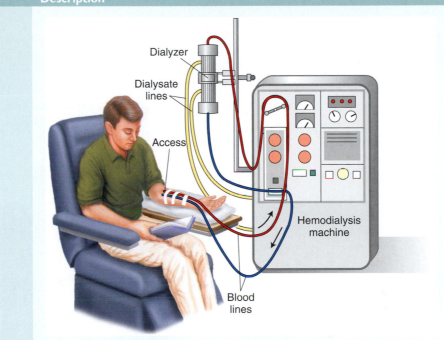

Figure 11-7 Hemodialysis.

peritoneal
pĕr-ĭ-tō-NĒ-ăl
peritone: peritoneum
-al: pertaining to

Type of dialysis in which toxic substances are removed from the body by using the peritoneal membrane as the filter by perfusing (flushing) the peritoneal cavity with a warm, sterile chemical solution. (See Figure 11-8.)

In peritoneal dialysis, the dialyzing fluid remains in the peritoneal cavity for 1 to 2 hours and is then removed.

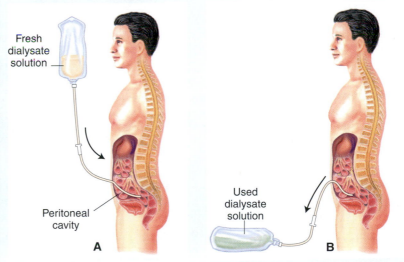

Figure 11-8 Peritoneal dialysis. **(A)** Introducing dialysis fluid into the peritoneal cavity. **(B)** Draining dialysate with waste products from the peritoneal cavity.

(continued)

Procedure	Description
Surgical	
kidney transplant	Replacement of a diseased kidney with one that is supplied by a compatible donor (usually a family member or a cadaver who has donated the kidney prior to death)
	The new kidney is usually placed below the diseased one for ease in attaching it to existing blood vessels. The diseased kidneys usually remain in place unless there is concern that they will cause infection, uncontrolled hypertension, or reflux to the kidneys. (See Figure 11-9.)

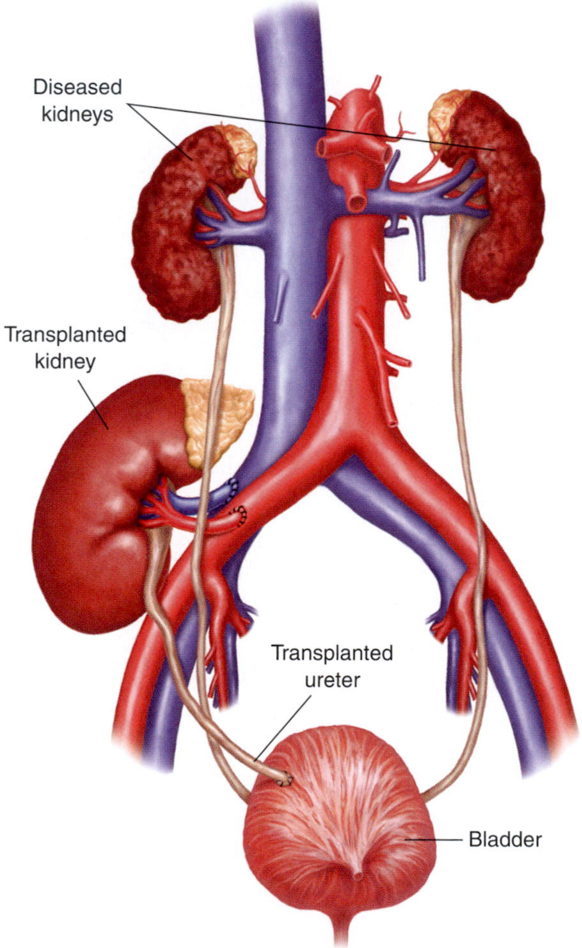

Figure 11-9 Kidney transplant with typical positioning of the new kidney placed beneath the diseased kidney.

Procedure	Description
nephropexy NĔF-rō-pĕks-ē *nephr/o:* kidney *-pexy:* fixation (of an organ)	Fixation of a floating or mobile kidney

Procedure	Description
nephrostomy nĕ-FRŎS-tō-mē *nephr/o:* kidney *-stomy:* forming an opening (mouth)	The passage of a tube through the skin and into the renal pelvis to drain urine to a collecting receptacle outside the body when the ureters are unable to do so *Besides providing for urine drainage, nephrostomy may be used to provide access to assess kidney structure or kidney function or deliver medications. (See Figure 11–10.)* **Posterior view** **Figure 11-10** Nephrostomy with the nephrostomy tube inserted into the renal pelvis with a catheter exiting an incision on the flank. From Williams and Hopper: *Understanding Medical-Surgical Nursing,* 4th ed. FA Davis, Philadelphia, 2011, p 848, with permission.

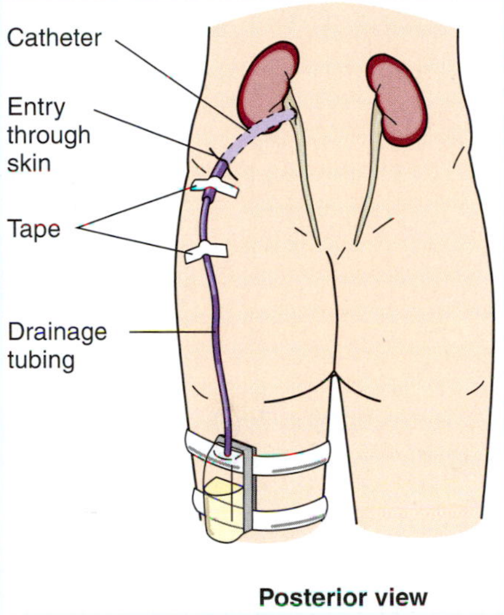

(continued)

Procedure	Description
stent placement	Insertion of a mesh tube into a natural passage conduit in the body to prevent, or counteract a disease-induced, localized flow constriction
ureteral ū-RĒ-tĕr-ăl	Insertion of a thin narrow tube into the ureter to prevent or treat obstruction of urine flow from the kidney *Indwelling stents require constant monitoring because they may lead to infections, blockages, or stone formations. To avoid complications, they must be removed or changed periodically. (See Figure 11-11.)* **Figure 11-11** Ureteral stent placement. From Williams and Hopper: *Understanding Medical-Surgical Nursing*, 4th ed. FA Davis, Philadelphia, 2011, p 848, with permission.
urethrotomy ū-rē-THRŎT-ō-mē *urethr/o:* urethra *-tomy:* incision	Incision of a urethral stricture *Urethrotomy corrects constrictions of the urethra that make voiding difficult.*
Diagnostic	
Clinical	
electromyography (EMG) ē-lĕk-trō-mī-ŎG-ră-fē *electr/o:* electricity *my/o:* muscle *-graphy:* process of recording	Measures the contraction of muscles that control urination using electrodes placed in the rectum and urethra *EMG determines whether incontinence is due to weak muscles or other causes.*

Procedure	Description
Endoscopic	
cystoscopy (cysto) sĭs-TŎS-kō-pē *cyst/o:* bladder *-scopy:* examination	Examination of the urinary bladder for evidence of pathology, obtaining biopsies of tumors or other growths, and removal of polyps using a specialized endoscope *In cystoscopy, a catheter can be inserted into the hollow channel in the cystoscope to collect tissue samples or introduce contrast media during radiography. (See Figure 11-12.)*

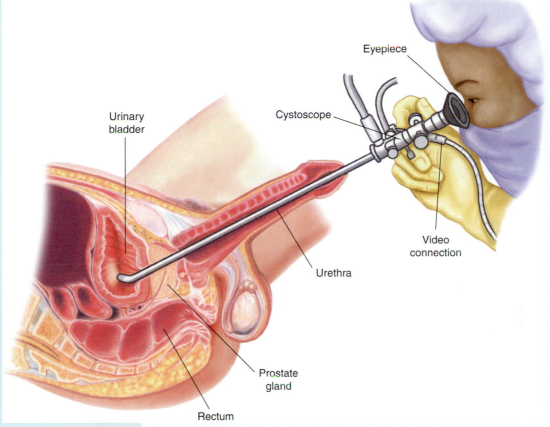

Eyepiece

Cystoscope

Urinary
bladder

Video
connection

Urethra

Prostate
gland

Rectum

Figure 11-12 Cystoscopy.

Procedure	Description
Laboratory	
blood urea nitrogen (BUN) ū-RĒ-ă NĪ-trō-jĕn	Determines the amount of nitrogen in blood that comes from urea, a waste product of protein metabolism *Because the kidneys clear urea from the bloodstream, the BUN test is used as an indicator of kidney function.*
culture and sensitivity (C&S)	Determines the causative organism of an infection and identifies how the organism responds to various antibiotics *A urine C&S test may be performed when bladder infections are chronic or unresponsive to treatment.*

(continued)

Procedure	Description
urinalysis (UA) ū-rĭ-NĂL-ĭ-sĭs	Urine screening test that includes physical observation, chemical tests, and microscopic evaluation *UA not only provides information on the urinary structures but may also be the first indicator of such system disorders as diabetes and liver and gallbladder disease.*

Imaging

Procedure	Description
ultrasonography (US) ŭl-tră-sōn-ŎG-ră-fē *ultra-:* excess, beyond *son/o:* sound *-graphy:* process of recording	High-frequency waves (ultrasound) are directed at soft tissue and reflected as "echoes" to produce an image on a monitor of an internal body structure; also called *ultrasound, sonography,* and *echo.* *Ultrasography is a noninvasive procedure that does not require a contrast medium. It is used to diagnose renal calculi and tumors, ureteral and bladder obstructions, hydronephrosis, and other urinary tract disorders.*
bladder	US produces images of the bladder to measure pre- and postvoid residual urine, thus determining bladder volume and, potentially, identifying incomplete bladder emptying (See Figure 11-13.) 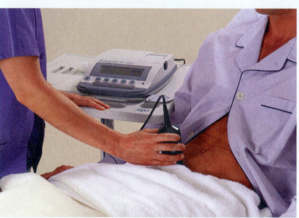 **Figure 11-13** Bladder ultrasonography. From Williams and Hopper: *Understanding Medical-Surgical Nursing,* 4th ed. FA Davis, Philadelphia, 2011, p 832, with permission.
intravenous pyelography (IVP) ĭn-tră-VĒ-nŭs pī-ĕ-LŎG-ră-fē *intra-:* in, within *ven:* vein *-ous:* pertaining to *pyel/o:* renal pelvis *-graphy:* process of recording	Imaging of the urinary tract after IV injection of a contrast medium; also called *excretory urography (EU)* *IVP detects kidney stones, enlarged prostate, internal injuries after an accident or trauma, and tumors in the kidneys, ureters, and bladder.*

Procedure	Description
nuclear scan NŪ-klē-ăr	Technique in which a radiopharmaceutical called a *tracer* is introduced into the body (inhaled, ingested, or injected) and a specialized camera (gamma camera) is used to produce images of organs and structures *A nuclear scan is the reverse of a conventional radiograph. Rather than being directed into the body, radiation comes from inside the body and is then detected by a specialized camera to produce an image.*
renal RĒ-năl *ren:* kidney *-al:* pertaining to	Nuclear scan of the kidneys used to determine their size, shape, and position *A renal nuclear scan is also used to determine the amount of blood the kidneys are able to filter over time, determine renal artery hypertension, and evaluate a kidney transplant to identify signs of rejection.*
voiding cystourethrography (VCUG) sĭs-tō-ū-rē-THRŎG-ră-fē *cyst/o:* bladder *urethr/o:* urethra *-graphy:* process of recording	X-ray of the bladder and urethra performed before, during, and after voiding using a contrast medium to enhance imaging *VCUG is performed to determine the cause of repeated bladder infections or stress incontinence and to identify congenital or acquired structural abnormalities of the bladder and urethra.*

Pharmacology

Pharmacological agents used to treat urinary tract disorders include antibiotics, diuretics, antidiuretics, urinary antispasmodics, and potassium supplements, which are commonly taken concurrently with many diuretics to counteract potassium depletion. (See Table 11-1.)

Table 11-1 Drugs Used to Treat Urinary Disorders

This table lists common drug classifications used to treat urinary disorders, their therapeutic actions, and selected generic and trade names.

Classification	Therapeutic Action	Generic and *Trade* Names
antibiotics ăn-tĭ-bī-ŎT-ĭks	Treat bacterial infections of the urinary tract by acting on the bacterial membrane or one of its metabolic processes *The type of antibiotic prescribed depends on the infecting organism and the type and extent of infection.*	**ciprofloxacin** sĭp-rō-FLŎX-ă-sĭn *Cipro* **sulfamethoxazole/ trimethoprim** sŭl-fă-mĕth-ŎX-ă-zol trī-MĔTH-ō-prĭm *Bactrim*
antispasmodics ăn-tĭ-spăz-MŎT-ĭks	Decrease spasms in the urethra and bladder by relaxing the smooth muscles lining their walls, thus allowing normal emptying of the bladder *Bladder spasms can result from such conditions as urinary tract infections and catheterization.*	**oxybutynin** ŏk-sē-BŪ-tĭ-nĭn *Ditropan*
diuretics dī-ū-RĔT-ĭks	Promote and increase the excretion of urine *Diuretics are grouped by their action and are used to treat edema, hypertension, heart failure, and various renal and hepatic diseases.*	**furosemide** fū-RŌ-sĕ-mīd *Lasix* **spironolactone** spī-rō-nō-LĂK-tōn *Aldactone*

(continued)

Table 11-1	Drugs Used to Treat Urinary Disorders—cont'd		
Classification	**Therapeutic Action**		**Generic and *Trade* Names**
potassium supplements pō-TĂS-ē-ŭm	Replace potassium due to depletion caused by diuretics *Dietary sources of potassium are usually not sufficient to replace potassium loss caused by diuretics.*		**potassium chloride** pō-TĂS-ē-ŭm KLŌ-rīd *K-Tab, Kaon Cl*

Abbreviations

This section introduces urinary-related abbreviations and their meanings.

Abbreviation	Meaning	Abbreviation	Meaning
ATN	acute tubular necrosis	**IVP**	intravenous pyelogram, intravenous pyelography
BNO	bladder neck obstruction	**pH**	symbol for degree of acidity or alkalinity
BUN	blood urea nitrogen	**PCNL**	percutaneous nephrolithotomy
C&S	culture and sensitivity	**PKD**	polycystic kidney disease
cysto	cystoscopy	**RP**	retrograde pyelogram, retrograde pyelography
EBT	external beam therapy	**TURBT**	transurethral resection of bladder tumor
EMG	electromyogram, electromyography	**UA**	urinalysis
ESRD	end-stage renal disease	**US**	ultrasound; ultrasonography
ESWL	extracorporeal shock-wave lithotripsy	**UTI**	urinary tract infection
EU	excretory urography	**VCUG**	voiding cystourethrography
IC	interstitial cystitis	**VUR**	vesicoureteral reflux

It is time to review procedures, pharmacology, and abbreviations by completing Learning Activity 11–4.

LEARNING ACTIVITIES

The following activities provide review of the urinary system terms introduced in this chapter. Complete each activity and review your answers to evaluate your understanding of the chapter.

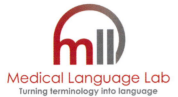

Medical Language Lab
Turning terminology into language

Visit the Medical Language Lab at the web site: medicallanguagelab.com. Use it to enhance your study and reinforcement of this chapter with the flash-card activity. We recommend you complete the flash-card activity before starting Learning Activities 11-1 and 11-2 below.

Learning Activity 11-1
Combining Forms, Suffixes, and Prefixes

Use the elements listed in the table to build medical words. You may use the elements more than once.

Combining Forms		Suffixes		Prefixes
azot/o	pyel/o	-cele	-plasty	an-
cyst/o	ureter/o	-ectasis	-sclerosis	dia-
glomerul/o		-emia	-scopy	poly-
hemat/o		-genesis	-tome	
lith/o		-gram	-tripsy	
meat/o		-lysis	-uria	
nephr/o		-pathy		

1. disease of the kidney _____
2. forming (producing) stones _____
3. surgical repair of the renal pelvis _____
4. without (producing) urine _____
5. hardening of the glomerulus _____
6. process of examining the bladder _____
7. separation across (a membrane) _____
8. blood in the urine _____
9. (producing) much urine _____
10. dilation of the ureters _____
11. instrument to cut (enlarge) the meatus _____
12. nitrogenous compounds in the blood _____
13. hernia of the kidney _____
14. crushing of a stone _____
15. (x-ray) record of the bladder _____

Check your answers in Appendix A. Review any material that you did not answer correctly.

Correct Answers _____ X 6.67 = _____ % Score

Learning Activity 11-2
Building Medical Words

Use *nephr/o* (kidney) to build words that mean:

1. stone in the kidney _____
2. abnormal condition of pus in the kidney _____
3. abnormal condition of water in the kidney _____

Use *pyel/o* (renal pelvis) to build words that mean:

4. process of recording the renal pelvis _____
5. disease of the renal pelvis _____

Use *ureter/o* (ureter) to build words that mean:

6. dilation of a ureter _____
7. calculus in a ureter _____
8. pain in the ureters _____

Use *cyst/o* (bladder) to build words that mean:

9. inflammation of the bladder _____
10. instrument to view the bladder _____
11. paralysis of the bladder _____

Use *vesic/o* (bladder) to build words that mean:

12. herniation of the bladder _____
13. pertaining to the bladder and urethra _____

Use *urethr/o* (urethra) to build words that mean:

14. narrowing or stricture of the urethra _____
15. instrument used to incise the urethra _____

Use *ur/o* (urine, urinary tract) to build words that mean:

16. study of the urinary tract _____
17. disease of the urinary tract _____

Use the suffix *-uria* (urine) to build words that mean:

18. difficult or painful urination _____
19. scanty urination _____
20. pus in the urine _____

Build surgical words that mean:

21. surgical repair of the ureters _____

22. excision of the bladder _____

23. suture of the urethra _____

24. forming a mouth in the renal pelvis _____

25. fixation of the bladder _____

Check your answers in Appendix A. Review material that you did not answer correctly.

Correct Answers _____ X 4 = _____ % Score

Learning Activity 11-3

Pathology, Diseases, and Conditions

Match the following terms with the definitions in the numbered list.

anuria	fistula	nephrotic syndrome	pyuria
azotemia	hesitancy	neurogenic bladder	pyelonephritis
cystocele	hydronephrosis	nocturia	urgency
dysuria	hypercalcemia	oliguria	urolithiasis
enuresis	nephrolithiasis	polycystic	Wilms tumor

1. need to void immediately _____
2. abnormal passage from a hollow organ to the surface or between organs _____
3. painful urination, usually a burning sensation _____
4. absence of urine production _____
5. nitrogenous wastes in blood _____
6. dilation of kidneys and calices, usually due to reflux _____
7. presence of a stone in any part of the urinary tract _____
8. difficulty in starting urination _____
9. scanty urine production _____
10. inflammation of the kidney and renal pelvis _____
11. herniation of the bladder _____
12. involuntary discharge of urine _____
13. kidney disease characterized by presence of fluid-filled sacs _____
14. impairment of bladder control due to brain or nerve conduction _____
15. pus in urine _____
16. loss of plasma protein due to increased permeability of the glomerulus _____
17. excessive urination at night _____
18. excessive calcium in the blood _____
19. rapidly developing malignant neoplasm of the kidney _____
20. presence of stones in the kidneys _____

Check your answers in Appendix A. Review any material that you did not answer correctly.

Correct Answers _____ X 5 = _____ % Score

Learning Activity 11-4

Procedures, Pharmacology, and Abbreviations

Match the following terms with the definitions in the numbered list.

antibiotics	electromyography	potassium
C&S	ESWL	renal nuclear scan
cystography	hemodialysis	stent insertion
cystoscopy	nephropexy	UA
diuretics	peritoneal	ultrasonography

1. fixation of a floating kidney _____

2. measures the contraction of urinary muscles _____

3. visual examination of the urinary bladder _____

4. drugs that inhibit or kill bacterial microorganisms _____

5. laboratory test that identifies and evaluates the effect of an antibiotic on an organism _____

6. drugs used to promote the excretion of urine _____

7. placement of a narrow tube into the ureter to treat obstruction of urine flow _____

8. noninvasive procedure used to pulverize urinary or bile stones _____

9. dialysis of toxic substances by perfusing the abdominopelvic cavity _____

10. use of a tracer to produce images of the kidney _____

11. dialysis of toxic products by shunting blood from the body _____

12. radiology of bladder after introduction of a radiopaque medium _____

13. imaging that uses sound waves to provide images of the bladder _____

14. supplements used to treat or prevent the hypokalemia commonly associated with the use of diuretics _____

15. test that includes physical observation as well as chemical and microscopic evaluation of urine _____

Check your answers in Appendix A. Review material that you did not answer correctly.

Correct Answers _____ X 6.67 = _____ % Score

Learning Activity 11-5
Medical Scenarios

To construct chart notes, replace the italicized terms in each of the two scenarios with one of the medical terms listed below.

glomerulonephritis	*lithotripsy*	*proteinuria*
hematuria	*oliguria*	*pyuria*
hydronephrosis	*prognosis*	*ureterolithiasis*
hypertension		

Mr. J. complains of intense pain in the abdomen and the side of the back with fever and chills. Urinalysis reveals (1) ***blood in the urine***, uric acid crystals, and (2) ***pus in the urine***. Radiology examination shows (3) ***the presence of a stone in the ureter***. Because of its size, urine is unable to pass to the bladder, causing (4) ***distention of the ureter***. It appears unlikely that the stone will pass through his urinary system. Due to its size and location, an ultrasound procedure will be used to (5) ***crush the stone***.

1. _____
2. _____
3. _____
4. _____
5. _____

Mr. K. was diagnosed with strep throat. Although on antibiotics, the infection is still present. Mr. K. now presents with (6) ***diminished urine output***, (7) ***elevated blood pressure***, and (8) ***protein in the urine***. The physician explained that the toxins from the strep infection caused (9) ***inflammation of the glomerulus***, impairing kidney function. The doctor's (10) ***anticipated outcome of this disease*** is full recovery once the strep infection is addressed and resolved.

6. _____
7. _____
8. _____
9. _____
10. _____

✓ *Check your answers in Appendix A. Review any material that you did not answer correctly.*

Correct Answers _____ X 10 = _____ % Score

MEDICAL RECORD ACTIVITIES

The two medical records included in the following activities use common clinical scenarios to show how medical terminology is used to document patient care. Complete the terminology and analysis sections for each activity to help you recognize and understand terms related to the urinary system.

Medical Record Activity 11-1

Operative Report: Ureterocele and Ureterocele Calculus

Terminology

Terms listed in the following table are taken from *Operative Report: Ureterocele and Ureterocele Calculus* that follows. Use a medical dictionary such as *Taber's Cyclopedic Medical Dictionary;* the appendices of *Systems*, 7th ed.; or other resources to define each term. Then review the pronunciations for each term and practice by reading the medical record aloud.

Term	Definition
calculus KĂL-kū-lŭs	
cystolithotripsy sĭs-tō-LĬTH- ō-trĭp-sē	
cystoscope SĬST-ō-skōp	
fulguration fŭl-gŭ-RĀ-shŭn	
hematuria hē-mă-TŪ-rē-ă	
resectoscope rē-SĔK-tō-skōp	
transurethral trăns-ū-RĒ-thrăl	
ureterocele ū-RĒ-tĕr-ō-sēl	
urethral sound ū-RĒ-thrăl	

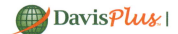

Visit the *Medical Terminology Systems* online resource center at Davis*Plus.* Use it to practice pronunciation and reinforce the meanings of the terms in this medical report.

OPERATIVE REPORT: URETEROCELE AND URETEROCELE CALCULUS

General Hospital

1511 Ninth Avenue ■■ **Sun City, USA 12345** ■■ **(555) 802-1887**

OPERATIVE REPORT

Date: May 14, 20xx   Physician: Elmer Augustino, MD
Patient: Motch, Edwin   Patient: ID#: 48778

PREOPERATIVE DIAGNOSIS: Hematuria with left ureterocele and ureterocele calculus.

POSTOPERATIVE DIAGNOSIS: Hematuria with left ureterocele and ureterocele calculus.

OPERATION: Cystoscopy, transurethral incision of ureterocele, extraction of stone, and cystolithotripsy.

ANESTHESIA: General.

COMPLICATIONS: None.

PROCEDURE: Patient was prepped and draped and placed in the lithotomy position. The urethra was calibrated with ease using a #26 French Van Buren urethral sound. A #24 resectoscope was inserted with ease. The prostate and bladder appeared normal, except for the presence of a left ureterocele, which was incised longitudinally; a large calculus was extracted from the ureterocele. There was minimal bleeding and no need for fulguration. The stone was crushed with the Storz stone-crushing instrument, and the fragments were evacuated. The bladder was emptied and the procedure terminated.

Patient tolerated the procedure well and was transferred to the postanesthesia care unit.

Elmer Augustino, MD
Elmer Augustino, MD

ea:bg

D: 5-14-20xx
T: 5-14-20xx

Analysis

Review the medical record *Operative Report: Ureterocele and Ureterocele Calculus* to answer the following questions.

1. What were the findings from the resectoscopy?

_____

_____

2. What was the name and size of the urethral sound used in the procedure?

_____

_____

3. What is the function of the urethral sound?

_____

_____

4. In what direction was the ureterocele incised?

_____

_____

5. Was fulguration required? Why or why not?

_____

_____

Operative Report: Extracorporeal Shock-Wave Lithotripsy

Terminology

Terms listed in the following table are taken from *Operative Report: Extracorporeal Shock-Wave Lithotripsy* that follows. Use a medical dictionary such as *Taber's Cyclopedic Medical Dictionary;* the appendices of *Systems*, 7th ed.; or other resources to define each term. Then review the pronunciations for each term and practice by reading the medical record aloud.

Term	Definition
calculus KĂL-kū-lŭs	
calyx KĀ-lĭx	
cystoscope SĬST-ō-skōp	
cystoscopy sĭs-TŎS-kō-pē	
dorsal lithotomy DOR-săl lĭth-ŎT-ō-mē	
ESWL	
extracorporeal ĕks-tră-kor-POR-ē-ăl	
fluoroscopy floo-or-ŎS-kō-pē	
lithotripsy LĬTH-ō-trĭp-sē	
shock-wave	
staghorn calculus STĂG-horn KĂL-kū-lŭs	
stent STĔNT	

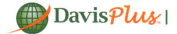

Visit the *Medical Terminology Systems* online resource center at Davis*Plus*. Use it to practice pronunciation and reinforce the meanings of the terms in this medical report.

OPERATIVE REPORT: EXTRACORPOREAL SHOCK-WAVE LITHOTRIPSY

General Hospital

1511 Ninth Avenue ■■ Sun City, USA 12345 ■■ (555) 802-1887

OPERATIVE REPORT

Date: April 1, 20xx   Physician: Elmer Augustino, MD
Patient: Marino, Julius   Room: 7201

PREOPERATIVE DIAGNOSIS: Left renal calculus.

POSTOPERATIVE DIAGNOSIS: Left renal calculus.

PROCEDURE: Extracorporeal shock-wave lithotripsy, cystoscopy with double-J stent removal

INDICATION FOR PROCEDURE: This 69-year-old male had undergone ESWL on 5/15/xx, with double-J stent placement to allow stone fragments to pass from the calyx to the bladder. At that time, approximately 50% of a partial staghorn calculus was fragmented. He now presents for the fragmenting of the remainder of the calculus and removal of the double-J stent.

ANESTHESIA: General.

COMPLICATIONS: None.

OPERATIVE TECHNIQUE: Patient was brought to the Lithotripsy Unit and placed in the supine position on the lithotripsy table. After induction of anesthesia, fluoroscopy was used to position the patient in the focal point of the shock waves. Being well positioned, he was given a total of 4,000 shocks with a maximum power setting of 3.0. After confirming complete fragmentation via fluoroscopy, the patient was transferred to the cystoscopy suite.

Patient was placed in the dorsal lithotomy position and draped and prepped in the usual manner. A cystoscope was inserted into the bladder through the urethra. Once the stent was visualized, it was grasped with the grasping forceps and removed as the scope was withdrawn.

Patient tolerated the procedure well and was transferred to recovery.

Elmer Augustino, MD
Elmer Augustino, MD

ea:bg

D: 5-14-20xx
T: 5-14-20xx

Analysis

Review the medical record *Operative Report: Extracorporeal Shock-Wave Lithotripsy* to answer the following questions.

1. What previous procedures were performed on the patient?

_____

_____

2. Why is this current procedure being performed?

_____

_____

3. What imaging technique was used for positioning the patient to ensure that the shock waves would strike the calculus?

_____

_____

4. In what position was the patient placed in the cystoscopy suite?

_____

_____

5. How was the double-J stent removed?

_____

_____

Female Reproductive System

Objectives

Upon completion of this chapter, you will be able to:

- Locate and describe the structures of the female reproductive system.
- Describe the functional relationship between the female reproductive system and other body systems.
- Pronounce, spell, and build words related to the female reproductive system.
- Describe diseases, conditions, and procedures related to the female reproductive system.
- Explain pharmacology related to the treatment of female reproductive disorders.
- Demonstrate your knowledge of this chapter by completing the learning and medical record activities.

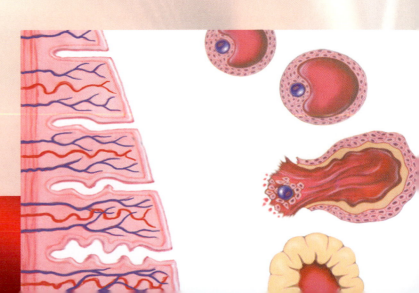

Anatomy and Physiology

The female reproductive system is designed to produce and transport ova (female sex cells), discharge ova from the body if fertilization does not occur, and nourish and provide a place for the developing fetus throughout pregnancy if fertilization occurs. The female reproductive system also produces the female sex hormones estrogen and progesterone, which play an important role in the reproductive process. These hormones are responsible for the development of secondary sex characteristics, such as breast development and regulation of the menstrual cycle.

Anatomy and Physiology Key Terms

This section introduces important female reproductive system terms and their definitions. Word analyses for selected terms are also provided.

Term	Definition
external genitalia jĕn-ĭ-TĀL-ē-ă	Sex, or reproductive, organs visible on the outside of the body; also called *genitals* *The external female genitalia are also called the* **vulva.** *Male genitalia include the penis, scrotum, and testicles.*
gestation jĕs-TĀ-shŭn *gest:* pregnancy *-ation:* process (of)	Length of time from conception to birth *The human gestational period typically extends approximately 280 days from the last menstrual period. Gestation (pregnancy) of less than 36 weeks is considered premature.*
lactation lăk-TĀ-shŭn *lact:* milk *-ation:* process (of)	Production and release of milk by mammary glands
orifice OR-ĭ-fĭs	Mouth; entrance, or outlet of any anatomical structure

Pronunciation Help — Long Sound: ā — rate, ē — rebirth, ī — isle, ō — over, ū — unite. Short Sound: ă — alone, ĕ — ever, ĭ — it, ŏ — not, ŭ — cut

Female Reproductive Structures

The female reproductive system is composed of internal organs of reproduction and the external genitalia. (See Figure 12-1.) The internal organs include the (1) **ovaries,** (2) **fallopian tubes,** (3) **uterus,** and (4) **vagina.** The **external genitalia** are collectively known as the **vulva.** Included in these structures are the (5) **labia minora,** (6) **labia majora,** (7) **clitoris,** (8) **Bartholin glands,** and **mons pubis,** an elevation of adipose tissue covered by skin and coarse pubic hair that cushions the **pubis (pubic bone).** The area between the vaginal orifice and the anus is known as the **perineum.**

Female Reproductive Organs

The female reproductive organs include the ovaries, fallopian tubes, uterus, and vagina. They are designed to produce female reproductive cells **(ova),** transport the cells to the site of fertilization, provide a favorable environment for a developing fetus through pregnancy and childbirth, and produce female sex hormones. Hormones play an important role in the reproductive process, providing their influence at critical times during preconception, fertilization, and gestation. (See Figure 12-2.)

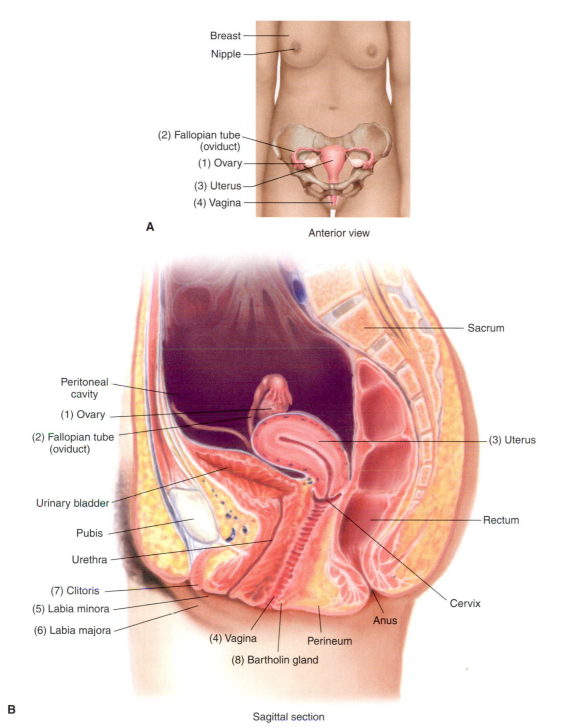

Breast

Nipple

(2) Fallopian tube
(oviduct)

(1) Ovary

(3) Uterus

(4) Vagina

A

Anterior view

Sacrum

Peritoneal
cavity

(1) Ovary

(2) Fallopian tube
(oviduct)

(3) Uterus

Urinary bladder

Rectum

Pubis

Urethra

(7) Clitoris

(5) Labia minora

(6) Labia majora

Cervix

Anus

(4) Vagina

Perineum

(8) Bartholin gland

B

Sagittal section

Figure 12-1 Female reproductive system. **(A)** Anterior view. **(B)** Lateral view showing the organs within the pelvic cavity.

Ovaries

The (1) **ovaries** are almond-shaped glands located in the pelvic cavity, one on each side of the uterus. Each ovary contains thousands of tiny, saclike structures called (2) **graafian follicles,** each containing an ovum. When an ovum ripens, the (3) **mature follicle** moves to the surface of the ovary, ruptures, and releases the ovum; this process is called **ovulation.** After ovulation, the empty follicle is transformed into a structure called the (4) **corpus luteum,** a small yellow mass that secretes estrogen and progesterone. The corpus luteum degenerates at the end of a nonfertile

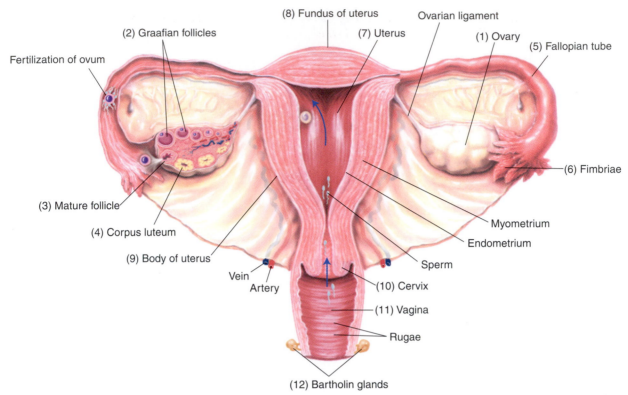

Figure 12-2 Anterior view of the female reproductive system with the developing follicles shown in the cross section of the right ovary.

cycle. Estrogen and progesterone influence the menstrual cycle and menopause. They also prepare the uterus for implantation of the fertilized egg, help maintain pregnancy, promote growth of the placenta, and play an important role in development of secondary sex characteristics. (See Chapter 14, Endocrine System.)

Fallopian Tubes

Two (5) **fallopian tubes (oviducts, uterine tubes)** extend laterally from superior angles of the uterus. The (6) **fimbriae** are fingerlike projections that create wavelike currents in fluid surrounding the ovary to move the ovum into the uterine tube. If the egg unites with a spermatozoon, the male reproductive cell, fertilization or conception takes place. The fertilized egg then continues its journey to the uterus where it implants on the uterine wall. If conception does not occur, the ovum disintegrates within 48 hours and is discharged through the vagina.

Uterus and Vagina

The (7) **uterus** contains and nourishes the embryo from the time the fertilized egg is implanted until the fetus is born. It is a muscular, hollow, inverted–pear-shaped structure located in the pelvic area between the bladder and rectum. The uterus is normally in a position of **anteflexion** (bent forward and consists of three parts: the (8) **fundus,** the upper, rounded part; the (9) **body,** the central part; and the (10) **cervix,** also called the **neck of the uterus** or **cervix uteri,** the inferior constricted portion that opens into the vagina.

The (11) **vagina** is a muscular tube that extends from the cervix to the exterior of the body. Its lining consists of folds of mucous membrane that give the organ an elastic quality. During sexual excitement, the vaginal **orifice** is lubricated by secretions from (12) **Bartholin glands.** In addition to serving as the organ of sexual intercourse and receptor of semen, the vagina discharges menstrual flow. It also acts as a passageway for the delivery of the fetus. The **clitoris,** located anterior to the vaginal orifice, is composed of erectile tissue that is richly innervated with sensory endings. The clitoris is similar in structure to the penis in the male, but is smaller and has no urethra.

The area between the vaginal orifice and the anus is known as the **perineum.** During childbirth, this area may be surgically incised **(episiotomy)** to enlarge the vaginal opening for delivery.

Mammary Glands

Although mammary glands (breasts) are present in both sexes, they function only in females. (See Figure 12-3.) The breasts are not directly involved in reproduction but become important after delivery. Their biological role is to secrete milk for the nourishment of the newborn, a process called lactation. Breasts begin to develop during puberty as a result of periodic stimulation of the

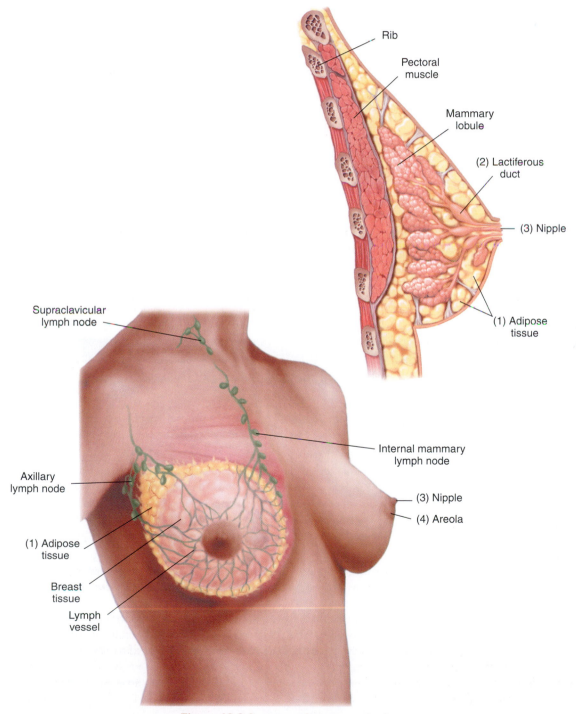

Figure 12-3 Structure of mammary glands.

ovarian hormones estrogen and progesterone and are fully developed by age 16. Estrogen is responsible for the development of (1) **adipose tissue,** which enlarges the size of the breasts until they reach full maturity. Breast size is primarily determined by the amount of fat around the glandular tissue but is not indicative of functional ability. Each breast is composed of 15 to 20 lobules of milk-producing glands that are drained by a (2) **lactiferous duct,** which opens on the tip of the raised (3) **nipple.** Circling the nipple is a border of slightly darker skin called the (4) **areola.** During pregnancy, the breasts enlarge and remain so until lactation ceases. At menopause, breast tissue begins to atrophy.

Menstrual Cycle

Menarche, the initial menstrual period, occurs at puberty (about age 12) and continues approximately 40 years, except during pregnancy. The menstrual cycle consists of a series of phases, during which the uterine endometrium changes as it responds to changing levels of ovarian hormones. (See Table 12-1.) The duration of the menstrual cycle is approximately 28 days. (See Figure 12-4.)

Pregnancy

During pregnancy, the uterus changes its shape, size, and consistency. It increases greatly in size and muscle mass; houses the growing placenta, which nourishes the embryo-fetus; and expels the fetus after gestation. To prepare and serve as the birth canal at the end of pregnancy, the vaginal canal elongates as the uterus rises in the pelvis. The mucosa thickens, secretions increase, and vascularity and elasticity of the cervix and vagina become more pronounced.

The average pregnancy **(gestation)** lasts approximately 9 months and is followed by childbirth **(parturition).** Up to the third month of pregnancy, the product of conception is referred to as the **embryo**. From the third month to the time of birth, the unborn offspring is referred to as the **fetus**.

Table 12-1	Phases of the Menstrual Cycle
	*The table below outlines the changes involved during the typical 28-day menstrual cycle.*
Phase	**Description**
Menstrual Days 1 to 5	Uterine endometrium sloughs off because of hormonal stimulation, a process accompanied by bleeding. The detached tissue and blood are discharged through the vagina as menstrual flow.
Ovulatory Days 6 to 14	When menstruation ceases, the endometrium begins to thicken as new tissue is rebuilt. As the estrogen level rises, several ova begin to mature in the graafian follicles, usually with only one ovum reaching full maturity. At about the 14th day of the cycle, the graafian follicle ruptures, releasing the egg, a process called *ovulation.* The egg then leaves the ovary and travels down the fallopian tube toward the uterus.
Postovulatory Days 15 to 28	The empty graafian follicle fills with a yellow material and is now called the *corpus luteum.* Secretions of estrogen and progesterone by the corpus luteum stimulate the building of the endometrium in preparation for implantation of an embryo. If fertilization does not occur, the corpus luteum begins to degenerate as estrogen and progesterone levels decrease.* With decreased hormone levels, the uterine lining begins to shed, the menstrual cycle starts over again, and the first day of menstruation begins.

*Some women experience a loose grouping of symptoms called **premenstrual syndrome (PMS).** These symptoms usually occur about 5 days after the decrease in hormone levels and include nervous tension, irritability, headaches, breast tenderness, and a feeling of depression.

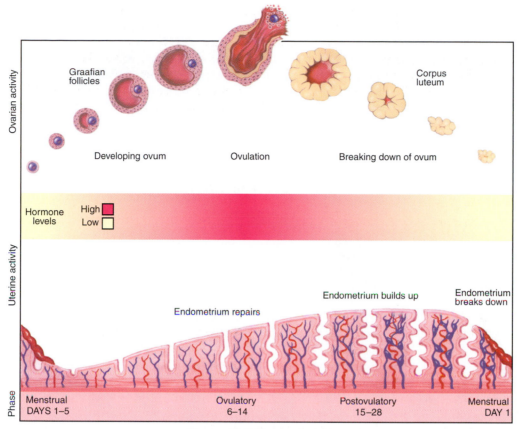

Figure 12-4 Menstrual cycle.

Pregnancy also causes enlargement of the breasts, sometimes to the point of pain. Many other changes occur throughout the body to accommodate the development and birth of the fetus. Toward the end of gestation, the myometrium begins to contract weakly at irregular intervals. At this time, the full-term fetus is usually positioned head down within the uterus.

Labor and Childbirth

Labor is the physiological process by which the fetus is expelled from the uterus. Labor occurs in three stages. The first is the **stage of dilation,** which begins with uterine contractions and terminates when there is complete dilation of the cervix (10 cm). The second is the **stage of expulsion,** the time from complete cervical dilation to birth of the baby. The last stage is the **placental stage,** or **afterbirth.** This stage begins shortly after childbirth when the uterine contractions discharge the placenta from the uterus. (See Figure 12-5.)

Menopause

Menopause is the cessation of ovarian activity and diminished hormone production that occurs at about age 50. Menopause is usually diagnosed if absence of menses (**amenorrhea)** has persisted for 1 year. The period in which symptoms of approaching menopause occur is also known as **change of life** or the **climacteric.**

Many women experience hot flashes and vaginal drying and thinning (**vaginal atrophy)** as estrogen levels fall. Although **hormone replacement therapy (HRT)** has become more controversial, it is still used to treat vaginal atrophy and porous bones (**osteoporosis),** and is believed to play a role in heart attack prevention. Restraint in prescribing estrogens for long periods in all menopausal women arises from concern that there is an increased risk that long-term usage will induce neoplastic changes in estrogen-sensitive aging tissue.

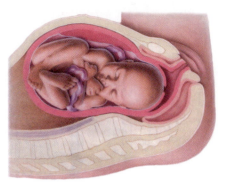

(1) Labor begins, membranes intact

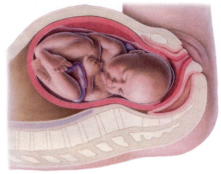

(2) Effacement of cervix,
which is now partially dilated

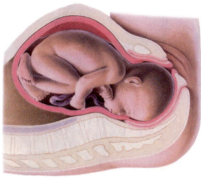

(3) When head reaches floor
of pelvis, it rotates

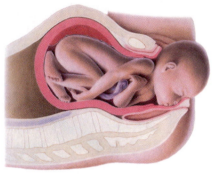

(4) Extension of the cervix allows head
to pass through

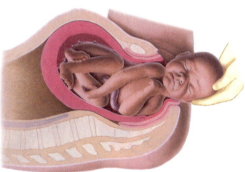

(5) Delivery of head, head rotates to
realign itself with body

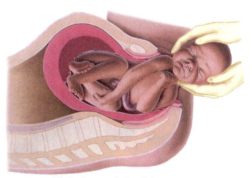

(6) Delivery of shoulders

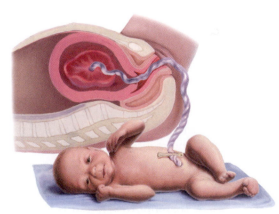

(7) Delivery of infant is complete,
uterus begins to contract

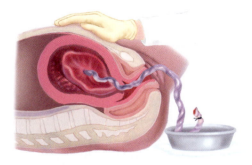

(8) Umbilical cord is cut, external massage
to uterus continues to stimulate
contractions, and placenta is delivered

Figure 12-5 Sequence of labor and childbirth.

Anatomy Review: Female Reproductive Structures (Lateral View)

To review the anatomy of the female reproductive system, label the illustration using the terms below.

Bartholin gland   *labia majora*   *perineum*

cervix   *labia minora*   *uterus*

clitoris   *ovary*   *vagina*

fallopian tube

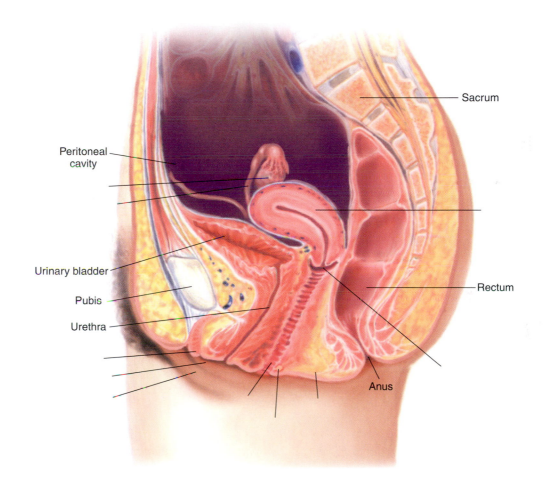

 Check your answers by referring to Figure 12–1 on page 387. Review material that you did not answer correctly.

Anatomy Review: Female Reproductive Structures (Anterior View)

To review the anatomy of the female reproductive system, label the illustration using the terms below.

Bartholin glands *fertilization of ovum* *ovarian ligament*

body of the uterus *fimbriae* *ovary*

cervix *fundus of uterus* *uterus*

corpus luteum *graafian follicles* *vagina*

fallopian tube *mature follicle*

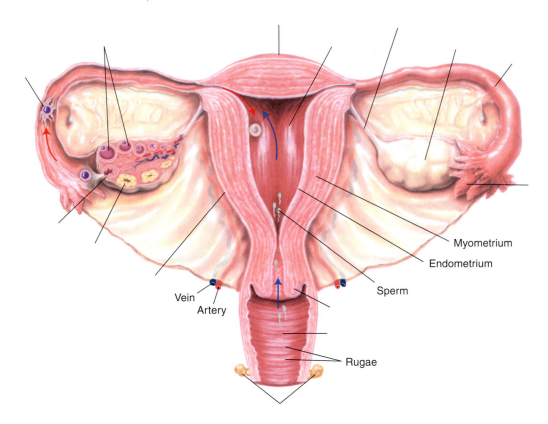

Myometrium

Endometrium

Vein

Artery

Sperm

Rugae

 Check your answers by referring to Figure 12-2 on page 388. Review material that you did not answer correctly.

CONNECTING BODY SYSTEMS—FEMALE REPRODUCTIVE SYSTEM

The main function of the female reproductive system is to produce hormones and to provide structures that support fertilization and development of a developing fetus. It also provides very limited support to the functions of other body systems. These limited functional relationships are summarized below.

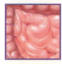

Blood, Lymph, and Immune
- Female immune system has special mechanisms that inhibit destruction of sperm cells.
- Female reproductive tract secretes enzymes and other substances that inhibit entry of pathogens into the internal reproductive structures.

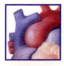

Cardiovascular
- Estrogens lower blood cholesterol levels and promote cardiovascular health in premenopausal women.

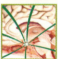

Digestive
- Estrogens have an effect on the metabolic rate.

Endocrine
- Estrogens provide a feedback mechanism, which influences pituitary function.
- Estrogens assist in the production of human chorionic gonadotropin (HCG) hormone.

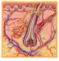

Integumentary
- Female hormones affect growth and distribution of body hair.
- Female hormones influence the activity of sebaceous glands.
- Female hormones influence skin texture and fat distribution.

Male Reproductive
- The female reproductive system provides the ovum needed to make fertilization by sperm possible.

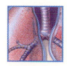

Musculoskeletal
- Estrogen influences muscle development and size.
- Estrogen influences bone growth, maintenance, and closure of epiphyseal plates.

Nervous
- Estrogen affects central nervous system development and sexual behavior.
- Estrogens provide antioxidants that have a neuroprotective function.

Respiratory
- Sexual arousal and pregnancy produce changes in rate and depth of breathing.
- Estrogen is believed to provide a beneficial effect on alveoli of the lungs.

Urinary
- Kidneys dispose of nitrogenous wastes and maintain homeostatic mechanisms of the mother and fetus.

Medical Word Elements

This section introduces combining forms, suffixes, and prefixes related to the female reproductive system. Word analyses are also provided.

Element	Meaning	Analysis
Combining Forms		
amni/o	amnion (amniotic sac)	**amni/o**/centesis (ăm-nē-ō-sĕn-TĒ-sĭs): surgical puncture of the amniotic sac *-centesis:* surgical puncture *Amniocentesis is a transabdominal puncture performed under ultrasound guidance using a needle and syringe to remove amniotic fluid.*

(continued)

Element	Meaning	Analysis
cervic/o	neck; cervix uteri (neck of uterus)	**cervic/**itis (sĕr-vĭ-SĪ-tĭs): inflammation of the cervix *-itis:* inflammation
colp/o	vagina	**colp/o/**scopy (kŏl-PŎS-kō-pē): visual examination of the vagina *-scopy:* visual examination
vagin/o		**vagin/o/**cele (VĂJ-ĭn-ō-sēl): vaginal hernia; also called *colpocele* *-cele:* hernia, swelling
galact/o	milk	**galact/o/**poiesis (gă-lăk-tō-poy-Ē-sĭs): production of milk *-poiesis:* formation, production
lact/o		**lact/o/**gen (LĂK-tō-jĕn): forming or producing milk *-gen:* forming, producing, origin *Lactogen refers to any substance that stimulates milk production, such as a hormone.*
gynec/o	woman, female	**gynec/o/**logist (gī-nĕ-KŎL-ō-jĭst): physician specializing in treating disorders of the female reproductive system *-logist:* specialist in the study of
hyster/o	uterus (womb)	**hyster/**ectomy (hĭs-tĕr-ĔK-tō-mē): excision of the uterus *-ectomy:* excision, removal
metri/o		endo/**metri/**al (ĕn-dō-MĒ-trē-ăl): pertaining to the lining of the uterus *endo-:* in, within *-al:* pertaining to
uter/o		**uter/o/**vagin/al (ū-tĕr-ō-VĂJ-ĭ-năl): relating to the uterus and vagina *vagin/o:* vagina *-al:* pertaining to
mamm/o	breast	**mamm/o/**gram (MĂM-ō-grăm): radiograph of the breast *-gram:* record, writing
mast/o		**mast/**o/pexy (MĂS-tō-pĕks-ē): surgical fixation of the breast(s) *-pexy:* fixation (of an organ) *Mastopexy is reconstructive, cosmetic surgery performed to affix sagging breasts in a more elevated position, commonly improving their shape.*
men/o	menses, menstruation	**men/o/**rrhagia (mĕn-ō-RĀ-jē-ă): bursting forth of the menses *-rrhagia:* bursting forth (of) *Menorrhagia is an excessive amount of menstrual flow over a longer duration than normal.*
metr/o	uterus (womb); measure	**metr/o/**ptosis (mē-trō-TŌ-sĭs): prolapse or downward displacement of the uterus *-ptosis:* prolapse, downward displacement

Element	Meaning	Analysis
nat/o	birth	pre/**nat**/al (prē-NĀ-tăl): pertaining to (the time period) before birth *pre-:* before, in front *-al:* pertaining to
oophor/o	ovary	**oophor**/oma (ō-ŏf-ō-RŌ-mă): ovarian tumor *-oma:* tumor
ovari/o		**ovari/o**/rrhexis (ō-vā-rē-ō-RĔK-sĭs): rupture of an ovary *-rrhexis:* rupture
perine/o	perineum	**perine/o**/rrhaphy (pĕr-ĭ-nē-OR-ă-fē): suture of the perineum *-rrhaphy:* suture *Perineorrhaphy is used to repair an episiotomy or a laceration that occurs during delivery of the fetus.*
salping/o	tube (usually fallopian or eustachian [auditory] tubes)	**salping/o**/plasty (săl-PĬNG-gō-plăs-tē): surgical repair of a fallopian tube *-plasty:* surgical repair

Suffixes		
-arche	beginning	men/**arche** (mĕn-ĂR-kē): beginning of menstruation *men:* menses, menstruation
-cyesis	pregnancy	pseudo/**cyesis** (soo-dō-sī-Ē-sĭs): false pregnancy *pseudo-:* false *Pseudocyesis, also called* **false pregnancy,** *is a condition in which a woman develops bodily changes consistent with pregnancy when she is not pregnant.*
-gravida	pregnant woman	multi/**gravida** (mŭl-tĭ-GRĂV-ĭ-dă): woman who has been pregnant more than once *multi-:* many, much *The term* gravida *may be followed by numbers, indicating the number of pregnancies, such as* gravida 1, gravida 2 *or* gravida I, gravida II, *and so forth.*
-para	to bear (offspring)	nulli/**para** (nŭl-ĬP-ă-ră): woman who has never produced a viable offspring *nulli-:* none *The term* para *followed by a Roman numeral or preceded by a Latin prefix (such as* primi-, quadri-, *and so forth) designates the number of times a pregnancy has culminated in a single or multiple birth. For example,* para I *and* primipara *refer to a woman who has given birth for the first time. Whether the births were multiple (twins, triplets) is irrelevant.*
-salpinx	tube (usually fallopian or eustachian [auditory] tubes)	hem/o/**salpinx** (hē-mō-SĂL-pĭnks): blood in a fallopian tube; also called *hematosalpinx* *hem/o:* blood

(continued)

Element	Meaning	Analysis
-tocia	childbirth, labor	dys/**tocia** (dĭs-TŌ-sē-ā): difficult childbirth *dys-:* bad; painful; difficult
-version	turning	retro/**version** (rĕt-rō-VĔR-shŭn): tipping or turning back (of an organ) *retro-:* backward, behind *Retroversion of the uterus occurs in one of every four otherwise healthy women.*

Prefixes

Element	Meaning	Analysis
ante-	before, in front of	**ante**/version (ăn-tē-VĔR-zhŭn): tipping or turning forward of an organ *-version:* turning
dys-	bad; painful; difficult	**dys**/men/o/rrhea (dĭs-mĕn-ō-RĒ-ă): painful menstruation *men/o:* menses, menstruation *-rrhea:* discharge, flow
endo-	in, within	**endo**/metr/itis (ĕn-dō-mē-TRĪ-tĭs): inflammation of (tissue) within the uterus *metr:* uterus (womb); measure *-itis:* inflammation
multi-	many, much	**multi**/para (mŭl-TĬP-ă-ră): woman who has delivered more than one viable infant regardless of whether the offspring was born alive *-para:* to bear (offspring)
post-	after	**post**/nat/al (pōst-NĀ-tăl): occurring after birth *nat:* birth *-al:* pertaining to
primi-	first	**primi**/gravida (prī-mĭ-GRĂV-ĭ-dă): woman during her first pregnancy *-gravida:* pregnant woman

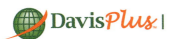 **DavisPlus** | Visit the *Medical Terminology Systems* online resource center at Davis*Plus* for an audio exercise of the terms in this table. Other activities are also available to reinforce content.

It is time to review medical word elements by completing Learning Activities 12–1 and 12–2.

Pathology

Female reproductive disorders may be caused by infection, injury, or hormonal dysfunction. Although some disorders may be mild and correct themselves over time, others, such as those caused by infection, may require medical attention. Pain, itching, lesions, and discharge are signs and symptoms commonly associated with sexually transmitted diseases and must not be ignored. Other common problems of the female reproductive system are related to hormonal dysfunction that may cause menstrual disorders.

As a preventive measure, a pelvic examination should be performed regularly throughout life. This diagnostic procedure helps identify many pelvic abnormalities and diseases. Cytological and bacteriological specimens are usually obtained at the time of examination.

Gynecology is the branch of medicine concerned with diseases of the female reproductive organs and breasts. **Obstetrics** is the branch of medicine that manages the health of a woman and her fetus during pregnancy and childbirth. It also includes the **puerperium,** which is the period of adjustment after childbirth during which the reproductive organs of the mother return to their normal nonpregnant state. Generally this period lasts six to eight weeks and ends with the first ovulation and the return of normal menstruation. Because of the obvious overlap between gynecology and obstetrics, many practices include both specialties. The physician who simultaneously practices these specialties is called an **obstetrician/gynecologist.**

Menstrual Disorders

Menstrual disorders are usually caused by hormonal dysfunction or pathological conditions of the uterus and may produce a variety of symptoms. Here are some common disorders:

- Menstrual pain and tension (**dysmenorrhea**) may be the result of uterine contractions, pathological growths, or such chronic disorders as anemia, fatigue, diabetes, and tuberculosis. The female hormone estrogen is used to treat dysmenorrhea and regulate menstrual abnormalities.
- Irregular uterine bleeding between menstrual periods (**metrorrhagia**) or after menopause is usually symptomatic of disease, including benign or malignant uterine tumors. Consequently, early diagnosis and treatment are warranted. Metrorrhagia is considered one of the most serious menstrual disorders.
- Profuse or prolonged bleeding during regular menstruation (**menorrhagia** or **hypermenorrhea**) may, during early life, be caused by endocrine disturbances. However, in later life, it is usually due to inflammatory diseases, fibroids, tumors, or emotional disturbances.
- **Premenstrual syndrome (PMS)** is a disorder with signs and symptoms that range from complaints of headache and fatigue to mood changes, anxiety, depression, uncontrolled crying spells, and water retention. Signs and symptoms involving almost every organ have been attributed to PMS. This syndrome occurs several days before the onset of menstruation and ends when menses begins or a short time after and appears to be related to hormonal changes. The reason most individuals with PMS seek medical assistance is related to mood change. Simple changes in behavior, such as an increase in exercise and a reduction in caffeine, salt, and alcohol use, may be beneficial.

Endometriosis

Endometriosis is the presence of functional endometrial tissue in areas outside the uterus. (See Figure 12-6.) The endometrial tissue develops into what are called **implants, lesions,** or **growths** and can cause pain, infertility, and other problems. The ectopic tissue is usually confined to the pelvic area but may appear anywhere in the abdominopelvic cavity. Like normal endometrial tissue, the ectopic endometrium responds to hormonal fluctuations of the menstrual cycle.

Pelvic and Vaginal Infections

Pelvic inflammatory disease (PID) is a general term for inflammation of the uterus, fallopian tubes, ovaries, and adjacent pelvic structures and is usually caused by bacterial infection. The infection may be confined to a single organ or it may involve all the internal reproductive organs. The disease-producing organisms (**pathogens**) generally enter through the vagina during coitus, induced abortion, childbirth, or the postpartum period. As an ascending infection, the pathogens spread from the vagina and cervix to the upper structures of the female reproductive tract. Two of the most common causes of PID are gonorrhea and chlamydial infection, which are sexually transmitted diseases (STDs). Unless treated promptly, PID may result in scarring of the narrow fallopian tubes and the ovaries, causing sterility. The widespread infection of reproductive structures can also lead to fatal **septicemia,** bacteria in the blood that often occurs with severe infections. Because regions of the uterine tubes have an internal diameter slightly larger than the width of a human hair, the scarring and closure of the tubes is one of the major causes of female infertility.

Vaginitis

The vagina is generally resistant to infection because of the acidity of vaginal secretions. Occasionally, localized infections and inflammations occur from viruses, bacteria, or yeast. If confined to the vagina, these infections are called **vaginitis.** Although symptoms may be numerous and

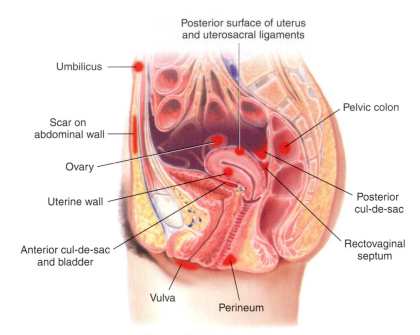

Figure 12-6 Endometriosis.

varied, the most common symptoms are genital itching, painful intercourse, and foul-smelling vaginal discharge. It is not uncommon for vaginitis to be accompanied by urethral inflammation **(urethritis)** because of the proximity of the urethra to the vagina. Two of the most common types of vaginitis are candidiasis and trichomoniasis.

Candidiasis, also called **moniliasis,** is caused by ***Candida albicans,*** a yeast that is present as part of the normal flora of the vagina. Steroid therapy, diabetes, or pregnancy may cause a change in the vaginal environment that disrupts the normal flora and promotes the overgrowth of this organism, resulting in a yeast **(fungal)** infection. The use of antibiotics may also disrupt the normal balance of microorganisms in the vagina by destroying "friendly bacteria," thus allowing the overpopulation of yeast. Antifungal agents **(mycostatics)** that suppress the growth of fungi are used to treat this disease.

Trichomoniasis, caused by the protozoan ***Trichomonas vaginalis,*** is now known to be one of the most common causes of sexually transmitted lower genital tract infections. Trichomoniasis is discussed more fully in the sexually transmitted disease section in Chapter 13, Male Reproductive System, page 440.

Oncology

The two most common forms of cancer (CA) involving the female reproductive system are breast cancer and cervical cancer.

Breast Cancer

Breast cancer, also called **carcinoma of the breast,** is the most common malignancy of women in the United States. This disease appears to be associated with ovarian hormonal function. In addition, a diet high in fats appears to increase the incidence of breast cancer. Other contributing factors include a family history of the disease and, possibly, the use of hormone replacement therapy (HRT). Women who have never borne children **(nulliparous)** or those who have had an early onset of menstruation **(menarche)** or late onset of menopause are also more likely to develop breast cancer. Because this type of malignancy is highly responsive to treatment when detected early, women are urged to practice breast self-examination monthly and to receive periodic mammograms after age 40. Many breast malignancies are detected by the patient.

Cervical Cancer

Cancer of the cervix most commonly affects women between ages 40 and 49. Statistics indicate that infection associated with sexual activity has some relationship to the incidence of cervical cancer. First coitus at a young age, a large number of sex partners, infection with certain sexually transmitted viruses, and frequent intercourse with men whose previous partners had cervical cancer are all associated with increased risk of developing cervical cancer.

The Pap test, a cytological examination, can detect cervical cancer before the disease becomes clinically evident. Abnormal cervical cytology routinely calls for colposcopy, which can detect the presence and extent of preclinical lesions requiring biopsy and histological examination. Treatment of cervical cancer consists of surgery, radiation, and chemotherapy. If left untreated, the cancer will eventually metastasize and lead to death.

Diseases and Conditions

This section introduces diseases and conditions of the female reproductive system along with their meanings and pronunciations. Word analyses for selected terms are also provided.

Term	Definition
Female Reproductive System	
atresia ă-TRĒ-zē-ă	Congenital absence or closure of a normal body opening, such as the vagina
choriocarcinoma kō-rē-ō-kăr-sĭ-NŌ-mă *chori/o:* chorion *carcin:* cancer *-oma:* tumor	Malignant neoplasm of the uterus or at the site of an ectopic pregnancy *Although its actual cause is unknown, choriocarcinoma is a rare tumor that may occur after pregnancy or abortion.*
dyspareunia dĭs-pă-RŪ-nē-ă	Occurrence of pain during sexual intercourse
endocervicitis ĕn-dō-sĕr-vĭ-SĪ-tĭs *endo-:* in, within *cervic:* neck; cervix uteri (neck of the uterus) *-itis:* inflammation	Inflammation of the mucous lining of the cervix uteri *Endocervicitis is usually chronic, commonly due to infection, and accompanied by cervical erosion.*
retroversion rĕt-rō-VĔR-shŭn *retro-:* backward, behind *-version:* turning	Turning or state of being turned back, especially an entire organ, such as the uterus, being tipped from its normal position
uterine fibroids Ū-tĕr-ĭn FĪ-broyds *fibr:* fiber, fibrous tissue *-oids:* resembling	Benign tumors composed of muscle and fibrous tissue that develop in the uterus; also called *leiomyomas, myomas,* or *fibroids* *Myomectomy or hysterectomy may be indicated if the fibroids grow too large, causing such symptoms as metrorrhagia, pelvic pain, and menorrhagia.*
sterility stĕr-ĬL-ĭ-tē	Inability of the female to become pregnant or the male to impregnate the female

(continued)

Term	Definition
Obstetrics	
abortion ă-BOR-shŭn	Termination of pregnancy before the embryo or fetus is capable of surviving outside the uterus
abruptio placentae ă-BRŬP-shē-ō plă-SĔN-tē	Premature separation of the placenta from the uterine wall before the third stage of labor; also called *placental abruption* *This condition results in uterine hemorrhage and threatens the life of the mother. It also disrupts blood flow and oxygen through the umbilical cord and threatens the life of the fetus.*
breech presentation	Common abnormality of delivery in which the fetal buttocks or feet present first rather than the head
Down syndrome DOWN SĬN-drōm	Genetic condition in which a person has 47 chromosomes instead of the usual 46 and occurs when there is an extra copy of chromosome 21 (trisomy), which causes delays in the way a child develops mentally and physically; also called *trisomy 21* *Symptoms vary from person to person and can range from mild to severe. However, children with Down syndrome have a widely recognized appearance. Down syndrome occurs in all human populations and is statistically more common with older parents due to increased mutagenic exposures on some older parents' reproductive cells.*
eclampsia ĕ-KLĂMP-sē-ă	Most serious form of toxemia during pregnancy *Signs of eclampsia include high blood pressure, edema, convulsions, renal dysfunction, proteinuria, and, in severe cases, coma.*
ectopic pregnancy ĕk-TŎP-ĭk PRĔG-năn-sē	Pregnancy in which the fertilized ovum does not reach the uterine cavity but becomes implanted on any tissue other than the lining of the uterine cavity, such as a fallopian tube, an ovary, the abdomen, or even the cervix uteri *Kinds of ectopic pregnancy include abdominal pregnancy, ovarian pregnancy, and tubal pregnancy. (See Figure 12-7.)*

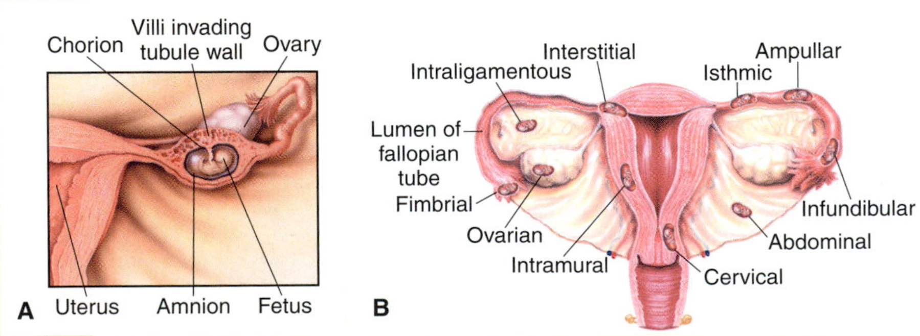

Figure 12-7 Tubal pregnancy **(A)** Other sites of ectopic pregnancy **(B)**.

Term	Definition
placenta previa plă-SĔN-tă PRĒ-vē-ă	Obstetric complication in which the placenta is attached close to or covers the cervical canal that results in bleeding during labor when the cervix dilates *Placenta previa is a leading cause of vaginal bleeding (spotting) that may lead to other complications. It may also necessitate a cesarean delivery.*

It is time to review pathology, diseases, and conditions by completing Learning Activity 12-3.

Medical, Surgical, and Diagnostic Procedures

This section introduces medical, surgical, and diagnostic procedures used to treat and diagnose female reproductive disorders. Descriptions are provided as well as pronunciations and word analyses for selected terms.

Procedure	Description
Medical	
intrauterine device (IUD) ĭn-tră-Ū-tĕr-ĭn	Small, T-shaped device inserted by a physician inside the uterus to prevent pregnancy *Two types of modern IUDs are available: a copper IUD, which releases copper particles to prevent pregnancy, and a hormonal IUD, which releases the hormone progestin to prevent pregnancy.*
Surgical	
cerclage sĕr-KLĂZH	Suturing of the cervix to prevent it from dilating prematurely during pregnancy, thus decreasing the chance of a spontaneous abortion *Cerclage is sometimes referred to as the* purse-string procedure. *The sutures are removed before delivery.*
cesarean section sē-SĀR-ē-ăn	Incision of the abdomen and uterus to remove the fetus; also called *C-section* *Cesarean section is most commonly used in the event of cephalopelvic disproportion, presence of sexually transmitted disease, fetal distress, and breech presentation.*
colpocleisis kŏl-pō-KLĪ-sĭs *colp/o:* vagina *-cleisis:* closure	Surgical closure of the vaginal canal
conization kŏn-ĭ-ZĀ-shŭn	Excision of a cone-shaped piece of tissue, such as mucosa of the cervix, for histological examination
cordocentesis kor-dō-sĕn-TĒ-sĭs	Sampling of fetal blood drawn from the umbilical vein and performed under ultrasound guidance *Cord blood is evaluated in the laboratory to identify hemolytic diseases or genetic abnormalities.*
cryosurgery krī-ō-SĔR-jĕr-ē	Process of freezing tissue to destroy cells; also called *cryocautery* *Cryosurgery is used for chronic cervical infections and erosions because offending organisms may be entrenched in cervical cells and glands. The process destroys these infected areas and, in the healing process, normal cells are replenished.*

(continued)

Procedure	Description
dilatation and curettage (D&C) dĭl-ă-TĀ-shŭn, kū-rĕ-TĂZH	Widening of the cervical canal with a dilator and scraping of the uterine endometrium with a curette *D&C is used to obtain a sample for cytological examination of tissue, control abnormal uterine bleeding, and treat incomplete abortion. (See Figure 12-8.)* 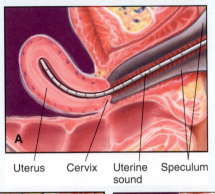 Uterus Cervix Uterine sound Speculum 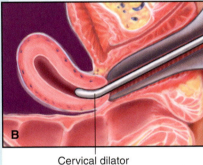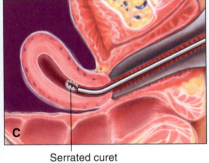 Cervical dilator Serrated curet **Figure 12-8** Dilatation and curettage. **(A)** Examination of the uterine cavity with a uterine sound. **(B)** Dilatation of the cervix with a series of cervical dilators. **(C)** Curettage (scraping) of the uterine lining with a serrated uterine curet.
hysterectomy hĭs-tĕr-ĔK-tō-mē *hyster:* uterus (womb) *-ectomy:* excision, removal	Excision of the uterus (See Figure 12-9.) *Indications for hysterectomy include abnormalities of the uterus and cervix (cancer, severe dysfunctional bleeding, large or bleeding fibroid tumors, prolapse of the uterus, or severe endometriosis). The approach to excision may be abdominal or vaginal.*
subtotal	Hysterectomy where the cervix, ovaries, and fallopian tubes remain
total	Hysterectomy where the cervix is removed but the ovaries and fallopian tubes remain; also called *complete hysterectomy*
total plus bilateral salpingo-oophorectomy bī-LĂT-ĕr-ăl săl-pĭng-gō-ō-ŏf-ō-RĔK-tō-mē	Total (complete) hysterectomy, including removal of the uterus, cervix, fallopian tubes, and ovaries

Procedure	Description

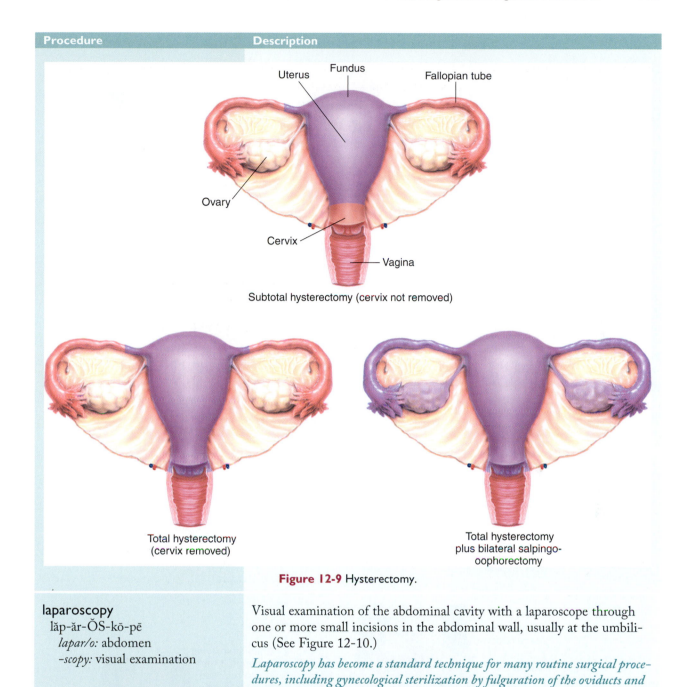

Uterus   Fundus   Fallopian tube

Ovary

Cervix

Vagina

Subtotal hysterectomy (cervix not removed)

Total hysterectomy
(cervix removed)

Total hysterectomy
plus bilateral salpingo-
oophorectomy

Figure 12-9 Hysterectomy.

laparoscopy
lăp-ăr-ŎS-kō-pē
lapar/o: abdomen
-scopy: visual examination

Visual examination of the abdominal cavity with a laparoscope through one or more small incisions in the abdominal wall, usually at the umbilicus (See Figure 12-10.)

Laparoscopy has become a standard technique for many routine surgical procedures, including gynecological sterilization by fulguration of the oviducts and tubal ligation.

(continued)

Procedure	Description

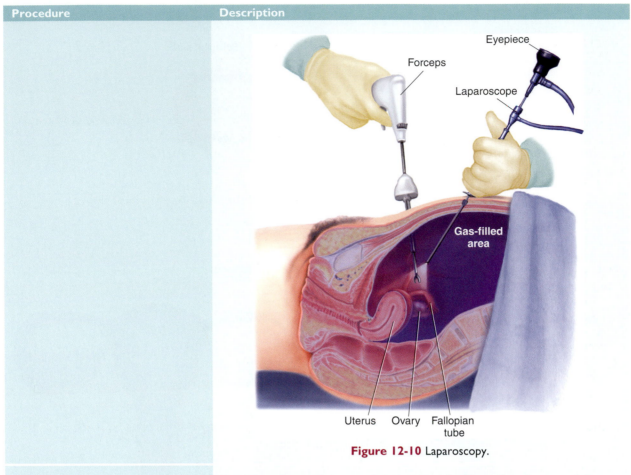

Figure 12-10 Laparoscopy.

lumpectomy
lŭm-PĔK-tō-mē

Excision of a small primary breast tumor (or "lump") and some of the normal tissue that surrounds it (See Figure 12-11.)

In lumpectomy, lymph nodes may also be removed because they are located within the breast tissue taken during surgery. Typically, the patient will undergo radiation therapy after lumpectomy.

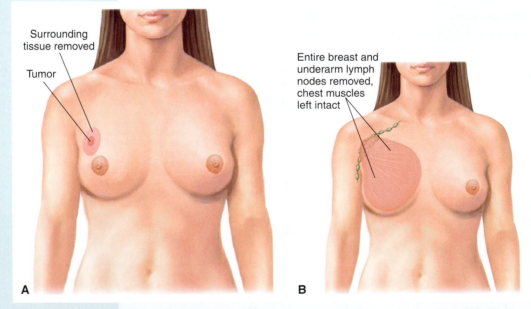

Figure 12-11 Lumpectomy and mastectomy. **(A)** Lumpectomy with the primary tumor in red and the surrounding tissue removed in pink. **(B)** Modified radical mastectomy.

Procedure	Description
mammoplasty MĂM-ō-plăs-tē *mamm/o:* breast *-plasty:* surgical repair	Surgical reconstruction of the breast(s) to change the size, shape, or position
augmentation	Insertion of a breast prosthesis (filled with silicone gel or saline) beneath the skin or beneath the pectoralis major muscle *Augmentation surgery is performed to increase breast size or replace one that has been surgically removed.*
reduction	Breast reduction to reduce the size of a large, pendulous breast *Breast reduction may be performed in conjunction with mastopexy, a surgery to uplift a sagging breast.*
mastectomy măs-TĔK-tō-mē *mast:* breast *-ectomy:* excision, removal	Excision of the entire breast
total (simple)	Excision of the entire breast, nipple, areola, and the involved overlying skin; also called *simple mastectomy* *In total mastectomy, lymph nodes are removed only if they are included in the breast tissue being removed.*
modified radical	Excision of the entire breast, including the lymph nodes in the underarm (axillary dissection) (See Figure 12-11B.) *Most women who have mastectomies today have modified radical mastectomies.*
radical	Excision of the entire breast, all underarm lymph nodes, and chest wall muscles under the breast
reconstructive breast surgery	Creation of a breast-shaped mound to replace a breast that has been removed due to cancer or other disease *Reconstruction is commonly possible immediately following mastectomy so the patient awakes from anesthesia with a breast mound already in place.*
tissue (skin) expansion	Common breast reconstruction technique in which a balloon expander is inserted beneath the skin and chest muscle, saline solution is gradually injected to increase size, and the expander is then replaced with a more permanent implant (See Figure 12-12.)

(continued)

Procedure	Description

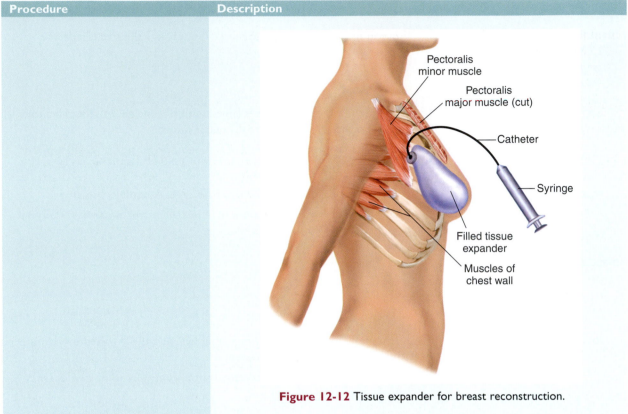

Figure 12-12 Tissue expander for breast reconstruction.

transverse rectus abdominis muscle (TRAM) flap

Surgical creation of a skin flap using skin and fat from the lower half of the abdomen, which is passed under the skin to the breast area, and then shaping the abdominal tissue (flap) into a natural-looking breast and suturing it into place (See Figure 12-13.)

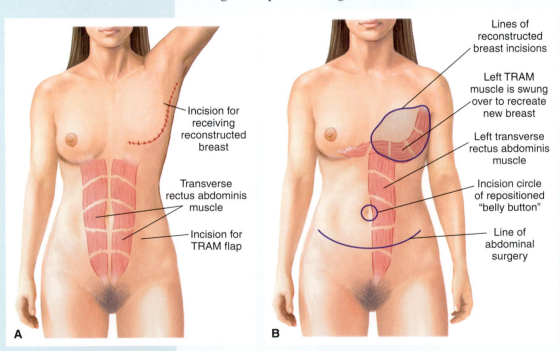

Figure 12-13 TRAM flap. **(A)** After mastectomy. **(B)** Process of TRAM reconstruction.

Procedure	Description
tubal ligation TŪ-băl lī-GĀ-shŭn	Procedure that ties (ligates) the fallopian tubes to prevent pregnancy *Tubal ligation is a form of sterilization surgery usually performed during laparoscopy.*

Diagnostic

Clinical

amniocentesis ăm-nē-ō-sĕn-TĒ-sĭs *amni/o:* amnion (amniotic sac) *-centesis:* surgical puncture	Transabdominal puncture of the amniotic sac under ultrasound guidance using a needle (position is verified by US on a monitor screen) and syringe to remove amniotic fluid (See Figure 12-14.) *The sample obtained in amniocentesis is chemically and cytologically studied to detect genetic and biochemical disorders and fetal maturity. The procedure also enables transfusion of blood to the fetus and instillation of drugs for treating the fetus.* **Figure 12-14** Amniocentesis.
colposcopy kŏl-PŎS-kō-pē *colp/o:* vagina *-scopy:* visual examination	Visual examination of the vagina and cervix with an optical magnifying instrument (colposcope) *Colposcopy is used chiefly to identify areas of cervical dysplasia in women with abnormal Papanicolaou tests and as an aid in biopsy or excision procedures, including cautery, cryotherapy, and loop electrosurgical excision.*
insufflation ĭn-sŭ-FLĀ-shŭn	Delivery of pressurized air or gas into a cavity, chamber, or organ to allow visual examination, remove an obstruction, or apply medication *Insufflation is performed to increase the distance between structures so the physician can see more clearly and better diagnose possible disorders.*
tubal TŪ-băl	Test for patency of the uterine tubes made by transuterine insufflation with carbon dioxide; also called *Rubin test*
pelvimetry pĕl-VĬM-ĕ-trē *pelv/i:* pelvis *-metry:* act of measuring	Measurement of pelvic dimensions to determine whether the head of the fetus will be able to pass through the bony pelvis to allow delivery *Pelvimetry is usually performed manually, by x-ray, or by ultrasound, depending on the stage of the pregnancy. The size of the pelvic outlet determines whether or not the baby is delivered vaginally or by cesarean section.*

(continued)

Procedure	Description
Laboratory	
chorionic villus sampling (CVS) kor-ē-ŎN-ĭk VĬL-ŭs SĂM-plĭng	Sampling of placental tissues for prenatal diagnosis of potential genetic defects *CVS involves insertion of a catheter into the uterus to obtain the sample. The advantage of CVS over amniocentesis is that it can be undertaken in the first trimester of pregnancy.*
endometrial biopsy ĕn-dō-MĒ-trē-ăl BĪ-ŏp-sē *endo-:* in, within *metri:* uterus (womb); measure *-al:* pertaining to	Removal of a sample of uterine endometrium for microscopic study *Endometrial biopsy is commonly used in fertility assessment to confirm ovulation and as a diagnostic tool to determine the cause of dysfunctional and postmenopausal bleeding.*
Papanicolaou (Pap) test pă-pă-NĪ-kō-lŏw	Cytological study used to detect abnormal cells sloughed from the cervix and vagina, usually obtained during routine pelvic examination (See Figure 12-15.) *A Pap test is commonly used to screen for and diagnose cervical cancer. It may also be used to evaluate cells from any organ, such as the pleura and peritoneum, to detect changes that indicate malignancy.*

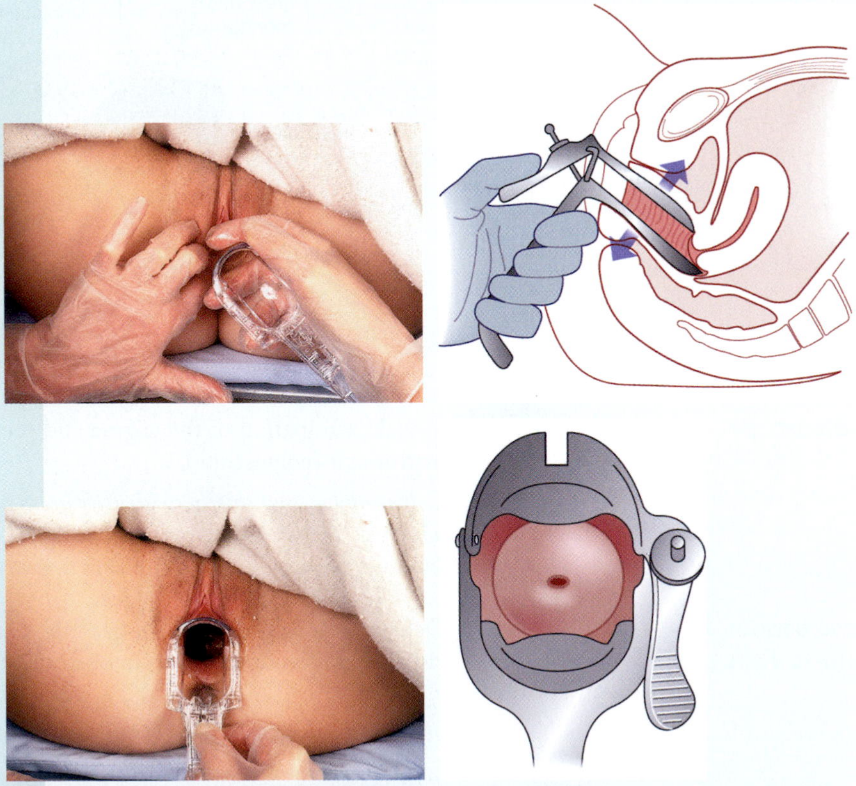

Figure 12-15 Pelvic examination with Papanicolaou (Pap) test. From Dillon: *Nursing Health Assessment,* 2nd ed. FA Davis, Philadelphia, 2007, pp 634-635, with permission.

Procedure	Description
Imaging	
hysterosalpingography (HSG) hĭs-tĕr-ō-săl-pĭn-GŎG-ră-fē *hyster/o:* uterus (womb) *salping/o:* tube (usually fallopian or eustachian [auditory] tube) *-graphy:* process of recording	Radiography and, usually, fluoroscopy of the uterus and uterine tubes (oviducts) following injection of a contrast medium *Hysterosalpingography is used to determine pathology in the uterine cavity, evaluate tubal patency, and determine the cause of infertility.*
mammography măm-ŎG-ră-fē *mamm/o:* breast *-graphy:* process of recording	Radiographic examination of the breast to screen for breast cancer *Mammography is used to detect tumors, cysts, and microcalcifications and may help locate a malignant lesion.*
ultrasonography (US) ŭl-tră-sŏn-ŎG-ră-fē *ultra-:* excess, beyond *son/o:* sound *-graphy:* process of recording	Use of high-frequency sound waves (ultrasound) directed at soft tissue and reflected as "echoes" to produce an image on a monitor of an internal body structure; also called *ultrasound, sonography,* and *echo* *A computer analyzes the reflected echoes and converts them into an image on a computer screen. Because US does not use ionizing radiation (x-ray), it is used to visualize the developing fetus during pregnancy, identify breast and uterine tumors, and perform amniocentesis.*

transvaginal
    trănz-VĂJ-ĭ-năl
    trans-: through, across
    vagin: vagina
    -al: pertaining to
	US of the pelvic area performed with a probe inserted into the vagina, which provides sharper images of pathological and normal structures within the pelvis

Pharmacology

Hormone replacement therapy (HRT) is the use of synthetic or natural estrogens or a combination of estrogen and progestin to replace the decline or lack of natural hormones, a condition that accompanies hysterectomy and menopause. (See Table 12-2.) Estrogen may be administered orally, transdermally, by injection, or as a topical cream (to treat vaginal symptoms only). Other hormones, including oxytocics and prostaglandins, are used for obstetrical applications. In addition, pharmacological agents are available for birth control and family planning. These include oral contraceptives, implants, and spermicides.

Table 12-2	**Drugs Used to Treat Obstetrical and Gynecological Disorders**	
Classification	**Therapeutic Action**	**Generic and *Trade* Names**
antifungals ăn-tĭ-FŬNG-găls	Treat vaginal yeast infection by altering the yeast cell membrane or interfering with a metabolic process *Most antifungals used to treat vaginal yeast infections are applied topically as ointments, suppositories, or vaginal tablets.*	**miconazole** mī-KŎN-ă-zōl *Monistat* **nystatin** NĬS-tă-tĭn *Mycostatin, Nilstat*
estrogens ĔS-trō-jĕns	Treat symptoms of menopause (hot flashes, vaginal dryness, fatigue) through hormone replacement therapy (HRT) *Long-term use of estrogen has been linked with an increased risk of thrombophlebitis and breast and endometrial cancers.*	**conjugated estrogens** KŎN-jū-gā-tĕd ĔS-trō-jĕnz *Cenestin, Premarin*
oral contraceptives kŏn-tră-SĔP-tĭvs	Synthetic hormones used to prevent pregnancy and treat menstrual disorders *Oral contraceptives, or birth control pills, contain a combination of estrogen and progestin and are highly effective in preventing pregnancy if taken as directed.*	**desogestrel/ethinyl estradiol** dĕz-ō-JĔS-trăl, ĔTH-ĭ-nĭl ĕs-tră-DĪ-ŏl *Desogen, Ortho-Cept* **ethinyl estradiol/norgestrel** ĔTH-ĭ-nĭl ĕs-tră-DĪ-ŏl, nor-JĔS-trĕl *Lo/Ovral-28*
oxytocics ŏk-sē-TŌ-sĭks	Induce labor at term by increasing the strength and frequency of uterine contractions *Oxytocics are also used during the postpartum period to control bleeding after the expulsion of the placenta.*	**oxytocin** ŏk-sē-TŌ-sĭn *Pitocin*
prostaglandins PRŎS-tă-glănd-ĭns	Terminate pregnancy *Large doses of certain prostaglandins can cause the uterus to contract strongly enough to spontaneously abort a fetus.*	**dinoprostone** dī-nō-PRŎS-tōn *Prostin E2, Cervidil* **mifepristone** mī-fĕ-PRĬS-tōn *Mifeprex*
spermicides SPĔR-mĭ-sīds	Chemically destroy sperm by creating a highly acidic environment in the uterus *Spermicides are available in foam, jelly, gel, and suppositories. They are used within the female vagina for contraception. Spermicides have a higher failure rate than other methods of birth control.*	**nonoxynol 9, octoxynol 9** nŏn-ŎK-sĭ-nŏl, ŏk-TŎKS-ĭ-nŏl *Semicid, Koromex, Ortho-Gynol*

Abbreviations

This section introduces female reproductive-related abbreviations and their meanings.

Abbreviation	Meaning	Abbreviation	Meaning
Gynecologic			
AB; Ab, ab	antibody; abortion	**LMP**	last menstrual period
CA	cancer; chronological age; cardiac arrest	**LSO**	left salpingo-oophorectomy
D&C	dilatation (dilation) and curettage	**OCPs**	oral contraceptive pills
DUB	dysfunctional uterine bleeding	**Pap**	Papanicolaou (test)
FSH	follicle-stimulating hormone	**PID**	pelvic inflammatory disease
GYN	gynecology	**STD**	sexually transmitted disease
HRT	hormone replacement therapy	**TRAM**	transverse rectus abdominis muscle (flap)
HSG	hysterosalpingography	**TVH**	total vaginal hysterectomy
IUD	intrauterine device	**US**	ultrasound, ultrasonography
LH	luteinizing hormone		
Fetal-Obstetrical			
CS, C-section	cesarean section	**IVF-ET**	in vitro fertilization and embryo transfer
CVS	chorionic villus sampling	**OB**	obstetrics
FECG, FEKG	fetal electrocardiogram	**para 1, 2, 3 and so on**	unipara, bipara, tripara (number of viable births)

It is time to review procedures, pharmacology, and abbreviations by completing Learning Activity 12–4.

LEARNING ACTIVITIES

The following activities provide review of the female reproductive system terms introduced in this chapter. Complete each activity and review your answers to evaluate your understanding of the chapter.

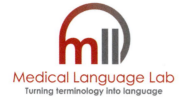

Medical Language Lab
Turning terminology into language

Visit the Medical Language Lab at the web site: medicallanguagelab.com. Use it to enhance your study and reinforcement of this chapter with the flash-card activity. We recommend you complete the flash-card activity before starting Learning Activities 12-1 and 12-2 below.

Learning Activity 12-1
Combining Forms, Suffixes, and Prefixes

Use the elements listed in the table to build medical words. You may use the elements more than once.

Combining Forms		Suffixes		Prefixes
amni/o	men/o	-al	-plasty	dys-
cervic/o	nat/o	-arche	-poiesis	multi-
colp/o	oophor/o	-centesis	-rrhaphy	pre-
galact/o	perine/o	-cyesis	-rrhexis	primi-
hem/o	salping/o	-gravida	-salpinx	pseudo-
hyster/o		-itis	-scopy	
		-oma	-tocia	
		-para		

1. visual examination of the vagina _____
2. pertaining to (the time) before birth _____
3. difficult childbirth _____
4. rupture of the uterus _____
5. tumor of the ovary _____
6. inflammation of the cervix uteri (neck of the uterus) _____
7. surgical puncture of the amnion (amniotic sac) _____
8. suture of the perineum _____
9. surgical repair of a fallopian tube _____
10. pregnant woman (for the) first (time) _____
11. false pregnancy _____
12. blood in a fallopian tube _____
13. to bear many (offspring) _____
14. beginning of menses or menstruation _____
15. formation or production of milk _____

✔ *Check your answers in Appendix A. Review any material that you did not answer correctly.*

Correct Answers _____ X 6.67 = _____ % Score

Learning Activity 12-2
Building Medical Words

Use *gynec/o* (woman, female) to build words that mean:

1. disease (specific to) women _____
2. physician who specializes in diseases of the female _____

Use *cervic/o* (neck; cervix uteri) to build words that mean:

3. inflammation of the cervix uteri and vagina _____
4. pertaining to the cervix uteri and bladder _____

Use *colp/o* (vagina) to build words that mean:

5. instrument used to examine the vagina _____
6. visual examination of the vagina _____

Use *vagin/o* (vagina) to build words that mean:

7. inflammation of the vagina _____
8. herniation of the vagina _____

Use *hyster/o* (uterus) to build words that mean:

9. myoma of the uterus _____
10. disease of the uterus _____
11. radiography of the uterus and oviducts _____

Use *metr/o* (uterus) to build words that mean:

12. hemorrhage from the uterus _____
13. inflammation around the uterus _____

Use *uter/o* (uterus) to build words that mean:

14. herniation of the uterus _____
15. relating to the uterus and cervix _____
16. pertaining to the uterus and bladder _____

Use *oophor/o* (ovary) to build words that mean:

17. inflammation of an ovary _____
18. inflammation of an ovary and oviduct _____

Use *salping/o* (fallopian tube) to build words that mean:

19. herniation of a fallopian tube _____
20. radiography of uterine tubes _____

Build surgical words that mean:

21. fixation of (a displaced) ovary _____

22. excision of the uterus and ovaries _____

23. suturing the perineum _____

24. excision of the uterus, oviducts, and ovaries _____

25. puncture of the amnion (amniotic sac) _____

Check your answers in Appendix A. Review material that you did not answer correctly.

Correct Answers _____ X 4 = _____ % Score

Pathology, Diseases, and Conditions

Match the following terms with the definitions in the numbered list.

atresia	dystocia	metrorrhagia	pyosalpinx
breech	eclampsia	oligomenorrhea	retroversion
choriocarcinoma	fibroids	pathogen	sterility
Down syndrome	gestation	primigravida	septicemia
dyspareunia	menarche	primipara	trichomoniasis

1. accumulation of pus in a uterine tube _____

2. woman who has had one pregnancy that has resulted in a viable offspring _____

3. average pregnancy; approximately 9 months _____

4. inability of the female to become pregnant _____

5. uterus that is tipped backward from its normal position _____

6. type of vaginitis that is a common cause of sexually transmitted lower genital
   tract infections _____

7. difficult labor or childbirth _____

8. congenital absence of a normal body opening, such as the vagina _____

9. trisomy 21 _____

10. bacteria in the blood that often occurs with severe infection _____

11. occurrence of pain during sexual intercourse _____

12. irregular uterine bleeding between menstrual periods _____

13. beginning of menstrual function _____

14. benign uterine tumor composed of muscle and fibrous tissue _____

15. infrequent menstrual flow _____

16. abnormal delivery in which fetal buttocks or feet present first rather than the head _____

17. most serious form of toxemia during pregnancy _____

18. malignant neoplasm of the uterus or at the site of an ectopic pregnancy _____

19. disease-producing organism _____

20. woman during her first pregnancy _____

 Check your answers in Appendix A. Review material that you did not answer correctly.

Correct Answers _____ X 5 = _____ % Score

Learning Activity 12-4

Procedures, Pharmacology, and Abbreviations

Match the following terms with the definitions in the numbered list.

amniocentesis	cryocautery	IUD	Pap test
antifungals	D&C	laparoscopy	PID
chorionic villus sampling	episiotomy	lumpectomy	prostaglandins
colpocleisis	estrogens	OCPs	TAH
cordocentesis	hysterosalpingography	oxytocins	tubal ligation

1. cytological study of tissue to detect cancer cells _____

2. radiography of the uterus and oviducts after injection of a contrast medium _____

3. puncture of the amniotic sac to remove amniotic fluid for biochemical and cytological study _____

4. drugs used to treat vaginal yeast infections _____

5. surgical closure of the vaginal canal _____

6. procedure that widens the cervical canal with a dilator and scrapes the uterine endometrium with a curet _____

7. excision of the uterus, including the cervix, through an abdominal incision _____

8. tying uterine tubes to prevent pregnancy _____

9. birth control pills taken orally _____

10. examination of the abdominal cavity using an endoscope _____

11. incision of the perineum to facilitate childbirth _____

12. inflammation of the uterus, fallopian tubes, ovaries, and adjacent pelvic structures, usually caused by bacterial infection _____

13. test to detect chromosomal abnormalities that can be done earlier than amniocentesis _____

14. hormone replacement to reduce adverse symptoms of menopause _____

15. agents used to induce labor and rid the uterus of an unexpelled placenta or a fetus that has died _____

16. freezing tissue to destroy cells _____

17. birth control method in which an object is placed inside the uterus to prevent pregnancy _____

18. sampling of fetal blood drawn from the umbilical vein _____

19. excision of a small primary breast tumor _____

20. agents used to terminate pregnancy _____

✓ *Check your answers in Appendix A. Review any material that you did not answer correctly.*

Correct Answers _____ X 5 = _____ % Score

Learning Activity 12-5

Medical Scenarios

To construct chart notes, replace the italicized terms in each of the two scenarios with one of the medical terms listed below.

dysmenorrhea	menopause	needle biopsy
gravida 3, para 3	menorrhagia	nullipara
mammography	metrorrhagia	uterine fibroids
menarche		

Ms. T. is a 32-year-old female who presents at our office with complaints of bleeding. Her past reproductive history includes (1) ***3 pregnancies resulting in 3 live births***. She is now experiencing (2) ***mid-cycle bleeding*** and complains of (3) ***excessively heavy periods***, commonly with blood clots. The patient further complains of (4) ***severe cramps, headache, and tension*** during her period. She is scheduled for a complete pelvic examination and a transvaginal ultrasound to establish the diagnosis of (5) ***benign tumors of the uterus***.

1. _____
2. _____
3. _____
4. _____
5. _____

Mrs. D. presents with a complaint of a small lump in her right breast and is concerned that this may be cancer. Her mother and sister are both cancer survivors. Besides a family history of the disease, she has several risk factors including (6) ***never giving birth*** and early (7) ***onset of menstruation***. She admits that she went through (8) ***change of life*** three years ago at age 53. She is scheduled for (9) ***breast x-ray*** and (10) ***an examination of a small piece of tissue obtained using a needle***, which will be performed under ultrasound guidance.

6. _____
7. _____
8. _____
9. _____
10. _____

✔ *Check your answers in Appendix A. Review any material that you did not answer correctly.*

Correct Answers _____ X 10 = _____ % Score

MEDICAL RECORD ACTIVITIES

The two medical records included in the following activities use common clinical scenarios to show how medical terminology is used to document patient care. Complete the terminology and analysis sections for each activity to help you recognize and understand terms related to the female reproductive system.

Medical Record Activity 12-1
SOAP Note: Primary Herpes 1 Infection

Terminology

Terms listed in the following table are taken from *SOAP Note: Primary Herpes 1 Infection* that follows. Use a medical dictionary such as *Taber's Cyclopedic Medical Dictionary;* the appendices of *Systems,* 7th ed.; or other resources to define each term. Then review the pronunciations for each term and practice by reading the medical record aloud.

Term	Definition
adenopathy ăd-ĕ-NŎP-ă-thē	
chlamydia klă-MĬD-ē-ă	
GC screen	
herpes lesions HĔR-pēz LĒ-zhŭnz	
introitus ĭn-TRŌ-ĭ-tŭs	
labia LĀ-bē-ă	
LMP	
monilial mō-NĬL-ē-ăl	
OCPs	

Term	Definition
pruritus proo-RĪ-tŭs	
R/O	
vulvar VŬL-văr	
Wet prep WĔT PRĔP	

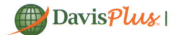 Visit the *Medical Terminology Systems* online resource center at Davis*Plus*. Use it to practice pronunciation and reinforce the meanings of the terms in this medical report.

SOAP NOTE: PRIMARY HERPES I INFECTION

PROGRESS NOTES

O'Malley, Roberta
09/01/xx

S: This 24-year-old patient started having some sore areas around the labia, both rt and lt side. She stated that the last few days she started having a brownish discharge. She has pruritus and pain of her vulvar area with adenopathy, p.m. fever, and blisters. Apparently, her partner had a cold sore and they had oral-genital sex. Patient has been using condoms since last seen in April. She has not missed any OCPs. LMP 5/15/xx.

O: Patient has what looks like herpes lesions and ulcers all over vulva and introitus area. Rt labia appears as an ulcerlike lesion; it appears to be almost like an infected follicle. Speculum inserted, a brown discharge noted. GC screen, chlamydia screen, and genital culture obtained from that. Wet prep revealed monilial forms. Viral culture obtained from the ulcerlike lesion on the right labia.

A: Primary herpes 1 infection; will rule out other infectious etiologies.

P: Patient advised to return next week for consultation with Dr. Abdu.

Joanna Masters, MD
Joanna Masters, MD

JM:st

Analysis

Review the medical record *SOAP Note: Primary Herpes 1 Infection* to answer the following questions.

1. Did the patient have any discharge? If so, describe it.

_____

2. What type of discomfort did the patient experience around the vulvar area?

_____

3. Has the patient been taking her oral contraceptive pills regularly?

_____

4. Where was the viral culture obtained?

_____

5. Even though the patient's partner used a condom, how do you think the patient became infected with herpes?

_____

Preoperative Consultation: Menometrorrhagia

Terminology

Terms listed in the following table are taken from *Preoperative Consultation: Menometrorrhagia* that follows. Use a medical dictionary such as *Taber's Cyclopedic Medical Dictionary;* the appendices of *Systems,* 7th ed.; or other resources to define each term. Then review the pronunciations for each term and practice by reading the medical record aloud.

Term	Definition
ablation ăb-LĀ-shŭn	
benign bē-NĪN	
cesarean section sē-SĀR-ē-ăn	
cholecystectomy kō-lē-sĭs- TĔK-tō-mē	
dysmenorrhea dĭs-mĕn-ō-RĒ-ă	
endometrial biopsy ĕn-dō-MĒ-trē-ăl BĪ-ŏp-sē	
fibroids FĪ-broyds	
gravida 2 GRĂV-ĭ-dă	
hysterectomy hĭs-tĕr-ĔK-tō-mē	
laparoscopic lăp-ă-rō-SKŎP-ĭk	
mammogram MĂM-ō-grăm	
menometrorrhagia mĕn-ō-mĕt-rō- RĀ-jē-ă	
palliative PĂL-ē-ā-tĭv	

(continued)

Term	Definition
para 1 PĂR-ă	
postoperative pōst-ŎP-ĕr-ă-tĭv	
Premarin PRĔM-ă-rĭn	
salpingo- oophorectomy săl-pĭng-gō-ō-ŏf-ō- RĔK-tō-mē	
therapeutic abortion thĕr-ă-PŪ-tĭk ă-BOR-shŭn	
thyroid function test THĪ-royd FŬNG-shŭn	

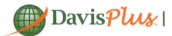

Visit the *Medical Terminology Systems* online resource center at Davis*Plus*. Use it to practice pronunciation and reinforce the meanings of the terms in this medical report.

PREOPERATIVE CONSULTATION: MENOMETRORRHAGIA

Physician Center
2422 Rodeo Drive ■■ Sun City, USA 12345 ■■ (555)788-2427

PREOPERATIVE CONSULTATION

Mazza, Rosemary   July 2, 20xx

CHIEF COMPLAINT: Dysmenorrhea and night sweats

HISTORY OF PRESENT ILLNESS: Patient is a 43-year-old gravida 2, para 1 with multiple small uterine fibroids, irregular menses twice a month, family history of ovarian cancer, benign endometrial biopsy, normal Pap, normal mammogram, and normal thyroid function tests. Negative cervical cultures. She has completed childbearing and desires definitive treatment of endometrial ablation, hormonal regulation.

SURGICAL HISTORY: Cesarean section, therapeutic abortion, and cholecystectomy.

ASSESSMENT: This is a patient with menometrorrhagia who declines palliative treatment and desires definitive treatment in the form of a hysterectomy.

PLAN: The plan is to perform a laparoscopic-assisted vaginal hysterectomy, as the patient has essentially no uterine prolapse, and she desires her ovaries to be taken out. She desires to be started on Premarin in the postoperative period. She has been counseled concerning the risks of surgery, including injury to bowel or bladder, infection, and bleeding. She voices understanding and agrees to the plan to perform a laparoscopic-assisted vaginal hysterectomy and bilateral salpingo-oophorectomy.

Julia Masters, MD
Julia Masters, MD

JM:st

Analysis

Review the medical record *Preoperative Consultation: Menometrorrhagia* to answer the following questions.

1. How many pregnancies did this patient have? How many viable infants did she deliver?

_____

2. What is a therapeutic abortion?

_____

3. Why did the physician propose to perform a hysterectomy?

_____

4. What is a vaginal hysterectomy?

_____

5. Does the surgeon plan to remove one or both ovaries and fallopian tubes?

_____

6. Why do you think the physician will use the laparoscope to perform the hysterectomy?

_____

Male Reproductive System

Objectives

Upon completion of this chapter, you will be able to:

- Locate and describe the structures of the male reproductive system.
- Describe the functional relationship between the male reproductive system and other body systems.
- Pronounce, spell, and build words related to the male reproductive system.
- Describe pathological conditions, diagnostic and therapeutic procedures, and other terms related to the male reproductive system.
- Explain pharmacology related to the treatment of male reproductive disorders.
- Demonstrate your knowledge of this chapter by completing the learning and medical record activities.

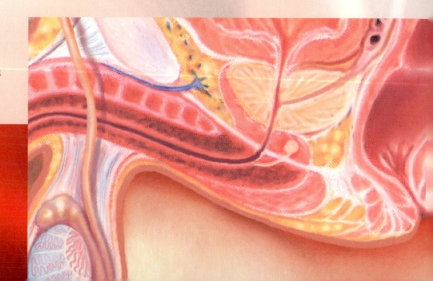

Anatomy and Physiology

The male reproductive system produces, maintains, and transports sperm, the male sex cell required for fertilization of the female egg. It is also responsible for the development of male secondary sex characteristics. (See Figure 13-1.)

Anatomy and Physiology Key Terms

This section introduces important male reproductive system terms and their definitions. Word analyses for selected terms are also provided.

Term	Definition
gamete GĂM-ēt	Reproductive cell (ovum or sperm) that contains one-half of the chromosomes required to produce an offspring of the species
libido lĭ-BĒ-dō	Psychological and physical drive for sexual activity
semen SĒ-mĕn	Fluid containing sperm and secretions from the prostate and other structures of the male reproductive system; also called *seminal fluid*
sphincter SFĬNGK-tĕr	Ringlike muscle that opens and closes a body opening to allow or restrict passage through the structure
testosterone tĕs-TŎS-tĕr-ōn	Androgenic hormone responsible for the development of the male sex organs, including the penis, testicles, scrotum, and prostate *Testosterone is also responsible for the development of secondary sex characteristics (musculature, hair patterns, thickened vocal cords, and so forth).*

Pronunciation Help	Long Sound	ā — rate	ē — rebirth	ī — isle	ō — over	ū — unite
	Short Sound	ă — alone	ĕ — ever	ĭ — it	ŏ — not	ŭ — cut

Male Reproductive Structures

The primary male reproductive organ consists of two (1) **testes** (singular, **testis**) located in an external sac called the (2) **scrotum.** The testes produce the hormone **testosterone**, which enables development of secondary sex characteristics. It also plays an important role in **libido**. Within the testes are numerous small tubes that twist and coil to form (3) **seminiferous tubules,** which produce sperm, the male **gamete**. Lying over the superior surface of each testis is a single, tightly coiled tube called the (4) **epididymis.** This structure stores sperm after it leaves the seminiferous tubules. The epididymis is the first duct through which sperm passes after its production in the testes. Tracing the duct upward, the epididymis forms the (5) **vas deferens** (also called the **seminal duct** or **ductus**

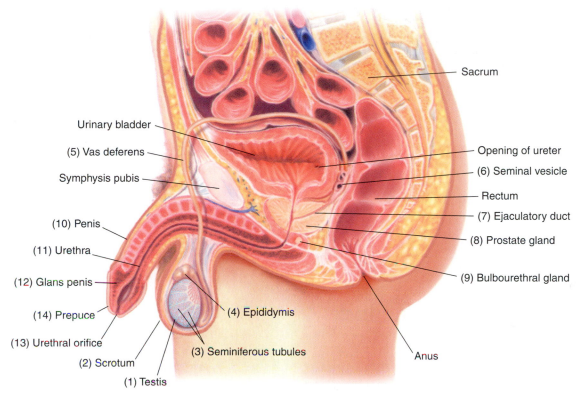

Sacrum

Urinary bladder

(5) Vas deferens

Symphysis pubis

Opening of ureter

(6) Seminal vesicle

Rectum

(7) Ejaculatory duct

(8) Prostate gland

(9) Bulbourethral gland

(10) Penis

(11) Urethra

(12) Glans penis

(14) Prepuce

(13) Urethral orifice

(2) Scrotum

(1) Testis

(4) Epididymis

(3) Seminiferous tubules

Anus

Figure 13-1 Midsaggital section of male reproductive structures shown through the pelvic cavity.

deferens), a narrow tube that passes through the inguinal canal into the abdominal cavity. The vas deferens extends over the top and down the posterior surface of the bladder, where it joins the (6) **seminal vesicle.** The union of the vas deferens with the duct from the seminal vesicle forms the (7) **ejaculatory duct.** The seminal vesicle contains nutrients that support sperm viability and produces approximately 60% of the seminal fluid that is ultimately ejaculated during sexual intercourse **(coitus).** The ejaculatory duct passes at an angle through the (8) **prostate gland,** a triple-lobed organ fused to the base of the bladder. The prostate gland secretes a thin, alkaline substance that accounts for about 30% of seminal fluid. Its alkalinity helps protect sperm from the acidic environments of the male urethra and the female vagina. Two pea-shaped structures, the (9) **bulbourethral (Cowper) glands,** are located below the prostate and are connected by a small duct to the urethra. The bulbourethral glands provide the alkaline fluid necessary for sperm viability. The (10) **penis** is the male organ of copulation. It is cylindrical and composed of erectile tissue that encloses the (11) **urethra.** The urethra expels semen and urine from the body. During ejaculation, the sphincter at the base of the bladder closes, which not only stops urine from being expelled with the semen, but also prevents semen from entering the bladder. The enlarged tip of the penis, the (12) **glans penis,** contains the (13) **urethral orifice (meatus).** A movable hood of skin, called the (14) **prepuce (foreskin)** covers the glans penis.

Anatomy Review

To review the anatomy of the male reproductive system, label the illustration using the terms listed below.

bulbourethral gland	*prepuce*	*testis*
ejaculatory duct	*prostate gland*	*urethra*
epididymis	*scrotum*	*urethral orifice*
glans penis	*seminal vesicle*	*vas deferens*
penis	*seminiferous tubules*	

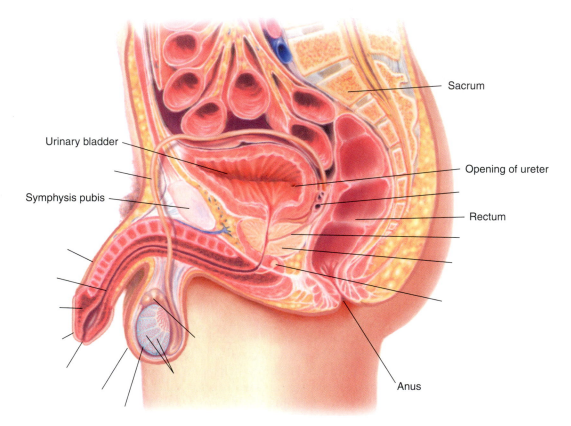

Sacrum

Urinary bladder

Opening of ureter

Symphysis pubis

Rectum

Anus

 Check your answers by referring to Figure 13-1 on page 429. Review material that you did not answer correctly.

CONNECTING BODY SYSTEMS—MALE REPRODUCTIVE SYSTEM

The main function of the male reproductive systems is to enable sexual reproduction. Specific functional relationships between the male reproductive system and other body systems are summarized below.

Blood, Lymph, and Immune
- Male reproductive system secretes testosterone into the extracellular fluids of the blood, lymph, and immune system for delivery throughout the body.
- Male reproductive system relies on increased blood supply to support erectile tissue needed for copulation.

Cardiovascular
- Male hormones are transported throughout the body by the vascular system.
- Increased heart rate maintains sexual excitement needed for ejaculation.

Digestive
- Male reproductive structures rely on a continuous supply of food and nourishment for proper functioning of the organs of reproduction.
- Male reproductive activities require food and nourishment for sexual behavior.

Endocrine
- Gonads produce hormones that provide feedback to influence pituitary function.
- Hormones produce and regulate the development of secondary sex characteristics.

Female Reproductive
- Male reproductive structures produce and deliver sperm, the cell that provides one-half of the genetic compliment required for the development of a fetus.
- Male organs of reproduction work in conjunction with the female reproductive system to enable fertilization of the ovum.

Integumentary
- Male hormones produce facial and body hair growth consistent with maleness.

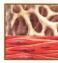
Musculoskeletal
- Male hormones produce skeletal and muscular structures consistent with a larger body frame than normally found in females.

Nervous
- Male reproductive structures rely on the nervous system to innervate the organs responsible for copulation.
- Mature male reproductive activities are regulated by the emotional aspects of the nervous system, especially the brain.

Respiratory
- Male reproductive system relies on increased respiratory activity required for sexual activity.
- The male organs of reproduction require a constant supply of oxygen and the removal of waste gases for healthy functioning.
- Male reproductive system causes laryngeal changes, resulting in a deepening of the voice.

Urinary
- Male reproductive system and the urinary system share common structures.
- Waste substances produced by the male reproductive organs are removed by the urinary system.

Medical Word Elements

This section introduces combining forms, suffixes, and prefixes related to the male reproductive system. Word analyses are also provided.

Element	Meaning	Word Analysis
Combining Forms		
andr/o	male	**andr/o**/gen/ic (ăn-drō-JĔN-ĭk): pertaining to maleness *gen:* forming, producing, origin *-ic:* pertaining to *Androgenic hormones include all natural or synthetic compounds that stimulate or maintain male characteristics. The most common androgenic hormone is testosterone.*
balan/o	glans penis	**balan/o**/plasty (BĂL-ă-nō-plăs-tē): surgical repair of the glans penis *-plasty:* surgical repair
crypt/o	hidden	**crypt**/orchid/ism (krĭpt-OR-kĭd-ĭzm): condition of hidden testes; also called *cryptorchism* *orchid:* testis (plural, testes) *-ism:* condition *Cryptorchidism is the failure of the testes to descend into the scrotum and is usually a congenital disorder.*
epididym/o	epididymis	**epididym/o**/tomy (ĕp-ĭ-dĭd-ĭ-MŎT-ō-mē): incision of the epididymis *-tomy:* incision
genit/o	genitalia	**genit/o**/urin/ary (jĕn-ĭ-tō-ŪR-ĭ-năr-ē): pertaining to the genitalia and urinary tract
gonad/o	gonads, sex glands	**gonad/o**/pathy (gŏn-ă-DŎP-ă-thē): disease of the sex glands *-pathy:* disease
olig/o	scanty	**olig/o**/sperm/ia (ŏl-ĭ-gō-SPĔR-mē-ă): scanty (decreased production) of sperm *sperm:* spermatozoa, sperm cells *-ia:* condition
orch/o	testis (plural, testes)	**orch**/itis (or-KĪ-tĭs): inflammation of testes *-itis:* inflammation *A common cause of orchitis in young boys is a mumps infection.*
orchi/o		**orchi**/algia (or-kē-ĂL-jē-ă): pain in the testes *-algia:* pain
orchid/o		**orchid/o**/ptosis (or-kĭd-ŏp-TŌ-sĭs): downward displacement of the testes *-ptosis:* prolapse, downward displacement
test/o		**test**/algia (tĕs-TĂL-jē-ă): pain of a testis *-algia:* pain

Element	Meaning	Word Analysis
perine/o	perineum (area between scrotum [or vulva in the female] and anus)	**perine**/al (pĕr-ĭ-NĒ-ăl): pertaining to the perineum *-al:* pertaining to
prostat/o	prostate gland	**prostat/o**/megaly (prŏs-tă-tŏ-MĔG-ă-lē): enlargement of the prostate gland *-megaly:* enlargement
spermat/o	spermatozoa, sperm cells	**spermat/o**/cele (spĕr-MĂT-ō-sēl): swelling containing spermatozoa *-cele:* hernia, swelling *A spermatocele is usually an epididymal cyst, commonly containing sperm.*
sperm/o		**sperm**/ic (SPĔR-mĭk): pertaining to sperm cells *-ic:* pertaining to
varic/o	dilated vein	**varic/o**/cele (VĂR-ĭ-kō-sēl): swelling of a dilated vein *-cele:* hernia, swelling *Varicocele is a dilation of the veins of the spermatic cord, the structure that supports the testicles.*
vas/o	vessel; vas deferens; duct	**vas**/ectomy (văs-ĔK-tō-mē): removal of (all or part of) the vas deferens *-ectomy:* excision, removal *Bilateral vasectomy is a surgical procedure to produce sterility in the male.*
vesicul/o	seminal vesicle	**vesicul**/itis (vĕ-sĭk-ū-LĪ-tĭs): inflammation of the seminal vesicle *-itis:* inflammation

Suffixes		
-cide	killing	sperm/i/**cide** (SPĔR-mĭ-sīd): (agents that) kill sperm; also called *spermaticide* *sperm/i:* spermatozoa, sperm cells
-genesis	forming, producing, origin	spermat/o/**genesis** (spĕr-măt-ō-JĔN-ĕ-sĭs): forming or producing sperm *spermat/o:* sperm

-ism	condition	an/orch/**ism** (ăn-OR-kĭzm): condition without testes
		  an-: without, not
		  orch: testis (plural, testes)
		
		Anorchism is the congenital or acquired absence of one or both testes.

-spadias	slit, fissure	hypo/**spadias** (hī-pō-SPĀ-dē-ăs): a fissure under (the penis) *hypo-:* under, below *Hypospadias is a congenital defect in which the urethra opens on the underside of the glans penis instead of the tip.*

(continued)

Element	Meaning	Word Analysis
Prefixes		
brachy-	short	**brachy**/therapy (brăk-ē-THĔR-ă-pē): treatment from a short (distance) *-therapy:* treatment *Treatment where radioactive seeds are implanted directly into the malignant tissue.*
epi-	above, upon	**epi**/spadias (ĕp-ĭ-SPĀ-dē-ăs): fissure upon (dorsum of penis) *-spadias:* slit, fissure

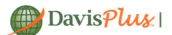 Visit the *Medical Terminology Systems* online resource center at Davis*Plus* for an audio exercise of the terms in this table. Other activities are also available to reinforce content.

 It is time to review medical word elements by completing Learning Activities 13-1 and 13-2.

Pathology

Signs and symptoms of male reproductive disorders include pain or swelling, erectile dysfunction, and loss of libido. Characteristics of sexually transmitted infections include pain, discharge, or development of lesions. A complete evaluation of the genitalia, reproductive history, and past and present genitourinary infections and disorders is necessary to identify disorders associated with male reproductive structures.

For diagnosis, treatment, and management of male reproductive disorders, the medical services of a specialist may be warranted. **Urology** is the branch of medicine concerned with the male reproductive system as well as urinary disorders in both males and females. The physician who specializes in diagnosis and treatment of genitourinary disorders is known as a **urologist.**

Sexually Transmitted Infections

Sexually transmitted infections (STIs), also called **sexually transmitted diseases (STDs),** include any contagious disease acquired as a result of sexual activity with an infected partner. In the United States, the widespread occurrence of STIs is regarded as an epidemic. As a group, STIs are the single most significant cause of reproductive disorders. The current STIs of medical concern include gonorrhea, syphilis, chlamydia, genital herpes, genital warts, trichomoniasis, and human immunodeficiency virus (HIV) and acquired immune deficiency syndrome (AIDS).

Gonorrhea

Gonorrhea is caused by the bacterium *Neisseria gonorrhoeae*. It involves the mucosal surface of the genitourinary tract and, possibly, the rectum and pharynx. This disease may be acquired through sexual intercourse and through orogenital and anogenital contact. The most common symptom of gonorrhea in men is pain upon urination **(dysuria)** and a white discharge **(leukorrhea).** Women are commonly asymptomatic; when symptoms are present, they include a vaginal discharge or pelvic pain. The organism may infect the eyes of the newborn during vaginal delivery, commonly leading to blindness. As a precaution, silver nitrate is instilled in the eyes of newborns immediately after delivery as a preventive measure to ensure that this infection does not occur. If gonorrhea is left untreated, the disease may infect the bladder **(cystitis)** and inflame joints **(arthritis).** In addition, sterility may result from formation of scars that close the reproductive tubes of both sexes, a disease called **pelvic inflammatory disease (PID).** Both sex partners must be treated for gonorrhea because the infection can recur. The usual treatment is antibiotics.

Chlamydia

Chlamydia, caused by infection with the bacterium *Chlamydia trachomatis*, is the most prevalent and one of the most damaging STIs in the United States. It is also called the "silent disease," because symptoms are commonly absent or mild. If present, men may produce a whitish discharge from the penis. In women there may be a mucopurulent discharge and inflammation of the cervix uteri **(cervicitis).** In both sexes, the disease may eventually affect the reproductive structures, leading to sterility. Chlamydia can be transmitted to the newborn baby during the birth process and cause a form of conjunctivitis or pneumonia. Chlamydia in men, women, and babies can be successfully treated with antibiotics. However, because many cases of chlamydia are asymptomatic (especially in women), the disease commonly remains untreated until irreversible damage to the reproductive structures has occurred.

Syphilis

Although less common than gonorrhea, syphilis is the more serious of the two diseases. It is caused by infection with the bacterium *Treponema pallidum*. If left untreated, syphilis may become a chronic, infectious, multisystemic disease. Syphilis is characterized by three distinct phases. In the first phase, a primary sore **(chancre)** develops at the point where the organism enters the body. The chancre is an ulcerated sore with hard edges that contains infectious organisms. The second phase produces a variety of symptoms that make diagnosis of the disease difficult. The third phase is the latent phase whereby the disease may remain dormant for years. Although there may be no symptoms of the disease during this time, the patient is nevertheless infectious. Symptoms of the latent stage may include blindness, mental disorders, and eventual death. Treatment with antibiotic therapy is effective.

Genital Herpes

Genital herpes causes red, blisterlike, painful lesions in the genital area that closely resemble fever blisters or cold sores that appear on the lips and around the mouth. Although both diseases are caused by the herpes simplex virus (HSV), genital herpes is associated with type 2 (HSV-2), and oral herpes is associated with type 1 (HSV-1). Regardless, both forms can cause oral and genital infections through oral-genital sexual activity. Fluid in the blisters is highly infectious and contains the active virus. However, this disease is associated with a phenomenon called **viral shedding.** During viral shedding, the virus is present on the skin of the infected patient, and can be transmitted to sexual partners, even when no lesions are present. The disease may be transmitted to a baby during the birth process and, although rare, may lead to death of the infant. In men, lesions appear on the glans, foreskin, or penile shaft. In females, lesions appear in the vaginal area, buttocks, and thighs. Individuals with a herpes infection may have only one episode or may have repeated attacks that usually lessen in severity over the years. Antiviral medication can relieve pain and discomfort during an outbreak by healing the sores more quickly but there is no cure available for this disease.

Genital Warts

Genital warts **(condylomata, condylomas)** are caused by the human papillomavirus (HPV). The warts may be very small and almost unnoticeable or may be large and appear in clusters. In females, the lesions may be found on the vulva, in the vagina, or on the cervix. In males, the lesions commonly appear on the penis or around the rectum. Many warts disappear without treatment, but there is no way to determine which ones will resolve. When treatment is required, surgical excision or freezing the wart is the usual method. HPV infection has been found to increase the risk of certain cancers, including penile, vaginal, cervical, and anal cancer. There is also a much greater incidence of miscarriages in women with HPV disease. HPV-16 is a specific type of HPV and is considered "high risk" insofar as it is very closely associated with cervical cancer and possibly penile cancer. Women diagnosed with this form of HPV require regular Pap smears. There is no treatment to eliminate the virus from the body, but various treatments are available to remove the warts. HPV vaccines are available for males and females to protect against the types of HPV that most commonly cause health problems. To be effective, it must be administered before the time the individual begins engaging in sexual activity.

Trichomoniasis

Trichomoniasis, caused by the protozoan *Trichomonas vaginalis,* affects males and females, but symptoms are more common in females. When symptoms are present in males, they include irritation inside the penis, mild discharge, or slight burning after urination **(dysuria)** or ejaculation. Treatment is generally effective, but reinfection is common if sexual partners are not treated simultaneously. In women, trichomonas causes vaginitis, urethritis, and cystitis. Signs and symptoms include a frothy, yellow-green vaginal discharge with a strong odor. The infection may also cause discomfort during intercourse and urination. Irritation and itching in the female genital area and, in rare cases, lower abdominal pain can also occur. It is important to treat both sex partners to avoid reinfection.

Benign Prostatic Hyperplasia

Benign prostatic hyperplasia (BPH), also called **benign prostatic hypertrophy,** is commonly associated with the aging process. As the prostate gland enlarges, it decreases the urethral lumen, and complete voiding of urine becomes difficult. (See Figure 13-2.) Urine that remains in the bladder commonly becomes a breeding ground for bacteria. Bladder infection **(cystitis)** and, ultimately, kidney infection **(nephritis)** may result. If medical management of BPH fails, it may be necessary to use surgical methods.

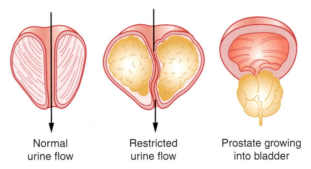

Normal urine flow   Restricted urine flow   Prostate growing into bladder

Figure 13-2 Benign prostatic hyperplasia showing restricted urine flow and the prostate growing into the bladder. From Tamparo: *Diseases of the Human Body,* 5th ed. FA Davis, Philadelphia, 2011, p 467, with permission.

Cryptorchidism

Failure of the testes to descend into the scrotal sac prior to birth is called **cryptorchidism.** In many infants born with this condition, the testes descend spontaneously by the end of the first year. If this does not occur, correction of the disorder involves surgical suspension of the testes **(orchiopexy)** in the scrotum. This procedure is usually done before the child reaches age 2. Because an inguinal hernia commonly accompanies cryptorchidism, the hernia may be sutured **(herniorrhaphy)** at the same time.

Oncology

Two of the most common forms of cancer associated with the male reproductive system are prostate cancer and testicular cancer.

Prostate Cancer

In the United States, prostate cancer is rarely found in men younger than age 50; however, the incidence dramatically increases with age. Symptoms include difficulty starting urination **(hesitancy)** and stopping the urinary stream, dysuria, urinary frequency, and hematuria. Early presymptomatic tests include a blood test for prostate-specific antigen (PSA) and periodic digital rectal examination (DRE).

Like other forms of cancer, prostate cancers are staged and graded to determine metastatic potential, response to treatment, chances of survival, and appropriate forms of therapy. Surgery and radiation therapy are the usual treatment methods, but other forms of treatment may also be used. Surgical treatment involves the removal of the entire prostate **(radical prostatectomy).** Two forms of radiation oncology include brachytherapy and external beam radiation. In **brachytherapy** (also called **internal radiation therapy**), radioactive "seeds" are placed directly in the malignant tissue. They remain in place for long or short periods of time, depending on the type of malignancy, its location, and other diagnostic criteria. (See Figure 13-3.) In **external beam radiation (EBR),** also called **external beam therapy (EBT),** or **teletherapy,** high-energy x-ray beams are generated by a machine and directed at the tumor from outside the body to destroy prostate tissue. Another treatment modality is the application of extreme cold **(cryosurgery),** which destroys prostate tissue. (See Figure 13-4.) This treatment is usually performed in early-stage prostate cancer or in cancer recurrence following other treatments. Administering antiandrogenic agents as well as hormones that deplete the body of testicular hormones **(combined hormonal therapy)** has been effective in treatment at the early stages of the disease. Because prostatic cancer is stimulated by testosterone, surgical removal of the testes **(bilateral orchiectomy,** also called **castration)** may be necessary.

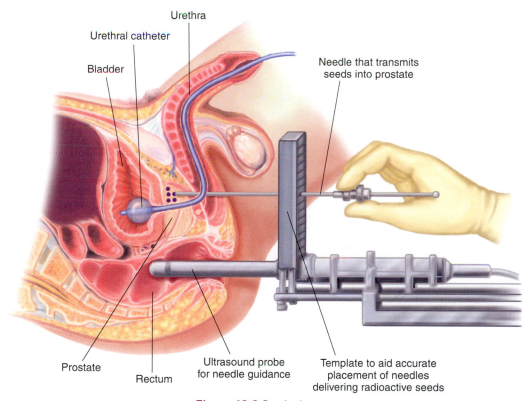

Urethra

Urethral catheter

Bladder

Needle that transmits
seeds into prostate

Prostate

Rectum

Ultrasound probe
for needle guidance

Template to aid accurate
placement of needles
delivering radioactive seeds

Figure 13-3 Brachytherapy.

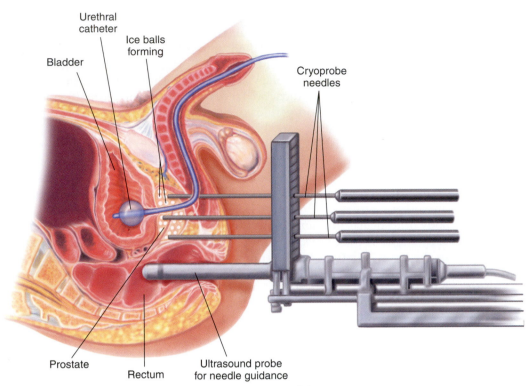

Figure 13-4 Cryosurgery of the prostate.

Testicular Cancer

Testicular cancer is the most common form of cancer in males between ages 15 and 34. Some forms of testicular cancer are asymptomatic during the early course of the disease. However, when present, signs and symptoms include swelling, enlargement or lump in the testes, testicular pain or discomfort, or lower back or abdominal pain. Enlargement of breast tissue **(gynecomastia)** may also occur. If the cancer has spread throughout the body **(metastasized),** various symptoms may also appear in the lungs, abdomen, back, or brain. Most forms of testicular cancer are responsive to treatment when found in the early stages. Accordingly, physicians encourage men to perform testicular self-examination (TSE) as a routine measure on a monthly basis. Ultrasound of the scrotum is a highly reliable test in the diagnosis of testicular cancer. If positive, the testes are removed and examined to determine the type of malignancy. The type of malignancy, stage, and grade will determine the various treatment methods, including orchiectomy, radiation therapy, and chemotherapy.

Diseases and Conditions

This section introduces diseases and conditions of the male reproductive system with their meanings and pronunciations. Word analyses for selected terms are also provided.

Term	Definition
balanitis băl-ă-NĪ-tĭs *balan:* glans penis *-itis:* inflammation	Inflammation of the skin covering the glans penis, caused by bacteria, fungi, or a virus *Uncircumcised men with poor personal hygiene are prone to this disorder.*
erectile dysfunction (ED) ĕ-RĔK-tĭl	Repeated inability to initiate or maintain an erection sufficient for sexual intercourse *Any disorder that causes injury to the nerves or impairs blood flow in the penis has the potential to cause ED.*

Term	Definition
hypogonadism hī-pō-GŌ-năd-ĭzm *hypo-:* under, below, deficient *gonad:* gonads, sex glands *-ism:* condition	Decrease or lack of hormones normally produced by the gonads *In the male reproductive system,* **hypogonadism** *refers to a decrease in or lack of testosterone, which plays a key role in masculine growth and development during puberty.*
hypospadias hī-pō-SPĀ-dē-ăs *hypo-:* under, below, deficient *-spadias:* slit, fissure	Congenital abnormality where the opening of the male urethra is on the undersurface of the penis, instead of at its tip
phimosis fī-MŌ-sĭs *phim:* muzzle *-osis:* abnormal condition; increase (used primarily with blood cells)	Stenosis or narrowing of foreskin so that it cannot be retracted over the glans penis
priapism PRĪ-ă-pĭzm	Prolonged and often painful erection of the penis, which occurs without sexual stimulation *Priapism is associated with sickle cell disease, leukemia, or spinal cord injury. It may also be caused by a side effect of drugs used to treat erectile dysfunction or by recreational drugs. Prompt treatment is usually needed to prevent tissue damage that could result in the inability to initiate or maintain an erection (erectile dysfunction).*
prostatitis prŏs-tă-TĪ-tĭs *prostat:* prostate *-itis:* inflammation	Acute or chronic inflammation of the prostate *Prostatitis is generally caused by a urinary tract infection or a sexually transmitted infection.*
testicular abnormalities tĕs-TĬK-ū-lăr	Any of the various disorders that affect the testes
anorchism ăn-OR-kĭzm *an-:* without, not *orch:* testis (plural, testes) *-ism:* condition	Absence of one or both testicles; also called *anorchia* or *anorchidism* *Treatment includes androgen (male hormone) supplementation, testicular prosthetic implantation, and psychological support.*
epididymitis ĕp-ĭ-dĭd-ĭ-MĪ-tĭs *epididym:* epididymis *-itis:* inflammation	Inflammation of the epididymis (See Figure 13-5A.) *Epididymitis is found most commonly in males between ages 14 and 35 and is usually associated with STIs, especially gonorrhea and chlamydia.*
hydrocele HĪ-drō-sēl *hydr/o:* water *-cele:* hernia, swelling	Swelling of the sac surrounding the testes that is typically harmless (See Figure 13-5B.) *Hydrocele in a neonate usually resolves without treatment within a year. In men and young boys, it is commonly caused by inflammation or injury to the scrotum.*
orchitis or-KĪ-tĭs *orch:* testis (plural, testes) *-itis:* inflammation	Painful swelling of one or both testes, commonly associated with mumps that develop after puberty (See Figure 13-5C.) *Other causes of orchitis include infection of the epididymis or STIs.*

(continued)

Term	Definition
spermatocele spĕr-MĂT-ō-sēl *spermat/o:* spermatozoa, sperm cells *-cele:* hernia, swelling	Abnormal, fluid-filled sac that develops in the epididymis and may or may not contain sperm; also called *spermatic cyst* (See Figure 13-5D.)
testicular mass tĕs-TĬK-ū-lăr	New tissue growth that appears on one or both testes and may be malignant or benign (See Figure 13-5E.)
testicular torsion tĕs-TĬK-ū-lăr TOR-shŭn	Spontaneous twisting of a testicle within the scrotum, leading to a decrease in blood flow to the affected testicle (See Figure 13-5F.) *Testicular torsion is a medical emergency, because interruption of blood supply may permanently damage the testicle.*
varicocele VĂR-ĭ-kō-sēl *varic/o:* dilated vein *-cele:* hernia, swelling	Swelling and distention of veins of the spermatic cord, somewhat resembling varicose veins of the legs (See Figure 13-5G.) *Some varicoceles cause sterility due to low sperm production or poor sperm quality. Varicoceles can be treated surgically.*

A B C D

Epididymitis   Hydrocele   Orchitis   Spermatocele

E F G

Testicular mass   Testicular torsion   Varicocele

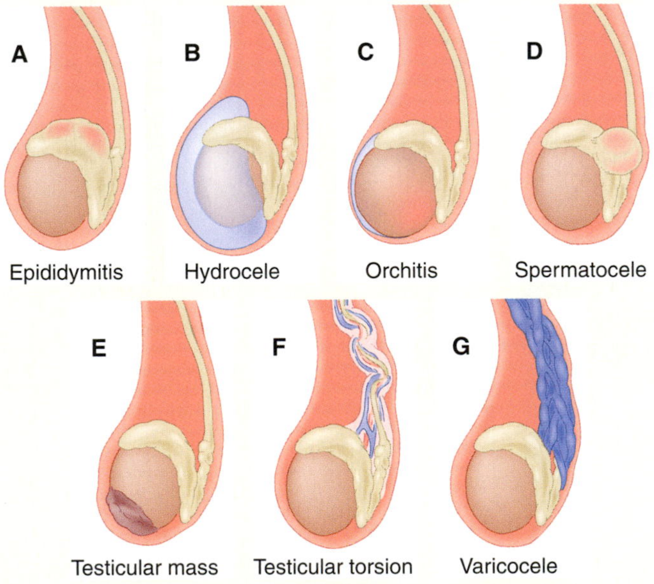

Figure 13-5 Testicular abnormalities. **(A)** Epididymitis. **(B)** Hydrocele. **(C)** Orchitis. **(D)** Spermatocele. **(E)** Testicular mass. **(F)** Testicular torsion. **(G)** Varicocele.

Term	Definition
sterility stĕr-ĬL-ĭ-tē	Inability to produce offspring; in the male, inability to fertilize the ovum

 It is time to review pathology, diseases, and conditions by completing Learning Activity 13–3.

Medical, Surgical, and Diagnostic Procedures

This section introduces medical, surgical, and diagnostic procedures used to treat and diagnose male reproductive disorders. Descriptions are provided as well as pronunciations and word analyses for selected terms.

Procedure	Description
Medical	
digital rectal examination (DRE) DĬJ-ĭt-ăl RĔK-tăl	Screening test that assesses the rectal wall surface for lesions or evaluates abnormalities of the pelvic area *In males, the physician also evaluates the size and consistency of the prostate. (See Figure 13-6.)* 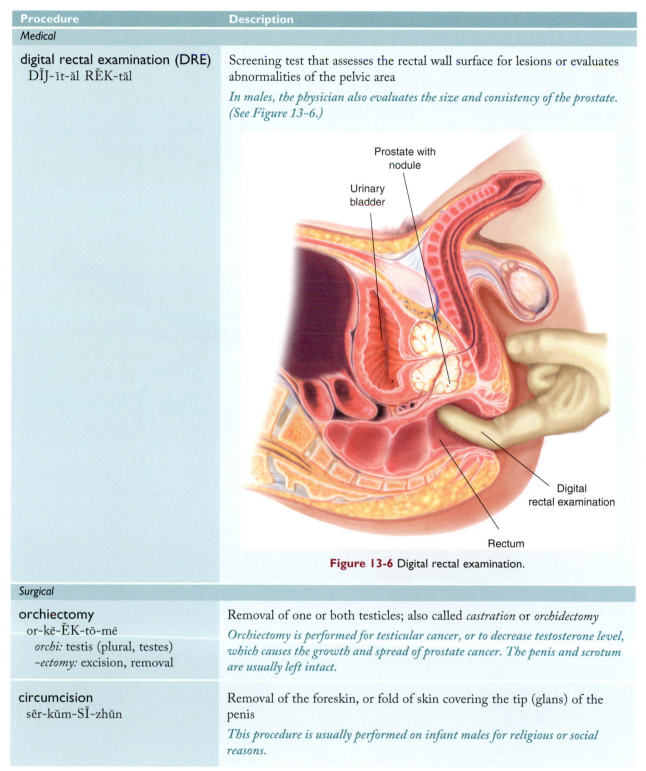 **Figure 13-6** Digital rectal examination.
Surgical	
orchiectomy or-kē-ĔK-tō-mē *orchi:* testis (plural, testes) *-ectomy:* excision, removal	Removal of one or both testicles; also called *castration* or *orchidectomy* *Orchiectomy is performed for testicular cancer, or to decrease testosterone level, which causes the growth and spread of prostate cancer. The penis and scrotum are usually left intact.*
circumcision sĕr-kŭm-SĬ-zhŭn	Removal of the foreskin, or fold of skin covering the tip (glans) of the penis *This procedure is usually performed on infant males for religious or social reasons.*

(continued)

Procedure	Description
orchiopexy or-kē-ō-PĔK-sē *orchi/o:* testis (plural, testes) *-pexy:* fixation (of an organ)	Fixation of the testes in the scrotum *This procedure is performed for undescended testicles (cryptorchidism), usually before age 2.*
prostatectomy prŏs-tă-TĔK-tō-mē *prostat:* prostate *-ectomy:* excision, removal	Removal of all or part of the prostate *Several prostatectomy procedures are possible, depending on the extent and reason for removal; however, transurethral resection of the prostate (TURP) is one of the most common.*
transurethral resection of prostate (TURP) trăns-ū-RĒ-thrăl rē-SĔK-shŭn, PRŎS-tāt *trans:* across, through *urethr:* urethra *-al:* pertaining to	Excision of the prostate gland by inserting a special endoscope (resectoscope) through the urethra and into the bladder to remove small pieces of tissue from the prostate gland (See Figure 13-7.) *The resectoscope is fitted with an electrically activated wire loop that removes tissue when dragged over the site and cauterizes it to minimize bleeding.*

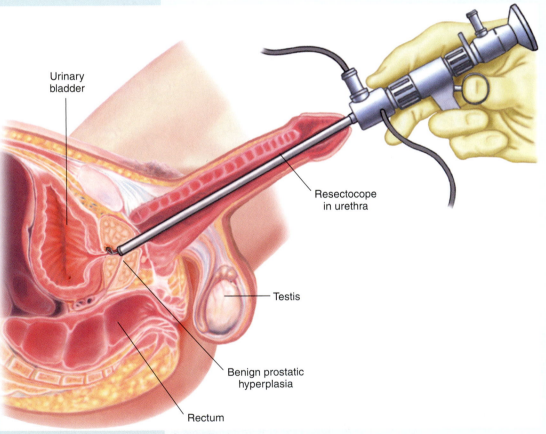

Urinary bladder

Resectocope in urethra

Testis

Benign prostatic hyperplasia

Rectum

Figure 13-7 Transurethral resection of the prostate (TURP).

urethroplasty ū-RĒ-thrō-plăs-tē *urethr/o:* urethra *-plasty:* surgical repair	Reconstruction of the urethra to relieve stricture or narrowing *Urethroplasty relieves pain and discomfort experienced during voiding and reduces the risk of contracting orchitis, prostatitis, and urinary tract infections.*

Procedure	Description
vasectomy văs-ĔK-tō-mē *vas:* vessel; vas deferens; duct *-ectomy:* excision, removal	Removal of all or a segment of the vas deferens for male sterilization *Vasectomy reversal* (**vasovasostomy**) *rejoins the two segments of the vas deferens. The reversal has the greatest chance of producing a pregnancy if performed within 3 years of the vasectomy. After 10 years, the success rate for producing pregnancy is less than 30%. (See Figure 13–8.)* **Figure 13-8** Vasectomy and vasovasostomy.

Diagnostic

Laboratory

Procedure	Description
prostate-specific antigen (PSA) PRŎS-tāt spĕ-SĬF-ĭk ĂN-tĭ-jĕn	Blood test used to detect prostatic disorders, especially prostate cancer; also called a *tumor marker test* *PSA is a substance produced by the prostate and is normally found in a blood sample in small quantities. The level is elevated in prostatitis, benign prostatic hyperplasia, and tumors of the prostate.*
semen analysis SĒ-mĕn ă-NĂL-ĭ-sĭs	Test that analyzes a semen sample for volume, sperm count, motility, and morphology to evaluate fertility or verify sterilization after a vasectomy

Imaging

Procedure	Description
ultrasound (US) ŬL-tră-sownd	High-frequency sound waves *(ultrasound)* are directed at soft tissue and reflected as "echoes" to produce an image on a monitor of an internal body structure; also called *ultrasound, sonography,* and *echo*
prostate	US using an ultrasound probe inserted through the rectum to evaluate the prostate; also called *transrectal ultrasound* *US of the prostate is used to detect abnormalities of the prostate, obtain biopsies, and aid in the diagnosis of infertility problems.*
scrotal SKRŌ-tăl	US used to assess the contents of the scrotum, including the testicles, epididymis, and vas deferens; also called *testicular ultrasound*

Pharmacology

Several classes of drugs are used to treat conditions of the male reproductive system, including antiviral and antibiotic agents to treat diseases and infections. In addition, hormones are used to treat hypogonadism and some reproductive disorders. (See Table 13-1.)

Table 13-1	**Drugs Used to Treat Disorders of the Male Reproductive System**	
	This table lists common drug classifications used to treat male reproductive disorders, their therapeutic actions, and selected generic and trade names	
Classification	**Therapeutic Action**	**Generic and *Trade* Names**
androgens ĂN-drō-jĕnz	Increase testosterone levels *Androgens are used to correct hormone deficiency in hypogonadism and treat delayed puberty in males.*	**testosterone base** tĕs-TŎS-tĕr-ōn *Androderm, Testim* **testosterone cypionate** tĕs-TŎS-tĕr-ōn SĬP-ē-ō-nāt *Depo-testosterone*
antiandrogens ăn-tĭ-ĂN-drō-jĕnz	Suppress the production of androgen *Antiandrogens may stop the growth of certain types of cancer cells, and may be used in the treatment of prostate cancer.*	**flutamide** FLOO-tă-mīd *Eulexin* **nilutamide** nī-LOO-tă-mīd *Nilandron*
anti-impotence agents ăn-tĭ-ĬM-pō-tĕnts	Treat erectile dysfunction (impotence) by increasing blood flow to the penis, resulting in an erection *Anti-impotence drugs should not be used by patients with coronary artery disease or hypertension.*	**sildenafil citrate** sĭl-DĔN-ă-fĭl SĬT-rāt *Viagra* **vardenafil** văr-DĔN-ă-fĭl *Levitra*
antivirals ăn-tĭ-VĪ-rălz	Treat viral disorders by inhibiting their development *Antivirals do not have the ability to destroy a virus. They are used to treat recurrent herpes in adults and lesions associated with chickenpox and shingles.*	**acyclovir** ā-SĪ-klō-vēr *Zovirax* **famciclovir** făm-SĪ-klō-vēr *Famvir*

Abbreviations

This section introduces male reproductive system–related abbreviations and their meanings.

Abbreviation	Meaning	Abbreviation	Meaning
BPH	benign prostatic hyperplasia; benign prostatic hypertrophy	HSV-2	herpes simplex virus type 2
DRE	digital rectal examination	PSA	prostate-specific antigen
EBR	external beam radiation	STD	sexually transmitted disease
EBT	external beam therapy	STI	sexually transmitted infection
ED	erectile dysfunction; emergency department	TSE	testicular self-examination
GC	gonorrhea; gonococci	TURP	transurethral resection of the prostate
HPV	human papillomavirus	US	ultrasound; ultrasonography

 It is time to review procedures, pharmacology, and abbreviations by completing Learning Activity 13-5.

LEARNING ACTIVITIES

The following activities provide review of the male reproductive system terms introduced in this chapter. Complete each activity and review your answers to evaluate your understanding of the chapter.

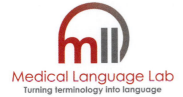

Visit the Medical Language Lab at the web site: medicallanguagelab.com. Use it to enhance your study and reinforcement of this chapter with the flash-card activity. We recommend you complete the flash-card activity before starting Learning Activities 13-1 and 13-2 below.

Learning Activity 13-1
Combining Forms, Suffixes, and Prefixes

Use the elements listed in the table to build medical words. You may use these elements more than once.

Combining Forms		Suffixes		Prefixes
andr/o	*prostat/o*	*-ary*	*-itis*	*an-*
balan/o	*scrot/o*	*-cele*	*-megaly*	*brachy-*
epididym/o	*sperm/i*	*-cide*	*-plasty*	*epi-*
genit/o	*urin/o*	*-ectomy*	*-rrhaphy*	
gonad/o	*varic/o*	*-gen*	*-spadias*	
orch/o	*vas/o*	*-graphy*	*-therapy*	
perine/o	*vesicul/o*	*-ism*		

1. killing sperm _____

2. swelling of a dilated vein _____

3. surgical repair of the scrotum _____

4. enlargement of the prostate _____

5. condition without testes _____

6. excision of a gonad _____

7. pertaining to genitals and the urinary tract _____

8. excision of the epididymis _____

9. treatment from a short (distance) _____

10. fissure upon (dorsum of penis) _____

11. inflammation of the glans penis _____

12. forming or producing a male _____

13. suture of the perineum _____

14. excision of the vas deferens _____

15. process of recording the seminal vesicle _____

Check your answers in Appendix A. Review any material that you did not answer correctly.

Correct Answers _____ X 6.67 = _____ % Score

Learning Activity 13-2

Building Medical Words

Use *orchid/o* (testis [plural, testes]) to build words that mean:

1. inflammation of the testes _____

2. prolapse or downward displacement of the testes _____

Use *balan/o* (glans penis) to build words that mean:

3. flow or discharge of the glans penis _____

4. hernia, swelling of the glans penis _____

Use *spermat/o* to build words that mean:

5. sperm cell _____

6. embryonic sperm (cell) _____

7. swelling or hernia (containing) sperm _____

Use *prostat/o* to build words that mean:

8. pain of the prostate _____

9. discharge of the prostate _____

10. enlargement of the prostate _____

11. stone or calculus of the prostate _____

Use the suffix *–spadias* (slit, fissure) to build words that mean:

12. fissure under (ventrum of penis) _____

13. fissure above (dorsum of penis) _____

Use *vesicul/o* (seminal vesicle) to build words that mean:

14. inflammation of the seminal vesicle _____

15. process of recording the seminal vesicle _____

Use *gonad/o* (gonads, sex glands) to build a word that means:

16. disease of the gonads _____

Build surgical words that mean:

17. surgical repair of glans penis _____

18. excision of (a segment of the) vas deferens _____

19. surgical repair of the scrotum _____

20. suture of the perineum _____

Check your answers in Appendix A. Review material that you did not answer correctly.

Correct Answers _____ X 4 = _____ % Score

Learning Activity 13-3
Pathology, Diseases, and Conditions

Match the following terms with the definitions in the numbered list.

anorchidism	*cryptorchidism*	*hesitancy*	*prostatitis*
balanitis	*cystitis*	*hypospadias*	*sterility*
chancre	*epispadias*	*leukorrhea*	*testicular torsion*
chlamydia	*genital herpes*	*phimosis*	*trichomoniasis*
condylomas	*gynecomastia*	*priapism*	*varicocele*

1. white discharge commonly associated with gonorrhea _____

2. disease characterized by blisterlike lesions around the genital area _____

3. failure of the testicles to descend into the scrotum before birth _____

4. condition where the urethra opens on the underside of the penis _____

5. stenosis of the foreskin so that it cannot be drawn over the glans _____

6. swelling and distention of the spermatic cord veins _____

7. condition where the urethra opens on the dorsum of the penis _____

8. twisting of the testicle within the scrotum _____

9. STI commonly known as *genital warts* _____

10. absence of one or both testicles _____

11. inflammation of the glans penis _____

12. persistent, painful erection lasting more than 4 hours _____

13. inflammation of the prostate _____

14. inflammation of the bladder commonly associated with an enlarged prostate _____

15. inability to produce offspring _____

16. STI caused by a protozoan, with symptoms that are more common in females than males _____

17. common STI called "silent disease" because symptoms are mild or absent _____

18. syphilitic lesion found at the point where the organism entered the body _____

19. difficulty starting urination _____

20. enlargement of breast tissue associated with testicular cancer _____

Check your answers in Appendix A. Review material that you did not answer correctly.

Correct Answers _____ X 5 = _____ % Score

Procedures, Pharmacology, and Abbreviations

Match the following terms with the definitions in the numbered list.

androgens	GC	semen analysis
antiandrogens	HPV	TURP
antivirals	orchiopexy	urethroplasty
BPH	PSA	vasectomy
circumcision	scrotal	vasovasostomy

1. test used to evaluate fertility or verify sterilization after vasectomy _____

2. agents used to increase testosterone levels _____

3. US procedure to assess the testicles, epididymis, and vas deferens for abnormalities _____

4. gonorrhea; gonococci _____

5. male sterilization procedure _____

6. reconstruction of the urethra to relieve a stricture or narrowing _____

7. reversal of a vasectomy _____

8. agents that suppress the production of an androgen _____

9. excision of the prostate through the urethra _____

10. blood test to detect prostate disorders, especially cancer _____

11. medications used to treat recurrent herpes _____

12. fixation of the testes in the scrotum _____

13. removal of the foreskin from the glans _____

14. virus causing genital warts _____

15. nonmalignant enlargement of the prostate that is usually associated with aging _____

Check your answers in Appendix A. Review any material that you did not answer correctly.

Correct Answers _____ X 6.67 = _____ % Score

Learning Activity 13-5
Medical Scenarios

To construct chart notes, replace the italicized terms in each of the two scenarios with one of the medical terms listed below.

dysuria	nocturia	pruritus
hesitancy	orchialgia	PSA
leukorrhea	prostatomegaly	urgency
meatus		

Mr. R. is a sexually active junior at State College. For the last six weeks, he was aware of a slight (1) *white discharge* from the tip of the penis but ignored this symptom. He now complains of (2) *pain upon urination* and (3) *intense itching* around the tip of the penis, and (4) *pain in the testicles.* Suspecting chlamydia, the physician will confirm his diagnosis with a swab taken from the urethral (5) *opening* and a urine test for the presence of chlamydia. In the meantime, the patient will begin a regimen of oral antibiotics and will return for a retest in 2 weeks. He was instructed on the benefits of condom use and advised to refrain from sexual activity until his infection resolves.

1. _____
2. _____
3. _____
4. _____
5. _____

Mr. L. is a 68-year-old male who presents to this office for his annual check-up. His blood test shows a slight elevation of the (6) *prostate tumor marker* test. He denies (7) *difficulty starting urination*, a (8) *need to void immediately*, or (9) *increased frequency of urination at night*. The digital rectal examination shows no evidence of nodules or lumps; however, there is a slight (10) *enlargement of the prostate*. Our diagnosis at this time is benign prostatic hypertrophy due to his age. He will be reexamined in 6 months.

6. _____
7. _____
8. _____
9. _____
10. _____

Check your answers in Appendix A. Review any material that you did not answer correctly.

Correct Answers _____ X 10 = _____ % Score

MEDICAL RECORD ACTIVITIES

The two medical records included in the following activities use common clinical scenarios to show how medical terminology is used to document patient care. Complete the terminology and analysis sections for each activity to help you recognize and understand terms related to the male reproductive system.

Medical Record Activity 13-1
Consultation Report: Benign Prostatic Hyperplasia

Terminology

Terms listed in the following table are taken from *Consultation Report: Benign Prostatic Hyperplasia* that follows. Use a medical dictionary such as *Taber's Cyclopedic Medical Dictionary;* the appendices of *Systems,* 7th ed.; or other resources to define each term. Then review the pronunciations for each term and practice by reading the medical record aloud.

Term	Definition
adhesions ăd-HĒ-zhŭnz	
benign bē-NĪN	
calculi KĂL-kū-lī	
catheter KĂTH-ĕ-tĕr	
culture and sensitivity KŬL-tūr, sĕn- sĭ-TĬV-ĭ-tē	
Darvocet DĂR-vō-sĕt	
Demerol DĔM-ĕ-rŏl	
dysuria dīs-Ū-rē-ă	
hematuria hē-mă-TŪ-rē-ă	
hernia HĔR-nē-ă	

(continued)

Term	Definition
hesitancy HĔS-ĭ-tăn-sē	
hyperlipidemia hī-pĕr-lĭp-ĭ-DĒ-mē-ă	
hyperplasia hī-pĕr-PLĀ-zē-ă	
incontinence ĭn-KŎNT-ĭn-ĕns	
Lipitor LĬP-ĭ-tor	
lysis LĪ-sĭs	
malignancies mă-LĬG-năn-sēz	
nocturia nŏk-TŪ-rē-ă	
Proscar PRŎS-kăr	
suprapubic soo-pră-PŪ-bĭk	

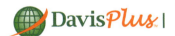

Visit the *Medical Terminology Systems* online resource center at Davis*Plus* to practice pronunciation and reinforce the meanings of the terms in this medical report.

CONSULTATION REPORT: BENIGN PROSTATIC HYPERPLASIA

General Hospital

1511 Ninth Avenue ■■ Sun City, USA 12345 ■■ (555) 802-1887

Patient: Smith, Milton   Consulting Physician: Richard Apper, MD
Birthdate: 05/10/xx   Patient ID#: 23-3444

CONSULTATION

DATE: 03/04/xx

REASON FOR CONSULTATION: Benign prostatic hyperplasia.

HISTORY OF PRESENT ILLNESS: This 82-year-old white male was admitted 03/04/xx for left inguinal hernia repair and ventral hernia repair. The patient has been seen by me in the past and is currently on Proscar. He had a Foley catheter in place postoperatively, which was removed this a.m., and since then, the patient has complained of dysuria, frequency, and a feeling of incomplete empty-ing with weak stream. The patient has a history of hesitancy, weak stream, and every 2-3 hour void-ing. He denies incontinence, nocturia, dysuria, hematuria, and only had microscopic hematuria and is being followed by me. History of urinary tract infection with catheter in the past. The patient recently voided 300 cc and then 250 cc again. He feels that he may have to void now. He has no history of any calculi or genitourinary malignancies.

PAST MEDICAL HISTORY: Benign prostatic hyperplasia and hyperlipidemia.

PAST SURGICAL HISTORY: Right inguinal hernia ×3, lysis of adhesions, ventral hernia repair as above.

SOCIAL HISTORY: Plus tobacco.

MEDICATIONS: Lipitor, Proscar, Demerol, and Darvocet.

ALLERGIES: No known drug allergies.

PHYSICAL EXAMINATION: Afebrile, and vital signs are stable. Urine output is good. Abdomen is soft, and there is plus suprapubic tenderness. The incision overlies the bladder area, and it is diffi-cult to assess for bladder distention. Rectal has a 4-5 cm prostate without nodules.

IMPRESSION: This is an 82-year-old white male with questionable urinary retention. Will hold on post-void residual check as patient is voiding well. Send a urinalysis and culture and sensitivity. Will pass a catheter if he has any difficulty voiding.

Richard Apper, MD
Richard Apper, MD

RC:kan

D: 03/04/xx
T: 03/05/xx

Analysis

1. What is the reason for the present admission?

_____

_____

2. What occurred when the Foley catheter was removed?

_____

_____

3. What did his previous history indicate regarding these symptoms?

_____

_____

4. Why was it difficult to assess for bladder distention?

_____

_____

5. Was there a definitive diagnosis identified in the impression?

_____

_____

6. What procedure will be performed if the patient has difficulty voiding?

_____

_____

Chart Note: Acute Epididymitis

Terminology

Terms listed in the following table are taken from *Chart Note: Acute Epididymitis* that follows. Use a medical dictionary such as *Taber's Cyclopedic Medical Dictionary;* the appendices of *Systems,* 7th ed.; or other resources to define each term. Then review the pronunciations for each term and practice by reading the medical record aloud.

Term	Definition
balanitis băl-ă-NĪ-tĭs	
erythematous ĕr-ĭ-THĔM-ă-tŭs	
hydrocele HĪ-drō-sēl	
hyperplasia hī-pĕr-PLĀ-zē-ă	
induration ĬN-dū-rā-shŭn	
inguinal ĬNG-gwĭ-năl	
meatus mē-Ā-tŭs	
prepuce PRĒ-pūs	
prostate-specific antigen PRŎS-tāt, ĂN-tĭ-jĕn	
scrotal SKRŌ-tăl	
torsion TOR-shŭn	

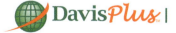

Visit the *Medical Terminology Systems* online resource center at Davis*Plus* to practice pronunciation and reinforce the meanings of the terms in this medical report.

CHART NOTE: ACUTE EPIDIDYMITIS

Homer, Aaron   **April 1, 20xx**
Age: 31

HISTORY OF PRESENT ILLNESS: Patient presents with complaints of severe left-sided groin pain, scrotal pain, and urethritis with a clear urethral discharge. He says it has developed over the last 2 days. He is sexually active, heterosexual, and says he had two sexual partners within the last month, the most recent being 4 days ago.

PHYSICAL EXAMINATION: The patient is uncircumcised and the prepuce is easily retractable. There are no observable lesions on the glans or shaft, and there is no balanitis. The urethral meatus is normal. A clear discharge is expressed upon compression of the glans and swabs are obtained for testing. The testes are descended bilaterally, smooth, and without masses. There is moderate pain and tenderness of the left testicle, which is alleviated with elevation of the testicles. There is no evidence of torsion of the spermatic cord. The scrotum is erythematous and there is a left-sided hydrocele. The left epididymis is palpable with significant induration and tenderness. The right epididymis is normal and nontender. No inguinal or femoral hernia is felt. There is enlargement of the left inguinal lymph nodes. Rectal examination reveals mild prostatic hyperplasia and tenderness. Urinalysis is positive for leukocytes and bacteria.

IMPRESSION: Acute epididymitis.

PLAN: Lab tests for chlamydia, gonorrhea, and prostate-specific antigen. Administer intravenous antibiotics, prescribe oral antibiotics and analgesics.

Julia Halm, MD
Julia Halm, MD

D: 04-01-20xx; T: 04-01-20xx

bcg

Analysis

Review the *Chart Note: Acute Epididymitis* to answer the following questions.

1. What were the complaints of the patient?

_____

_____

2. What procedure was performed regarding the urethral discharge?

_____

_____

3. What information is provided regarding the left testicle?

_____

_____

4. How was the left epididymis described?

_____

_____

5. What did the rectal examination reveal?

_____

_____

Endocrine System

CHAPTER

14

Chapter Outline

Objectives

Upon completion of this chapter, you will be able to:

- Locate and describe the structures of the endocrine system.
- Describe the functional relationship between the endocrine system and other body systems.
- Pronounce, spell, and build words related to the endocrine system.
- Describe diseases, conditions, and procedures related to the endocrine system.
- Explain pharmacology related to the treatment of endocrine disorders.
- Demonstrate your knowledge of this chapter by completing the learning and medical record activities.

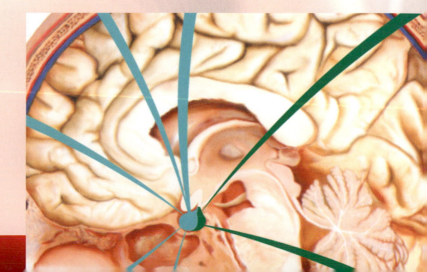

Anatomy and Physiology

The primary function of the endocrine system is to produce specialized chemicals called **hormones** that directly enter the bloodstream and travel to specific tissues or organs of the body called **targets.** Some hormonal actions cause short-term changes, such as a faster heartbeat or sweaty palms during a panic situation. Others control long-term changes, such as bone and muscle development. Still other hormones help maintain continuous body functions, such as a balance of body fluids, and a normal metabolism. The endocrine system also maintains an internal state of equilibrium in the body **(homeostasis)** so all body systems function effectively. The ductless glands of the endocrine system include the **pituitary, thyroid, parathyroid, adrenal, pancreatic, pineal,** and **thymus glands** as well as the **ovaries** and **testes.** (See Figure 14-1.)

Anatomy and Physiology Key Terms

This section lists important terms found in the anatomy and physiology section as well as their definitions and pronunciations.

Term	Definition
antagonistic ăn-TĂG-ō-nĭst-ĭk	Acting in opposition; mutually opposing
electrolyte ē-LĔK-trō-līt	Mineral salt (sodium, potassium, and calcium) that carries an electrical charge in solution *A proper balance of electrolytes is essential to the normal functioning of the entire body.*
glucagon GLOO-kă-gŏn	Hormone produced by pancreatic alpha cells that stimulates the liver to change stored glycogen (a starch form of sugar) to glucose *Glucagon opposes the action of insulin. It is used to reverse hypoglycemic reactions in insulin shock.*
glucose GLOO-kōs	Simple sugar that is the end product of carbohydrate digestion *Glucose is found in many foods, especially fruits, and is a major source of energy for living organisms. Analysis of blood glucose levels is an important diagnostic test in diabetes and other disorders.*
insulin ĬN-sŭ-lĭn	Hormone produced by pancreatic beta cells that allows body cells to use glucose for energy or store it in the liver as glycogen
sympathomimetic sĭm-pă-thō-mĭm-ĔT-ĭk	Agent that mimics the effects of the sympathetic nervous system *Epinephrine and norepinephrine are sympathomimetic hormones because they produce effects that mimic those brought about by the sympathetic nervous system.*

Pronunciation Help	Long Sound	ā — rate	ē — rebirth	ī — isle	ō — over	ū — unite
	Short Sound	ă — alone	ĕ — ever	ĭ — it	ŏ — not	ŭ — cut

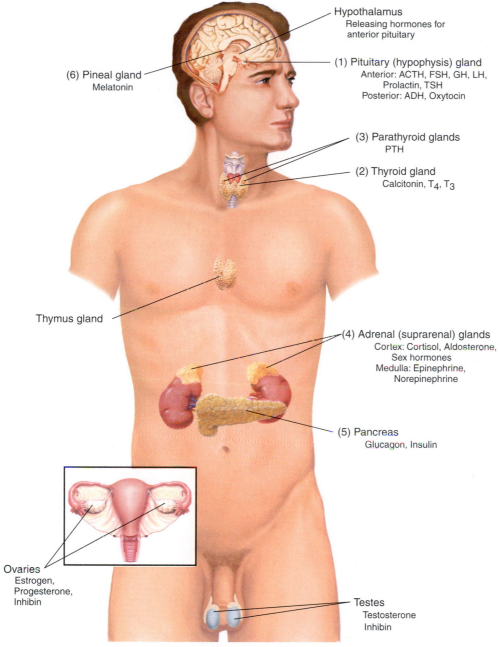

Hypothalamus
Releasing hormones for
anterior pituitary

(6) Pineal gland
Melatonin

(1) Pituitary (hypophysis) gland
Anterior: ACTH, FSH, GH, LH,
Prolactin, TSH
Posterior: ADH, Oxytocin

(3) Parathyroid glands
PTH

(2) Thyroid gland
Calcitonin, T_4, T_3

Thymus gland

(4) Adrenal (suprarenal) glands
Cortex: Cortisol, Aldosterone,
Sex hormones
Medulla: Epinephrine,
Norepinephrine

(5) Pancreas
Glucagon, Insulin

Ovaries
Estrogen,
Progesterone,
Inhibin

Testes
Testosterone
Inhibin

Figure 14-1 Locations of major endocrine glands.

Although hormones travel throughout the body in blood and lymph, they affect only the target tissues or organs that have specific receptors for the hormone. Once bound to the receptor, the hormone initiates a specific biological effect. For example, thyroid-stimulating hormone (TSH) binds to receptors on cells of the thyroid gland causing it to secrete thyroxine, but it does not bind to cells of the ovaries because ovarian cells do not have TSH receptors. Some hormones, such as insulin and thyroxine, have many target organs. Other hormones, such as calcitonin and some pituitary gland hormones, have only one or a few target organs. In general, hormones regulate growth, metabolism, reproduction, energy level, and sexual characteristics.

Pituitary Gland

The (1) **pituitary gland,** or **hypophysis**, is a pea-sized organ located at the base of the brain. It is known as the **master gland** because it regulates many body activities and stimulates other glands to secrete their own specific hormones. (See Figure 14-2.) The pituitary gland consists of two distinct portions, an anterior lobe **(adenohypophysis)** and a posterior lobe **(neurohypophysis).** The anterior lobe, triggered by the action of the hypothalamus, produces at least six hormones. The posterior lobe stores and secretes two hormones produced by the hypothalamus: antidiuretic hormone (ADH) and oxytocin. These hormones are released into the bloodstream as needed. (See Table 14-1.)

Thyroid Gland

The (2) **thyroid gland** is the largest gland of the endocrine system. An H-shaped organ located in the neck just below the larynx, this gland is composed of two large lobes that are separated by a strip of tissue called an **isthmus.** Thyroid hormone (TH) is the body's major metabolic hormone. TH increases the rate of oxygen consumption and, thus, the rate at which carbohydrates,

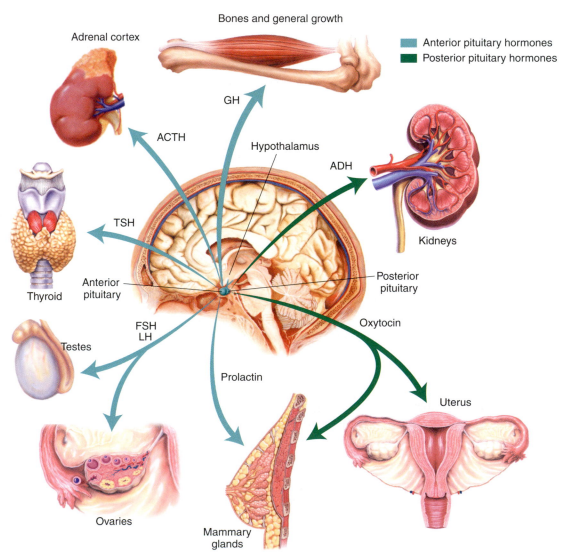

Figure 14-2 Hormones secreted by the anterior and posterior pituitary gland, along with target organs.

Table 14-1 **Pituitary Hormones**

This table identifies pituitary hormones, their target organs and functions, and associated disorders.

Hormone	Target Organ and Functions	Disorders
Anterior Pituitary Hormones (Adenohypophysis)		
Adrenocorticotropic hormone (ACTH)	• Adrenal cortex—promotes secretion of corticosteroids, especially cortisol	• Hyposecretion is rare. • Hypersecretion causes Cushing disease.
Follicle-stimulating hormone (FSH)	• Ovaries—in females, stimulates egg production (ova); increases secretion of estrogen • Testes—in males, stimulates sperm production	• Hyposecretion causes failure of sexual maturation. • Hypersecretion has no known significant effects.
Growth hormone (GH) or somatotropin	• Regulates growth of bone, muscle, and other body tissues • Increases use of fats for energy	• Hyposecretion during childhood and puberty causes pituitary dwarfism. • Hypersecretion during childhood and puberty causes gigantism; hypersecretion during adulthood causes acromegaly.
Luteinizing hormone (LH)	• Ovaries—in females, promotes ovulation; stimulates production of estrogen and progesterone • Testes—in males, promotes secretion of testosterone	• Hyposecretion in nursing mothers causes poor lactation. •Hyposecretion causes failure of sexual maturation. • Hypersecretion has no known significant effects.
Prolactin (PRL)	• Breast—in conjunction with other hormones, promotes lactation	• Hypersecretion in nursing mothers causes excessive secretion of milk (**galactorrhea**).
Thyroid-stimulating hormone (TSH) or thyrotropin	• Thyroid gland—stimulates secretion of thyroid hormones	• Hyposecretion in infants causes cretinism; hyposecretion in adults causes myxedema. • Hypersecretion causes Graves disease, which results in exophthalmos.
Posterior Pituitary Hormones (Neurohypophysis)		
Antidiuretic hormone (ADH)	• Kidney—increases water reabsorption (water returns to the blood)	• Hyposecretion causes diabetes insipidus (DI). • Hypersecretion causes syndrome of inappropriate antidiuretic hormone (SIADH).
Oxytocin	• Uterus—stimulates uterine contractions; initiates labor • Breast—promotes milk secretion from the mammary glands	• Unknown

proteins, and fats are metabolized. TH is actually two active iodine-containing hormones: **thyroxine (T_4)** and **triiodothyronine (T_3).** T_4 is the major hormone secreted by the thyroid; most T_3 is formed at the target tissues by conversion of T_4 to T_3. Except for the adult brain, spleen, testes, uterus, and the thyroid gland itself, thyroid hormone affects virtually every cell in the body. TH also influences growth hormone and plays an important role in maintaining blood pressure. (See Table 14-2.)

Table 14-2	**Thyroid Hormones**	
This table identifies thyroid hormones, their functions, and associated disorders.		
Hormone	**Target Organs and Functions**	**Disorders**
Calcitonin	• Regulates calcium levels in the blood in conjunction with parathyroid hormone • Decreases the reabsorption of calcium and phosphate from bones to blood	• The most significant effects are exerted in childhood when bones are growing and changing dramatically in mass, size, and shape. • At best, calcitonin is a weak hypocalcemic agent in adults.
Thyroxine (T_4) and triiodothyronine (T_3)	• Increases energy production from all food types • Increases rate of protein synthesis	• Hyposecretion in infants causes cretinism; hyposecretion in adults causes myxedema. • Hypersecretion causes Graves disease, which results in exophthalmos.

Parathyroid Glands

The (3) **parathyroid glands** consist of at least four separate glands located on the posterior surface of the lobes of the thyroid gland. The only hormone known to be secreted by the parathyroid glands is parathyroid hormone (PTH). PTH helps to regulate calcium balance by stimulating three target organs: bones, kidneys, and intestines. (See Table 14-3.) Because of PTH stimulation, calcium and phosphates are released from bones, increasing concentration of these substances in blood. Thus, calcium that is necessary for the proper functioning of body tissues is available in the bloodstream. At the same time, PTH enhances the absorption of calcium and phosphates from foods in the intestine, causing a rise in blood levels of calcium and phosphates. PTH causes the kidneys to conserve blood calcium and increase the excretion of phosphates in urine.

Table 14-3	**Parathyroid Hormones**	
This table identifies the target organs and functions of parathyroid hormone as well as disorders associated with it.		
Hormone	**Target Organ and Functions**	**Disorders**
Parathyroid hormone (PTH)	• Bones—increases the reabsorption of calcium and phosphate from bone to blood • Kidneys—increases calcium absorption and phosphate excretion • Small intestine—increases absorption of calcium and phosphate	• Hyposecretion causes tetany. • Hypersecretion causes osteitis fibrosa cystica.

Adrenal Glands

The (4) **adrenal glands** are paired organs covering the superior surface of the kidneys. Because of their location, the adrenal glands are also known as **suprarenal glands.** Each adrenal gland is divided into two sections, each having its own structure and function. The outer adrenal cortex makes up the bulk of the gland and the adrenal medulla makes up the inner portion. Although these regions are not sharply divided, they represent distinct glands that secrete different hormones.

Adrenal Cortex

The adrenal cortex secretes three types of steroid hormones:

1. **Mineralocorticoids,** mainly aldosterone, are essential to life. These hormones act mainly through the kidneys to maintain the balance of **electrolytes** (sodium and potassium) in the body. More specifically, aldosterone causes the kidneys to conserve sodium and excrete potassium (K). At the same time, it promotes water conservation by reducing urine output.
2. **Glucocorticoids,** mainly cortisol, influence the metabolism of carbohydrates, fats, and proteins. The glucocorticoid with the greatest activity is cortisol. It helps regulate the concentration of **glucose** in the blood, protecting against low blood sugar levels between meals. Cortisol also stimulates the breakdown of fats in adipose tissue and releases fatty acids into the blood. The increase in fatty acids causes many cells to use relatively less glucose.
3. **Sex hormones,** including androgens, estrogens, and progestins, help maintain secondary sex characteristics, such as development of the breasts in females and distribution of body hair in adults.

Adrenal Medulla

The cells of the adrenal medulla secrete two closely related hormones, epinephrine **(adrenaline)** and norepinephrine **(noradrenaline).** Both hormones are activated when the body responds to crisis situations, and are considered **sympathomimetic** agents because they produce effects that mimic those brought about by the sympathetic nervous system. Because hormones of the adrenal medulla merely intensify activities set into motion by the sympathetic nervous system, their deficiency does not cause dysfunction.

Of the two hormones, epinephrine is secreted in larger amounts. In the physiological response to stress, epinephrine is responsible for maintaining blood pressure and cardiac output, dilating airways, and raising blood glucose levels. All these functions are useful for frightened, traumatized, injured, or sick persons. Norepinephrine reduces the diameter of blood vessels in the periphery (vasoconstriction), thereby raising blood pressure. (See Table 14-4.)

Table 14-4	**Adrenal Hormones**	

This table identifies adrenal hormones, their target organs and functions, and associated disorders.

Hormone	Target Organ and Functions	Disorders
Adrenal Cortex Hormones		
Glucocorticoids (mainly cortisol)	• Body cells—promote gluconeogenesis; regulate metabolism of carbohydrates, proteins, and fats; and help depress inflammatory and immune responses	• Hyposecretion causes Addison disease. • Hypersecretion causes Cushing syndrome.
Mineralocorticoids (mainly aldosterone)	• Kidneys—increase blood levels of sodium and decrease blood levels of potassium in the kidneys	• Hyposecretion causes Addison disease. • Hypersecretion causes aldosteronism.
Sex hormones (any of the androgens, estrogens, or related steroid hormones produced by the ovaries, testes, and adrenal cortices)	• In females, possibly responsible for female libido and source of estrogen after menopause (otherwise, insignificant effects in adults)	• Hypersecretion of adrenal androgen in females leads to virilism (development of male secondary sex characteristics). • Hypersecretion of adrenal estrogen and progestin secretion in males leads to feminization (development of female secondary sex characteristics). • Hyposecretion has no known significant effect.
Adrenal Medullary Hormones		
Epinephrine and norepinephrine	• Sympathetic nervous system target organs—hormone effects mimic sympathetic nervous system activation (sympathomimetic), increase metabolic rate and heart rate, and raise blood pressure by promoting vasoconstriction	• Hyposecretion has no known significant effect. • Hypersecretion causes prolonged "fight-or-flight" reaction and hypertension.

Pancreas

The (5) **pancreas** lies inferior to the stomach in a bend of the duodenum. It functions as an exocrine and endocrine gland. In its exocrine role, it carries digestive secretions from the pancreas to the small intestine through a large pancreatic duct. The digestive secretions assist in the break-down of proteins, starches, and fats in the small intestine. In its endocrine role, the pancreas secretes two other hormones through the **islets of Langerhans: glucagon**, which is produced by the alpha cells, and **insulin**, which is produced by the beta cells. Both hormones play important roles in regulating blood glucose (sugar) levels:

- **Glucagon** stimulates the release of glucose from storage sites in the liver when blood glucose levels are low **(hypoglycemia),** thereby raising the blood glucose level.
- **Insulin** clears glucose molecules from the blood by promoting their storage in tissues as carbohydrates when blood glucose levels are high **(hyperglycemia),** thereby lowering the blood glucose level and enabling the cells to use glucose for energy.

Insulin and glucagon function **antagonistically**, so that normal secretion of both hormones ensures a blood glucose level that fluctuates within normal limits. (See Table 14-5.)

Table 14-5	**Pancreatic Hormones**	
This table identifies pancreatic hormones, their target organs and functions, and associated disorders.		
Hormone	**Target Organ and Functions**	**Disorders**
Glucagon	• Liver and blood—raises the blood glucose level by accelerating conversion of glycogen into glucose in the liver (glycogenolysis) and other nutrients into glucose in the liver (gluconeogenesis) and releasing glucose into blood (glycogen to glucose)	• A deficiency in glucagon may cause persistently low blood glucose levels (hypoglycemia).
Insulin	• Tissue cells—lowers blood glucose level by accelerating glucose transport into cells and the use of that glucose for energy production (glucose to glycogen)	• Hyposecretion of insulin causes diabetes mellitus. • Hypersecretion of insulin causes hyperinsulinism.

Pineal Gland

The (6) **pineal gland,** which is shaped like a pine cone, is attached to the posterior part of the third ventricle of the brain. Although the exact functions of this gland have not been established, there is evidence that it secretes the hormone melatonin. It is believed that melatonin may inhibit the activities of the ovaries. When melatonin production is high, ovulation is blocked, and there may be a delay in puberty.

Anatomy Review

To review the anatomy of the endocrine system, label the following illustration using the terms listed below.

adrenal (suprarenal) glands   *parathyroid glands*   *testes*

ovaries   *pineal gland*   *thymus gland*

pancreas   *pituitary (hypophysis) gland* *thyroid gland*

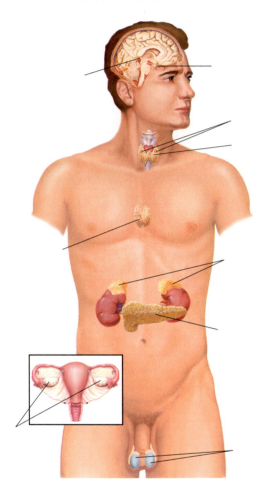

 Check your answers by referring to Figure 14–1 on page 461. Review material that you did not answer correctly.

CONNECTING BODY SYSTEMS—ENDOCRINE SYSTEM

The main function of the endocrine system is to secrete hormones that have a diverse effect on cells, tissues, organs, and organ systems. Specific functional relationships between the endocrine system and other body systems are summarized below.

Blood, Lymph, and Immune

- Hormones from the thymus stimulate lymphocyte production.
- Glucocorticoids depress the immune response and inflammation.

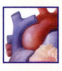

Cardiovascular

- Hormones influence heart rate, contraction strength, blood volume, and blood pressure.
- Estrogen helps maintain vascular health in women.

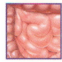

Digestive

- Hormones help control digestive system activity.
- Hormones influence motility and glandular activity of the digestive tract, gallbladder secretion, and secretion of enzymes from the pancreas.
- Insulin and glucagon adjust glucose metabolism in the liver.

Female Reproductive

- Hormones play a major role in the development and function of the reproductive organs.
- Hormones influence the menstrual cycle, pregnancy, parturition, and lactation.
- Sex hormones play a major role in the development of secondary sex characteristics.
- Hormone oxytocin triggers contraction of the pregnant uterus and then later stimulates the release of breast milk.

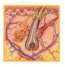

Integumentary

- Hormones regulate activity of the sebaceous glands, distribution of subcutaneous tissue, and hair growth.
- Hormones stimulate melanocytes to produce skin pigment.
- Hormone estrogen increases skin hydration.

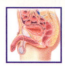

Male Reproductive

- Hormones play a major role in the development and function of the reproductive organs.
- Sex hormones play a major role in the development of secondary sex characteristics.
- Hormones play a role in sexual development, sex drive, and sperm production.

Musculoskeletal

- Hormone secretions influence blood flow to muscles during exercise.
- Hormones influence muscle metabolism, mass, and strength.
- Hormones from the pituitary and thyroid glands and the gonads stimulate bone growth.
- Hormones govern blood calcium balance.

Nervous

- Several hormones play an important role in the normal maturation and function of the nervous system.

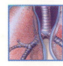

Respiratory

- Hormones stimulate red blood cell production when the body experiences a decrease in oxygen.
- Epinephrine influences ventilation by dilating the bronchioles; epinephrine and thyroxine stimulate cell respiration.

Urinary

- Hormones regulate water and electrolyte balance in the kidneys.

Medical Word Elements

This section introduces combining forms, suffixes, and prefixes related to the endocrine system. Word analyses are also provided.

Element	Meaning	Word Analysis
Combining Forms		
adren/o	adrenal glands	**adren/o**/megaly (ăd-rēn-ō-MĔG-ă-lē): enlargement of adrenal glands *-megaly:* enlargement
adrenal/o		**adrenal**/ectomy (ăd-rē-năl-ĔK-tō-mē): excision of (one or both) adrenal glands *-ectomy:* excision, removal
calc/o	calcium	hyper/**calc**/emia (hī-pĕr-kăl-SĒ-mē-ă): excessive calcium in the blood *hyper-:* excessive, above normal *-emia:* blood condition
crin/o	secrete	endo/**crin/o**/logy (ĕn-dō-krĭn-ŎL-ō-jē): study of endocrine glands (and their functions) *endo-:* in, within *-logy:* study of
gluc/o	sugar, sweetness	**gluc/o**/genesis (gloo-kō-JĔN-ĕ-sĭs): forming or producing glucose *-genesis:* forming, producing, origin
glyc/o		hypo/**glyc**/emia (hī-pō-glī-SĒ-mē-ă): abnormally low level of glucose in the blood *hypo-:* under, below *-emia:* blood condition *Hypoglycemia is usually caused by administration of too much insulin, excessive secretion of insulin by the islet cells of the pancreas, or dietary deficiency.*
glycos/o		**glycos**/uria (glī-kō-SŪ-rē-ă): abnormal amount of glucose in the urine *-uria:* urine
home/o	same, alike	**home/o**/stasis (hō-mē-ō-STĀ-sĭs): state of equilibrium in the internal environment of the body *-stasis:* standing still
kal/i	potassium (an electrolyte)	**kal**/emia (kă-LĒ-mē-ă): potassium in the blood *-emia:* blood condition
pancreat/o	pancreas	**pancreat/o**/tomy (păn-krē-ă-TŎT-ō-mē): incision of the pancreas *-tomy:* incision
parathyroid/o	parathyroid glands	**parathyroid**/ectomy (păr-ă-thī-royd-ĔK-tō-mē): excision of (one or more of the) parathyroid glands *-ectomy:* excision, removal
thym/o	thymus gland	**thym**/oma (thī-MŌ-mă): tumor of the thymus gland *-oma:* tumor *A thymoma is a rare neoplasm of the thymus gland. Treatment includes surgical removal, radiation therapy, or chemotherapy.*

Element	Meaning	Word Analysis
thyr/o	thyroid gland	**thyr/o**/megaly (thī-rō-MĔG-ă-lē): enlargement of the thyroid gland *-megaly:* enlargement
thyroid/o		hyper/**thyroid**/ism (hī-pĕr-THĪ-royd-ĭzm): condition of excessive thyroid gland (function) *hyper-:* excessive, above normal *-ism:* condition
toxic/o	poison	**toxic/o**/logist (tŏks-ĭ-KŎL-ō-jĭst): specialist in the study of poisons *-logist:* specialist in the study of *Toxicologists also study the effects of toxins and antidotes used for treatment of toxic disorders.*

Suffixes

Element	Meaning	Word Analysis
-crine	secrete	endo/**crine** (ĔN-dō-krĭn): secrete within *endo-:* in, within
-dipsia	thirst	poly/**dipsia** (pŏl-ē-DĬP-sē-ă): excessive thirst *poly-:* many, much *Polydipsia is one of the three "polys" (as well as* **polyphagia** *and* **polyuria***) associated with diabetes.*
-gen	forming, producing, origin	andr/o/**gen** (ĂN-drō-jĕn): any steroid hormone that increases masculinization *andr/o:* male
-toxic	pertaining to poison	thyr/o/**toxic** (thī-rō-TŎKS-ĭk): pertaining to poison (associated with) the thyroid gland *thyr/o:* thyroid gland
-uria	urine	glycos/**uria** (glī-kō-SŪ-rē-ă): glucose in the urine *glycos:* sugar, sweetness

Prefixes

Element	Meaning	Word Analysis
eu-	good, normal	**eu**/thyr/oid (ū-THĪ-royd): resembling a normal thyroid gland *thyr/o:* thyroid gland *-oid:* resembling
exo-	outside, outward	**exo**/crine (ĔKS-ō-krĭn): secretes outside (of bloodstream) *-crine:* secrete *Exocrine glands (sweat and oil glands) secrete their products outwardly through excretory ducts. Endocrine glands are ductless glands that secrete their hormones directly into the bloodstream.*
hyper-	excessive, above normal	**hyper**/glyc/emia (hī-pĕr-glī-SĒ-mē-ă): excessive glucose in the blood *glyc:* sugar, sweetness *-emia:* blood condition *Abnormally high blood glucose levels are found in patients with diabetes mellitus or those treated with such drugs as prednisone.*

(continued)

Element	Meaning	Word Analysis
hypo-	under, below	**hypo**/insulin/ism (hī-pō-ĬN-sŭ-lĭn-ĭzm): condition of deficiency of insulin *-ism:* condition *Hypoinsulinism is a characteristic of type 1 diabetes mellitus.*
poly-	many, much	**poly**/uria (pŏl-ē-Ū-rē-ă): excessive urination *-uria:* urine *Some causes of polyuria are diabetes, use of diuretics, excessive fluid intake, and hypercalcemia.*

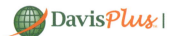 Visit the *Medical Terminology Systems* online resource center at Davis*Plus* for an audio exercise of the terms in this table. Other activities are also available to reinforce content.

 It is time to review medical word elements by completing Learning Activities 14-1 and 14-2.

Pathology

Disorders of the endocrine system are caused by underproduction **(hyposecretion)** or overproduction **(hypersecretion)** of hormones. In general, hyposecretion is treated with drug therapy in the form of hormone replacement. Hypersecretion is generally treated by surgery. Most hormone deficiencies result from genetic defects in the glands, surgical removal of the glands, or production of poor-quality hormones.

For diagnosis, treatment, and management of endocrine disorders, the medical services of a specialist may be warranted. **Endocrinology** is the branch of medicine concerned with endocrine disorders. The physician who specializes in diagnoses and treatment of endocrine disorders is known as an **endocrinologist.**

Pituitary Disorders

Pituitary disorders are related to hypersecretion or hyposecretion of **growth hormone (GH),** which leads to body-size abnormalities. Abnormal variations of **antidiuretic hormone (ADH)** makes it more difficult for the body to remove water. This causes fluid to build up in the body and also low blood sodium levels **(hyponatremia)** can occur. An ADH test is used to aid in the diagnosis of diabetes insipidus or the syndrome of inappropriate antidiruretic hormone (SIADH).

Thyroid Disorders

Thyroid gland disorders are common and may occur at any time during life. They may be the result of a developmental problem, injury, disease, or dietary deficiency. One form of hypothyroidism that develops in infants is called **cretinism.** If not treated, this disorder leads to mental retardation, impaired growth, low body temperatures, and abnormal bone formation. Usually these symptoms do not appear at birth because the infant has received thyroid hormones from the mother's blood during fetal development. When hypothyroidism develops during adulthood, it is known as **myxedema.** The signs and symptoms of this disease include edema, low blood levels of T_3 and T_4, weight gain, cold intolerance, fatigue, depression, muscle or joint pain, and sluggishness.

Hyperthyroidism results from excessive secretions of T_3, T_4, or both. Two of the most common disorders of hyperthyroidism are Graves disease and toxic goiter. **Graves disease** is considerably more prevalent with signs and symptoms of an elevated metabolic rate, abnormal weight loss, excessive perspiration, muscle weakness, and emotional instability. Also, the eyes are likely to protrude **(exophthalmos)** because of edematous swelling in the tissues behind them. (See Figure 14-3.) At the same time, the thyroid gland is likely to enlarge, producing **goiter.** (See Figure 14-4.)

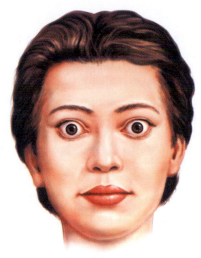

Figure 14-3 Exophthalmos caused by Graves disease.

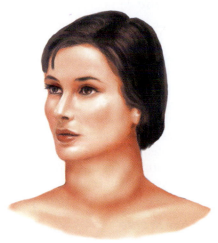

Figure 14-4 Enlargement of the thyroid gland in goiter.

It is believed that **toxic goiter** may occur because of excessive release of thyroid-stimulating hormone (TSH) from the anterior lobe of the pituitary gland. Overstimulation by TSH causes thyroid cells to enlarge and secrete extra amounts of hormones. Treatment for **hyperthyroidism** may involve drug therapy to block the production of thyroid hormones or surgical removal of all or part of the thyroid gland. Another method for treating this disorder is to administer a sufficient amount of radioactive iodine to destroy the thyroid secretory cells.

Parathyroid Disorders

As with the thyroid gland, dysfunction of the parathyroids is usually characterized by inadequate or excessive hormone secretion. Insufficient production of parathyroid hormone (PTH), called **hypoparathyroidism,** may be caused by primary parathyroid dysfunction or elevated blood calcium levels. This condition can result from an injury or from surgical removal of the glands, sometimes in conjunction with thyroid surgery. The primary effect of hypoparathyroidism is a decreased blood calcium level **(hypocalcemia).** Decreased calcium causes muscle twitches and spasms **(tetany).**

Excessive production of PTH, called **hyperparathyroidism,** is commonly caused by a benign tumor. The increase in PTH secretion leads to demineralization of bones **(osteitis fibrosa cystica),** making them porous **(osteoporosis)** and highly susceptible to fracture and deformity. When this condition is the result of a benign glandular tumor **(adenoma)** of the parathyroid, the tumor is removed. Excess PTH also causes calcium deposits in the kidneys. When the disease is generalized and all bones are affected, this disorder is known as *von Recklinghausen* **disease.** Renal symptoms and kidney stones **(nephrolithiasis)** may also develop.

Adrenal Gland Disorders

The adrenal cortex and adrenal medulla have their own structures and functions as well as their own sets of associated disorders.

Adrenal Cortex

The adrenal cortex is mainly associated with Addison disease and Cushing syndrome.

Addison Disease

Addison disease, a relatively uncommon chronic disorder caused by a deficiency of cortical hormones, results when the adrenal cortex is damaged or atrophied. Atrophy of the adrenal glands is probably the result of an autoimmune process in which circulating adrenal antibodies slowly destroy the gland. The gland usually suffers 90% destruction before clinical signs of adrenal insufficiency appear. Hypofunction of the adrenal cortex interferes with the body's ability to handle internal and external stress. In severe cases, the disturbance of sodium and potassium metabolism may be marked by depletion of sodium and water through urination, resulting in severe chronic dehydration. Other clinical manifestations include muscle weakness, anorexia, gastrointestinal symptoms, fatigue, hypoglycemia, hypotension, low blood sodium **(hyponatremia),** and high serum potassium **(hyperkalemia).** If treatment for this condition begins early (usually with adrenocortical hormone therapy), the prognosis is excellent. If untreated, the disease will continue a chronic course with progressive but relatively slow deterioration. In some patients, the deterioration may be rapid.

Cushing Syndrome

Cushing syndrome is a cluster of symptoms produced by excessive amounts of cortisol, adrenocorticotropic hormone (ACTH), or both circulating in the blood. (See Figure 14-5.)

Causes of this excess secretion include:

- long-term administration of steroid drugs (glucocorticoids) in treating such diseases as rheumatoid arthritis, lupus erythematosus, and asthma
- adrenal tumor, resulting in excessive production of cortisol
- Cushing disease, a pituitary disorder caused by hypersecretion of ACTH from an adenoma in the anterior pituitary gland.

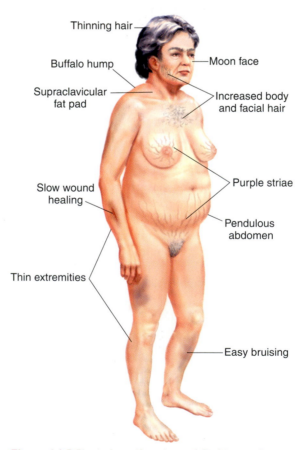

Figure 14-5 Physical manifestations of Cushing syndrome.

Regardless of the cause, Cushing syndrome alters carbohydrate and protein metabolism and electrolyte balance. Overproduction of mineralocorticoids and glucocorticoids causes blood glucose concentration to remain high, depleting tissue protein. In addition, sodium retention causes increased fluid in tissues, leading to edema. These metabolic changes produce weight gain and may cause structural changes, such as a moon-shaped face, grossly exaggerated head and trunk, and pencil-thin arms and legs. Other symptoms include fatigue, high blood pressure, and excessive hair growth in unusual places **(hirsutism),** especially in women. The treatment goal for this disease is to restore serum cortisol to normal levels. Nevertheless, treatment varies with the cause and may necessitate radiation, drug therapy, surgery, or a combination of these methods.

Adrenal Medulla

No specific diseases can be traced directly to a deficiency of hormones from the adrenal medulla. However, medullary tumors sometimes cause excess secretions. The most common disorder is a neoplasm known as **pheochromocytoma,** which produces excessive amounts of epinephrine and norepinephrine. Most of these tumors are encapsulated and benign. These hypersecretions produce high blood pressure, rapid heart rate, stress, fear, palpitations, headaches, visual blurring, muscle spasms, and sweating. Typical treatment consists of antihypertensive drugs and surgery.

Pancreatic Disorders

Diabetes is a general term that, when used alone, refers to diabetes mellitus (DM). It is by far the most common pancreatic disorder. DM is a chronic metabolic disorder of impaired carbohydrate, protein, and fat metabolism due to insufficient production of insulin or the body's inability to use insulin properly. When body cells are deprived of glucose, their principal energy fuel, they begin to metabolize proteins and fats. Fat metabolism produces ketones, which enter the blood, causing a condition called **ketosis.** Hyperglycemia and ketosis are responsible for the host of troubling and, commonly, life-threatening symptoms of diabetes mellitus. (See Table 14-6.)

Insulin is an essential hormone that prepares body cells to absorb and use glucose as an energy source. When insulin is lacking, sugar does not enter cells but returns to the bloodstream with a subsequent rise in its concentration in the blood **(hyperglycemia).** When blood glucose levels elevate beyond a level tolerated by the kidneys, glucose "spills" into the urine **(glucosuria)** and is expelled from the body along with electrolytes, particularly sodium. Sodium and potassium losses

Table 14-6	**Clinical Manifestations of Diabetes**

According to the American Diabetes Association, the following signs and symptoms are manifestations of type 1 and type 2 diabetes.

Type 1 Diabetes

Type 1 diabetes may be suspected if any one of the associated signs and symptoms appears. Children usually exhibit dramatic, sudden symptoms and must receive prompt treatment. Signs and symptoms that signal type 1 diabetes can be remembered using the mnemonic **CAUTION** as outlined below. Type 1 diabetes is characterized by the sudden appearance of:

• **C**onstant urination (polyuria) and glycosuria

• **A**bnormal thirst (polydipsia)

• **U**nusual hunger (polyphagia)

• **T**he rapid loss of weight

• **I**rritability

• **O**bvious weakness and fatigue

• **N**ausea and vomiting.

(continued)

Table 14-6	Clinical Manifestations of Diabetes—cont'd

Type 2 Diabetes

Many adults may have type 2 diabetes with none of the associated signs or symptoms. The disease is commonly discovered during a routine physical examination. In addition to any of the signs and symptoms associated with type 1 diabetes, those for type 2 diabetes can be remembered using the acronym *DIABETES*:

• **D**rowsiness

• **I**tching

• **A** family history of diabetes

• **B**lurred vision

• **E**xcessive weight

• **T**ingling, numbness, and pain in the extremities

• **E**asily fatigued

• **S**kin infections and slow healing of cuts and scratches, especially of the feet.

result in muscle weakness and fatigue. Because glucose is unavailable to cells, cellular starvation results and leads to hunger and an increased appetite **(polyphagia).**

Although genetics and environmental factors, such as obesity and lack of exercise, seem significant in the development of this disease, the cause of diabetes is not always clear. Diabetes mellitus occurs in two primary forms: type 1 and type 2.

Type 1 Diabetes

Type 1 diabetes is usually diagnosed in children and young adults. In type 1 diabetes, the body does not produce sufficient insulin. Treatment consists of a balanced diet, exercise, and insulin. Daily injections of insulin are commonly required to maintain a normal blood glucose level.

The patient monitors his blood glucose levels several times a day to determine the amount of insulin he requires. To determine the need for insulin injections, the patient pricks the skin to draw a blood sample and places it in a **glucometer.** This instrument determines the amount of sugar in the blood sample so that insulin can be injected if needed. Insulin injections should be administered in a different subcutaneous site each time to avoid injury to the tissues. A sample rotation chart is shown in Figure 14-6.

Besides injecting insulin into the abdomen, thighs, buttocks, or arms, type 1 diabetics who desire tighter control of blood glucose levels may choose to use an **insulin pump.** (See Figure 14-7.) This small device administers insulin via a portable pump, which infuses insulin continuously in small (basal) amounts through an indwelling needle under the skin. Basal insulin is delivered continuously over 24 hours and mimics the normal pancreatic secretion. The patient can also add a bolus of insulin with the push of a button before meals or snacks. This provides insulin levels to cover a specific amount of starch or sugar that will be ingested.

Type 2 Diabetes

Type 2 diabetes is the most common form and is distinctively different from type 1. Its onset is typically later in life; however, it has become more prevalent in children as the incidence of obesity has increased. Risk factors include a family history of diabetes and obesity. In type 2 diabetes, the body is deficient in producing sufficient insulin or the body's cells are resistant to insulin action in target tissues. Hyperglycemia that results may damage the kidneys, eyes, nerves, or heart. Treatment for type 2 diabetes includes exercise, diet, weight loss, and, if needed, insulin or oral antidiabetic agents. Oral antidiabetic agents activate the release of pancreatic insulin and improve the body's sensitivity to insulin.

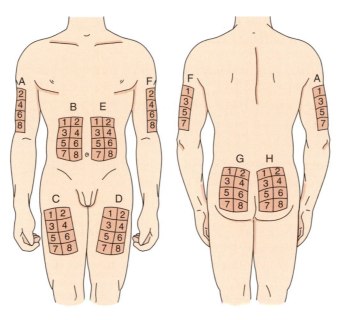

Rotation sites for injection of insulin.

Figure 14-6 Rotation sites for injection of insulin. From Williams and Hopper: *Understanding Medical-Surgical Nursing,* 4th ed. FA Davis, Philadelphia, 2011, p 922, with permission.

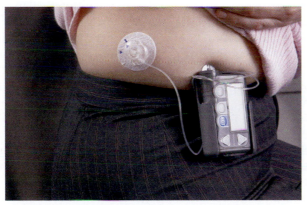

Figure 14-7 Insulin pump attached to the abdomen. From Williams and Hopper: *Understanding Medical-Surgical Nursing,* 4th ed. FA Davis, Philadelphia, 2011, p 923, with permission.

Complications

Diabetes is associated with a number of primary and secondary complications. Patients with type 1 diabetes usually report rapidly developing symptoms. With type 2 diabetes, the patient's symptoms are commonly vague, long standing, and develop gradually.

Primary complications of type 1 diabetes include **diabetic ketoacidosis (DKA).** DKA, also referred to as **diabetic acidosis** or **diabetic coma,** may develop over several days or weeks. It can be caused by too little insulin, failure to follow a prescribed diet, physical or emotional stress, or undiagnosed diabetes.

Secondary complications due to long-standing diabetes emerge years after the initial diagnosis **(Dx, dx).** Common chronic complications include diabetic retinopathy and diabetic nephropathy. In diabetic retinopathy, the retina's blood vessels are destroyed, causing vision loss and, eventually, blindness. In diabetic nephropathy, destruction of the kidneys causes renal insufficiency and commonly requires hemodialysis or renal transplantation.

Gestational diabetes may occur in women who are not diabetic, but develop diabetes during pregnancy. That is, they develop an inability to metabolize carbohydrates (glucose intolerance) with resultant hyperglycemia. Gestational diabetes most often resolves after childbirth (parturition). This places women at risk of developing type 2 diabetes.

Oncology

Oncological disorders of the endocrine system vary based on the organ involved and include pancreatic cancer, pituitary tumors, and thyroid carcinoma.

Pancreatic Cancer

Most carcinomas of the pancreas arise as epithelial tumors **(adenocarcinomas)** and make their presence known by obstruction and local invasion. Because the pancreas is richly supplied with nerves, pain is a prominent feature of pancreatic cancer, whether it arises in the head, body, or tail of the organ.

The prognosis in pancreatic cancer is poor, with only a 2% survival rate in 5 years. Pancreatic cancer is the fourth leading cause of cancer death in the United States. The highest incidence is among people ages 60 to 70. The etiology is unknown, but cigarette smoking, exposure to occupational chemicals, a diet high in fats, and heavy coffee intake are associated with an increased incidence of pancreatic cancer.

Pituitary Tumors

Pituitary tumors are abnormal growths that develop in the pituitary gland. Some pituitary tumors cause excessive production of hormones that regulate important functions of the body. Other pituitary tumors can restrict normal function of the pituitary gland, causing it to produce lower levels of hormones. The vast majority of pituitary tumors are noncancerous **(benign)** growths known as **adenomas.** Adenomas remain confined to the pituitary gland or surrounding tissues and do not spread to other parts of the body. As the tumor grows, it can cause a variety of symptoms including compression of nearby nerves, resulting in vision problems. Treatment involves removing the tumor, especially if it is pressing on the optic nerves, which could cause blindness. Pituitary tumors are frequently removed through the nose and sphenoid sinuses **(transsphenoidal hypophysectomy).** Other treatment modalities include restoring normal hormone levels or radiation therapy to shrink the tumor. These treatments are used either in combination with surgery or for patients who cannot tolerate surgery.

Thyroid Carcinoma

Cancer of the thyroid gland, or **thyroid carcinoma,** is classified according to the specific tissue that is affected. In general, however, all types share many predisposing factors, including radiation, prolonged TSH stimulation, familial disposition, and chronic goiter. The malignancy usually begins with a painless, commonly hard nodule or a nodule in the adjacent lymph nodes accompanied with an enlarged thyroid. When the tumor is large, it typically destroys thyroid tissue, which results in symptoms of hypothyroidism. Sometimes the tumor stimulates the production of thyroid hormone, resulting in symptoms of hyperthyroidism. Treatment includes surgical removal, radiation, or both.

Diseases and Conditions

This section introduces diseases and conditions of the endocrine system with their meanings and pronunciations. Word analyses for selected terms are also provided.

Term	Definition
acromegaly ăk-rō-MĔG-ă-lē *acr/o:* extremity *-megaly:* enlargement	Rare hormonal disorder in adulthood, usually caused by a GH-secreting pituitary tumor (adenoma) that promotes the soft tissue and bones of the face, hands, and feet to grow larger than normal *Treatment includes radiation, pharmacological agents, or surgery, to supress secretion of GH. This surgery involves partial resection of the pituitary gland.*
diuresis dī-ū-RĒ-sĭs *di-:* double *ur:* urine *-esis:* condition	Increased formation and secretion of urine *Diuresis occurs in such conditions as diabetes mellitus, diabetes insipidus, and acute renal failure. Alcohol and coffee are common diuretics that increase formation and secretion of urine.*
glycosuria glī-kō-SŪ-rē-ă *glycos:* sugar, sweetness *-uria:* urine	Abnormal amount of glucose in the urine
Graves disease	Multisystem autoimmune disorder characterized by pronounced hyperthyroidism usually associated with enlarged thyroid gland (goiter) and exophthalmos (abnormal protrusion of the eyeball)
hirsutism HĬR-sū-tĭzm	Excessive distribution of body hair, especially in women *Hirsutism in women is usually caused by abnormalities of androgen production or metabolism.*
hypercalcemia hī-pĕr-kăl-SĒ-mē-ă *hyper-:* excessive, above normal *calc:* calcium *-emia:* blood	Condition in which the calcium level in the blood is higher than normal *The main cause of hypercalcemia is overactivity in one or more parathyroid glands (which regulate blood calcium levels). Other causes include cancer, other medical disorders, medications, and excessive use of calcium and vitamin D supplements.*
hyperkalemia hī-pĕr-kă-LĒ-mē-ă *hyper-:* excessive, above normal *kal:* potassium (an electrolyte) *-emia:* blood	Condition in which the potassium level in the blood is higher than normal *Potassium is a critical nutrient in the proper functioning of nerve and muscle cells, including the heart. It is also important for normal transmission of electrical signals throughout the nervous system. Severe hyperkalemia requires immediate treatment because it is a potentially life-threatening illness that can lead to cardiac arrest and death.*
hypervolemia hī-pĕr-vŏl-Ē-mē-ă *hyper-:* excessive, above normal *vol:* volume *-emia:* blood	Abnormal increase in the volume of blood plasma (liquid part of the blood and lymphatic fluid) in the body *Hypervolemia commonly results from retention of large amounts of sodium and water by the kidneys.*

(continued)

Term	Definition
hyponatremia hī-pō-nă-TRĒ-mē-ă *hypo-:* under, below, deficient *natr:* sodium (an electrolyte) *-emia:* blood	Lower than normal level of sodium in the blood *Hyponatremia is caused by an excessive amount of fluid in the body, thereby diluting the amount of sodium when exercising (especially in the heat) without replacing the water and electrolytes lost through perspiration.*
insulinoma ĭn-sū-lĭn-Ō-mă *insulin:* insulin *-oma:* tumor	Tumor of the islets of Langerhans of the pancreas
obesity ō-BĒ-sĭ-tē	Excessive accumulation of fat that exceeds the body's skeletal and physical standards, usually an increase of 20 percent or more above ideal body weight *Obesity may be due to excessive intake of food (exogenous) or metabolic or endocrine abnormalities (endogenous).*
morbid obesity ō-BĒ-sĭ-tē	Body mass index (BMI) of 40 or greater, which is generally 100 or more pounds over ideal body weight *Morbid obesity is a disease with serious psychological, social, and medical ramifications and one that threatens necessary body functions such as respiration.*
panhypopituitarism păn-hī-pō-pĭ-TŪ-ĭ-tăr-ĭzm *pan-:* all *hyp/o:* under, below, deficient *pituitar:* pituitary gland *-ism:* condition	Total pituitary impairment that brings about a progressive and general loss of hormone activity
pheochromocytoma fē-ō-krō-mō-sī-TŌ-mă	Small chromaffin cell tumor, usually located in the adrenal medulla, causing elevated heart rate and blood *Pheochromocytoms may be life threatening if not treated.*
thyroid storm THĪ-royd *thyr:* thyroid gland *-oid:* resembling	Crisis of uncontrolled hyperthyroidism caused by the release into the bloodstream of an increased amount of thyroid hormone; also called *thyroid crisis* or *thyrotoxic crisis* *Thyroid storm may occur spontaneously or be precipitated by infection, stress, or thyroidectomy performed on a patient who is inadequately prepared with antithyroid drugs. Thyroid storm is considered a medical emergency and, if left untreated, may be fatal.*
virilism VĬR-ĭl-ĭzm	Masculinization or development of male secondary sex characteristics in a woman

 It is time to review diseases and conditions by completing Learning Activity 14–3.

Medical, Surgical, and Diagnostic Procedures

Procedure	Description
Medical	

exophthalmometry
ĕk-sŏf-thăl-MŎM-ĕ-trē
  ex-: out, out from
  ophthalm/o: eye
  -metry: act of measuring
	Measures the degree of forward displacement of the eyeball (exophthalmos) as seen in Graves disease
	Exophthalmometry is performed with an instrument called an exophthalmometer, *which enables measurement of the distance from the center of the cornea to the lateral orbital rim.*

Surgical	

parathyroidectomy
păr-ă-thī-royd-ĔK-tō-mē
  para-: near, beside; beyond
  thyroid: thyroid gland
  -ectomy: excision, removal
	Excision of one or more of the parathyroid glands, usually to control hyperparathyroidism

transsphenoidal hypophysectomy trăns-sfē-NOY-dăl hī-pŏf-ĭ-SĔK-tō-mē	Endoscopic procedure to surgically remove a pituitary tumor through an incision in the sphenoid sinus (transsphenoidal) without disturbing brain tissue (See Figure 14-8.) *This is a minimally invasive procedure commonly performed to remove abnormal pituitary gland tissue or pituitary tumors. It is also performed to treat Cushing syndrome due to a pituitary tumor.*

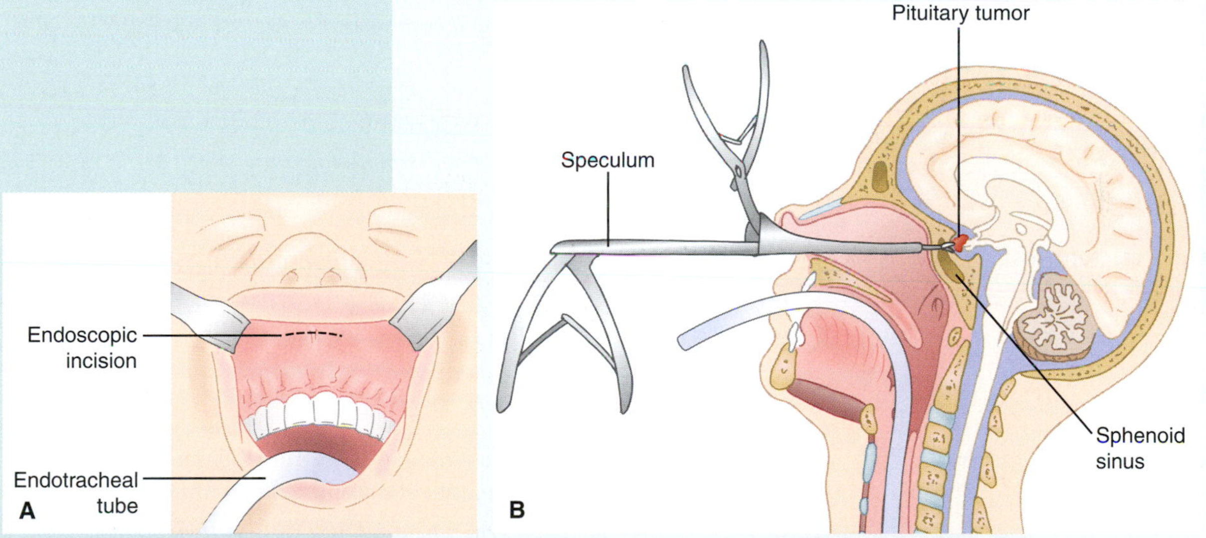

Figure 14-8 Hypophysectomy. **(A)** Incision made beneath the upper lip to enter the nasal cavity and gain access to the pituitary gland. **(B)**. Insertion of a speculum and special forceps used to remove the pituitary tumor.

Procedure	Description

thymectomy
thī-MĔK-tō-mē
  thym: thymus gland
  -ectomy: excision, removal
	Excision of the thymus gland
	Thymectomy is used to remove tumors of the thymus. It is also performed in treatment of myasthenia gravis (MG) as this disease commonly causes abnormalities of the thymus. Once the thymus is removed, remission of MG is common.

(continued)

Procedure	Description
thyroidectomy thī-royd-ĔK-tō-mē *thyroid:* thyroid gland *-ectomy:* excision, removal	Excision of the entire thyroid gland (thyroidectomy), a part of it (subtotal thyroidectomy), or a single lobe (thyroid lobectomy) *Thyroidectomy is performed for goiter, tumors, or hyperthyroidism that does not respond to iodine therapy and antithyroid drugs.*

Diagnostic

Laboratory

fasting blood sugar	Test that measures glucose levels in a blood sample following a fast of at least 8 hours *This test helps diagnose diabetes and monitor glucose levels in diabetic patients.*
glucose tolerance test (GTT) GLOO-kōs	Screening test in which a dose of glucose is administered and blood samples are taken afterward at regular intervals to determine how quickly glucose is cleared from the blood *GTT is performed after the patient has fasted at least 8 hours. It is used to diagnose pre-diabetes and gestational diabetes.*
insulin tolerance test (ITT) ĬN-sŭ-lĭn	Diagnostic test in which insulin is injected into the vein to assess pituitary function, adrenal function, and to determine insulin sensitivity *Insulin injections are used to evaluate pituitary function. The symptoms of low blood sugar will cause the release of growth hormone and cortisol. The growth hormone and cortisol will be measured at specified intervals through blood work.*
thyroid function test (TFT) THĪ-royd	Test that detects an increase or decrease in thyroid function *The TFT measures levels of thyroid-stimulating hormone (TSH), triiodothyronine (T_3), and thyroxine (T_4).*
total calcium test KĂL-sē-ŭm	Test that measures calcium to detect bone and parathyroid disorders *Hypercalcemia can indicate primary hyperparathyroidism; hypocalcemia can indicate hypoparathyroidism.*

Imaging

computed tomography (CT) kŏm-PŪ-tĕd tō-MŎG-ră-fē *tom/o:* to cut *-graphy:* process of recording	Imaging technique that rotates an x-ray emitter around the area to be scanned and measures the intensity of transmitted rays from different angles *In a CT scan, the computer generates a detailed cross-sectional image that appears as a slice. CT scan is used to detect disease and tumors in soft body tissues, such as the pancreas, thyroid, and adrenal glands, and may be used with or without a contrast medium.*
magnetic resonance imaging (MRI) măg-NĔT-ĭk RĔZ-ĕn-ăns ĬM-ĭj-ĭng	Noninvasive imaging technique that uses radio waves and a strong magnetic field, rather than an x-ray beam, to produce multiplanar cross-sectional images *MRI is the method of choice for diagnosing a growing number of diseases because it provides superior soft-tissue contrast, allows multiple plane views, and avoids the hazards of ionizing radiation. MRI is used to identify abnormalities of the pancreas and the pituitary, adrenal, and thyroid glands.*

Procedure	Description
radioactive iodine uptake (RAIU) rā-dē-ō-ĂK-tĭv Ī-ō-dīn	Administration of a radioactive iodine (RAI) in pill or liquid form is used as a tracer to test how quickly the thyroid gland takes up (uptake) iodine from the blood *The RAIU test is used to determine thyroid function and thyroid abnormalities, especially to assess an overactive thyroid gland (hyperthyroidism). An RAIU test may also be done at the same time as a thyroid scan.*
thyroid scan THĪ-royd *thyr:* thyroid gland *-oid:* resembling	Images of the thyroid gland are obtained after oral or intravenous administration of a small dose of radioactive iodine *Thyroid scanning is used to identify such pathologies as nodules and tumors, or to determine the cause of an overactive thyroid. A thyroid scan may also be performed with a radioactive iodine uptake test (RAIU) to check thyroid gland function.*

Pharmacology

Common disorders associated with endocrine glands include hyposecretion and hypersecretion of hormones. When deficiencies of this type occur, natural and synthetic hormones, such as insulin and thyroid agents, are prescribed. These agents normalize hormone levels to maintain proper functioning and homeostasis. Therapeutic agents are also available to regulate various substances in the body, such as glucose levels in diabetic patients. Hormone replacement therapy (HRT), such as synthetic thyroid and estrogen, treat these hormone deficiencies. Although specific drugs are not covered in this section, hormone chemotherapy drugs are used to treat certain cancers, such as testicular, ovarian, breast, and endometrial cancer. (See Table 14-7.)

Table 14-7 Drugs Used to Treat Endocrine Disorders

This table lists common drug classifications used to treat endocrine disorders, their therapeutic actions, and selected generic and trade names.

Classification	Therapeutic Action	Generic and *Trade* Names
antidiuretics ăn-tĭ-dī-ū-RĔT-ĭks	Reduce or control excretion of urine	**vasopressin** văs-ō-PRĔS-ĭn *Pitressin, Pressyn*
antithyroids ăn-tĭ-THĪ-roydz	Treat hyperthyroidism by impeding the formation of T_3 and T_4 hormone *Antithyroids are administered in preparation for a thyroidectomy and in thyrotoxic crisis.*	**methimazole** mĕth-ĬM-ă-zōl *Tapazole* **strong iodine solution** Ī-ō-dīn *Lugol's solution*
corticosteroids kor-tĭ-kō-STĔR-oydz	Replace hormones lost in adrenal insufficiency (Addison disease) *Corticosteroids are also widely used to suppress inflammation, control allergic reactions, reduce rejection in transplantation, and treat some cancers.*	**cortisone** KOR-tĭ-sōn *Cortisone acetate* **hydrocortisone** hī-drō-KOR-tĭ-sōn *A-Hydrocort, Cortef*

(continued)

Table 14-7	Drugs Used to Treat Endocrine Disorders—cont'd		
Classification	**Therapeutic Action**	**Generic and *Trade* Names**	

Classification	Therapeutic Action	Generic and Trade Names
growth hormone replacements	Increase skeletal growth in children and growth hormone deficiencies in adults *Growth hormones increase spinal bone density and help manage growth failure in children.*	**somatropin (recombinant)** sō-mă-TRŌ-pĭn *Humatrope, Norditropin*
insulins	Lower blood glucose levels by promoting its entrance into body cells and converting glucose to glycogen (a starch-storage form of glucose) *Type 1 diabetes must always be treated with insulin. Insulin can also be administered through an implanted pump, which infuses the drug continuously. Type 2 diabetes that cannot be controlled with oral antidiabetics may require insulin to maintain a normal level of glucose in the blood.*	**regular insulin** ĬN-sŭ-lĭn *Humulin R*, Novolin R* **NPH insulin** ĬN-sŭ-lĭn *Humulin N, Novolin N, Humulin* **insulin aspart** ĬN-sŭ-lĭn *Novolog*
oral antidiabetics ăn-tĭ-dī-ă-BĔT-ĭks	Treat type 2 diabetes mellitus by stimulating the pancreas to produce more insulin and decrease peripheral resistance to insulin *Antidiabetic drugs are not insulin and they are not used in treating type 1 diabetes mellitus.*	**glipizide** GLĬP-ĭ-zīd *Glucotrol, Glucotrol XL* **metformin** mĕt-FOR-mĭn *Glucophage*
thyroid supplements	Replace or supplement thyroid hormones *Each thyroid supplement contains T_3, T_4, or a combination of both. Thyroid supplements are also used to treat some types of thyroid cancer.*	**levothyroxine** lē-vō-thī-RŎK-sēn *Levo-T, Levoxyl, Synthroid* **liothyronine** lī-ō-THĪ-rō-nēn *Cytomel, Triostat*

*The trade name for all human genetically produced insulins is *Humulin*. Traditionally, insulin has been derived from beef or pork pancreas. Human insulin is genetically produced using recombinant DNA techniques to avoid the potential for allergic reaction.

Abbreviations

This section introduces endocrine-related abbreviations and their meanings.

Abbreviation	Meaning	Abbreviation	Meaning
ACTH	adrenocorticotropic stimulating hormone	**LH**	luteinizing hormone
ADH	antidiuretic hormone (vasopressin)	**NPH**	neutral protamine Hagedorn (insulin)
DI	diabetes insipidus; diagnostic imaging	**PRL**	prolactin
DKA	diabetic ketoacidosis	**PGH**	pituitary growth hormone
DM	diabetes mellitus	**PTH**	parathyroid hormone; also called *parathormone*
FBS	fasting blood sugar	**RAI**	radioactive iodine
FSH	follicle-stimulating hormone	**RAIU**	radioactive iodine uptake
GH	growth hormone	**T$_3$**	triiodothyronine (thyroid hormone)
GTT	glucose tolerance test	**T$_4$**	thyroxine (thyroid hormone)
HRT	hormone replacement therapy	**TFT**	thyroid function test
K	potassium (an electrolyte)	**TSH**	thyroid-stimulating hormone

It is time to review procedures, pharmacology, and abbreviations by completing Learning Activity 14–4.

LEARNING ACTIVITIES

The following activities provide a review of the endocrine system terms introduced in this chapter. Complete each activity and review your answers to evaluate your understanding of the chapter.

Learning Activity 14-1

Combining Forms, Suffixes, and Prefixes

Use the elements listed below to build medical words. You may use elements more than once.

Combining Forms		Suffixes		Prefixes
acr/o	thym/o	-crine	-megaly	a-
adrenal/o	thyr/o	-dipsia	-oma	endo-
calc/o		-ectomy		exo-
glyc/o		-emia		hyper-
kal/i		-graphy		hypo-
lith/o		-itis		poly-
pancreat/o		-lysis		

1. tumor of the thymus _____

2. destruction of glucose (by enzymes) _____

3. much thirst _____

4. removal of a stone from the pancreas _____

5. (glands that) secrete within (the blood) _____

6. without thirst _____

7. (glands that) secrete outward (through ducts) _____

8. blood condition of excessive sugar _____

9. destruction of the thymus _____

10. enlargement of the thyroid gland _____

11. inflammation of the adrenal glands _____

12. blood condition of below (normal) calcium _____

13. blood condition of excessive potassium (an electrolyte) _____

14. enlargement of the extremities _____

15. process of recording (x-ray) the pancreas _____

Check your answers in Appendix A. Review any material that you did not answer correctly.

Correct Answers _____ X 6.67 = _____ % Score

Learning Activity 14-2
Building Medical Words

Use *glyc/o* (sugar) to build words that mean:

1. blood condition of excessive glucose _____
2. blood condition of deficiency of glucose _____
3. formation of glycogen _____

Use *pancreat/o* (pancreas) to build words that mean:

4. inflammation of the pancreas _____
5. destruction of the pancreas _____
6. disease of the pancreas _____

Use *thyr/o* or *thyroid/o* (thyroid gland) to build words that mean:

7. inflammation of the thyroid gland _____
8. enlargement of the thyroid _____

Build surgical words that mean:

9. excision of a parathyroid gland _____
10. removal of the adrenal gland _____

   ✓ *Check your answers in Appendix A. Review material that you did not answer correctly.*

Correct Answers _____ X 10 = _____ % Score

Learning Activity 14-3
Diseases and Conditions

Match the following terms with the definitions in the numbered list.

acromegaly	*exophthalmic goiter*	*myxedema*
Addison disease	*glycosuria*	*pheochromocytoma*
cretinism	*hirsutism*	*type 1 diabetes*
Cushing syndrome	*hyperkalemia*	*type 2 diabetes*
diuresis	*hyponatremia*	*thyroid storm*

1. hypersecretion of GH that causes soft tissue and bones of the face, hands, and feet to grow larger than normal _____

2. hypothyroidism acquired in adulthood _____

3. increased excretion of urine _____

4. excessive growth of hair in unusual places, especially in women _____

5. hypothyroidism that appears as a congenital condition and is commonly associated with other endocrine abnormalities _____

6. crisis of uncontrolled hyperthyroidism _____

7. caused by deficiency in the secretion of adrenocortical hormones _____

8. characterized by protrusion of the eyeballs, increased heart action, enlargement of the thyroid gland, weight loss, and nervousness _____

9. excessive amount of potassium in the blood _____

10. small chromaffin cell tumor, usually located in the adrenal medulla _____

11. insulin-dependent diabetes mellitus; occurs most commonly in children and adolescents (juvenile onset) _____

12. decreased concentration of sodium in the blood _____

13. abnormal presence of glucose in the urine _____

14. metabolic disorder caused by hypersecretion of the adrenal cortex resulting in excessive production of glucocorticoids, mainly cortisol _____

15. non-insulin-dependent diabetes mellitus; occurs later in life (maturity onset) _____

✓ *Check your answers in Appendix A. Review material that you did not answer correctly.*

Correct Answers _____ X 6.67 = _____ % Score

Learning Activity 14-4

Procedures, Pharmacology, and Abbreviations

Match the following terms with the definitions in the numbered list.

antithyroids	*growth hormone*	*oral antidiabetics*
corticosteroids	*GTT*	*RAIU*
CT scan	*Humulin*	*T_3*
exophthalmometry	*hypophysectomy*	*T_4*
FBS	*MRI*	*thyroid scan*

1. measures circulating glucose level after a 12-hour fast _____

2. measures thyroid function and monitors how quickly ingested iodine is taken into the thyroid gland _____

3. replacement hormones for adrenal insufficiency (Addison disease) _____

4. increases skeletal growth in children _____

5. thyroid gland images are taken following administration of a small dose of radioactive iodine in order to detect thyroid abnormalities _____

6. thyroxine _____

7. used to treat type 2 diabetes _____

8. test commonly used to help diagnose diabetes or other disorders that affect carbohydrate metabolism _____

9. used to treat hyperthyroidism by impeding the formation of T_3 and T_4 hormone _____

10. partial or complete excision of the pituitary gland _____

11. triiodothyronine _____

12. noninvasive imaging technique that uses radio waves and a strong magnetic field to produce multiplanar cross-sectional images _____

13. test that measures the degree of forward displacement of the eyeball as seen in Graves disease _____

14. imaging technique achieved by rotating an x-ray emitter around the area to be scanned and measuring the intensity of transmitted rays from different angles; used to detect disease in soft body tissues, such as the pancreas, thyroid, and adrenal glands _____

15. trade name for all human genetically produced insulins _____

✔ *Check your answers in Appendix A. Review any material that you did not answer correctly.*

Correct Answers _____ X 6.67 = _____ % Score

Learning Activity 14-5
Medical Scenarios

To construct chart notes, replace the italicized terms in each of the scenarios with one of the medical terms listed below.

bradycardia	*hypopnea*	*polyphagia*
constipation	*lethargy*	*polyuria*
glycosuria	*polydipsia*	*triiodothyronine and thyroxine*
hyperglycemia		

Ms. H., a 20-year-old nursing student, presents with complaints of (1) ***excessive thirst***, (2) ***excessive urination***, and (3) ***excessive hunger***. She has headaches and occasional blurred vision. Because of her training as a health-care provider, she recognizes that these symptoms are associated with diabetes. She is further concerned since her mother and sister are diabetic. Her laboratory tests indicate (4) ***high blood sugar*** and (5) ***sugar in the urine***. She will be seen by Dr. M. for a more complete work-up and he will begin management of her condition.

1. _____
2. _____
3. _____
4. _____
5. _____

Ms. C., a 56-year-old female, presents with complaints of (6) ***lack of energy***, (7) ***difficulty passing stool***, and "always feeling cold." Although she has decreased appetite, she has slowly gained 12 lb over the last two years. Her hair appears thin and brittle. Her physical examination was unremarkable except for a (8) ***slow heart rate*** and (9) ***shallow breathing***. The physician schedules her for a CBC, metabolic blood panel, lipid panel, and (10) T_3 ***and*** T_4 tests.

6. _____
7. _____
8. _____
9. _____
10. _____

✓ *Check your answers in Appendix A. Review any material that you did not answer correctly.*

Correct Answers _____ X 10 = _____ % Score

MEDICAL RECORD ACTIVITIES

The two medical records included in the activities that follow use common clinical scenarios to show how medical terminology is used to document patient care. Complete the terminology and analysis sections for each activity to help you recognize and understand terms related to the endocrine system.

Medical Record Activity 14-1
Consultation Note: Hyperparathyroidism

Terminology

Terms listed in the following table are taken from *Consultation Note: Hyperparathyroidism* that follows. Use a medical dictionary such as *Taber's Cyclopedic Medical Dictionary;* the appendices of *Systems,* 7th ed.; or other resources to define each term. Then review the pronunciations for each term and practice by reading the medical record aloud.

Term	Definition
adenoma ăd-ĕ-NŌ-mă	
claudication klăw-dĭ-KĀ-shŭn	
diabetes mellitus dī-ă-BĒ-tēz MĔ-lĭ-tŭs	
endocrinologist ĕn-dō-krĭn-OL-ō-jĭst	
hypercalciuria hī-pĕr-kăl-sē-Ū-rē-ă	
hyperparathyroidism hī-pĕr-păr-ă-THĪ-roy-dĭzm	
impression ĭm-PRĔSH-ŭn	
osteoarthritis ŏs-tē-ō-ăr-THRĪ-tĭs	
parathyroid păr-ă-THĪ-royd	
peripheral vascular disease pĕr-ĬF-ĕr-ăl VĂS-kū-lăr	

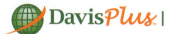

Visit the *Medical Terminology Systems* online resource center at Davis*Plus.* Use it to practice pronunciation and reinforce the meanings of the terms in this medical report.

CONSULTATION NOTE: HYPERPARATHYROIDISM

Consultation Note

Day, Phyllis   5/25/xx   Med Record: P25882

HISTORY OF PRESENT ILLNESS: This 66-year-old former blackjack dealer is under evaluation for hyperparathyroidism. Surgery evidently has been recommended, but there is confusion as to how urgent this is. She has a 13-year history of type 1 diabetes mellitus, a history of shoulder pain, osteoarthritis of the spine, and peripheral vascular disease with claudication. She states her 548-pack/year smoking history ended 3-1/2 years ago. Her first knowledge of parathyroid disease was about 3 years ago when laboratory findings revealed an elevated calcium level. This subsequently led to the diagnosis of hyperparathyroidism. She was further evaluated by an endocrinologist in the Lake Tahoe area, who determined that she also had hypercalciuria, although there is nothing to suggest a history of kidney stones.

IMPRESSION: Hyperparathyroidism and hypercalciuria, probably a parathyroid adenoma

PLAN: Patient advised to make a follow-up appointment with her endocrinologist.

Juan Perez, MD
Juan Perez, MD

D: 05-25-xx
T: 05-25-xx

jp:lg

Analysis

Review the medical record *Consultation Note: Hyperparathyroidism* to answer the following questions.

1. What is an adenoma?

_____

2. What does the physician suspect caused the patient's hyperparathyroidism?

_____

3. What type of laboratory findings revealed parathyroid disease?

_____

4. What is hypercalciuria?

_____

5. If the patient smoked 548 packs of cigarettes per year, how many packs did she smoke in an average day?

_____

Medical Record Activity 14-2
SOAP Note: Diabetes Mellitus

Terminology

Terms listed in the following table are taken from *SOAP Note: Diabetes Mellitus* that follows. Use a medical dictionary such as *Taber's Cyclopedic Medical Dictionary;* the appendices of *Systems,* 7th ed.; or other resources to define each term. Then review the pronunciations for each term and practice by reading the medical record aloud.

Term	Definition
Accu-chek ĂK-ū-chĕk	
morbid obesity MOR-bĭd ō-BĒ-sĭ-tē	
obesity, exogenous ō-BĒ-sĭ-tē, ĕks-ŎJ-ĕ-nŭs	
polydipsia pŏl-ē-DĬP-sē-ă	
polyphagia pŏl-ē-FĀ-jē-ă	
polyuria pŏl-ē-Ū-rē-ă	

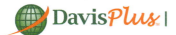

Visit the *Medical Terminology Systems* online resource center at Davis*Plus.* Use it to practice pronunciation and reinforce the meanings of the terms in this medical report.

SOAP NOTE: DIABETES MELLITUS

Emergency Department Record

Date: 2/4/xx
Patient: Pleume, Roberta
Age: 68

Time Registered: 1445 hours
Physician: Samara Batichara, MD
Patient ID#: 22258

Chief Complaint: Frequent urination, increased hunger and thirst.

S: This 200-pound patient was admitted to the hospital because of a 10-day history of polyuria, polydipsia, and polyphagia. She has been very nervous, irritable, and very sensitive emotionally and cries easily. During this period, she has had headaches and has become very sleepy and tired after eating. On admission, her Accu-Chek was 540 mg/dL. Family history is significant in that both parents and two sisters have type 1 diabetes.

O: Physical examination was essentially negative. The abdomen was difficult to evaluate because of morbid obesity.

A: Diabetes mellitus; obesity, exogenous.

P: Patient admitted to the hospital for further evaluation.

Samara Batichara, MD
Samara Batichara, MD

D: 02-04-xx
T: 02-04-xx

sb:lb

Analysis

Review the medical record *SOAP Note: Diabetes Mellitus* to answer the following questions.

1. How long has this patient been experiencing voracious eating?

_____

2. Was the patient's obesity due to overeating or metabolic imbalance?

_____

3. Why did the doctor experience difficulty in examining the patient's abdomen?

_____

4. Was the patient's blood glucose above or below normal on admission?

_____

5. What is the reference range for fasting blood glucose?

_____

Nervous System

Chapter Outline

Objectives

Upon completion of this chapter, you will be able to:

- Locate and describe the structures of the nervous system.
- Describe the functional relationship between the nervous system and other body systems.
- Pronounce, spell, and build words related to the nervous system.
- Describe diseases, conditions, and procedures related to the nervous system.
- Explain pharmacology related to the treatment of nervous disorders.
- Demonstrate your knowledge of this chapter by completing the learning and medical record activities.

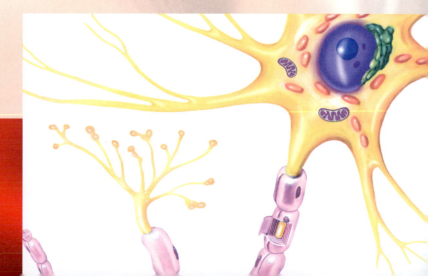

Anatomy and Physiology

The nervous system is one of the most complicated systems of the body in structure and function. It senses physical and chemical changes in the internal and external environments, processes them, and then responds to maintain homeostasis. Voluntary activities, such as walking and talking, and involuntary activities, such as digestion and circulation, are coordinated, regulated, and integrated by the nervous system. The entire neural network of the body relies on the transmission of electro-chemical impulses that travel from one area of the body to another. The speed at which this transmission occurs is almost instantaneous, thus providing an immediate response to change.

Anatomy and Physiology Key Terms

This section introduces important nervous system terms and their definitions. Word analyses for selected terms are also provided.

Term	Definition
afferent ĂF-ĕr-ĕnt	Carry or move inward or toward a central structure *In the nervous system, afferent impulses travel toward the central nervous system.*
blood–brain barrier	Protective mechanism that blocks specific substances found in the bloodstream from entering delicate brain tissue
efferent ĔF-ĕ-rĕnt	Carry or move away from a central structure *In the nervous system, efferent impulses travel away from the central nervous system.*
limbic system LĬM-bĭk	Complex neural system located beneath the cerebrum that controls basic emotions and drives and plays an important role in memory *The limbic system is primarily related to survival and includes such emotions as fear, anger, and pleasure (food and sexual behavior).*
neurilemma nū-rĭ-LĔM-ă	Additional external myelin sheath that is formed by Schwann cells and found only on axons in the peripheral nervous system *Because the neurilemma does not disintegrate after injury to the axon, its enclosed hollow tube provides an avenue for regeneration of injured axons.*
ventricle VĔN-trĭk-l *ventr:* belly, belly side *-ical:* pertaining to	Organ chamber or cavity that receives or holds fluid *In the nervous system, cerebrospinal fluid flows through the ventricles into the spinal cavity and back toward the brain, where it is absorbed into the blood.*

Pronunciation Help	Long Sound	ā — rate	ē — rebirth	ī — isle	ō — over	ū — unite
	Short Sound	ă — alone	ĕ — ever	ĭ — it	ŏ — not	ŭ — cut

Cellular Structure of the Nervous System

Despite its complexity, the nervous system is composed of only two principal cell types: neurons and neuroglia. Together, neurons and neuroglia constitute the nervous tissue of the body.

Neurons

Neurons transmit impulses. They are commonly identified as by the direction the impulse travels: **afferent** when the direction is toward the brain or spinal cord, or **efferent** when the direction is away from the brain or spinal cord. The three major structures of the neuron are the cell body, axon, and dendrites. (See Figure 15-1.) The (1) **cell body** is the enlarged structure of the neuron that contains the (2) **nucleus** of the cell and various organelles. Its branching cytoplasmic projections are (3) **dendrites** that carry impulses to the cell body and (4) **axons** that carry impulses from the cell body. Dendrites resemble tiny branches on a tree, providing additional surface area for receiving impulses from other neurons. Axons are threadlike extensions of nerve cells that transmit impulses to dendrites of other neurons as well as muscles and glands.

Axons possess a white, lipoid covering called a (5) **myelin sheath.** This covering acts as an electrical insulator that reduces the possibility of an impulse stimulating adjacent nerves. It also accelerates impulse transmission through the axon. On nerves in the **peripheral nervous system,**

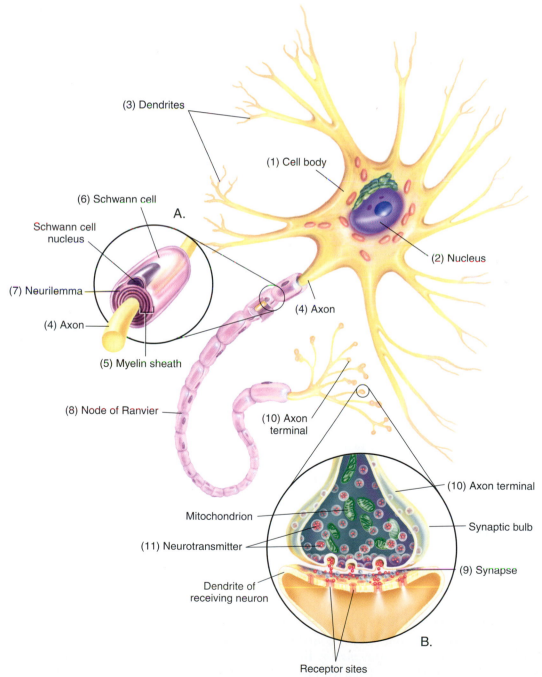

Figure 15-1 Neuron. **(A)** Schwann cell. **(B)** Axon terminal synapse.

the myelin sheath is formed by a neuroglial cell called a (6) **Schwann cell** that wraps tightly around the axon. Its exterior surface forms a thin tube called the (7) neurilemma, or **neurolemma.** The neurilemma does not disintegrate after an axon has been crushed or severed, as does the axon and myelin sheath, but remains intact. This intact sheath provides a pathway for possible neuron regeneration after injury.

The myelin sheath covering the axons in the **central nervous system** is formed by oligodendrocytes, rather than Schwann cells. Oligodendrocytes do not produce neurilemma, thus injury or damage to neurons located in the central nervous system is irreparable. The short, unmyelinated spaces between adjacent segments of the myelin sheath are called (8) **nodes of Ranvier.** These nodes help speed the transmission of impulses down the axon, because an impulse jumps across the nodes at a faster rate than it is able to travel through the myelinated axon.

The functional connection between two neurons or between a neuron and its effector organ (muscle or gland) is a gap or space called a (9) **synapse.** Impulses must travel from the (10) **axon terminal** of one neuron to the dendrite of the next neuron or to its effector organ by crossing this synapse. The impulse within the transmitting axon causes a chemical substance called a (11) **neurotransmitter** to be released at the end of its axon. The neurotransmitter diffuses across the synapse and attaches to the receiving neuron at specialized receptor sites. When sufficient receptor sites are occupied, it signals an acceptance "message" and the impulse passes to the receiving neuron. The receiving neuron immediately inactivates the neurotransmitter and prepares the site to receive another impulse.

Neuroglia

Neuroglia are cells that support neurons and bind them to other neurons or other tissues of the body. Although they do not transmit impulses, they provide a variety of activities essential to the proper functioning of neurons. The term **neuroglia** literally means *nerve glue* because these cells were originally believed to serve only to bind neurons to each other and to other structures. They are now known to supply nutrients and oxygen to neurons and assist in other metabolic activities. They also play an important role when the nervous system suffers injury or infection. The four major types of neuroglia are astrocytes, oligodendrocytes, microglia, and ependyma. (See Figure 15-2.)

Astrocytes, as their name suggests, are star-shaped neuroglia. They provide three-dimensional mechanical support for neurons and form tight sheaths around the capillaries of the brain. These sheaths provide an obstruction, called the blood–brain barrier, that keeps large molecular substances from entering the delicate tissue of the brain. Even so, small molecules, such as water, carbon dioxide, oxygen, and alcohol, readily pass from blood vessels through the barrier and enter the interstitial spaces of the brain. Researchers must take the blood–brain barrier into consideration when developing drugs for treatment of brain disorders. Astrocytes also perform mildly phagocytic functions in the brain and spinal cord. **Oligodendrocytes,** also called **oligodendroglia,** are responsible for developing myelin on axons of neurons in the central nervous system. **Microglia,** the smallest of the neuroglia, possess phagocytic properties and may become very active during times of infection. **Ependyma** are ciliated cells that line fluid-filled cavities of the central nervous system, especially the ventricles of the brain. They assist in the circulation of cerebrospinal fluid (CSF).

Nervous System Divisions

The two major divisions of the nervous system are the central nervous system and the peripheral nervous system. The central nervous system consists of the brain and spinal cord. The peripheral nervous system consists of 12 pairs of cranial nerves and 31 pairs of spinal nerves. (See Table 15-1.)

Central Nervous System

The **central nervous system (CNS)** consists of the brain and spinal cord. Its nervous tissue is classified as *white matter* or *gray matter.* Bundles of axons with their white lipoid myelin sheath constitute white matter. Unmyelinated fibers, dendrites, and nerve cell bodies make up the gray matter of the brain and spinal cord.

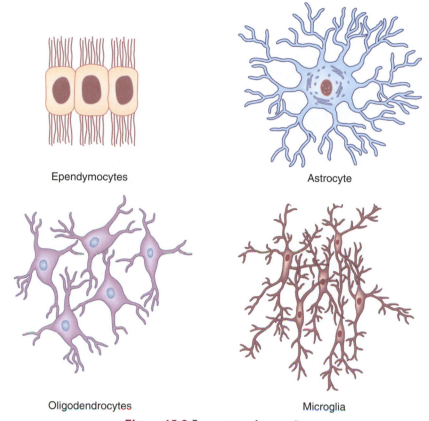

Ependymocytes

Astrocyte

Oligodendrocytes

Microglia

Figure 15-2 Four types of neuroglia.

Table 15-1	**Nervous System Structures and Functions**
This table lists the structures of the nervous system along with their functions.	
Structures	**Function**
Central	
Brain	Center for thought and emotion, interpretation of sensory stimuli, and coordination of body functions
Spinal cord	Main pathway for transmission of information between the brain and body
Peripheral	
Cranial nerves	12 pairs of nerves that emerge from the base of the skull and may act in a motor capacity, sensory capacity, or both
Spinal nerves	31 pairs of nerves that emerge from the spine and act in both motor and sensory capacities

Brain

In addition to being one of the largest organs of the body, the brain is highly complex in structure and function. (See Figure 15-3.) It integrates almost every physical and mental activity of the body and is the center for memory, emotion, thought, judgment, reasoning, and consciousness. The four major structures of the brain are:

- cerebrum
- cerebellum
- diencephalon
- brainstem.

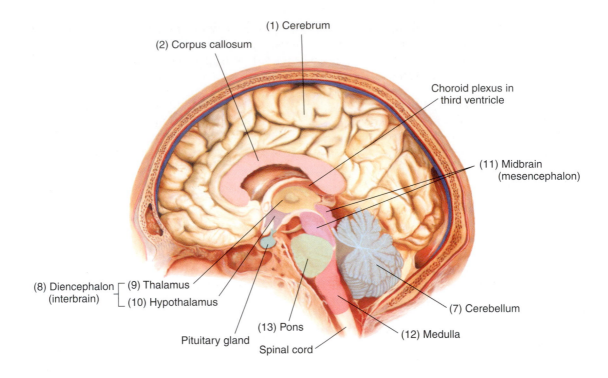

(1) Cerebrum

(2) Corpus callosum

Choroid plexus in third ventricle

(11) Midbrain (mesencephalon)

(8) Diencephalon (interbrain)
(9) Thalamus
(10) Hypothalamus

(7) Cerebellum

(13) Pons

Pituitary gland

Spinal cord

(12) Medulla

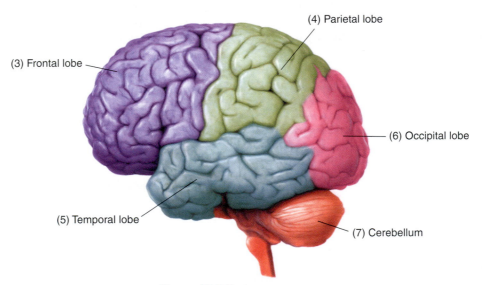

(4) Parietal lobe

(3) Frontal lobe

(6) Occipital lobe

(5) Temporal lobe

(7) Cerebellum

Figure 15-3 Brain structures.

Cerebrum

The (1) **cerebrum** is the largest, uppermost portion of the brain. It consists of two hemispheres divided by a deep longitudinal fissure, or groove. The fissure does not completely separate the hemispheres. A structure called the (2) **corpus callosum** joins these hemispheres, permitting communication between the right and left sides of the brain. Each hemisphere is divided into five lobes. Four of these lobes are named for the bones that lie directly above them: (3) **frontal,** (4) **parietal,** (5) **temporal,** and (6) **occipital.** The fifth lobe, the **insula** (not shown in Figure 15-3), is hidden from view and can be seen only upon dissection.

The cerebral surface consists of numerous folds, or convolutions, called **gyri.** The gyri are separated by furrows, or fissures, called **sulci.** A thin layer called the **cerebral cortex** covers the entire cerebrum and is composed of gray matter. Most information processing occurs in the cerebral cortex.

The remainder of the cerebrum is primarily composed of white matter (myelinated axons). Major functions of the cerebrum include sensory perception and interpretation, language, voluntary movement, and memory. Beneath the cerebrum is a primitive "emotional brain" called the limbic system. The limbic system is essential for survival and works in conjunction with the "thinking brain." It controls such behaviors as rage, fear, and anger and the emotional aspects such as food enjoyment and sexual behavior. Mental and emotional illnesses are commonly the result of an imbalance in brain chemicals or electrical activity in the limbic system.

Cerebellum

The second largest structure of the brain, the (7) **cerebellum,** occupies the posterior portion of the skull. Most functions of the cerebellum involve movement, posture, or balance. When the cerebrum initiates muscular movement, the cerebellum coordinates and refines it.

Diencephalon

The (8) **diencephalon** (also called the **interbrain**) is composed of many smaller structures, including the thalamus and the hypothalamus. The (9) **thalamus** receives all sensory stimuli except olfactory and processes and transmits them to the appropriate centers in the cerebral cortex. In addition, the thalamus receives impulses from the cerebrum and relays them to efferent nerves. The (10) **hypothalamus** regulates involuntary activities, such as heart rate, body temperature, and fluid balance. It also controls many endocrine functions.

Brainstem

The brainstem completes the last major section of the brain. It is composed of three structures: the (11) **midbrain** (also called the **mesencephalon**), separating the cerebrum from the brainstem; the (12) **medulla,** which attaches to the spinal cord; and (13) the **pons,** or "bridge," connecting the midbrain to the medulla. In general, the brainstem is a pathway for impulse conduction between the brain and spinal cord. The brainstem is the origin of 10 of the 12 pairs of cranial nerves and controls respiration, blood pressure, and heart rate. The brainstem is the site that controls the beginning of life (initiation of the beating heart in a fetus) and the end of life (the cessation of respiration and heart activity).

Spinal Cord

The **spinal cord** transmits sensory impulses from the body to the brain and motor impulses from the brain to muscles and organs of the body. The sensory nerve tracts are called **ascending tracts** because the direction of the impulse is upward. Conversely, motor nerve tracts are called **descending tracts** because they carry impulses in a downward direction to muscles and organs. A cross-sectional view of the spinal cord reveals an inner gray matter composed of cell bodies and dendrites and an outer white matter area composed of myelinated tissue of the ascending and descending tracts.

The entire spinal cord is located within the spinal cavity of the vertebral column, with spinal nerves exiting between the intervertebral spaces throughout almost the entire length of the spinal column. Unlike the cranial nerves, which have specific names, the spinal nerves are identified by the region of the vertebral column from which they exit.

Meninges

The brain and spinal cord receive limited protection from three coverings called **meninges** (singular, **meninx**). These coverings are the dura mater, arachnoid, and pia mater.

The **dura mater** is the outermost covering of the brain and spinal cord. It is tough, fibrous, and dense and composed primarily of connective tissue. Because of its thickness, this membrane is also called the **pachymeninges.** Beneath the dura mater is a cavity called the **subdural space,** which is filled with serous fluid.

The **arachnoid** is the middle covering and, as its name suggests, has a spider-web appearance. It fits loosely over the underlying structures. A **subarachnoid space** contains **cerebrospinal fluid,** a colorless fluid that contains proteins, glucose, urea, salts, and some white blood cells. This fluid circulates around the spinal cord and brain and through ventricles located within the inner portion of the brain. It provides nutritive substances to the central nervous system and adds additional protection for the brain and spinal cord by acting as a shock absorber. Normally, cerebrospinal fluid is absorbed as rapidly as it is formed, maintaining a constant fluid volume.

Any interference with its absorption results in a collection of fluid in the brain, a condition called **hydrocephalus.**

The **pia mater** is the innermost meninx. This membrane directly adheres to the brain and spinal cord. As it passes over the brain, it follows the contours of the gyri and sulci. It contains numerous blood vessels and lymphatics that nourish the underlying tissues. Because of the thinness and delicacy of the arachnoid and pia mater, these two meninges are collectively called the **leptomeninges.**

Peripheral Nervous System

The **peripheral nervous system (PNS)** is composed of all nervous tissue located outside the spinal column and skull. It consists of sensory neurons, which carry impulses from the body to the CNS (afferent), and motor neurons, which carry impulses from the brain and spinal cord to muscles and glands (efferent). It is further divided into the somatic nervous system and the autonomic nervous system, which is subdivided into the sympathetic and parasympathetic divisions. (See Figure 15-4.)

The PNS includes the cranial nerves and the spinal nerves. Its anatomical structures consist of 12 pairs of cranial nerves and 31 pairs of spinal nerves.

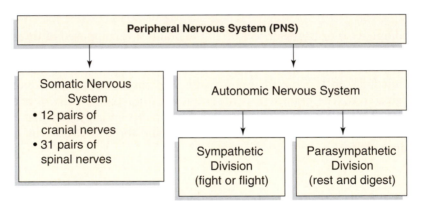

Figure 15-4 Divisions of the peripheral nervous system.

Cranial Nerves

The cranial nerves originate in the base of the brain and emerge though openings in the base of the skull. They are designated by name or number. (See Figure 15-5.) Cranial nerves may be sensory, motor, or a mixture of both. **Sensory nerves** are afferent, and receive impulses from the sense organs, including the eyes, ears, nose, tongue, and skin and transmit them to the CNS. **Motor nerves** are efferent and conduct impulses to muscles and glands. Some cranial nerves are composed of sensory and motor fibers. They are called **mixed nerves.** An example of a mixed nerve is the facial nerve. It acts in a motor capacity by transmitting impulses for smiling or frowning. However, it also acts in a sensory capacity by transmitting taste impulses from the tongue to the brain.

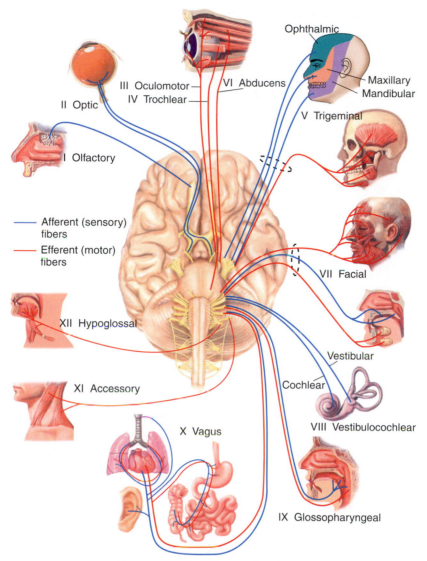

Figure 15-5 Cranial nerve distribution.

Spinal Nerves

The spinal nerves emerge from the intervertebral spaces in the spinal column and extend to various locations of the body. All 31 pairs of spinal nerves are mixed nerves. (See Figure 15-6.) Each of them is identified according to the vertebra from which they exit. Each of them has two points of attachment to the spinal cord: an anterior (ventral) root and a posterior (dorsal) root. The **anterior root** contains motor fibers and the **posterior root** contains sensory fibers. These two roots unite to form the spinal nerve that has afferent and efferent qualities.

Somatic and Autonomic Nervous Systems

Motor impulses transmitted to muscles under conscious control (walking and talking) belong to the **somatic nervous system.** Motor impulses transmitted to glands and muscles not under conscious control (heart rate, respiration, digestion, pupil diameter, and so forth) belong to the **autonomic nervous system.**

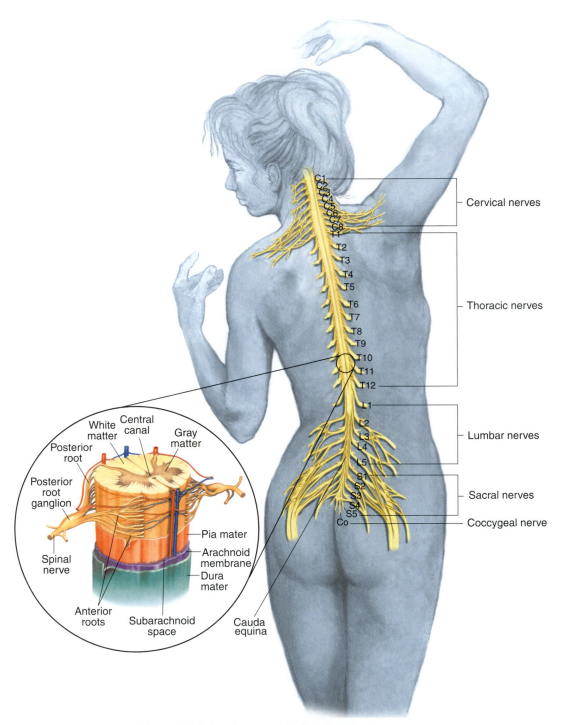

C1
C2
C3
C4
C5
C6
C7
C8
T1
T2
T3
T4
T5
T6
T7
T8
T9
T10
T11
T12
L1
L2
L3
L4
L5
S1
S2
S3
S4
S5
Co

Cervical nerves

Thoracic nerves

Lumbar nerves

Sacral nerves

Coccygeal nerve

White matter
Central canal
Gray matter
Posterior root
Posterior root ganglion
Spinal nerve
Pia mater
Arachnoid membrane
Dura mater
Anterior roots
Subarachnoid space
Cauda equina

Figure 15-6 Spinal nerves. **(A)** Spinal cord enlargement.

The autonomic nervous system divides further into the **sympathetic** and **parasympathetic** divisions. In general, these divisions typically bring about opposite effects on the activity of the same organs. Ordinarily, what one division stimulates, the other inhibits. The sympathetic division regulates body activities when an immediate action is required. It increases heart rate, depth of breathing, and muscle strength, preparing the body for "fight-or-flight" responses. Conversely, the parasympathetic division decreases the rate and intensity of these processes. It results in slowing the heart, dilating visceral blood vessels, and an increasing the activity of the digestive tract, preparing the body for "rest-and-digest" responses. (See Table 15-2.)

Table 15-2	**Sympathetic and Parasympathetic Actions**

This table shows opposing actions between the sympathetic and the parasympathetic divisions of the peripheral nervous system.

Sympathetic Division	Parasympathetic Division
Dilates the pupils to increase the amount of light entering the eye to optimize vision	Decreases or increases the diameter of the pupils in response to changing levels of light
Decreases the flow of saliva	Increases the flow of saliva
Dilates the bronchi	Constricts the bronchi
Increases heart rate and metabolic rate	Decreases heart rate, blood pressure, and metabolic rate
Decreases digestive activities	Increases digestive activities
Constricts visceral blood vessels	Dilates visceral blood vessels

Anatomy Review

To review the anatomy of the nervous system, label the illustration using the terms listed below.

cerebellum

cerebrum

corpus callosum

diencephalon (interbrain)

frontal lobe

hypothalamus

medulla

midbrain (mesencephalon)

occipital lobe

parietal lobe

pons

temporal lobe

thalamus

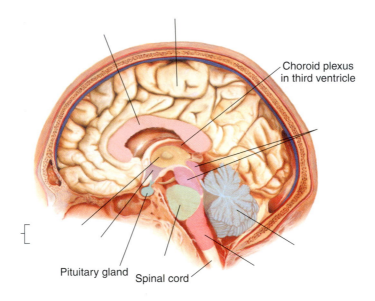

Choroid plexus
in third ventricle

Pituitary gland   Spinal cord

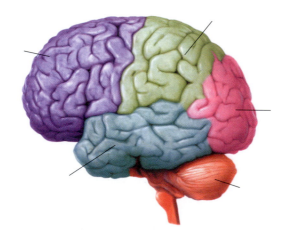

 Check your answers by referring to Figure 15–3 on page 500. Review material that you did not answer correctly.

CONNECTING BODY SYSTEMS—NERVOUS SYSTEM

The main function of the nervous system is to identify and respond to internal and external changes in the environment to maintain homeostasis. Specific functional relationships between the nervous system and other body systems are discussed below.

Blood, Lymph, and Immune
- Nervous system identifies changes in blood and lymph composition and provides the stimuli to maintain homeostasis.
- Nervous system identifies pathologically altered tissue and assists the immune system in containing injury and promoting healing.

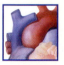

Cardiovascular
- Nervous tissue, especially the conduction system of the heart, transmits a contraction impulse.
- Nervous system identifies pressure changes on vascular walls and responds to regulate blood pressure.

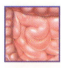

Digestive
- Nervous stimuli of digestive organs propel food by peristalsis.
- Nerve receptors in the lower colon identify the need to defecate.

Endocrine
- The hypothalamus regulates hormone production.

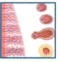

Female Reproductive
- Nervous system transmits contraction impulses needed for delivery of a fetus.
- Nervous system provides stimuli needed for lactation.
- Nervous system regulates hormones needed for the menstrual cycle.

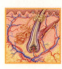

Integumentary
- Sensory nervous system supplies receptors in the skin that respond to environmental stimuli.
- Autonomic nervous system regulates body temperature by controlling shivering and sweating.

Male Reproductive
- Nervous system regulates sexual responses.
- Nervous tissue in reproductive organs provides pleasure responses.

Musculoskeletal
- Nervous system provides impulses for contraction, resulting in voluntary and involuntary movement of muscles.
- Autonomic nervous tissue responds to positional changes.

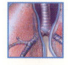

Respiratory
- Nervous system stimulates muscle contractions that create pressure changes necessary for ventilation.
- Nervous system regulates rate and depth of breathing.

Urinary
- Nervous system stimulates the thirst reflex when body fluid levels are low.
- Nervous system regulates all aspects of urine formation.

Medical Word Elements

This section introduces combining forms, suffixes, and prefixes related to the nervous system. Word analyses are also provided.

Element	Meaning	Word Analysis
Combining Forms		
cerebr/o	cerebrum	**cerebr/o**/tomy (sĕr-ĕ-BRŎT-ō-mē): incision of the cerebrum *-tomy:* incision
crani/o	cranium (skull)	**crani/o**/malacia (krā-nē-ō-mă-LĀ-shē-ă): softening of the cranium *-malacia:* softening

(continued)

Element	Meaning	Word Analysis
encephal/o	brain	**encephal/o**/cele (ĕn-SĔF-ă-lō-sēl): herniation of the brain *-cele:* hernia, swelling *Encephalocele is a condition in which portions of the brain and meninges protrude through a bony midline defect in the skull.*
gangli/o	ganglion (knot or knotlike mass)	**gangli**/ectomy (găng-glē-ĔK-tō-mē): excision of a ganglion *-ectomy:* excision, removal *A ganglion is a mass of nerve cell bodies (gray matter) in the peripheral nervous system.*
gli/o	glue; neuroglial tissue	**gli**/oma (glī-Ō-mă): tumor (composed of) neuroglial tissue *-oma:* tumor
kinesi/o	movement	brady/**kines**/ia (brăd-ē-kĭ-NĒ-sē-ă): condition of slow movement *brady-:* slow *-ia:* condition
lept/o	thin, slender	**lept/o**/mening/o/pathy (lĕp-tō-mĕn-ĭn-GŎP-ă-thē): disease of the thin meninges *-mening/o:* meninges (membranes covering the brain and spinal cord) *-pathy:* disease *The leptomeninges include the pia mater and arachnoid, both of which are thin and delicate in structure, as opposed to the dura mater.*
lex/o	word, phrase	dys/**lex**/ia (dĭs-LĔK-sē-ă): difficulty using words *dys-:* bad; painful; difficult *-ia:* condition *Dyslexia is a difficulty with reading or an inability to read, including the tendency to reverse letters or words when reading or writing.*
mening/o	meninges (membranes covering the brain and spinal cord)	**mening/o**/cele (mĕn-ĬN-gō-sēl): herniation of the meninges *-cele:* hernia, swelling
meningi/o		**meningi**/oma (mĕn-ĭn-jē-Ō-mă): tumor in the meninges *-oma:* tumor
myel/o	bone marrow; spinal cord	poli/o/**myel**/itis (pōl-ē-ō-mī-ĕl-Ī-tĭs): inflammation of the gray matter of the spinal cord *poli/o:* gray; gray matter (of brain or spinal cord) *-itis:* inflammation
narc/o	stupor; numbness; sleep	**narc/o**/tic (năr-KŎT-ĭk): relating to sleep *-tic:* pertaining to *Narcotics depress the central nervous system, thus relieving pain and producing sleep.*

Element	Meaning	Word Analysis
neur/o	nerve	**neur/o**/lysis (nū-RŎL-ĭs-ĭs): destruction of a nerve *-lysis:* separation; destruction; loosening *Neurolysis is sometimes performed using cryoablation or radio-frequency techniques to relieve intractable pain as a temporary or permanent measure.*
radicul/o	nerve root	**radicul**/algia (ră-dĭk-ū-LĂL-jē-ă): pain in the nerve root *-algia:* pain
sthen/o	strength	hyper/**sthen**/ia (hī-pĕr-STHĒ-nē-ă): condition of excessive strength *hyper-:* excessive, above normal *-ia:* condition *Hypersthenia is a condition of excessive strength or tonicity of the body or a body part.*
thalam/o	thalamus	**thalam/o**/tomy (thăl-ă-MŎT-ō-mē): incision of the thalamus *-tomy:* incision *Thalamotomy is performed to treat intractable pain or psychoses.*
thec/o	sheath (usually refers to meninges)	intra/**thec**/al (ĭn-tră-THĒ-kăl): pertaining to the space within a sheath *intra-:* in, within *-al:* pertaining to
ton/o	tension	dys/**ton**/ia (dĭs-TŌ-nē-ă): poor (muscle) tone *dys-:* bad; painful; difficult *-ia:* condition *Dystonia usually refers to a movement disorder characterized by sustained muscle contractions, resulting in a persistently abnormal posture.*
ventricul/o	ventricle (of the heart or brain)	**ventricul**/itis (vĕn-trĭk-ū-L Ī-tĭs): inflammation of the ventricles (of the heart or brain) *-itis:* inflammation
Suffixes		
-algesia	pain	an/**algesia** (ăn-ăl-JĒ-zē-ă): absence of (a normal sense of) pain *an-:* without, not
-algia		syn/**algia** (sĭn-ĂL-jē-ă): joined (referred) pain *syn-:* union, together, joined *Synalgia is pain experienced in a part of the body other than the place of pathology. For example, right shoulder pain is commonly associated with gallstones.*
-asthenia	weakness, debility	my/**asthenia** (mī-ăs-THĒ-nē-ă): muscle weakness *my:* muscle
-esthesia	feeling	hyper/**esthesia** (hī-pĕr-ĕs-THĒ-zē-ă): increased feeling *hyper-:* excessive, above normal *Hyperesthesia involves a marked sensitivity to touch, pain, or other sensory stimuli.*

(continued)

Element	Meaning	Word Analysis
-kinesia	movement	hyper/**kinesia** (hī-pĕr-kĭ-NĒ-zē-ă): excessive movement; also called *hyperactivity* *hyper–:* excessive, above normal
-lepsy	seizure	narc/o/**lepsy** (NĂR-kō-lĕp-sē): seizure of sleep *narc/o:* sleep *In narcolepsy, the individual has a sudden and uncontrollable urge to sleep at an inappropriate time, such as when driving.*
-paresis	partial paralysis	hemi/**paresis** (hĕm-ē-pă-RĒ-sĭs): partial paralysis of one-half (of the body) *hemi–:* one-half *When used alone, the term* paresis *means* partial paralysis *or* motor weakness.
-phasia	speech	a/**phasia** (ă-FĀ-zē-ă): without speech *a–:* without, not
-plegia	paralysis	quadri/**plegia** (kwŏd-rĭ-PLĒ-jē-ă): paralysis of four (extremities) *quadri–:* four
-taxia	order, coordination	a/**taxia** (ă-TĂK-sē-ă): without coordination *a–:* without, not *Ataxia refers to poor muscle coordination, especially when voluntary movements are attempted.*

Prefixes		
pachy-	thick	**pachy**/mening/itis (păk-ē-mĕn-ĭn-JĪ-tĭs): inflammation of the dura mater *mening:* meninges (membranes covering the brain and spinal cord) *-itis:* inflammation *The dura mater is a thick membrane that provides protection for the brain and spinal cord.*
para-	near, beside; beyond	**para**/plegia (păr-ă-PLĒ-jē-ă): paralysis of the lower body and limbs **-plegia:** paralysis
syn-	union, together, joined	**syn**/algia (sĭn-ĂL-jē-ă): referred pain *-algia:* pain *Pain in a deteriorated hip commonly causes referred pain in a healthy knee.*
uni-	one	**uni**/later/al (ū-nĭ-LĂT-ĕr-ăl): pertaining to one side *later:* side, to one side *-al:* pertaining to

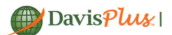

Visit the *Medical Terminology Systems* online resource center at Davis*Plus* for an audio exercise of the terms in this table. Other activities are also available to reinforce content.

It is time to review medical word elements by completing Learning Activities 15–1 and 15–2.

Pathology

Damage to the brain and spinal cord invariably causes signs and symptoms in other parts of the body. Common signs and symptoms for many neurological disorders include headache, insomnia, back or neck pain, weakness, and involuntary movement **(dyskinesia).** Careful observation of the patient during the history and physical examination may provide valuable clues about mental status and cognitive and motor ability.

For diagnosis, treatment, and management of neurological disorders, the medical services of a specialist may be warranted. **Neurology** is the branch of medicine concerned with neurological diseases. The physician who specializes in the diagnoses and treatment of nervous system disorders is known as a **neurologist. Psychiatry** is the branch of medicine concerned with mental illnesses. The physician who specializes in diagnosing and treating mental illnesses is a **Psychiatrist.**

Radiculopathy

Radiculopathy, also called **radiculitis,** is an inflammation of the nerve root associated with the spinal column. Spinal nerves exit the spinal column at each level along the length of the spine. When pressure is applied to the nerve root **(compression),** the patient experiences tingling, numbness, weakness, or a radiating pain starting in the spine and moving outward. Pressure can be the result of a herniated disk, degenerative changes, arthritis, fractures, bone spurs, or tumors. The areas most commonly affected are the neck **(cervical radiculopathy)** and the lower back **(lumbar radiculopathy, sciatica),** commonly with pain radiating down the leg.

Rest and antiinflammatory medications are the usual method of treatment. However, for disabling pain that lasts for several months or is accompanied by loss of bowel or bladder control, surgery to remove the cause of the pressure **(decompression surgery)** may be the only option.

Cerebrovascular Disease

Cerebrovascular disease is any functional abnormality of the cerebrum caused by disorders of the blood vessels of the brain. It is most commonly associated with a **stroke,** also called **cerebrovascular accident (CVA).** The three major types of stroke are ischemic stroke, intracerebral hemorrhage, and subarachnoid hemorrhage. The most common type, which accounts for about 80% of all strokes, is ischemic stroke. **Ischemic stroke** is caused by a narrowing of the arteries of the brain or the arteries of the neck **(carotid),** generally due to atherosclerosis. This narrowing causes insufficient oxygen delivery to the brain tissue and within a few minutes the tissue begins to die. Occasionally, pieces of plaque break loose and travel to the narrower vessels of the brain, causing occlusion, also resulting in ischemia. An **intracerebral hemorrhage** is caused by the sudden rupture of an artery within the brain. After the rupture, released blood compresses brain structures and destroys them. In a **subarachnoid hemorrhage,** blood is released into the space surrounding the brain. This condition is commonly caused by a ruptured aneurysm and is usually fatal.

Signs and symptoms of stroke include weakness in one-half of the body **(hemiparesis),** paralysis in one-half of the body **(hemiplegia),** inability to speak **(aphasia),** lack of muscle coordination **(ataxia),** stupor, loss of consciousness (LOC), coma, or even death. If the stroke is mild, the patient may experience a brief "blackout," visual impairment, difficulty in speaking or understanding speech, or loss of balance and may be unaware of the "minor stroke." Stroke symptoms that resolve within 24 hours are known as a **transient ischemic attack (TIA).** About one-third of all strokes are preceded by a TIA. A family history of cerebrovascular disease and high blood pressure appear to be contributing factors to stroke. Computed tomography (CT) is usually performed to determine the type of stroke. If a "clot buster" **(thrombolytic)** medication is administered within 3 hours of symptom onset, it can usually prevent permanent disability. Antihypertensives may also be administered to control blood pressure. Treatment for disabilities caused by stroke involves speech, physical, and occupational therapy and various medications, depending on the type of stroke.

Seizure Disorders

Seizure disorders include any medical condition characterized by sudden changes in behavior or consciousness as a result of uncontrolled electrical activity in the brain. However, chronic or recurring seizure disorders are called **epilepsies.** Causes of epilepsy include brain injury, congenital anomalies, metabolic disorders, brain tumors, vascular disturbances, and genetic disorders.

Seizures are characterized by sudden bursts of abnormal electrical activity in neurons, resulting in temporary changes in brain function. Patients may experience a warning signal **(aura)** of an imminent seizure. Auras vary considerably and may include sensory phenomena without a precipitating stimulus such as a strange taste in the mouth, the sound of a ringing bell, or an inability to react properly to usual situations. Auras provide time for preparation so that injuries are minimized.

Two major seizure types are partial and generalized. In **partial seizures,** only a portion of the brain is involved. There is a short alteration of consciousness of about 10 to 30 seconds with repetitive, unusual movements and confusion. In a **generalized seizure,** the entire brain is involved. The most common type of generalized seizure is the **tonic-clonic seizure,** also called **grand mal seizure.** In the **tonic phase,** the entire body becomes rigid; in the **clonic phase,** there is uncontrolled jerking caused by alternate muscle contraction and relaxation. Recovery may take minutes to hours and usually leaves the patient weak. In **status epilepticus,** a life-threatening emergency, tonic-clonic seizures follow one after another without an intervening period of recovery. It involves the entire cortex and emergency medical attention is essential. Diagnosis and evaluation of epilepsies commonly rely on electroencephalography and magnetic source imaging (MSI) to locate the affected area of the brain. Epilepsy can usually be controlled by antiepileptic medications.

Parkinson Disease

Parkinson disease, also called **shaking palsy,** is a progressive neurological disorder affecting the portion of the brain responsible for controlling movement. As neurons degenerate, the patient develops uncontrollable nodding of the head, slow movement **(bradykinesia, hypokinesia),** tremors, large joint stiffness, and a shuffling gait. Muscle rigidity causes facial expressions to appear fixed and masklike with unblinking eyes. Sometimes the patient exhibits "pill rolling," in which he or she inadvertently rubs the thumb against the index finger.

In patients with Parkinson disease, dopamine (a neurotransmitter that facilitates the transmission of impulses at synapses) is lacking in the brain. Management involves the administration of L-dopa, which can cross the blood–brain barrier, and is converted to dopamine in the brain. Even so, this treatment only reduces symptoms; it is not a cure for Parkinson disease.

Multiple Sclerosis

Multiple sclerosis (MS) is a progressive, degenerative disease of the central nervous system. MS is characterized by inflammation, hardening, and, finally, loss of myelin **(demyelination)** throughout the spinal cord and brain. Myelin deterioration impedes the transmission of electrical impulses from one neuron to another. In effect, the conduction pathway develops "short circuits."

Signs and symptoms of MS include tremors, muscle weakness, and bradykinesia. Occasionally, visual disturbances exist. During remissions, symptoms temporarily disappear, but progressive hardening of myelin areas leads to other attacks. Ultimately, most voluntary motor control is lost and the patient becomes bedridden. Death occurs anywhere from 7 to 30 years after the onset of the disease. Young adults, usually women, between ages 20 and 40 are the most common victims of MS. The etiology of the disease is unclear, but autoimmune disease or a slow viral infection is believed to be the most probable cause.

Alzheimer Disease

Alzheimer disease (AD) is a progressive neurological disorder that causes memory loss and serious mental deterioration. Small lesions called **plaques** develop in the cerebral cortex and disrupt the passage of electrochemical signals between cells. The clinical manifestations of Alzheimer disease include memory loss and cognitive decline. There is also a decline in social skills and the ability to carry out activities of daily living. Most patients undergo personality, emotional, and behavioral changes. As the disease progresses, loss of concentration and increased fatigue, restlessness, and anxiety are common. Alzheimer disease was once considered rare but is now identified as a leading cause of senile dementia. Although there is no specific treatment, moderate relief has been associated with medications that prevent a breakdown of brain chemicals required for neurotransmission.

Mental Illness

Mental illness includes an array of psychological disorders, syndromes, and behavioral patterns that cause alterations in mood, behavior, and thinking. Its forms range from mild to serious. For example, anxiety may manifest as a slight apprehension or uneasiness lasting a few days, to a more severe form involving intense fears lasting for months and even years. The various forms of mental illnesses commonly result in a diminished capacity for coping with the ordinary demands of life.

Diagnosis and treatment of serious mental disorders usually require the skills of a medical specialist called a **psychiatrist.** In the capacity of a physician, the psychiatrist is licensed to prescribe medications and perform medical procedures not available to those who do not hold a medical license. Psychiatrists commonly work in association with **clinical psychologists,** individuals trained in evaluating human behavior, intelligence, and personality.

Psychosis refers to a mental disorder in which there is severe loss of contact with reality and commonly characterized by false beliefs despite overwhelming evidence to the contrary **(delusions).** The psychotic patient typically "hears voices" and "sees visions" in the absence of an actual stimulus **(hallucinations).** The patient's speech is usually incoherent and disorganized and behavior is erratic.

Neurosis is a mental disorder caused by an emotion experienced in the past that overwhelmingly interferes or affects a present emotion. For example, a child bitten by a dog may show irrational fear of animals as an adult. Many mental disorders are forms of neuroses, including irrational fears **(phobias),** exaggerated emotional and reflexive behaviors **(hysterias),** or irrational, uncontrolled performance of ritualistic actions for fear of a dire consequence **(obsessive-compulsive disorders).** (See Table 15-3.)

Research and education have removed much of the stigma attached to mental illness. Today, mental illness is becoming a more recognizable and treatable disorder. Many psychological disorders can be effectively treated or managed by family physicians, school psychologists, marriage counselors, family counselors, and even such support groups as grief support groups and Alcoholics Anonymous.

Table 15-3	**Common Terms Associated with Mental Illness**
Term	**Definition**
affective disorder	Psychological disorder in which the major characteristic is an abnormal mood, usually mania or depression
anorexia nervosa ăn-ō-RĔK-sē-ă nĕr-VŌS-ă	Eating disorder characterized by a refusal to maintain adequate weight for age and height and an all-consuming desire to remain thin
anxiety	Psychological "worry" disorder characterized by excessive pondering or thinking "what if..." *Feelings of worry, dread, lack of energy, and a loss of interest in life are common signs associated with anxiety.*
attention deficit–hyperactivity disorder (ADHD) hī-pĕr-ăk-TĬV-ĭ-tē	Disorder affecting children and adults characterized by impulsiveness, overactivity, and the inability to remain focused on a task *Behavioral modification with or without medical management is commonly used in the treatment of ADHD.*

(continued)

Table 15-3	Common Terms Associated with Mental Illness—cont'd

Term	Definition
autism AW-tĭzm	Developmental disorder characterized by extreme withdrawal and an abnormal absorption in fantasy, usually accompanied by an inability to communicate even on a basic level *A person with autism may engage in repetitive behavior, such as rocking or repeating words.*
bipolar disorder bī-PŌL-ăr	Mental disorder that causes unusual shifts in mood, emotion, energy, and the ability to function; also called *manic-depressive illness*
bulimia nervosa bū-LĒM-ē-ă nĕr-VŌS-ă	Eating disorder characterized by binging (overeating) and purging (vomiting or use of laxatives)
depression dē-PRĔSH-ŭn	Mood disorder associated with sadness, despair, discouragement, and, commonly, feelings of low self-esteem, guilt, and withdrawal
mania MĀ-nē-ă	Mood disorder characterized by mental and physical hyperactivity, disorganized behavior, and excessively elevated mood
neurosis nū-RŌ-sĭs	Nonpsychotic mental illness that triggers feelings of distress and anxiety and impairs normal behavior *A child who has consistently been warned of "germs" by an overprotective parent may later develop an irrational fear of such things as using public restrooms and touching doorknobs or phones.*
panic attack PĂN-ĭk	Sudden, intense feeling of fear that comes without warning and is not attributable to any immediate danger *A key symptom of a panic attack is the fear of its recurrence.*
psychosis sī-KŌ-sĭs	Major emotional disorder in which contact with reality is lost to the point that the individual is incapable of meeting the challenges of daily life

Oncology

Intracranial tumors that originate directly in brain tissue are called **primary intracranial tumors.** They are commonly classified according to histological type and include those that originate in neurons and those that develop in glial tissue. A major symptom of intracranial tumors is headache, especially upon arising in the morning, during coughing episodes, and upon bending or sudden movement. Occasionally, the optic disc in the back of the eyeball swells **(papilledema)** because of increased intracranial pressure. Personality changes are common and include depression, anxiety, and irritability.

Intracranial tumors can arise from any structure within the cranial cavity, including the pituitary and pineal glands, cranial nerves, and the arachnoid and pia mater **(leptomeninges).** In addition, all of these tissues may be the sites of metastatic spread from primary malignancies that occur outside the nervous system. Metastatic tumors of the cranial cavity tend to exhibit growth characteristics similar to those of the primary malignancy but tend to grow more slowly than the parent tumor. Metastatic tumors of the cranial cavity are usually easier to remove than primary intracranial tumors.

Computed tomography (CT) scans and magnetic resonance imaging (MRI) help establish a diagnosis but are not definitive. Surgical removal relieves pressure and confirms or rules out malignancy. Even after surgery, most intracranial tumors require radiation therapy as a second line of treatment. Chemotherapy combined with radiation therapy usually provides the best chance for survival and quality of life.

Diseases and Conditions

This section introduces diseases and conditions of the nervous system with their meanings and pronunciations. Word analyses for selected terms are also provided.

Term	Definition

agnosia
ăg-NŌ-zē-ă
  a-: without, not
  gnos: knowing
  -ia: condition
	Inability to comprehend auditory, visual, spatial, olfactory, or other sensations, even though the sensory sphere is intact
	The type of agnosia is usually identified by the sense or senses affected, such as visual agnosia. Agnosia is common in parietal lobe tumors.

asthenia
ăs-THĔ-nē-ă
  a-: without, not
  sthen: strength
  -ia: condition
	Weakness, debility, or loss of strength
	Asthenia is a characteristic of multiple sclerosis (MS).

ataxia
ă-TĂK-sē-ă
  a-: without, not
  tax: order, coordination
  -ia: condition
	Lack of muscle coordination in the execution of voluntary movement
	Ataxia may be the result of head injury, stroke, MS, alcoholism, or a variety of hereditary disorders.

closed head trauma TRAW-mă	Injury to the head in which the dura mater remains intact and brain tissue is not exposed *In closed head trauma, the injury site may occur at the impact site, where the brain hits the inside of the skull (coup) or at the rebound site, where the opposite side of the brain strikes the skull (contrecoup).*
coma KŌ-mă	Abnormally deep unconsciousness with an absence of voluntary response to stimuli
concussion kŏn-KŬSH-ŭn	Injury to the brain, occasionally with transient loss of consciousness, as a result of trauma to the head *Delayed symptoms of concussion may include headache, nausea, vomiting, and blurred vision.*
convulsion kŏn-VŬL-shŭn	Any sudden and violent contraction of one or more voluntary muscles

dementia
dĭ-MĔN-shē-ă
  de-: cessation
  ment: mind
  -ia: condition
	Broad term that refers to cognitive deficit, including memory impairment

dyslexia
dĭs-LĔK-sē-ă
  dys-: bad; painful; difficult
  lex: word, phrase
  -ia: condition
	Inability to learn and process written language, despite adequate intelligence, sensory ability, and exposure

(continued)

Term	Definition
Guillain-Barré syndrome gē-YĂ băr-RĀ SĬN-drōm	Autoimmune condition that causes acute inflammation of the peripheral nerves in which myelin sheaths on the axons are destroyed, resulting in decreased nerve impulses, loss of reflex response, and sudden muscle weakness *This disease usually follows a viral gastrointestinal or respiratory infection, stress, or trauma. The muscle weakness involves the entire body and the patient may temporarily require respiratory support until the inflammation subsides.*
herpes zoster HĔR-pēz ZŎS-tĕr	Acute inflammatory eruption of highly painful vesicles on the trunk of the body or, occasionally, the face; also called *shingles* (See Figure 15-7.) *Herpes zoster is caused by the same virus that causes chickenpox. The first symptom is pain along the course of the affected nerve, usually occurring 1 to 3 days before appearance of the lesions. The skin eruption begins as an erythematous maculopapular rash that develops rapidly into vesicles.* **Figure 15-7** Herpes zoster (shingles). From Goldsmith, Lazarus, and Tharp: *Adult and Pediatric Dermatology: A Color Guide to Diagnosis and Treatment.* FA Davis, Philadelphia, 1997, p 307, with permission.
Huntington chorea HŬNT-ĭng-tŭn kō-RĒ-ă	Inherited disease of the CNS characterized by quick, involuntary movements, speech disturbances, and mental deterioration *Onset of Huntington chorea commonly occurs between ages 30 and 50.*
hydrocephalus hī-drō-SĔF-ă-lŭs *hydr/o:* water *cephal:* head *-us:* condition; structure	Accumulation of fluid in the ventricles of the brain, causing increased intracranial pressure (ICP), thinning of brain tissue, and separation of cranial bones
acquired	Hydrocephalus that develops at birth or any time afterward as a result of injury or disease
congenital kŏn-JĔN-ĭ-tăl	Hydrocephalus caused by factors that occur during fetal development or as a result of genetic abnormalities
lethargy LĔTH-ăr-jē	Abnormal inactivity or lack of response to normal stimuli

Term	Definition
anencephaly ăn-ĕn-SĔF-ă-lē *an-:* without, not, loss *encephal:* brain *-y:* noun ending	Congenital deformity in which some or all of fetal brain is missing *With this defect, the infant is usually stillborn or dies shortly after birth. This deformity can be detected through amniocentesis or ultrasonography early in pregnancy.*
spina bifida SPĪ-nă BĬ-fĭ-dă	Congenital deformity of the neural tube (embryonic structure that becomes the fetal brain and spinal cord), which fails to close during fetal development; also called *neural tube defect* *The most common forms of spina bifida include meningocele, meningomyelocele, and occulta. (See Figure 15–8.)*
meningocele mĕn-ĬN-gō-sēl *mening/o:* meninges (membranes covering the brain and spinal cord) *-cele:* hernia, swelling	Form of spina bifida in which the spinal cord develops properly but the meninges protrude through the spine
myelomeningocele mī-ĕ-lō-mĕn-ĬN-gō-sēl *myel/o:* bone marrow; spinal cord *mening/o:* meninges (membranes covering the brain and spinal cord) *-cele:* hernia, swelling	Most severe form of spina bifida in which the spinal cord and meninges protrude through the spine
occulta ŏ-KŬL-tă	Form of spina bifida in which one or more vertebrae are malformed and the spinal cord is covered with a layer of skin

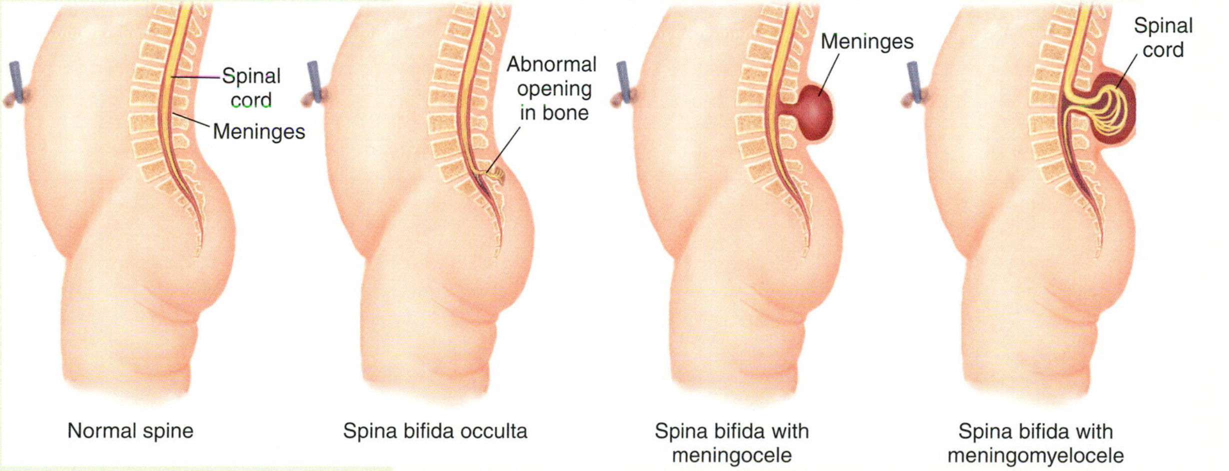

Normal spine   Spina bifida occulta   Spina bifida with meningocele   Spina bifida with meningomyelocele

Figure 15-8 Spina bifida.

(continued)

Term	Definition
palsy PAWL-zē	Paralysis, usually partial, and commonly characterized by weakness and shaking or uncontrolled tremor
Bell	Facial paralysis caused by a functional disorder of the seventh cranial nerve *Bell palsy is self-limiting and usually spontaneously resolves in 3 to 5 weeks. It is associated with herpes virus.*
cerebral sĕ-RĒ-brăl *cerebr:* cerebrum *-al:* pertaining to	Type of paralysis that affects movement and body position and, sometimes, speech and learning ability *Cerebral palsy (CP) commonly occurs as a result of trauma to the brain during the birthing process.*
paralysis pă-RĂL-ĭ-sĭs *para-:* near, beside; beyond *-lysis:* separation, destruction, loosening	Loss of voluntary motion in one or more muscle groups with or without loss of sensation *Strokes and spinal cord injuries are the common causes of paralysis. Strokes usually affect only one side of the body. Spinal cord injuries result in paralysis below the site of the injury. (See Figure 15-9.)*
hemiplegia hĕm-ē-PLĒ-jē-ă *hemi-:* one-half *-plegia:* paralysis	Paralysis of one side of the body, typically as the result of a stroke; also called *unilateral paralysis*
paraplegia păr-ă-PLĒ-jē-ă *para-:* near, beside; beyond *-plegia:* paralysis	Paralysis of both lower limbs, typically as a result of trauma or disease of the lower spinal cord
quadriplegia kwŏd-rĭ-PLĒ-jē-ă *quadri-:* four *-plegia:* paralysis	Paralysis of both arms and legs, commonly resulting in bowel, bladder, and sexual dysfunction

Term	Definition

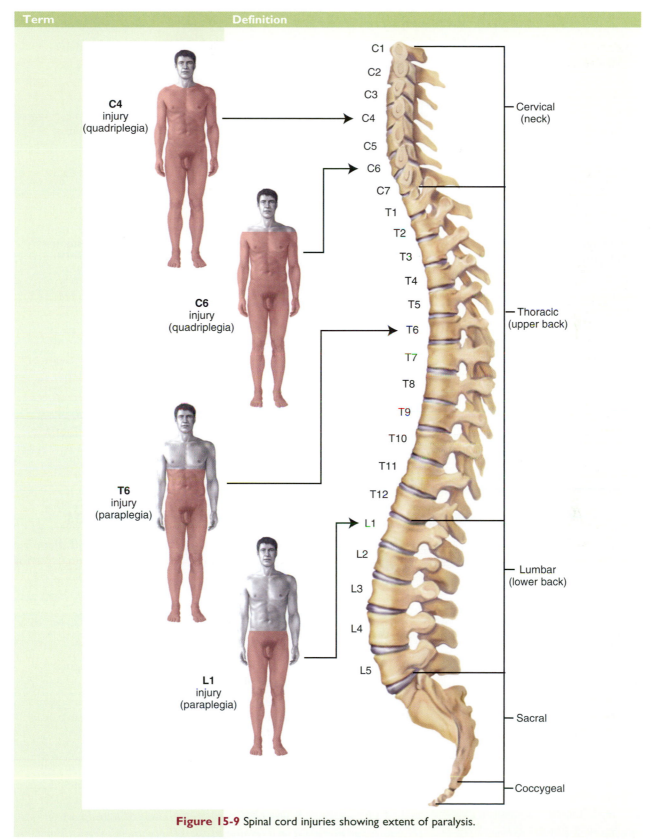

Figure 15-9 Spinal cord injuries showing extent of paralysis.

(continued)

Term	Definition
paresthesia păr-ĕs-THĒ-zē-ă	Sensation of numbness, prickling, tingling, or heightened sensitivity *Paresthesia can be caused by disorders affecting the central nervous system, such as stroke, transient ischemic attack, multiple sclerosis, transverse myelitis, and encephalitis.*
poliomyelitis pŏl-ē-ō-mī-ĕl-Ī-tĭs *poli/o:* gray; gray matter (of the brain or spinal cord) *myel:* bone marrow; spinal cord *–itis:* inflammation	Inflammation of the gray matter of the spinal cord caused by a virus, commonly resulting in spinal and muscle deformity and paralysis *Polio is preventable with standard vaccinations administered to children.*
Reye syndrome RĪ SĬN-drōm	Acute encephalopathy and fatty infiltration of the brain, liver, and, possibly, the pancreas, heart, kidney, spleen, and lymph nodes *Reye syndrome is usually seen in children younger than age 15 who had an acute viral infection. Mortality in Reye syndrome may be as high as 80%. The use of aspirin by children experiencing chickenpox or influenza may induce Reye syndrome.*
syncope SĬN-kō-pē	Brief loss of consciousness and posture caused by a temporary decrease of blood flow to the brain; also called *fainting* *Syncope may be associated with a sudden decrease in blood pressure, a decrease in heart rate, or changes in blood volume or distribution. The person usually regains consciousness and becomes alert right away, but may experience a brief period of confusion.*

 It is time to review pathology, diseases, and conditions by completing Learning Activity 15–3.

Medical, Surgical, and Diagnostic Procedures

This section introduces medical, surgical, and diagnostic procedures used to treat and diagnose neurological disorders. Descriptions are provided as well as pronunciations and word analyses for selected terms.

Procedure	Description
Medical	
electroencephalography (EEG) ē-lĕk-trō-ĕn-sĕf-ă-LŎG-ră-fē *electr/o:* electricity *encephal/o:* brain *-graphy:* process of recording	Recording of electrical activity in the brain, whose cells emit distinct patterns of rhythmic electrical impulses *Different wave patterns in the EEG are associated with normal and abnormal waking and sleeping states. They help diagnose such conditions as tumors and infections and help locate seizure focus or areas of inactivity.*
electromyography (EMG) ē-lĕk-trō-mī-ŎG-ră-fē *electr/o:* electricity *my/o:* muscle *-graphy:* process of recording	Recording of electrical signals (action potentials) that occur in a muscle when it is at rest and during contraction to assess muscular disease or nerve damage *In an EMG, an electrode inserted into a muscle transmits electrical activity of the muscle and displays it on a monitor to assess the health of the muscle and the motor neurons that control it.*

Procedure	Description
lumbar puncture (LP) LŬM-băr PŬNK-chūr	Needle puncture of the spinal cavity to extract spinal fluid for diagnostic purposes, introduce anesthetic agents into the spinal canal, or remove fluid to allow other fluids (such as radiopaque substances) to be injected; also called *spinal puncture* and *spinal tap* (See Figure 15-10.)

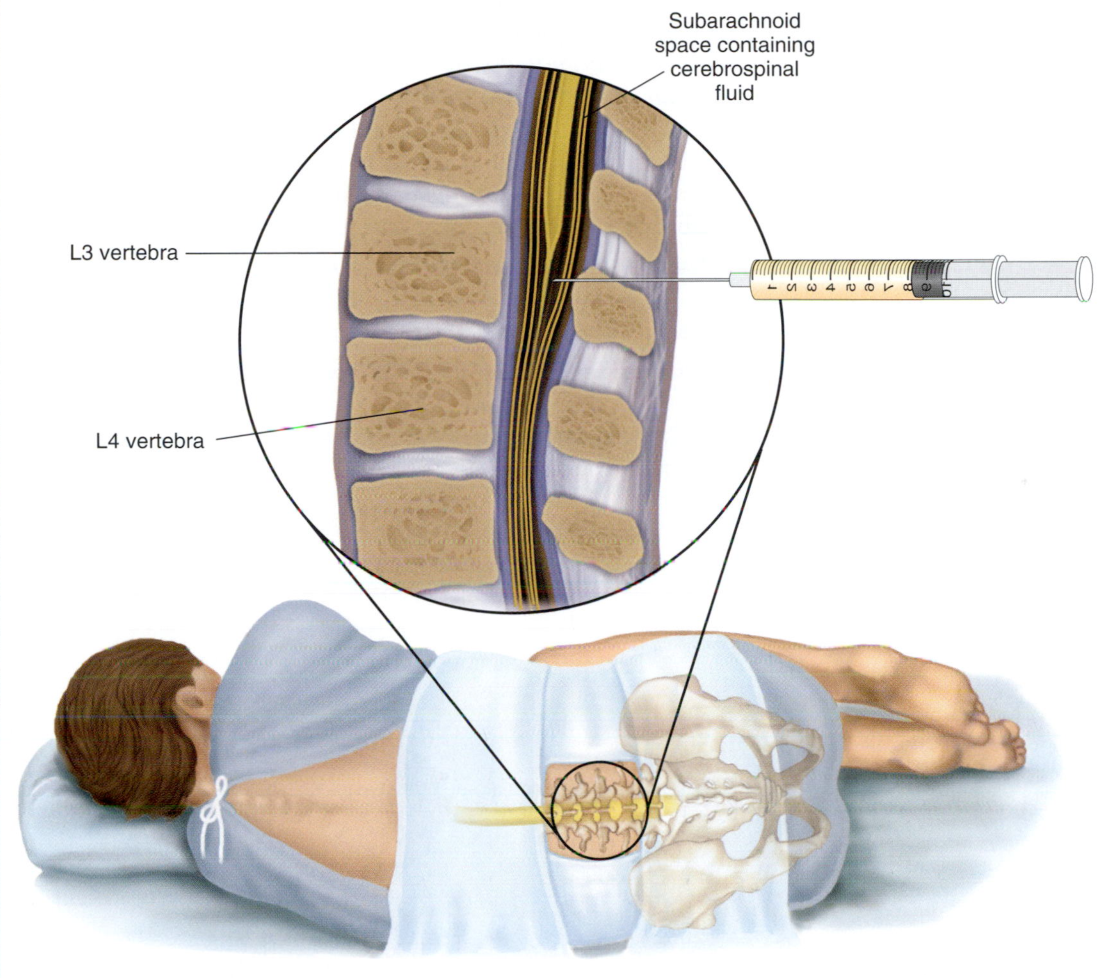

Subarachnoid space containing cerebrospinal fluid

L3 vertebra

L4 vertebra

Figure 15-10 Lumbar puncture.

nerve conduction velocity (NCV) NĔRV kŏn-DŬK-shŭn vĕ-LŎ-sĭ-tē	Test that measures the speed at which impulses travel through a nerve *In NCV, one electrode stimulates a nerve while other electrodes, placed over different areas of the nerve record an electrical signal (action potential) as it travels through the nerve. This test is used for diagnosing muscular dystrophy and neurological disorders that destroy myelin.*

Surgical

cryosurgery krī-ō-SĔR-jĕr-ē	Technique that exposes abnormal tissue to extreme cold to destroy it *Cryosurgery is sometimes used to destroy malignant tumors of the brain.*

(continued)

Procedure	Description
stereotactic radiosurgery (SRS) stĕr-ē-ō-TĂK-tĭk rā-dē-ō-SŬR-jĕr-ē	Precisely focused (stereotactic) radiation beams are used to treat tumors and other abnormal growths in the brain, spinal column and other body sites, and delivers high doses of radiation to the tumor with minimal exposure to surrounding healthy tissue *SRS is used to treat a variety of brain tumors that are malignant (gliomas, metastases) or benign (meningiomas, pituitary adenomas). It also has an enhanced ability to control intracranial disease coupled with a reduction in the risk of side effects from radiation therapy.*
thalamotomy thăl-ă-MŎT-ō-mē *thalam/o:* thalamus *-tomy:* incision	Partial destruction of the thalamus to treat intractable pain; involuntary movements, including tremors in Parkinson disease; or emotional disturbances *Thalamotomy produces few neurological deficits or changes in personality.*
tractotomy trăk-TŎT-ō-mē	Transection of a nerve tract in the brain stem or spinal cord *Tractotomy is sometimes used to relieve intractable pain.*
trephination trĕf-ĭn-Ā-shŭn	Technique that cuts a circular opening into the skull to reveal brain tissue and decrease intracranial pressure
ventriculoperitoneal shunting vĕn-trĭk-ū-lō-pĕr-ĭ-tō-NĒ-ăl SHŬNT-ĭng *ventricul/o:* ventricle *peritone:* peritoneum *-al:* pertaining to	Relieves intracranial pressure due to hydrocephalus by diverting (shunting) excess cerebrospinal fluid from the ventricles into the peritoneal or thoracic cavity (See Figure 15-11.) 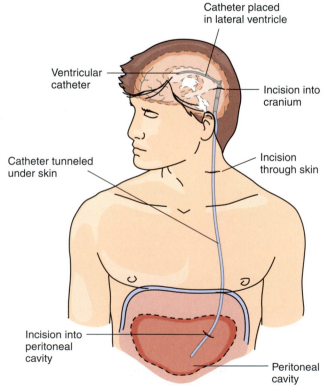 **Figure 15-11** Ventriculoperitoneal shunt. From Williams and Hopper: *Understanding Medical-Surgical Nursing,* 4th ed. FA Davis, Philadelphia, 2011, p 1199, with permission.

Procedure	Description
Diagnostic	

Laboratory

Procedure	Description

cerebrospinal fluid (CSF) analysis
sĕr-ē-brō-SPĪ-năl
  cerebr/o: cerebrum
  spin: spine
  -al: pertaining to
	Laboratory test to examine a sample of the fluid surrounding the brain and spinal cord; used to diagnose disorders of the central nervous system, including viral and bacterial infections, tumors, and hemorrhage
	The fluid is withdrawn through a needle in the procedure called lumbar puncture.

Imaging

Procedure	Description

angiography
ăn-jē-ŎG-ră-fē
  angi/o: vessel (usually blood or lymph)
  -graphy: process of recording
	Radiographic image (angiogram) of the inside of a blood vessel after injection of a contrast medium; also called *arteriography*
	Angiography is used to diagnose vascular disorders, especially blockages, narrowed areas, and aneurysms.

computed tomography angiography (CTA)
  kŏm-PŪ-tĕd tŏ-MŎG-ră-fē
  ăn-jē-ŎG-ră-fē
    tom/o: to cut
    -graphy: process of recording
    angi/o: vessel (usually blood or lymph)
    -graphy: process of recording
	Angiography in combination with a CT scan to produce high-resolution, three-dimensional vascular images of the blood vessels
	CTA, or CT angiography, identifies blocked blood vessels, aneurysms, and buildup of plaque in a blood vessel. It also aids in differentiating hemorrhagic stroke and ischemic stroke.

discography dĭs-KŎG-ră-fē	CT scan of the lumbar region after injection of a contrast medium to detect problems with the spine and spinal nerve roots

echoencephalography
ĕk-ō-ĕn-sĕf-ă-LŎG-ră-fē
  echo-: repeated sound
  encephal/o: brain
  -graphy: process of recording
	Ultrasound technique used to study intracranial structures of the brain and diagnose conditions that cause a shift in the midline structures of the brain
	This bedside procedure is especially useful in detecting hemorrhage and hydrocephalus in children less than 2 years of age and infants in the neonatal unit but has largely been replaced by CT for older children and adults.

magnetic source imaging (MSI)	Noninvasive neuroimaging technique to pinpoint the specific location where seizure activity originates and enable custom surgical treatment for tumor and epileptic tissue resection; also called *magnetoencephalography* (MEG) *MSI is medically necessary for presurgical evaluation of persons with epilepsy to identify and localize areas of epileptic activity.*

myelography
mī-ĕ-LŎG-ră-fē
  myel/o: bone marrow; spinal cord
  -graphy: process of recording
	Radiographic examination to detect pathology of the spinal cord, including the location of a spinal cord injury, cysts, and tumors following injection of a contrast medium

positron emission tomography (PET) PŎZ-ĭ-trŏn ē-MĬSH-ŭn tŏ-MŎG-ră-fē	Computed tomography that records the positrons (positively charged particles) emitted from a radiopharmaceutical and produces a cross-sectional image of metabolic activity of body tissues to determine the presence of disease *PET is particularly useful in scanning the brain and nervous system to diagnose disorders that involve abnormal tissue metabolism, such as schizophrenia, brain tumors, epilepsy, stroke, and Alzheimer disease, as well as cardiac and pulmonary disorders.*

Pharmacology

Neurological agents are used to relieve or eliminate pain, suppress seizures, control tremors, and reduce muscle rigidity. (See Table 15-4.) Hypnotics, a class of drugs used as sedatives, depress CNS function to relieve agitation and induce sleep. Anesthetics are capable of producing a complete or partial loss of feeling and are used for surgery. Psychotherapeutic agents alter brain chemistry to treat mental illness. These drugs are used as mood stabilizers in various mental disorders. They also reduce symptoms of depression and treat ADHD and narcolepsy.

Table 15-4 | **Drugs Used to Treat Neurological and Psychiatric Disorders**

This table lists common drug classifications used to treat neurological and psychiatric disorders along with their therapeutic actions, and selected generic and trade names.

Classification	Therapeutic Action	Generic and *Trade* Names
Neurological		
anesthetics ăn-ĕs-THĔT-ĭks	Produce partial or complete loss of sensation, with or without loss of consciousness *Forms of anesthetics include general, local, and nerve block.*	
general	Act upon the brain to produce complete loss of feeling with loss of consciousness *General anesthetics affect all areas of the body including the brain. Because they suppress all reflexes, including coughing and swallowing, breathing tubes are usually required during their administration.*	**propofol** PRŎ-pō-fŏl *Diprivan*
local	Act upon nerves or nerve tracts to affect only a local area *Local anesthetics are injected directly into the area involved in the local surgery. Patients may remain fully alert unless additional medications to induce sleep are given.*	**procaine** PRŌ-kān *Novocain* **lidocaine** LĪ-dō-kān *Xylocaine*
nerve block	Type of regional anesthetic to block pain from the area supplied by that nerve *A nerve block is usually used for procedures on the arms, legs, hands, feet, and face.*	**levobupivacaine** lĕv-ō-bū-PĪ-vă-kān *Chirocaine*
anticonvulsants ăn-tĭ-kŏn-VŬL-sănts	Prevent uncontrolled neuron activity associated with seizures by altering electrical transmission along neurons or altering the chemical composition of neurotransmitters; also called *antiepileptics* *Many anticonvulsants are also used as mood stabilizers.*	**carbamazepine** kăr-bă-MĂZ-ĕ-pēn *Tegretol* **valproate** văl-PRŌ-āt *Depacon* **phenytoin** FĔN-ĭ-tō-ĭn *Dilantin*
antiparkinsonian agents ăn-tĭ-păr-kĭn-SŌN-ē-ăn	Control tremors and muscle rigidity associated with Parkinson disease by increasing dopamine in the brain	**levodopa** lē-vō-DŌ-pă *l-dopa, Larodopa* **levodopa/carbidopa** kăr-bĭ-DŌ-pă *Sinemet, Sinemet CR*

Table 15-4	Drugs Used to Treat Neurological and Psychiatric Disorders—cont'd	
Classification	**Therapeutic Action**	**Generic and *Trade* Names**
Psychiatric		
antipsychotics ăn-tĭ-sī-KŎT-ĭks	Treat psychosis, paranoia, and schizophrenia by altering chemicals in the brain, including the limbic system (group of brain structures), which controls emotions	**clozapine** CLŌ-ză-pēn *Clozaril* **risperidone** rĭs-PĔR-ĭ-dōn *Risperdal*
antidepressants ăn-tĭ-dē-PRĔS-săntz	Treat multiple symptoms of depression by increasing levels of specific neurotransmitters *Antidepressants fall under different classifications and some are also used to treat anxiety and pain.*	**citalopram** sī-TĂL-ō-prăm *Celexa* **fluoxetine** floo-ŎK-sĕ-tēn *Prozac*
hypnotics hĭp-NŎT-ĭks	Depress central nervous system (CNS) functions, promote sedation and sleep, and relieve agitation, anxiousness, and restlessness *Hypnotics may be nonbarbiturates or barbiturates. Barbiturate hypnotics carry a risk of addiction.*	**secobarbital** sē-kō-BĂR-bĭ-tŏl *Seconal* **temazepam** tĕ-MĂZ-ĕ-păm *Restoril*
psychostimulants sī-kō-STĬM-ū-lăntz	Reduce impulsive behavior by increasing the level of neurotransmitters *Psychostimulants have a calming effect on people with attention deficit–hyperactivity disorder (ADHD) and are also used to treat narcolepsy.*	**dextroamphetamine** dĕks-trō-ăm-FĔT-ă-mēn *Dexedrine* **methylphenidate** mĕth-ĭl-FĔN-ĭ-dāt *Ritalin*

Abbreviations

This section introduces nervous system–related abbreviations and their meanings.

Abbreviation	Meaning	Abbreviation	Meaning
AD	Alzheimer disease	**LOC**	loss of consciousness
ADHD	attention deficit–hyperactivity disorder	**LP**	lumbar puncture
CNS	central nervous system	**MEG**	magnetoencephalography
CP	cerebral palsy	**MRI**	magnetic resonance imaging
CSF	cerebrospinal fluid	**MS**	musculoskeletal; multiple sclerosis; mental status; mitral stenosis
CT	computed tomography	**MSI**	magnetic source imaging
CTA	computed tomography angiography	**NCV**	nerve conduction velocity
CVA	cerebrovascular accident	**PET**	positron emission tomography
EEG	electroencephalography	**PNS**	peripheral nervous system
EMG	electromyography	**SRS**	stereotactic radiosurgery
ICP	intracranial pressure	**TIA**	transient ischemic attack

⌖ *It is time to review procedures, pharmacology, and abbreviations by completing Learning Activity 15–4.*

LEARNING ACTIVITIES

The following activities provide review of the nervous system terms introduced in this chapter. Complete each activity and review your answers to evaluate your understanding of the chapter.

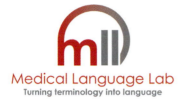
Medical Language Lab
Turning terminology into language

Visit the Medical Language Lab at the web site: medicallanguagelab.com. Use it to enhance your study and reinforcement of this chapter with the flash-card activity. We recommend you complete the flash-card activity before starting Learning Activities 15-1 and 15-2 below.

Learning Activity 15-1
Combining Forms, Suffixes, and Prefixes

Use the elements listed below to build medical words. You may use elements more than once.

Combining Forms		Suffixes		Prefixes
cerebr/o	myel/o	-al	-oma	hyper-
encephal/o	narc/o	-algia	-pathy	intra-
gangli/o	neur/o	-asthenia	-plegia	quadri-
kinesi/o	radicul/o	-cele	-rrhaphy	uni-
later/o	thec/o	-itis	-stomy	
mening/o	ventricul/o	-kinesia	-therapy	
my/o		-lepsy		

1. forming an opening (mouth) in the ventricle _____

2. tumor of a nerve _____

3. pain in a nerve root _____

4. inflammation of a ganglion _____

5. seizure of sleep _____

6. pertaining to one side _____

7. inflammation of the meninges _____

8. paralysis of four (extremities) _____

9. movement that is excessive _____

10. weakness or debility of muscles _____

11. disease of the cerebrum _____

12. pertaining to within the sheath _____

13. hernia(tion) or swelling of the brain _____

14. treatment (using) movement _____

15. suture of the spinal cord _____

 Check your answers in Appendix A. Review any material that you did not answer correctly.

Correct Answers _____ X 6.67 = _____ % Score

Learning Activity 15-2
Building Medical Words

Use *encephal/o* (brain) to build words that mean:

1. disease of the brain _____
2. herniation of the brain _____
3. radiography of the brain _____

Use *cerebr/o* (cerebrum) to build words that mean:

4. disease of the cerebrum _____
5. inflammation of the cerebrum _____

Use *crani/o* (cranium [skull]) to build words that mean:

6. herniation (through the) cranium _____
7. instrument for measuring the skull _____

Use *neur/o* (nerve) to build words that mean:

8. pain in a nerve _____
9. specialist in the study of the nervous system _____
10. crushing a nerve _____

Use *myel/o* (bone marrow; spinal cord) to build words that mean:

11. herniation of the spinal cord _____
12. paralysis of the spinal cord _____

Use *psych/o* (mind) to build words that mean:

13. pertaining to the mind _____
14. abnormal condition of the mind _____

Use the suffix *-kinesia* (movement) to build words that mean:

15. movement that is slow _____
16. painful or difficult movement _____

Use the suffix *-plegia* (paralysis) to build words that mean:

17. paralysis of one half (of the body) _____
18. paralysis of four (limbs) _____

Use the suffix *-phasia* (speech) to build words that mean:

19. difficult speech _____
20. lacking or without speech _____

Build surgical terms that mean:

21. destruction of a nerve _____

22. incision of the skull _____

23. surgical repair of the skull _____

24. suture of a nerve _____

25. incision of the brain _____

    Check your answers in Appendix A. Review material that you did not answer correctly.

Correct Answers _____ X 4 = _____ % Score

Learning Activity 15-3
Pathology, Diseases, and Conditions

Match the following terms with the definitions in the numbered list.

Alzheimer	clonic	Guillain-Barré	paraplegia
ataxia	concussion	hemiparesis	Parkinson
autism	convulsion	ischemic	poliomyelitis
bipolar disorder	dementia	multiple sclerosis	radiculopathy
bulimia	epilepsies	myelomeningocele	shingles

1. weakness in one-half of the body _____
2. cognitive deficit, including memory impairment _____
3. disease associated with formation of small plaques in the cerebral cortex _____
4. eating disorder characterized by binging and purging _____
5. phase of the grand mal seizure characterized by uncontrolled jerking of the body _____
6. autoimmune syndrome that causes acute inflammation of peripheral nerves _____
7. defective muscle coordination _____
8. mental disorder that causes unusual shifts in mood, emotion, and energy _____
9. chronic or recurring seizure disorders _____
10. stroke caused by narrowing of the carotid arteries _____
11. disease caused by the same organism that causes chickenpox in children _____
12. disease of the nerve root associated with the spinal cord _____
13. paralysis of the lower portion of the trunk and both legs _____
14. disease that causes inflammation of the gray matter of the spinal cord _____
15. sudden and violent contraction of one or more voluntary muscles _____
16. most severe form of spina bifida, where the spinal cord and meninges protrude though the spine _____
17. mental disorder characterized by extreme withdrawal and abnormal absorption in fantasy _____
18. disease characterized by head nodding, bradykinesia, tremors, and shuffling gait _____
19. disease characterized by demyelination in the spinal cord and brain _____
20. loss of consciousness caused by trauma to the head _____

✔ *Check your answers in Appendix A. Review any material that you did not answer correctly.*

Correct Answers _____ X 5 = _____ % Score

Learning Activity 15-4

Procedures, Pharmacology, and Abbreviations

Match the following terms with the definitions in the numbered list.

antipsychotics	electromyography	myelography	TIA
cryosurgery	general anesthetics	NCV	tractotomy
CSF analysis	hypnotics	psychostimulants	trephination
echoencephalography	lumbar puncture	thalamotomy	

1. tests the speed at which impulses travel through a nerve _____

2. treat attention deficit hyperactivity disorder and narcolepsy _____

3. treat psychosis, paranoia, and schizophrenia by altering chemicals in the brain, including the limbic system, which controls emotions _____

4. act upon the brain to produce complete loss of feeling with loss of consciousness _____

5. ultrasound technique used to study the intracranial structures of the brain _____

6. technique that uses extreme cold to destroy tissue _____

7. radiological examination of the spinal canal, nerve roots, and spinal cord _____

8. stroke whose symptoms resolve in about 24 hours _____

9. laboratory analysis used to diagnose infections, tumors, and intracranial hemorrhage _____

10. recording of electrical signals when a muscle is at rest and during contraction to assess nerve damage _____

11. procedure to extract spinal fluid for diagnostic purposes, introduce anesthetic agents, or remove fluid _____

12. surgical treatment for intractable pain; involuntary movements, including tremors in Parkinson disease; or emotional disturbances _____

13. transection of a nerve tract in the brain stem or spinal cord _____

14. agents that depress central nervous system functions, promote sedation and sleep, and relieve agitation, anxiousness, and restlessness _____

15. incision of a circular opening into the skull to reveal brain tissue and decrease intracranial pressure _____

Check your answers in Appendix A. Review any material that you did not answer correctly.

Correct Answers _____ X 6.67 = _____ % Score

Learning Activity 15-5
Medical Scenarios

To construct chart notes, replace the italicized terms in each of the scenarios with one of the medical terms listed below.

bradykinesia	*neuralgia*	*Parkinson disease*
bradyphasia	*neuropathy*	*sciatica*
dysphagia	*osteophyte*	*tremor*
herniation		

Mr. K., a 58-year-old male, works at a local newspaper. He has been tying and lifting bundles of papers, and placing them in trucks for delivery throughout the city, for most of his life. He complains of (1) *nerve pain* of the lower back and, when standing, (2) *pain that radiates down the nerve* of his right leg, causing his foot to "tingle." The results of an MRI show a (3) *protrusion* of the disc at the L3-L4, compressing the nerve. The MRI also reveals a small (4) *bone spur* impinging on the same nerve. A nerve conduction velocity will be ordered to assess (5) *nerve disease*.

1. _____
2. _____
3. _____
4. _____
5. _____

Mr. M. is an 82-year-old man who was brought to our office by his daughter. She expresses concern because her father frequently has a "far away stare," and his left hand has developed a noticeable (6) *shake*. His (7) *slow speech* and "word slurring" makes it difficult for her to understand and respond to him, causing him further frustration. The daughter notes that her father has (8) *slow movement* and (9) *difficulty in swallowing*, often gagging on his food. The results of a complete medical history, examination, and full neurological workup indicate that this gentleman is suffering from (10) *shaking palsy*. The plan is to begin treatment with Levodopa. This medication increases dopamine in the brain and helps control tremors and muscle rigidity.

6. _____
7. _____
8. _____
9. _____
10. _____

✓ *Check your answers in Appendix A. Review any material that you did not answer correctly.*

Correct Answers _____ X 10 = _____ % Score

MEDICAL RECORD ACTIVITIES

The two medical records included in the following activities use common clinical scenarios to show how medical terminology is used to document patient care. Complete the terminology and analysis sections for each activity to help you recognize and understand terms related to the nervous system.

Medical Record Activity 15-1
Discharge Summary: Subarachnoid Hemorrhage

Terminology

Terms listed in the following table are taken from *Discharge Summary: Subarachnoid Hemorrhage* that follows. Use a medical dictionary such as *Taber's Cyclopedic Medical Dictionary;* the appendices of *Systems,* 7th ed.; or other resources to define each term. Then review the pronunciations for each term and practice by reading the medical record aloud.

Term	Definition
aneurysm ĂN-ū-rĭzm	
cerebral MRI sĕ-RĒ-brăl	
cisterna subarachnoidalis sĭs-TĔR-nă sŭb-ă- răk-NOYD-ă-lĭs	
CSF	
CT	
hydrocephalus hī-drō-SĔF-ă-lŭs	
lumbar puncture LŬM-băr PŬNK-chūr	
meningismus mĕn-ĭn-JĬS-mŭs	
occipital ŏk-SĬP-ĭ-tăl	
R/O	
subarachnoid sŭb-ă-RĂK-noyd	

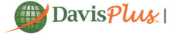

Visit the *Medical Terminology Systems* online resource center at Davis*Plus* to practice pronunciation and reinforce the meanings of the terms in this medical report.

DISCHARGE SUMMARY: SUBARACHNOID HEMORRHAGE

General Hospital
1511 Ninth Avenue ■■ Sun City, USA 12345 ■■ (555) 802-1887

DISCHARGE SUMMARY

ADMISSION DATE: July 5, 20xx   **DISCHARGE DATE:** July 16, 20xx

ADMITTING DIAGNOSIS: Severe headaches associated with nausea and vomiting.

DISCHARGE DIAGNOSIS: Subarachnoid hemorrhage.

HISTORY OF PRESENT ILLNESS: Patient is a 61-year-old woman who presents at this time complaining of an "extreme severe headache while swimming." She also complains of associated neck pain, occipital pain, nausea, and vomiting.

A CT scan was obtained that showed blood in the cisterna subarachnoidalis consistent with subarachnoid hemorrhage. The patient also had mild acute hydrocephalus. Neurologically, the patient was found to be within normal limits. A cerebral MRI was performed and no aneurysm was noted.

HOSPITAL COURSE: The patient was hospitalized on 7/5/xx. On 7/7/xx, she had sudden worsening of her headache, associated with nausea and vomiting. Also, she was noted to have meningismus on examination. A lumbar puncture was performed to R/O possible rebleed. At the time of the lumbar puncture, CSF in four tubes was read as consistent with recurrent subarachnoid hemorrhage. A repeat MRI was performed without evidence of an aneurysm.

PROCEDURE: On 7/9/xx, the patient underwent repeat MRI, which again showed no aneurysm. The patient was deemed stable for discharge on 7/10/xx.

ACTIVITY: Patient instructed to avoid any type of activity that could result in raised pressure in the head. The patient was advised that she should undergo no activity more vigorous than walking.

Michael R. Saadi, MD
Michael R. Saadi, MD

MRS:dp

D: 7-16-20xx
T: 7-16-20xx

Analysis

Review the medical record *Discharge Summary: Subarachnoid Hemorrhage* to answer the following questions.

1. In what part of the head did the patient feel pain?

   _____

2. What imaging tests were performed, and what was the finding in each test?

   _____

3. What was the result of the lumbar puncture?

   _____

4. What was the result of the repeat MRI?

   _____

5. Regarding activity, what limitations were placed on the patient?

   _____

Consultation Report: Acute-Onset Paraplegia

Terminology

Terms listed in the following table are taken from *Consultation Report: Acute–Onset Paraplegia* that follows. Use a medical dictionary such as *Taber's Cyclopedic Medical Dictionary*; the appendices of *Systems*, 7th ed.; or other resources to define each term. Then review the pronunciations for each term and practice by reading the medical record aloud.

Term	Definition
abscess ĂB-sĕs	
acute ă-KŪT	
clonidine KLŌ-nĭ-dēn	
epidural ĕp-ĭ-DOO-răl	
fluoroscopy floo-or-ŎS-kō-pē	
infarct ĬN-fărkt	
L2-3	
lumbar LŬM-băr	
methadone MĔTH-ă-dōn	
myelitis mī-ĕ-LĪ-tĭs	
paraplegia păr-ă-PLĒ-jē-ă	
paresthesia păr-ĕs-THĒ-zē-ă	

Term	Definition
subarachnoid sŭb-ă-RĂK-noyd	
T10-11	
transverse trăns-VĔRS	

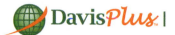 Visit the *Medical Terminology Systems* online resource center at Davis*Plus* to practice pronunciation and reinforce the meanings of the terms in this medical report.

CONSULTATION REPORT: ACUTE-ONSET PARAPLEGIA

Physician Center
2422 Rodeo Drive ■■ Sun City, USA 12345 ■■ (555)788-2427

CONSULTATION

Jacobs, Elaine   **August 15, 20xx**

CHIEF COMPLAINT: Low back pain and lower extremity weakness.

HISTORY OF PRESENT ILLNESS: This is a 41-year-old, right-handed white female with a history of low back pain for the past 15 to 20 years after falling at work. She has had four subsequent lumbar surgeries, with the most recent on 7/20/xx. She was admitted to the hospital for pain management. The patient had a subarachnoid catheter placement for pain control and management on 7/28/xx, at the L10-11 level. This was followed by trials of clonidine for hypertension and methadone for pain control, with bladder retention noted after clonidine administration. Upon catheter removal, the patient noted the subacute onset of paresis, paresthesias, and pain in the legs approximately 2-½ to 3 hours later. We were consulted neurologically for assessment of the lower extremity weakness.

IMPRESSION: Patient has symptoms of acute-onset paraplegia. Differential diagnoses include a subarachnoid hemorrhage, epidural abscess, and transverse myelitis.

PLAN: Patient will be placed on IV steroids with compression stockings for lymphedema should physical therapy be cleared by cardiology for manipulation of that region. Documentation of spinal fluid will be obtained under fluoroscopy. Her glucose and blood pressures must be carefully monitored.

Jake S. Domer, MD
Jake S. Domer, MD

JSD:st

Analysis

Review the medical record *Consultation Report: Acute-Onset Paraplegia* to answer the following questions.

1. What was the original cause of the patient's current problems and what treatments were provided?

_____

2. Why was the patient admitted to the hospital?

_____

3. What medications did the patient receive and why was each given?

_____

4. What was the cause of bladder retention?

_____

5. What occurred after the catheter was removed?

_____

6. What three disorders were listed in the differential diagnosis?

_____

Special Senses

Chapter Outline

Objectives

Upon completion of this chapter, you will be able to:

- Locate and describe the structures of the eye and ear.
- Pronounce, speii, and build words related to the special senses.
- Describe diseases, conditions, and procedures related to the special senses.
- Explain pharmacology related to the treatment of eye and ear disorders.
- Demonstrate your knowledge of this chapter by completing the learning and medical record activities.

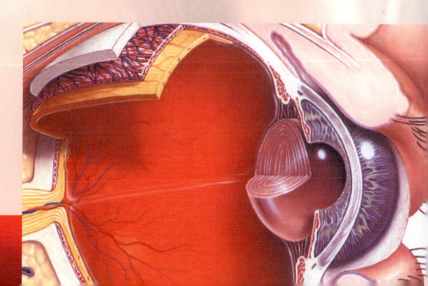

Anatomy and Physiology

General sensations perceived by the body include touch, pressure, pain, and temperature. These sensations are not identified with any specific site of the body. Specific sensations include smell, taste, vision, hearing, and equilibrium. Each specific sensation is connected to a specific organ or structure in the body. This chapter presents information on the sense of vision provided by the eye and senses of hearing and equilibrium provided by the ear.

Anatomy and Physiology Key Terms

This section introduces important terms associated with the special senses and their definitions. Word analyses for selected terms are also provided.

Term	Definition
accommodation ă-kŏm-ō-DĀ-shŭn	Adjustment of the eye for various distances so that images fall on the retina of the eye
acuity ă-KŪ-ĭ-tē	Clearness or sharpness of a sensory function
adnexa ăd-NĔK-să	Tissues or structures in the body adjacent to or near a related structure *The adnexa of the eye include the extraocular muscles, orbits, eyelids, conjunctiva, and lacrimal apparatus.*
humor	Any fluid or semifluid of the body
labyrinth LĂB-ĭ-rĭnth	Series of intricate communicating passages *The labyrinth of the ear includes the cochlea, semicircular canals, and vestibule.*
opaque ō-PĀK	Substance or surface that neither transmits nor allows the passage of light
perilymph PĔR-ĭ-lĭmf	Fluid that very closely resembles spinal fluid but found in the cochlea
photopigment fō-tō-PĬG-mĕnt	Light-sensitive pigment in the retinal cones and rods that absorbs light and initiates the visual process; also called *visual pigment*
refractive rĕ-FRĂK-tĭv	Ability to bend light rays as they pass from one medium to another
tunic TŪ-nĭk	Layer or coat of tissue; also called *membrane layer* *The fibrous, vascular, and sensory tunics are the three layers that comprise the eyeball.*

Pronunciation Help	Long Sound	ā — rate	ē — rebirth	ī — isle	ō — over	ū — unite
	Short Sound	ă — alone	ĕ — ever	ĭ — it	ŏ — not	ŭ — cut

Eye

The eye is a globe-shaped organ composed of three distinct tunics, or layers: the fibrous tunic, the vascular tunic, and the sensory tunic. (See Figure 16-1.)

Fibrous Tunic

The outermost layer of the eyeball, the **fibrous tunic,** serves as a protective coat for the more sensitive structures beneath. It includes the (1) **sclera,** (2) **cornea,** and (3) **conjunctiva.** The sclera, or "white of the eye," provides strength, shape, and structure to the eye. As the sclera passes in front of the eye, it bulges forward to become the cornea. Rather than being opaque, the cornea is transparent, allowing light to enter the interior of the eye. The cornea is one of the few body structures that does not contain capillaries and must rely on eye fluids for nourishment. The conjunctiva covers the outer surface of the eye and lines the eyelids.

Vascular Tunic

The middle layer of the eyeball, the **vascular tunic,** is also known as the *uvea.* The **uvea** consists of the choroid, iris, and ciliary body. The (4) **choroid** provides the blood supply for the entire eye. It contains pigmented cells that prevent extraneous light from entering the inside of the eye. An opening in the choroid allows the optic nerve to enter the inside of the eyeball. The anterior portion of the choroid contains two modified structures, the (5) **iris** and the (6) **ciliary body.** The iris is a colored, contractile membrane with a perforated center called the (7) **pupil.** The iris regulates the amount of light passing through the pupil to the interior of the eye. As environmental light increases, the pupil constricts; as light decreases, the pupil dilates. The ciliary body is a circular muscle that produces aqueous humor. The ciliary body is attached to a capsular bag that holds the (8) **lens** between the (9) **suspensory ligaments.** As the ciliary muscle contracts and relaxes, it

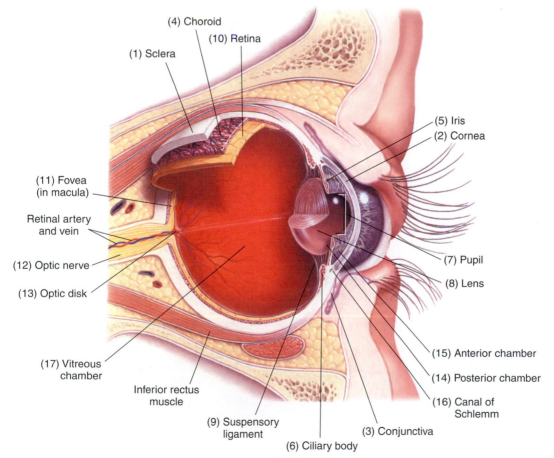

Figure 16-1 Eye structures.

alters the shape of the lens making it thicker or thinner. These changes in shape allow the eye to focus on an image, a process called **accommodation** (Acc).

Sensory Tunic

The innermost **sensory tunic** is the delicate, double-layered (10) **retina.** It consists of a thin, outer **pigmented layer** lying over the choroid and a thick, inner **nervous layer,** or visual portion. The retina is responsible for the reception and transmission of visual impulses to the brain. It has two types of visual receptors: rods and cones. **Rods** function in dim light and produce black-and-white vision. **Cones** function in bright light and produce color vision. In the central portion of the retina is a highly sensitive structure called the **macula.** In the center of the macula is the (11) **fovea.** When the eye focuses on an object, light rays from that object are directed to the fovea. Because the fovea is composed of only cones that lie very close to each other, it provides the greatest **acuity** for color vision.

Rods and cones contain a chemical called **photopigment,** or **visual pigment.** As light strikes the photopigment, a chemical change occurs that stimulates rods and cones. The chemical changes produce impulses that are transmitted through the (12) **optic nerve** to the brain, where they are interpreted as vision. The optic nerve and blood vessels of the eye enter at the (13) **optic disc.** Its center is referred to as the **blind spot,** because the area has neither rods nor cones for vision.

One of two major fluids **(humors)** of the eye is **aqueous humor.** It is found in the (14) **posterior chamber** and (15) **anterior chamber** of the anterior portion of the eye, and provides nourishment for the lens and the cornea. The ciliary body continually produces aqueous humor, which drains from the eye through a small opening called the (16) **canal of Schlemm.** If aqueous humor fails to drain from the eye at the rate at which it is produced, a condition called **glaucoma** results. The second major humor of the eye is **vitreous humor,** a jellylike substance that fills the interior of eye, the (17) **vitreous chamber.** The vitreous humor, lens, and aqueous humor are the **refractive** structures of the eye, focusing light rays sharply on the retina. If any one of these structures does not function properly, vision is impaired.

Adnexa

The **adnexa** of the eye includes all supporting structures of the eye globe. Six extraocular muscles control the movement of the eye: the superior, inferior, lateral, and medial rectus muscles and the superior and inferior oblique muscles. These muscles coordinate the eyes so that they move in a synchronized manner.

Two movable folds of skin constitute the eyelids, each with eyelashes that protect the front of the eye. (See Figure 16-2.) The (1) **conjunctiva** lines the inner surface of the eyelids and the cornea. Lying superior and to the outer edge of each eye are the (2) **lacrimal glands,** which produce tears that bathe and lubricate the eyes. The tears collect at the inner edges of the eyes, the **canthi** (singular, **canthus**), and pass through pinpoint openings, the (3) **lacrimal canals,** to the mucous membranes that line the inside of the (4) **nasal cavity.**

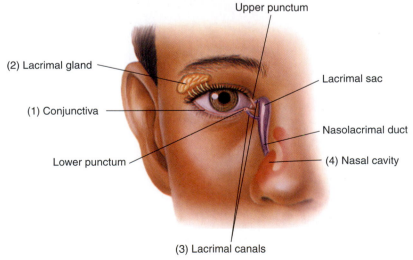

Figure 16-2 Lacrimal apparatus.

Ear

The ear is the sense receptor organ for two senses: hearing and equilibrium. Hearing is a function of the cochlea. Equilibrium is a function of the semicircular canals and vestibule.

Hearing

The ear consists of three major sections: the outer ear, or **external ear;** the middle ear, or **tympanic cavity;** and the inner ear, or **labyrinth**. (See Figure 16-3.) The external ear conducts sound waves through air; the middle ear, through bone; and the inner ear, through fluid. This series of transmissions ultimately generates impulses that are sent to the brain and interpreted as sound.

An (1) **auricle** (or *pinna*) collects waves traveling through air and channels them to the (2) **external auditory canal,** also called the **ear canal.** The ear canal is a slender tube lined with glands that produce a waxy secretion called **cerumen.** Its stickiness traps tiny foreign particles and prevents them from entering the deeper areas of the canal. The (3) **tympanic membrane** (also called the **tympanum** or **eardrum**) is a flat, membranous structure drawn over the end of the ear canal. Sound waves entering the ear canal strike against the tympanic membrane, causing it to vibrate. These vibrations cause movement of the three smallest bones of the body, collectively called the **ossicles.** These tiny articulating bones, the (4) **malleus** (or **hammer**), the (5) **incus** (or **anvil**), and the (6) **stapes** (or **stirrups**), are located within the tympanic cavity and form a connection between the tympanic membrane and the (7) **cochlea,** the first structure of the inner ear. The cochlea is a snail-shaped structure filled with a fluid called **perilymph**. Its inner surfaces are lined with a highly sensitive hearing structure called the **organ of Corti,** which contains tiny nerve endings called the **hair cells.** A membrane-covered opening on the external surface of the cochlea called the (8) **oval window** provides a place for attachment of

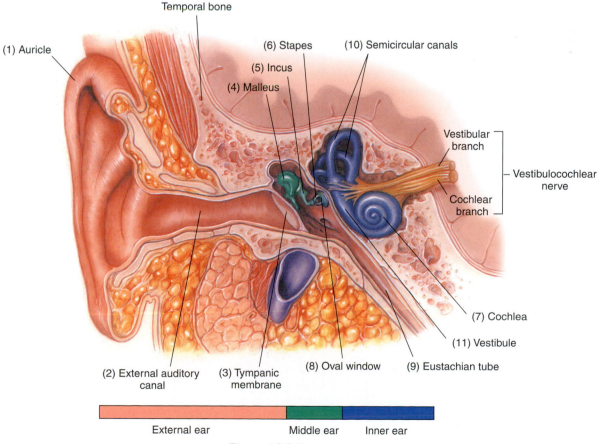

Figure 16-3 Ear structures.

the stapes. The movement of the ossicles in the middle ear causes the stapes to exert a gentle pumping action against the oval window. The pumping action forces the perilymph to disturb the hair cells, generating impulses that are transmitted to the brain by way of the auditory nerve, where they are interpreted as sound. The (9) **eustachian tube** connects the middle ear to the pharynx. It equalizes pressure on the outer and inner surfaces of the eardrum. When pressure on either side of the membrane changes, a deliberate swallow will commonly correct the inequality.

Equilibrium

The inner ear consists of a system of fluid-filled tubes and sacs as well as nerves that connect these structures to the brain. Because of its mazelike design, it is referred to as the **labyrinth.** The labyrinth, which rests inside the skull bones, includes not only the cochlear system (the organ devoted to hearing) but also the vestibular system, which is devoted to the control of balance and eye movements. The vestibular system contains the (10) **semicircular canals** and the (11) **vestibule.** The vestibule joins the cochlea and the semicircular canals. Many complex structures located in this maze are responsible for maintaining both static and dynamic equilibrium.

Anatomy Review: The Eye

To review the anatomy of the eye, label the illustration using the terms listed below.

anterior chamber	*cornea*	*optic disc*	*retina*
canal of Schlemm	*fovea*	*optic nerve*	*sclera*
choroid	*iris*	*posterior chamber*	*suspensory ligaments*
ciliary body	*lens*	*pupil*	*vitreous chamber*
conjunctiva			

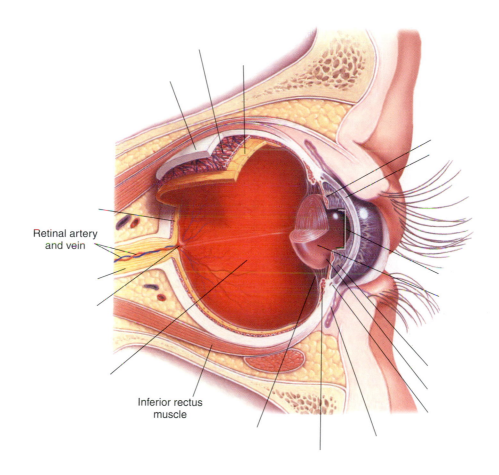

Retinal artery
and vein

Inferior rectus
muscle

Check your answers by referring to Figure 16–1 on page 541. Review material that you did not answer correctly.

Anatomy Review: The Ear

To review the anatomy of the ear, label the illustration using the terms listed below.

auricle	*incus*	*stapes*
cochlea	*malleus*	*tympanic membrane*
eustachian tube	*oval window*	*vestibule*
external auditory canal	*semicircular canals*	

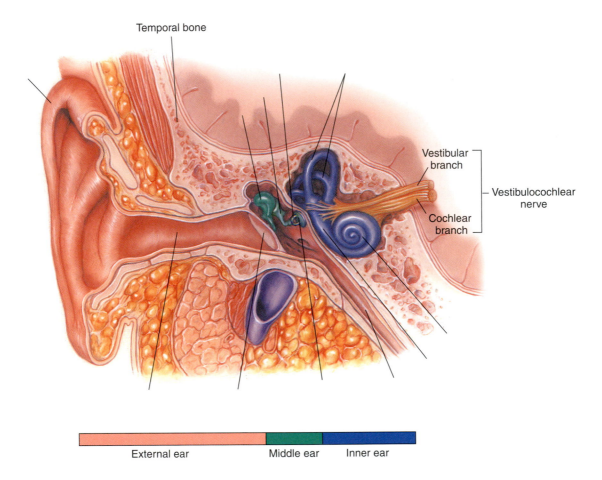

Temporal bone

Vestibular branch

Vestibulocochlear nerve

Cochlear branch

External ear   Middle ear   Inner ear

 Check your answers by referring to Figure 16–2 on page 543. Review material that you did not answer correctly.

Medical Word Elements

This section introduces combining forms, suffixes, and prefixes related to the special senses. Word analyses are also provided.

Element	Meaning	Word Analysis
Combining Forms		
Eye		
ambly/o	dull, dim	**ambly**/opia (ăm-blē-Ō-pē-ă): dimness of vision *-opia:* vision *In amblyopia, visual stimulation through the optic nerve of one eye (lazy eye) is impaired, thus resulting in poor or dim vision.*
aque/o	water	**aque**/ous (Ā-kwē-ŭs): pertaining to water *-ous:* pertaining to
blephar/o	eyelid	**blephar/o**/ptosis (blĕf-ă-rō-TŌ-sĭs): prolapse or downward displacement of the eyelid *-ptosis:* prolapse, downward displacement
choroid/o	choroid	**choroid/o**/pathy (kō-roy-DŎP-ă-thē): disease of the choroid *-pathy:* disease
conjunctiv/o	conjunctiva	**conjunctiv**/al (kŏn-jŭnk-TĪ-văl): pertaining to the conjunctiva *-al:* pertaining to
core/o	pupil	**core/o**/meter (kō-rē-ŎM-ĕ-tĕr): instrument for measuring the pupil *-meter:* instrument for measuring
pupill/o		**pupill/o**/graphy (pū-pĭ-LŎG-ră-fē): process of recording (movement of) the pupil *-graphy:* process of recording
corne/o	cornea	**corne**/al (KOR-nē-ăl): pertaining to the cornea *-al:* pertaining to
cycl/o	ciliary body of the eye; circular; cycle	**cycl/o**/plegia (sī-klō-PLĒ-jē-ă): paralysis of the ciliary body *-plegia:* paralysis
dacry/o	tear; lacrimal apparatus (duct, sac, or gland)	**dacry**/oma (dăk-rē-Ō-mă): tumorlike swelling of the lacrimal duct *-oma:* tumor
lacrim/o		**lacrim/o**/tomy (lăk-rĭ-MŎT-ō-mē): incision of the lacrimal duct or sac *-tomy:* incision
dacryocyst/o	lacrimal sac	**dacryocyst/o**/ptosis (dăk-rē-ō-sĭs-tŏp-TŌ-sĭs): prolapse of the lacrimal sac *-ptosis:* prolapse, downward displacement

(continued)

Element	Meaning	Word Analysis
glauc/o	gray	**glauc**/oma (glaw-KŌ-mă): gray tumor -*oma:* tumor *If not treated, glaucoma results in increased intraocular pressure (IOP) that destroys the retina and optic nerve.*
goni/o	angle	**goni/o**/scopy (gŏ-nē-ŎS-kŏ-pē): visual examination of the irideocorneal angle -*scopy:* visual examination *Gonioscopy is used to differentiate the two forms of glaucoma (open- and closed-angle).*
irid/o	iris	**irid/o**/plegia (ĭr-ĭd-ō-PLĒ-jē-ă): paralysis of (the sphincter of) the iris -*plegia:* paralysis
kerat/o	horny tissue; hard; cornea	**kerat/o**/tomy (kĕr-ă-TŎT-ō-mē): incision of the cornea -*tomy:* incision
ocul/o	eye	**ocul/o**/myc/osis (ŏk-ū-lō-mī-KŌ-sĭs): fungal infection of the eye (or its parts) *myc:* fungus -*osis:* abnormal condition; increase (used primarily with blood cells)
ophthalm/o		**opthalm/o**/logist (ŏf-thăl-MŎL-ō-jĭst): specialist in the study of the eye -*logist:* specialist in the study of *Ophthalmologists are physicians who specialize in the medical and surgical management of diseases and disorders of the eyes.*
opt/o	eye, vision	**opt/o**/metry (ŏp-TŎM-ĕ-trē): act of measuring vision -*metry:* act of measuring *Optometry is the science of diagnosing, managing, and treating nonsurgical conditions and diseases of the eye and visual system.*
optic/o		**optic**/al (ŎP-tĭ-kăl): pertaining to the eye or vision -*al:* pertaining to
phac/o	lens	**phac/o**/cele (FĀK-ō-sēl): herniation (displacement) of the lens into the interior chamber of the eye -*cele:* hernia, swelling *The usual cause of phacocele is blunt trauma to the eye.*
phot/o	light	**phot/o**/phobia (fō-tō-FŌ-bē-ă): abnormal fear of (intolerance to) light -*phobia:* fear *Intolerance to light is associated with people who suffer from migraines or have light-colored eyes or glaucoma. Some medications also cause a marked intolerance to light.*
presby/o	old age	**presby**/opia (prĕz-bē-Ō-pē-ă): (poor) vision (associated with) old age -*opia:* vision *Presbyopia is the loss of accommodation due to weakening of the ciliary muscles as a result of the aging process.*

Element	Meaning	Word Analysis
retin/o	retina	**retin/o**/sis (rĕt-ĭ-NŌ-sĭs): abnormal condition of the retina *-osis:* abnormal condition; increase (used primarily with blood cells) *Retinosis includes any degenerative process of the retina not associated with inflammation.*
scler/o	hardening; sclera (white of eye)	**scler/o**/malacia (sklĕ-rō-mă-LĀ-shē-ă): softening of the sclera *-malacia:* softening
scot/o	darkness	**scot/o**/ma (skō-TŌ-mă): dark, tumorlike spot *-oma:* tumor *Scotoma is an area of diminished vision in the visual field.*
vitr/o	vitreous body (of the eye)	**vitr**/ectomy (vĭ-TRĔK-tō-mē): removal of the (contents of the) vitreous chamber *-ectomy:* excision, removal *The removal of the vitreous body allows surgical procedures that would otherwise be impossible, including repair of macular holes and tears in the retina.*
Ear		
audi/o	hearing	**audi/o**/meter (aw-dē-ŎM-ĕ-tĕr): instrument for measuring hearing *-meter:* instrument for measuring
labyrinth/o	labyrinth (inner ear)	**labyrinth/o**/tomy (lăb-ĭ-rĭn-THŎT-ō-mē): incision of the labyrinth *-tomy:* incision
mastoid/o	mastoid process	**mastoid**/ectomy (măs-toyd-ĔK-tō-mē): removal of the mastoid process *-ectomy:* excision, removal
ot/o	ear	**ot/o**/py/o/rrhea (ō-tō-pī-ō-RĒ-ă): discharge of pus from the ear *py/o:* pus *-rrhea:* discharge, flow
salping/o	tubes (usually fallopian or eustachian [auditory] tubes)	**salping/o**/pharyng/eal: (săl-pĭng-gō-fă-RĬN-jē-ăl): pertaining to the eustachian (auditory) tube and pharynx *-al:* pertaining to *pharyng:* pharynx
staped/o	stapes	**staped**/ectomy (stā-pĕ-DĔK-tō-mē): excision of the stapes *-ectomy:* excision, removal *Stapedectomy is performed to improve hearing, especially in cases of otosclerosis.*
myring/o	tympanic membrane (eardrum)	**myring/o**/myc/osis (mĭr-ĭn-gō-mī-KŌ-sĭs): abnormal condition due to fungal infection of the tympanic membrane *myc:* fungus *-osis:* abnormal condition; increase (used primarily with blood cells)

(continued)

Element	Meaning	Word Analysis
tympan/o		**tympan/o**/stomy (tǐm-pǎ-NŎS-tō-mē): forming an opening in the tympanic membrane *-stomy:* forming an opening (mouth) *This procedure is usually performed to insert small pressure-equalizing (PE) tubes through the tympanum.*

Suffixes		
-acusia	hearing	an/**acusia** (ăn-ă-KŪ-sē-ă): not hearing (deafness) *an-:* without, not
-cusis		presby/**cusis** (prěz-bǐ-KŪ-sǐs): hearing (loss) associated with old age *presby:* old age *Presbycusis generally occurs in both ears and primarily affects perception of high-pitched tones.*
-opia	vision	dipl/**opia** (dǐp-LŌ-pē-ă): double vision *dipl-:* double, twofold
-opsia		heter/**opsia** (hět-ěr-ŎP-sē-ă): inequality of vision (in the two eyes) *heter-:* different
-tropia	turning	eso/**tropia** (ěs-ō-TRŌ-pē-ă): turning inward (of the eyes); also called *convergent strabismus* or *crossed eyes* *eso-:* inward

Prefixes		
exo-	outside, outward	**exo**/tropia (ěks-ō-TRŌ-pē-ă): abnormal turning outward of (one or both eyes); also called *divergent strabismus* *-tropia:* turning
hyper-	excessive, above normal	**hyper**/opia (hī-pěr-Ō-pē-ă): excess (farsighted) vision *-opia:* vision

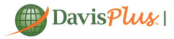 | Visit the *Medical Terminology Systems* online resource center at Davis*Plus* for an audio exercise of the terms in this table. Other activities are also available to reinforce content.

 It is time to review medical word elements by completing Learning Activities 16–1 and 16–2.

Pathology

Common signs and symptoms of eye disorders include a decrease in visual acuity, headaches, and pain in the eye or adnexa. However, many disorders of the eye are serious but asymptomatic; therefore, regular eye checkups are necessary. For diagnosis, treatment, and management of visual disorders, the medical services of a specialist may be warranted. **Ophthalmology** is the medical specialty concerned with disorders of the eye. The physician who treats these disorders is called an **ophthalmologist.** Optometrists work with ophthalmologists in a medical practice or practice independently. **Optometrists** are not medical doctors, but are doctors of optometry (O.D.). They diagnose vision problems and eye diseases, prescribe eyeglasses and contact lenses, and prescribe drugs to treat eye disorders. Although they cannot perform surgery, they commonly provide preoperative and postoperative care.

Common signs and symptoms of ear disorders include hearing impairment, ringing in the ears, pain or drainage from the ears, loss of balance, dizziness, or nausea. For diagnosis, treatment, and management of hearing disorders, the medical services of a specialist may be warranted. **Otolaryngology** is the medical specialty concerned with disorders of the ear, nose, and throat. The physician who treats these disorders is called an **otolaryngologist.** Many otolaryngologists employ audiologists. The **audiologist** specializes in non-medical management of the auditory and balance systems. Using various testing strategies (e.g. hearing tests, otoacoustic emission measurements, and elecytrophysiologic tests), the audiologist aims to determine whether someone can hear within the normal range, and if not, which portions of hearing (high, middle, or low frequencies) are affected and to what degree. If an audiologist determines there is a hearing loss or vestibular abnormality, they may recommend a hearing aid, cochlear implant, surgery, or an appropriate medical referral.

Eye Disorders

Eye disorders include not only visual deficiencies associated with refractive errors, but also disorders of associated structures, such as the eye muscles, nerves, and blood vessels. A complete examination of the eyes and their adnexa is necessary to identify the source of any disorder. Next, visual acuity (VA) and visual field (VF) are assessed. Then the eyelids, pupils, cornea, and lacrimal structures are examined and intraocular pressure is assessed as well. If infection is detected, it must be located and identified by culturing eye and nasal discharge and performing computed tomography (CT) of the sinuses. Occasionally, the patient may be referred for dental examination to determine if abscesses in the mouth are the source of infection. Family history is important because many eye disorders have a genetic predisposition, including glaucoma. Common eye disorders include errors of refraction, cataracts, glaucoma, strabismus, and macular degeneration.

Errors of Refraction

An error of refraction **(ametropia)** exists when light rays fail to focus sharply on the retina. This may be due to a defect in the lens, cornea, or shape of the eyeball. If the eyeball is too long, the image falls in front of the retina, causing nearsightedness. (See Figure 16-4.) In farsightedness **(hyperopia, hypermetropia),** the opposite of myopia, the eyeball is too short and the image falls

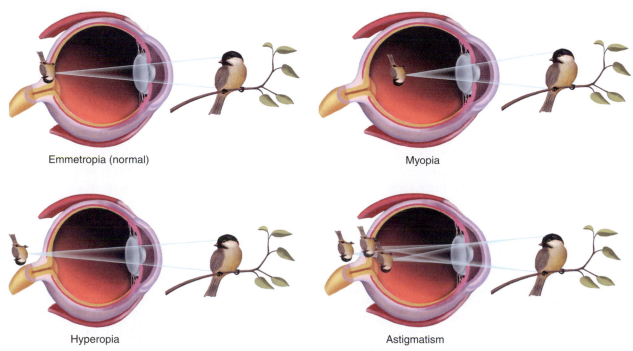

Emmetropia (normal) Myopia

Hyperopia Astigmatism

Figure 16-4 Errors of refraction.

behind the retina. A form of farsightedness is **presbyopia,** a defect associated with the aging process. The onset of presbyopia usually occurs between ages 40 and 45. Distant objects are seen clearly, but near objects are not in proper focus. In another form of ametropia called **astigmatism (Ast),** the cornea or lens has a defective curvature. This curvature causes light rays to diffuse over a large area of the retina rather than being sharply focused.

Corrective lenses usually compensate for the various types of ametropia. An alternative to corrective lenses is **laser-assisted in situ keratomileusis (LASIK)** surgery. This procedure changes the shape of the cornea and, in most instances, the change is permanent. A small incision is made in the cornea to produce a flap. The flap is lifted to the side while a laser reshapes the underlying corneal tissue. At the completion of the procedure, the corneal flap is replaced. The procedure usually takes less than 15 minutes. However, not all people are candidates for this surgery. Some medical conditions, certain medications, or the shape and structure of the eye may preclude this procedure as a viable alternative to corrective lenses.

Cataracts

Cataracts are opacities that form on the lens and impair vision. These opacities are commonly produced by protein that slowly builds up over time until vision is affected. The most common form of cataract is age-related. More than one-half of Americans older than age 65 have cataracts to some degree. Congenital cataracts found in children are usually a result of genetic defects or maternal rubella during the first trimester of pregnancy. This rare form of cataract is treated in the same manner as age-related cataract. The usual treatment is removal of the clouded lens by emulsifying it using ultrasound or a laser probe **(phacoemulsification, phaco).** An ultrasonic device breaks apart the cataract and the fragments are aspirated. An artificial, bendable intraocular lens (IOL) is then inserted into the capsule. Once in position, the lens unfolds. The surgery is usually performed using a topical anesthetic, and the incision normally does not require stitches. This is one of the safest and most effective surgical procedures performed in medicine.

Glaucoma

Glaucoma is characterized by increased intraocular pressure (IOP) caused by the failure of aqueous humor to drain from the eye through a tiny duct called the **canal of Schlemm.** (See Figure 16-5.) The increased pressure on the optic nerve destroys it, and vision is permanently lost.

Although there are various forms of glaucoma, all of them eventually lead to blindness unless the condition is detected and treated in its early stages. Glaucoma may occur as a primary or congenital disease or secondary to other causes, such as injury, infection, surgery, or prolonged topical corticosteroid use. Primary glaucoma can be chronic or acute. The **chronic form** is also called **open-angle, simple,** or **wide-angle glaucoma.** The **acute form** is called **angle-closure** or **narrow-angle glaucoma.** Chronic glaucoma may produce no symptoms except gradual loss of peripheral vision over a period of years. Headaches, blurred vision, and dull pain in the eye may also be present. Cupping of the optic discs may be noted on ophthalmoscopic examination. Acute glaucoma is accompanied by extreme ocular pain, blurred vision, redness of the eye, and dilation of the pupil. Nausea and vomiting may also occur. If untreated, acute glaucoma causes complete and permanent blindness within 2 to 5 days.

The more common and chronic form of glaucoma is open-angle glaucoma, which is slow to develop and is usually painless. By the time the patient seeks medical attention, it may be too late to restore vision. The rarer form of glaucoma is closed-angle glaucoma. Because of pain and the rapid decrease in vision, the patient generally seeks medical attention before visual field is lost or blindness has occurred. Treatment for glaucoma includes medications that cause the pupils to constrict **(miotics),** which permits aqueous humor to escape from the eye, thereby relieving pressure. If miotics are ineffective, surgery may be necessary.

Strabismus

Strabismus, also called **heterotropia** or **tropia,** is a condition in which one eye is misaligned with the other and the eyes do not focus simultaneously when viewing an object. This misalignment may be in any direction—inward **(esotropia [ST]),** outward **(exotropia [XT]),** up, down, or a

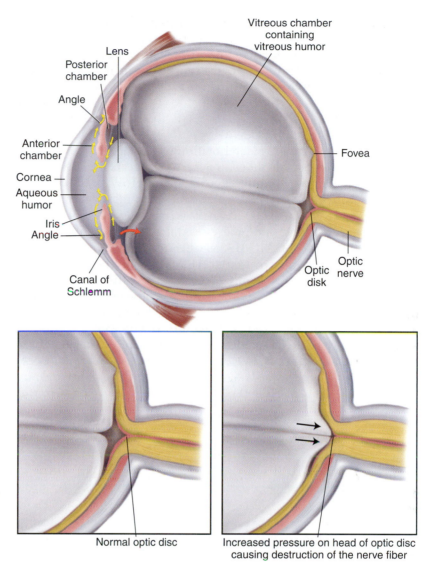

Figure 16-5 Glaucoma, with the eye showing a normal flow of aqueous humor (*yellow arrows*) and an abnormal flow of aqueous humor (*red arrow*), causing destruction of the optic nerve.

Normal optic disc

Increased pressure on head of optic disc causing destruction of the nerve fiber

combination. The deviation may be a constant condition or may arise intermittently with stress, exhaustion, or illness. (See Figure 16-6.) In normal vision, each eye views an image from a somewhat different vantage point, thus transmitting a slightly different image to the brain. The result is binocular perception of depth or three-dimensional space, a phenomenon known as **stereopsis.** Strabismus commonly causes a loss of stereopsis. In children, strabismus is commonly, but not always, associated with "lazy-eye syndrome" **(amblyopia).** Vision is suppressed in the "lazy" eye so that the child uses only the "good" eye for vision. The vision pathway fails to develop in the "lazy" eye.

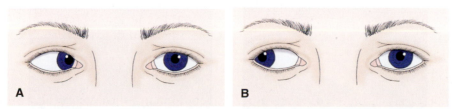

A B

Figure 16-6 Types of strabismus. **(A)** Esotropia (affected eye turning inward). **(B)** Exotropia (affected eye turning outward).

There is a critical period during which amblyopia must be corrected, usually before age 6. If not detected and treated early in life, amblyopia can cause a permanent loss of vision in the affected eye, with associated loss of stereopsis. Treatment for strabismus depends on the cause. It commonly consists of covering the normal eye, forcing the child to use the deviated, or lazy, eye. Eye exercises and corrective lenses may be prescribed, or surgical correction may be necessary.

Macular Degeneration

Macular degeneration is a deterioration of the macula, the most sensitive portion of the retina. The macula is responsible for central, or "straight-ahead," vision required for reading, driving, detail work, and recognizing faces. (See Figure 16-7.) Although deterioration of the macula is associated with toxic effects of some drugs, the most common type is **age-related macular degeneration (ARMD, AMD).** ARMD is a leading cause of visual loss in the United States. The disease is unpredictable and progresses differently in each individual.

So far, two forms of ARMD have been identified: wet and dry. The less common, but more severe, form is **wet,** or **neovascular ARMD.** It affects about 10% of those afflicted with the disease. Small blood vessels form under the macula. Blood and other fluids leak from these vessels and destroy the visual cells, leading to severe loss of central vision and permanent visual impairment. If identified in its early stages, laser surgery can be used to destroy the newly forming vessels. This treatment is called **laser photocoagulation.** It is successful in about one-half of the patients with wet ARMD. However, the effects of the procedure commonly do not last and new vessels begin to form.

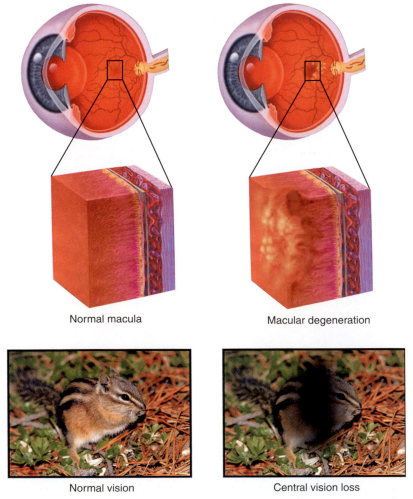

Normal macula   Macular degeneration

Normal vision   Central vision loss

Figure 16-7 Macular degeneration.

The more common form of macular degeneration is **dry ARMD.** Small, yellowish deposits called **drusen** develop on the macula and interfere with central vision. Drusen are dried retinal pigment epithelial cells that form granules on the macula. Although some vision is lost, this form of the disease rarely leads to total blindness. Patients with dry ARMD are encouraged to see their ophthalmologist frequently and perform a simple at-home test that identifies visual changes that may indicate the development of the more serious neovascular ARMD.

Ear Disorders

Common signs and symptoms of ear disorders include hearing loss, earache, vertigo, and tinnitus. Hearing tests are important in diagnosing hearing loss as well as aiding in localizing the source and nature of the hearing deficiency. In addition, many infections of the nose and throat refer pain **(synalgia)** to the ear. Therefore, an examination of the nose and throat is usually essential in identifying the cause of ear pain. Common ear disorders include otitis media and otosclerosis.

Otitis Media

Otitis media (OM) is an inflammation of the middle ear. This infection may be caused by a virus or bacterium. However, the most common culprit is *Streptococcus pneumoniae*. Otitis media is found most commonly in infants and young children, especially in the presence of an upper respiratory infection (URI). Symptoms may include earache and draining of pus from the ear **(otopyorrhea).** In its most severe form, otitis media may lead to infection of the mastoid process **(mastoiditis)** or inflammation of brain tissue near the middle ear **(otoencephalitis).** Recurrent episodes of otitis media may cause scarring of the tympanic membrane, leading to hearing loss. Treatment consists of bed rest, medications to relieve pain **(analgesics),** and antibiotics. Occasionally, an incision of the eardrum **(myringotomy, tympanotomy)** may be necessary to relieve pressure and promote drainage.

The usual treatment for children with recurrent infection is the use of **pressure-equalizing tubes (PE tubes)** that are passed through the tympanic membrane. These tubes help drain fluid from the middle ear.

Otosclerosis

Otosclerosis is a disorder characterized by an abnormal hardening **(ankylosis)** of bones of the middle ear that causes hearing loss. The ossicle most commonly affected is the stapes, the bone that attaches to the oval window of the cochlea. The formation of a spongy growth at the footplate of the stapes decreases its ability to move the oval window, resulting in hearing loss. Occasionally, the patient perceives a ringing sound **(tinnitus)** within the ear, along with dizziness and a progressive loss of hearing, especially of low tones. Development of otosclerosis is typically closely tied to genetic factors; if one or both parents have the disorder, the child is at high risk for developing the disease. Surgical correction involves removing part of the stapes **(stapedectomy** or, more commonly, **stapedotomy)** and implanting a prosthetic device that allows sound waves to pass to the inner ear. The procedure requires only a local anesthetic and usually lasts only 45 minutes. Hearing is immediately restored.

Oncology

Oncological disorders can occur in almost any structure of the eye or ear as a primary malignancy or from other areas of the body to the eye or ear via metastasis.

Eye

Two major **neoplastic diseases** account for more than 90% of all primary intraocular diseases: **retinoblastoma,** found primarily in children, and **melanoma,** found primarily in adults. Most retinoblastomas tend to be familial. The cell involved is the retinal neuron. Vision is impaired and, in about 30% of patients, the disease is found in both eyes **(bilateral).** Melanoma may occur in the orbit, the bony cavity of the eyeball, the iris, or the ciliary body, but it arises most commonly in the pigmented cells of the choroid. The disease is usually asymptomatic until there is a hemorrhage into the anterior chamber. Any discrete, fleshy mass on the iris should be examined by an ophthalmologist. If malignancy occurs in the choroid, it usually appears as a brown or gray mushroom-shaped lesion.

Treatment for retinoblastoma usually involves the removal of the affected eye(s) **(enucleation),** followed by radiation. In melanoma where the lesion is on the iris, an iridectomy is performed. For melanoma of the choroid, enucleation is necessary. Many eye tumors are noninvasive and are not necessarily life threatening.

Ear

Both malignant and nonmalignant tumors can arise in the external **ear,** the canal, or the middle ear. Malignant tumors of the ear include **basal cell carcinoma** and squamous cell tumors. The most common ear malignancy is basal cell carcinoma, which usually occurs on the top of the pinna as the result of sun exposure. It is found more commonly in elderly patients or those with fair skin. Small, craterlike ulcers form as the disease progresses. Basal cell carcinoma does not readily metastasize; however, failure to treat it in a timely manner may result in the need for extensive surgery to remove the tumor. **Squamous cell carcinoma,** on the other hand, is much more invasive. However, it is a very rare type of ear tumor. In appearance, it closely resembles basal cell carcinoma, and biopsy is required to make a definitive diagnosis. Squamous cell carcinoma grows more slowly than basal cell carcinoma; however, because of its tendency to metastasize to the surrounding nodes and the nodes of the neck, it must be removed. Surgery combined with radiation therapy is the most effective treatment for squamous cell carcinoma.

Diseases and Conditions

This section introduces diseases and conditions of the eye and ear with their meanings and pronunciation. Word analyses for selected terms are also provided.

Term	Definition
Eye	
achromatopsia ă-krō-mă-TŎP-sē-ă *a-:* without, not *chromat:* color *-opsia:* vision	Severe congenital deficiency in color perception; also called *complete color blindness*
chalazion kă-LĀ-zē-ōn	Small, hard tumor developing on the eyelid, somewhat similar to a sebaceous cyst
conjunctivitis kŏn-jŭnk-tĭ-VĪ-tĭs *conjunctiv:* conjunctiva *-itis:* inflammation	Inflammation of the conjunctiva with vascular congestion that produces a red or pink eye and may be secondary to allergy or viral, bacterial, or fungal infections
ectropion ĕk-TRŌ-pē-ŏn	Eversion, or outward turning, of the edge of the lower eyelid
entropion ĕn-TRŌ-pē-ŏn	Inversion, or inward turning, of the edge of the lower eyelid
epiphora ĕ-PĬF-ō-ră	Abnormal overflow of tears *Epiphora is sometimes caused by obstruction of the tear ducts.*

Term	Definition
hordeolum hor-DĒ-ō-lŭm	Localized, circumscribed, inflammatory swelling of one of the several sebaceous glands of the eyelid, generally caused by a bacterial infection; also called *stye*
metamorphopsia mĕt-ă-mor-FŎP-sē-ă *meta-*: change; beyond *morph*: form, shape, structure *-opsia*: vision	Visual distortion of objects *Metamorphopsia is commonly associated with errors of refraction, retinal disease, choroiditis, detachment of the retina, and tumors of the retina or choroid.*
nyctalopia nĭk-tă-LŌ-pē-ă *nyctal*: night *-opia*: vision	Impaired vision in dim light; also called *night blindness* *Common causes of nyctalopia include cataracts, vitamin A deficiency, certain medications, and hereditary causes.*
nystagmus nĭs-TĂG-mŭs	Type of involuntary eye movements that appear jerky and may reduce vision or be associated with other, more serious conditions that limit vision
papilledema păp-ĭl-ĕ-DĒ-mă	Swelling and hyperemia of the optic disc, usually associated with increased intracranial pressure; also called *choked disc*
photophobia fō-tō-FŌ-bē-ă *phot/o*: light *-phobia*: fear	Unusual intolerance and sensitivity to light *Photophobia commonly occurs in such diseases as meningitis, inflammation of the eyes, measles, and rubella.*
presbyopia prĕz-bē-Ō-pē-ă *presby*: old age *-opia*: vision	Loss of accommodation of the crystalline lens associated with the aging process *During the aging process, proteins in the lens become harder and less elastic and muscle fibers surrounding the lens lose strength. These changes cause a decreased ability to focus, especially at close range.*
retinopathy rĕt-ĭn-ŎP-ă-thē *retin/o*: retina *-pathy*: disease	Any disorder of retinal blood vessels
diabetic dī-ă-BĔT-ĭk	Disorder that occurs in patients with diabetes and manifests as small hemorrhages, edema, and formation of new vessels on the retina, leading to scarring and eventual loss of vision
trachoma trā-KŌ-mă	Chronic, contagious form of conjunctivitis that typically leads to blindness
Ear	
anacusis ăn-ă-KŪ-sĭs *an-*: without, not *-acusis*: hearing	Complete deafness; also called *anacusia* *Anacusis may be unilateral or bilateral. Anacusis should not be confused with hearing loss. Hearing loss refers to impairment in hearing and the individual may be able to respond to auditory stimuli, including speech.*

(continued)

Term	Definition
conduction impairment kŏn-DŬK-shŭn	Blocking of sound waves as they pass through the external and middle ear (conduction pathway)
labyrinthitis lăb-ĭ-rĭn-THĪ-tĭs *labyrinth:* labyrinth (inner ear) *-itis:* inflammation	Inflammation of the inner ear that usually results from an acute febrile process *Labyrinthitis may lead to progressive vertigo.*
Ménière disease mĕn-ē-ĀR	Disorder of the labyrinth that leads to progressive loss of hearing *Ménière disease is characterized by vertigo, sensorineural hearing loss, and tinnitus.*
noise-induced hearing loss (NIHL)	Condition caused by the destruction of hair cells, the organs responsible for hearing, as a result of sounds that are "too long, too loud, or too close" *Target shooting, leaf blowing, motorcycle engines, rock concerts, woodworking, and other such environmental noises all produce sounds that may, over time, cause NIHL.*
otitis externa ō-TĪ-tĭs ĕks-TĔR-nă *ot:* ear *-itis:* inflammation	Infection of the external auditory canal *Common causes of otitis externa include exposure to water when swimming (swimmer's ear), bacterial or fungal infections, seborrhea, eczema, and such chronic conditions as allergies.*
presbyacusis prĕz-bē-ă-KŪ-sĭs *presby:* old age *-acusis:* hearing	Impairment of hearing resulting from old age; also called *presbyacusia* *In presbyacusis, patients are generally able to hear low tones but lose the ability to hear higher tones. This condition usually affects speech perception, especially in the presence of background noise, as in a restaurant or a large crowd. This type of hearing loss is irreversible.*
tinnitus tĭn-Ī-tŭs	Perception of ringing, hissing, or other sounds in the ears or head when no external sound is present *Tinnitus may be caused by a blow to the head, ingestion of large doses of aspirin, anemia, noise exposure, stress, impacted wax, hypertension, and certain types of medications and tumors.*
vertigo VĔR-tĭ-gō	Sensation of a spinning motion either of oneself or of the surroundings *Vertigo usually results from damage to inner ear structures associated with balance and equilibrium. It may be caused by labyrinthitis or from the nerves that carry messages from the semicicurlar canals to the brain.*

 It is time to review pathology, diseases, and conditions by completing Learning Activity 16–3.

Medical, Surgical, and Diagnostic Procedures

This section introduces medical, surgical and diagnostic procedures used to treat and diagnose eye and ear disorders. Descriptions are provided as well as pronunciations and word analyses for selected terms.

Procedure	Description
Medical	
ear irrigation	Flushing of the ear canal with water or saline to dislodge foreign bodies or impacted cerumen (earwax) (See Figure 16-8.) **Figure 16-8** Ear irrigation. From Williams and Hopper: *Understanding Medical-Surgical Nursing,* 4th ed. FA Davis, Philadelphia, 2011, p 1275, with permission.
slit-lamp examination (SLE)	Stereoscopic magnified view of the anterior eye structures in detail, which includes the cornea, lens, iris, sclera, and vitreous humor *The application of fluorescein dye during a slit-lamp examination makes it easier to detect and remove foreign bodies and treat infection, corneal ulcers, and abrasions.*
Surgical	
blepharoplasty BLĔF-ă-rō-plăs-tē *blephar/o:* eyelid *-plasty:* surgical repair	Cosmetic surgery that removes fatty tissue above and below the eyes that commonly form as a result of the aging process or excessive exposure to the sun

(continued)

Procedure	Description
pressure-equalizing (PE) tube placement	Insertion of tubes through the tympanic membrane, commonly used to treat chronic otitis media; also called *tympanostomy tubes* or *ventilation tubes* *PE tubes remain in the ear several months, and then fall out on their own or are removed surgically. (See Figure 16-9.)*

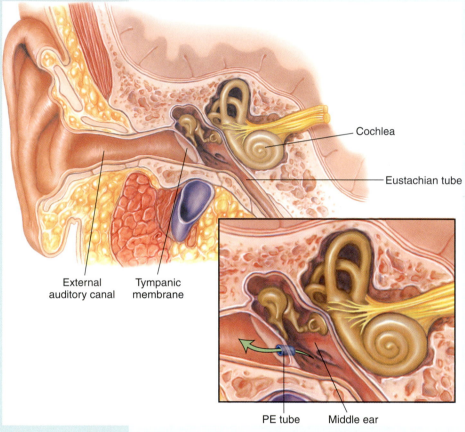

Cochlea

Eustachian tube

External auditory canal

Tympanic membrane

PE tube   Middle ear

Figure 16-9 Placement of a pressure-equalizing (PE) tube.

Procedure	Description
cochlear implant insertion KŎK-lē-ăr ĬM-plănt *cochle:* cochlea *-ar:* pertaining to	Placement of an artificial hearing device that produces hearing sensations by electrically stimulating nerves inside the inner ear; also called *bionic ear*
cyclodialysis sī-klō-dī-ĂL-ĭ-sĭs *cycl/o:* ciliary body of the eye; circular, cycle *dia:* through, across *-lysis:* separation; destruction; loosening	Formation of an opening between the anterior chamber and the supra-choroidal space for the draining of aqueous humor in glaucoma
enucleation ē-nū-klē-Ā-shŭn	Removal of the eyeball from the orbit *Enucleation is performed to treat cancer of the eye when the tumor is large and fills most of the structure.*

Procedure	Description
evisceration ē-vĭs-ĕr-Ā-shŭn	Removal of the contents of the eye while leaving the sclera and cornea intact *Evisceration is performed when the blind eye is painful or unsightly. The eye muscles are left intact, and a thin prosthesis called a* **cover shell** *is fitted over the sclera and cornea.*
mastoid antrotomy MĂS-toyd ăn-TRŎT-ō-mē	Surgical opening of a cavity within the mastoid process
otoplasty Ō-tō-plăs-tē *ot/o:* ear *–plasty:* surgical repair	Corrective surgery for a deformed or excessively large or small pinna *Otoplasty is also performed to rebuild new ears for those who lost them through burns or other trauma or were born without them.*
phacoemulsification fā-kō-ē-mŭl-sĭ-fĭ-KĀ-shŭn	Method of treating cataracts by using ultrasonic waves to disintegrate a cloudy lens, which is then aspirated and removed (See Figure 16-10.)

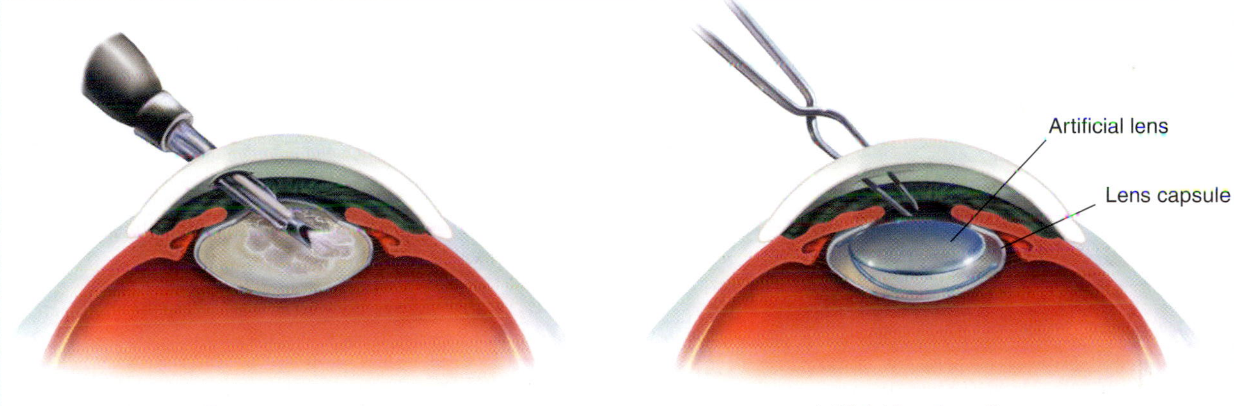

Cataract removal   Artificial lens insertion

Artificial lens

Lens capsule

Figure 16-10 Phacoemulsification.

Procedure	Description
radial keratotomy (RK) kĕr-ă-TŎT-ō-mē *kerat/o:* horny tissue; hard; cornea *–tomy:* incision	Incision of the cornea for treatment of nearsightedness or astigmatism *In RK, hairline radial incisions are made on the outer portion of the cornea that allow the cornea to be flattened to correct nearsightedness or to reshape an irregular curvature of the cornea in astigmatism.*
sclerostomy sklē-RŎS-tō-mē *scler/o:* hardening; sclera (white of the eye) *–stomy:* forming an opening (mouth)	Surgical formation of an opening in the sclera *Sclerostomy is commonly performed on the anterior chamber in conjunction with surgery for glaucoma for relief of pressure.*
tympanoplasty tĭm-păn-ō-PLĂS-tē *tympan/o:* tympanic membrane (eardrum) *–plasty:* surgical repair	Reconstruction of the eardrum, commonly due to perforation; also called *myringoplasty* *Connective tissue located beneath the skin directly behind the ear is used for the tympanic graft.*

(continued)

Procedure	Description
Diagnostic	
Clinical	
audiometry aw-dē-ŎM-ĕ-trē *audi/o:* hearing *-metry:* act of measuring	Measurement of hearing acuity at various sound-wave frequencies *In audiometry, pure tones of controlled intensity are delivered through earphones to each ear individually while the patient indicates if the tone was heard. The minimum intensity (volume) required to hear each tone is graphed.*
caloric stimulation test	Test that uses different water temperatures to assess the vestibular portion of the nerve of the inner ear (acoustic nerve) to determine if nerve damage is the cause of vertigo *In the caloric stimulation test, cold and warm water are separately introduced into each ear while electrodes placed around the eye record nystagmus. Eyes move in a predictable pattern when the water is introduced, except with acoustic nerve damage.*
electronystagmography (ENG) ē-lĕk-trō-nĭs-tăg-MŎG-ră-fē	Method of assessing and recording eye movements by measuring the electrical activity of the extraocular muscles *In ENG, electrodes are placed above, below, and to the side of each eye. A ground electrode is placed on the forehead. The electrodes record eye movement relative to the position of the ground electrode.*
gonioscopy gō-nē-ŎS-kō-pē *goni/o:* angle *-scopy:* visual examination	Examination of the angle of the anterior chamber of the eye to determine ocular motility and rotation and diagnose and manage glaucoma
ophthalmodynamometry ŏf-thăl-mō-dī-nă-MŎM-ĕ-trē	Measurement of the blood pressure of the retinal vessels *Ophthalmodynamometry is a screening test used to determine reduction of blood flow in the carotid artery.*
ophthalmoscopy ŏf-thăl-MŎS-kō-pē *ophthalm/o:* eye *-scopy:* visual examination	Visual examination of the interior of the eye using a handheld instrument called an *ophthalmoscope*, which has various adjustable lenses for magnification and a light source to illuminate the interior of the eye *Ophthalmoscopy is used to detect eye disorders as well as other disorders that cause changes in the eye.*
otoscopy ō-TŎS-kō-pē *ot/o:* ear *-scopy:* visual examination	Visual examination of the external auditory canal and the tympanic membrane using an otoscope
pneumatic nū-MĂT-ĭk	Procedure that assesses the ability of the tympanic membrane to move in response to a change in air pressure *In pneumatic otoscopy, a tight seal is created in the ear canal and then a very slight positive pressure and then a negative pressure is applied by squeezing and releasing a rubber bulb attached to the pneumatic otoscope. The fluctuation in air pressure causes movement of a normal tympanic membrane.*

Procedure	Description
retinoscopy rĕt-ĭn-ŎS-kō-pē *retin/o:* retina *-scopy:* visual examination	Evaluation of refractive errors of the eye by projecting a light into the eyes and determining the movement of reflected light rays *Retinoscopy is especially important in determining errors of refraction in babies and small children who cannot be refracted by traditional methods.*
tonometry tōn-ŎM-ĕ-trē *ton/o:* tension *-metry:* act of measuring	Evaluation of intraocular pressure by measuring the resistance of the eyeball to indentation by an applied force *Tonometry is used to detect glaucoma. The applanation method of tonometry uses a sensor to depress the cornea and is considered the most accurate method of tonometry. (See Figure 16–11.)*

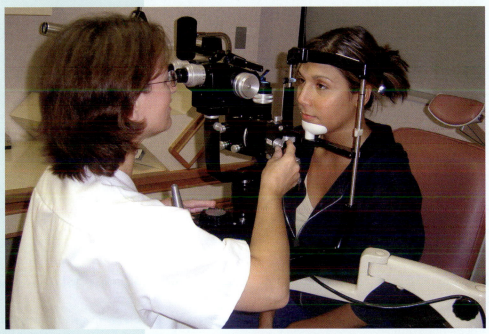

Figure 16-11 Applanation tonometry. (Courtesy of Richard H. Koop, MD.)

tuning fork test	Evaluation of sound conduction using a vibrating tuning fork
Rinne RĬN-nē	Tuning fork test that evaluates bone conduction (BC) versus air conduction (AC) of sound *In the Rinne test, a vibrating fork is placed against the mastoid bone (bone conduction) and in front of the auditory meatus (air conduction). If the sound is louder when the tuning fork is next to the ear, hearing in that ear is normal. If the sound is louder when the tuning fork touches the mastoid process, it is an indication of conductive hearing loss. (See Figure 16–12.)*
Weber	Tuning fork test that evaluates bone conduction of sound in both ears at the same time *In the Weber test, the vibrating tuning fork is placed on the center of the forehead. If sound perception is equal in both ears, hearing is normal.*

(continued)

Procedure	Description

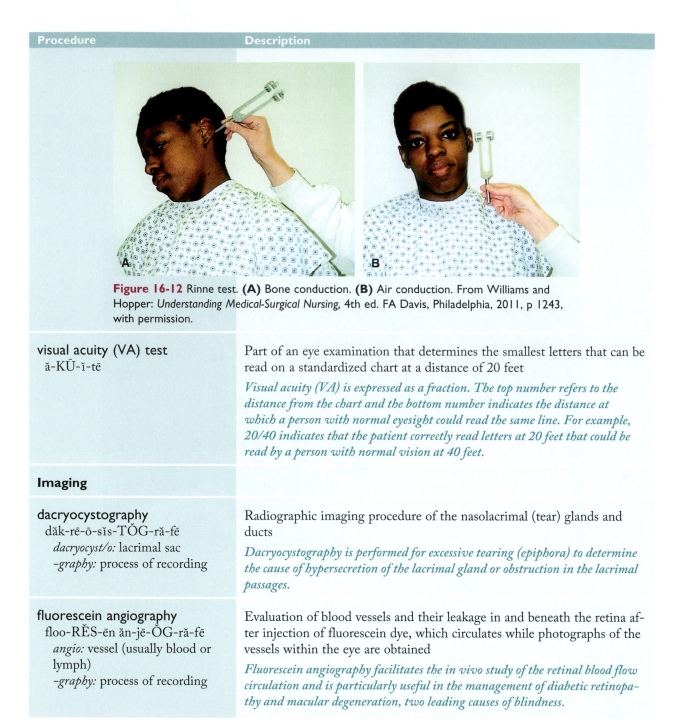

Figure 16-12 Rinne test. **(A)** Bone conduction. **(B)** Air conduction. From Williams and Hopper: *Understanding Medical-Surgical Nursing*, 4th ed. FA Davis, Philadelphia, 2011, p 1243, with permission.

Procedure	Description
visual acuity (VA) test ă-KŪ-ĭ-tē	Part of an eye examination that determines the smallest letters that can be read on a standardized chart at a distance of 20 feet *Visual acuity (VA) is expressed as a fraction. The top number refers to the distance from the chart and the bottom number indicates the distance at which a person with normal eyesight could read the same line. For example, 20/40 indicates that the patient correctly read letters at 20 feet that could be read by a person with normal vision at 40 feet.*
Imaging	
dacryocystography dăk-rē-ō-sĭs-TŎG-ră-fē *dacryocyst/o:* lacrimal sac *-graphy:* process of recording	Radiographic imaging procedure of the nasolacrimal (tear) glands and ducts *Dacryocystography is performed for excessive tearing (epiphora) to determine the cause of hypersecretion of the lacrimal gland or obstruction in the lacrimal passages.*
fluorescein angiography floo-RĔS-ēn ăn-jē-ŎG-ră-fē *angio:* vessel (usually blood or lymph) *-graphy:* process of recording	Evaluation of blood vessels and their leakage in and beneath the retina after injection of fluorescein dye, which circulates while photographs of the vessels within the eye are obtained *Fluorescein angiography facilitates the in vivo study of the retinal blood flow circulation and is particularly useful in the management of diabetic retinopathy and macular degeneration, two leading causes of blindness.*

Pharmacology

Disorders of the eyes and ears are commonly treated with instillation of drops onto the surface of the eye or into the cavity of the ear. The eyes and ears are typically irrigated with liquid solution to remove foreign objects and to provide topical application of medications. Pharmacological agents used to treat eye disorders include antibiotics for bacterial eye infections, beta blockers and carbonic anhydrase inhibitors for glaucoma, and ophthalmic decongestants and moisturizers for irritated eyes. Mydriatics and miotics are used not only to treat eye disorders but also to dilate (mydriatics) and contract (miotics) the pupil during eye examinations. Ear medications include antiemetics to relieve nausea associated with inner ear infections, products to loosen and remove wax buildup in the ear canal, and local anesthetics to relieve pain associated with ear infections. (See Table 16-1.)

Table 16-1 Drugs Used to Treat Eye and Ear Disorders

This table lists common drug classifications used to treat eye and ear disorders, their therapeutic actions, and selected generic and trade names.

Classification	Therapeutic Action	Generic and *Trade* Names
Eye		
antibiotics, ophthalmic ăn-tĭ-bī-ŎT-ĭks, ŏf-THĂL-mĭk	Inhibit growth of microorganisms that infect the eye *Ophthalmic antibiotics are dispensed as topical ointments and solutions to treat various bacterial eye infections such as conjunctivitis (pinkeye).*	**tobramycin** TŌ-bră-mī-sĭn *Tobrex*
antiglaucoma agents ăn-tĭ-glaw-KŌ-mă	Decrease aqueous humor production by constricting the pupil to open the angle between the iris and cornea	**timolol** TĪ-mō-lŏl *Betimol* **acetazolamide** ăs-ĕt-ă-ZŌL-ă-mīd *Diamox*
mydriatics mĭd-rē-ĂT-ĭks	Disrupt parasympathetic nerve supply to the eye or stimulate the sympathetic nervous system, causing the pupil to dilate *Mydriatics are commonly used to dilate the pupil to treat inflammatory conditions or in preparation for internal examinations of the eye.*	**atropine sulfate** ĂT-rō-pēn SŬL-fāt
decongestants, ophthalmic dē-kŏn-JĔST-ănts, ŏf-THĂL-mĭk	Constrict the small arterioles of the eye, decreasing redness and relieving conjunctival congestion *Ophthalmic decongestants are over-the-counter products that temporarily relieve the itching and minor irritation commonly associated with allergy.*	**tetrahydrozoline** tĕt-ră-hī-DRŎZ-ō-lēn *Murine, Visine*
moisturizers, ophthalmic MOYST-ūr-ī-zĕrz, ŏf-THĂL-mĭk	Soothe eyes that are dry due to environmental irritants and allergens *Ophthalmic moisturizers are administered topically and may also be used to facilitate ophthalmoscopic examination in gonioscopy and ophthalmoscopy.*	**buffered isotonic solutions** BŬ-fĕrd ī-sō-TŎN-ĭk *Akwa Tears, Moisture Eyes*
Ear		
antiemetics ăn-tĭ-ĕ-MĔT-ĭks	Treat and prevent nausea, vomiting, dizziness, and vertigo by reducing the sensitivity of the inner ear to motion or inhibiting stimuli from reaching the part of the brain that triggers nausea and vomiting *Antiemetics are commonly used to treat vertigo.*	**meclizine** MĔK-lĭ-zēn *Antivert, Bonine, Meni-D*
otic analgesics Ō-tĭk ăn-ăl-JĒ-zĭks	Provide temporary relief from pain and inflammation associated with otic disorders *Otic analgesics may be prescribed for otitis media, otitis externa, and swimmer's ear. Some otic analgesics are also wax emulsifiers.*	**antipyrine and benzocaine** ăn-tĭ-PĪ-rēn, BĔN-zō-kān *Allergan Ear Drops, A/B Otic*
wax emulsifiers ē-MŬL-sĭ-fī-ĕrz	Loosen and help remove impacted cerumen (ear wax) *Excessive wax may be washed out, vacuumed out, or removed using special instruments.*	**carbamide peroxide** KĂR-bă-mīd pĕr-ŎK-sīd *Debrox Drops, Murine Ear Drops*

Abbreviations

This section introduces abbreviations related to the eye and ear along with their meanings.

Abbreviation	Meaning	Abbreviation	Meaning
Eye			
Acc	accommodation	**O.D.**	Doctor of optometry
ARMD, AMD	age-related macular degeneration	**RK**	radial keratotomy
Ast	astigmatism	**SLE**	slit-lamp examination; systemic lupus erythematosus
ENG	electronystagmography	**ST**	esotropia
IOL	intraocular lens	**VA**	visual acuity
IOP	intraocular pressure	**VF**	visual field
LASIK	laser-assisted in situ keratomileusis	**XT**	exotropia
Ear			
AC	air conduction	**OM**	otitis media
BC	bone conduction	**PE**	physical examination; pulmonary embolism; pressure-equalizing (tube)
ENT	ears, nose, and throat	**URI**	upper respiratory infection
NIHL	noise-induced hearing loss		

It is time to review procedures, pharmacology, and abbreviations by completing Learning Activity 16–4.

LEARNING ACTIVITIES

The following activities provide review of the special senses terms introduced in this chapter. Complete each activity and review your answers to evaluate your understanding of the chapter.

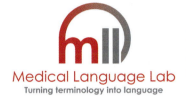

Visit the Medical Language Lab at the web site: medicallanguagelab.com. Use it to enhance your study and reinforcement of this chapter with the flash-card activity. We recommend you complete the flash-card activity before starting Learning Activities 16-1 and 16-2 below.

Learning Activity 16-1
Combining Forms, Suffixes, and Prefixes

Use the elements listed in the table to build medical words. You may use these elements more than once.

Combining Forms		Suffixes		Prefixes
ambly/o	myring/o	-acusia	-plasty	an-
audi/o	ocul/o	-ar	-ptosis	dipl-
blephar/o	ot/o	-cele	-rrhea	intra-
goni/o	phac/o	-itis	-tomy	
kerat/o	presby/o	-meter		
labyrinth/o	scler/o	-opia		
mastoid/o		-osis		

1. dimness of vision _____
2. herniation of the lens _____
3. double vision _____
4. downward displacement of the eyelid _____
5. instrument for measuring the (iridocorneal) angle _____
6. pertaining to within the eye _____
7. incision of the cornea _____
8. discharge from the ear _____
9. instrument for measuring hearing _____
10. total deafness _____
11. inflammation of the labyrinth of the inner ear _____
12. abnormal condition of hardening of (bones of) the ear _____
13. inflammation of the mastoid _____
14. surgical repair of the eardrum _____
15. (poor) hearing (associated with) old age _____

 Check your answers in Appendix A. Review any material that you did not answer correctly.

Correct Answers _____ X 6.67 = _____ % Score

Learning Activity 16-2
Building Medical Words

Use *ophthalm/o* (eye) to build words that mean:

1. paralysis of the eye _____
2. study of the eye _____

Use *pupill/o* (pupil) to build a word that means:

3. examination of the pupil _____

Use *kerat/o* (cornea) to build words that mean:

4. softening of the cornea _____
5. instrument for measuring the cornea _____

Use *scler/o* (sclera) to build words that mean:

6. inflammation of the sclera _____
7. softening of the sclera _____

Use *irid/o* (iris) to build words that mean:

8. paralysis of the iris _____
9. herniation of the iris _____

Use *retin/o* (retina) to build words that mean:

10. disease of the retina _____
11. inflammation of the retina _____

Use *blephar/o* (eyelid) to build words that mean:

12. paralysis of the eyelid _____
13. prolapse of the eyelid _____

Use *ot/o* (ear) to build a word that means:

14. flow of pus from the ear _____

Use *audi/o* (hearing) to build a word that means:

15. instrument for measuring hearing _____

Use *myring/o* (tympanic membrane [eardrum]) to build a word that means:

16. instrument for cutting the eardrum _____

Use the suffix *-opia* (vision) to build words that mean:

17. dim or dull vision _____

18. excessive (farsighted) vision _____

Use the suffix *-acusis* (hearing) to build words that mean:

19. without hearing _____

20. excessive (sensitivity to) hearing _____

Build surgical words that mean:

21. removal of the stapes _____

22. incision of the labyrinth _____

23. removal of the mastoid process _____

24. surgical repair of the eardrum _____

25. incision of the cornea _____

Check your answers in Appendix A. Review material that you did not answer correctly.

Correct Answers _____ X 4 = _____ % Score

Learning Activity 16-3
Pathology, Diseases, and Conditions

Match the following terms with the definitions in the numbered list.

achromatopsia	drusen	nyctalopia	otosclerosis
amblyopia	epiphora	otitis externa	presbyacusis
anacusis	exotropia	otitis media	retinoblastoma
cataract	hordeolum	otoencephalitis	tinnitus
chalazion	neovascular	otopyorrhea	vertigo

1. opacity that forms on the lens and impairs vision _____

2. severe congenital form of color blindness _____

3. impaired vision in dim light _____

4. impaired hearing due to old age _____

5. complete deafness _____

6. infection of the external auditory canal _____

7. ankylosis of the middle ear bones resulting in hearing loss _____

8. middle ear infection commonly found in infants and children _____

9. discharge of pus from the ear _____

10. abnormal overflow of tears _____

11. localized, circumscribed swelling of a sebaceous gland of the eyelid; stye _____

12. inflammation of the brain tissue near the middle ear _____

13. the wet form of macular degeneration _____

14. feeling of dizziness or spinning _____

15. outward deviation of the eye _____

16. small, yellowish deposits that develop on macula in age-related macular degeneration _____

17. tumor of the eyelid similar to a sebaceous cyst _____

18. "lazy-eye" syndrome _____

19. neoplastic disease of the eye found primarily in children _____

20. perception of ringing in the ears with no external stimuli _____

✅ *Check your answers in Appendix A. Review any material that you did not answer correctly.*

Correct Answers _____ X 5 = _____ % Score

Learning Activity 16-4

Matching Procedures, Pharmacology, and Abbreviations

Match the following terms with the definitions in the numbered list.

antiemetics	evisceration	ophthalmoscopy	ST
audiometry	fluorescein angiography	otic analgesics	tonometry
caloric stimulation	gonioscopy	otoplasty	visual acuity
cochlear implant	mydriatics	otoscopy	wax emulsifiers
enucleation	ophthalmic decongestants	radial keratotomy	XT

1. test that uses different temperatures to assess the vestibular portion of the nerve _____

2. visual examination of the interior of the eye _____

3. artificial device that produces hearing sensations by electrically stimulating nerves inside the inner ear _____

4. assesses blood vessels and retinal circulation using a colored dye while photographs are taken _____

5. corrective surgery for large, small, or deformed ears _____

6. agents that dilate the pupils and paralyze the eye muscles of accommodation _____

7. measurement of the intraocular pressure for detecting glaucoma _____

8. test that determines the smallest letters that can be read on a standardized chart _____

9. removal of the contents of the eyeball, leaving the sclera and cornea _____

10. treat and prevent nausea, vomiting, dizziness, and vertigo _____

11. loosen and help remove impacted cerumen _____

12. removal of the entire eyeball from its orbit _____

13. esotropia _____

14. constrict small arterioles of the eye to decrease redness and conjunctival congestion _____

15. exotropia _____

16. visual examination of the angle of the anterior chamber of the eye _____

17. visual examination of the external auditory canal _____

18. measurement of hearing acuity at various frequencies _____

19. surgical treatment for nearsightedness that uses small incisions to flatten the cornea _____

20. provide temporary relief from earache _____

Check your answers in Appendix A. Review any material that you did not answer correctly.

Correct Answers _____ X 5 = _____ % Score

Learning Activity 16-5
Medical Scenarios

To construct chart notes, replace the italicized terms in each of the scenarios with one of the medical terms listed below.

asymptomatic	otorrhea	tonometry
gonioscopy	pediatrician	trabeculoplasty
hyperopia	pharyngalgia	tympanorrhexis
otalgia		

Mrs. B. is an established patient and presents for her annual eye examination. Although she is (1) *without symptoms*, in 20xx the results of the (2) *pressure measurement* of the eyes were normal. She was subsequently diagnosed with glaucoma. For the last three years she was effectively managed with medications. The patient now complains of losing "side vision." Results of her eye refraction shows there has been no changes in her (3) *farsightedness*. A (4) *visual examination of the angle* of the anterior chamber of the eye indicates bilateral open-angle glaucoma. The plan is to schedule Mrs. B. for (5) *surgical repair of the trabecula* using a low-level laser.

1. _____
2. _____
3. _____
4. _____
5. _____

Johnny K. was seen at this clinic by Dr. Roberts, a (6) *specialist in children's disorders.* His mother said that for the past three days he complains of an (7) *earache* and (8) *sore throat.* Earlier today his mother noted an (9) *ear discharge* from the left ear. Upon examination a (10) *ruptured eardrum* was clearly evident in the left ear. The right eardrum was intact. His tonsillar area showed evidence of strep throat, which was confirmed with a rapid strep test. The patient will begin a regimen of erythromycin with follow-up in 10 days.

6. _____
7. _____
8. _____
9. _____
10. _____

✓ *Check your answers in Appendix A. Review any material that you did not answer correctly.*

Correct Answers _____ X 10 = _____ % Score

MEDICAL RECORD ACTIVITIES

The two medical records included in the following activities use common clinical scenarios to show how medical terminology is used to document patient care. Complete the terminology and analysis sections for each activity to help you recognize and understand terms related to the special senses.

Medical Record Activity 16-1

Operative Report: Retained Foreign Bodies

Terminology

Terms listed in the following table are taken from *Operative Report: Retained Foreign Bodies* that follows. Use a medical dictionary such as *Taber's Cyclopedic Medical Dictionary;* the appendices of *Systems*, 7th ed.; or other resources to define each term. Then review the pronunciations for each term and practice by reading the medical record aloud.

Term	Definition
bilateral bī-LĂT-ĕr-ăl	
cerumen sĕ-ROO-mĕn	
perforation pĕr-fō-RĀ-shŭn	
supine sū-PĪN	
tympanostomy tĭm-pă-NŎS- tō-mē	

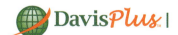 | Visit the *Medical Terminology Systems* online resource center at Davis*Plus* to practice pronunciation and reinforce the meanings of the terms in this medical report.

OPERATIVE REPORT: RETAINED FOREIGN BODIES

Physicians Day Surgery

1514 Ninth Avenue ▪▪ Sun City, USA 12345 ▪▪ (555) 936-1933

OPERATIVE REPORT

Date: 5/13/xx   Surgeon: Richard Roake, MD
Patient: Hirsch, Annie   Patient ID#: 33328

PREOPERATIVE DIAGNOSIS: Foreign body, ears.

POSTOPERATIVE DIAGNOSIS: Foreign body, ears.

OPERATIVE INDICATIONS: Patient is a 9-year-old girl who presents with bilateral retained tympanostomy tubes. The tubes had been placed for more than 2-½ years.

ANESTHESIA: General.

COMPLICATIONS: None.

OPERATIVE FINDINGS: Retained tympanostomy tubes, bilateral.

PROCEDURE: Removal of foreign bodies from ears with placement of paper patches.

INFORMED CONSENT: The risks and alternatives were explained to the mother, and she consented to the surgery.

In the supine position under satisfactory general anesthesia via mask, the patient was draped in a routine fashion.

The operating microscope was used to inspect the right ear. A previously placed tympanostomy tube was found to be in position and was surrounded with hard cerumen. The cerumen and the tube were removed, resulting in a very large perforation. The edges of the perforation were freshened sharply with a pick, and a paper patch was applied.

Patient tolerated the surgery very well, and was sent to recovery in stable condition.

Richard Roake, MD
Richard Roake, MD

rk:bg

D: 5-14-20xx
T: 5-14-20xx

Analysis

Review the medical record *Operative Report: Retained Foreign Bodies* to answer the following questions.

1. Did the surgery involve one or both ears?

   _____

2. What was the nature of the foreign body in the patient's ears?

   _____

3. What ear structure was involved?

   _____

4. What instrument was used to locate the tubes?

   _____

5. What was the material in which the tubes were embedded?

   _____

6. What occurred when the cerumen and tubes were removed?

   _____

7. How was the perforation treated?

   _____

Medical Record Activity 16-2
Operative Report: Phacoemulsification and Lens Implant

Terminology

Terms listed in the following table are taken from *Operative Report: Phacoemulsification and Lens Implant* that follows. Use a medical dictionary such as *Taber's Cyclopedic Medical Dictionary;* the appendices of *Systems*, 7th ed.; or other resources to define each term. Then review the pronunciations for each term and practice by reading the medical record aloud.

Term	Definition
blepharostat BLĔF-ă-rō-stăt	
capsulorrhexis kăp-sū-lō-RĔK-sĭs	
cataract KĂT-ă-răkt	
conjunctival kŏn-jŭnk-TĪ-văl	
diopter dī-ŎP-tĕr	
keratome KĔR-ă-tōm	
peritomy pĕr-ĬT-ō-mē	
phacoemulsification fă-kō-ē-mŭl-sĭ-fĭ-KĀ-shŭn	
posterior chamber pŏs-TĒR-ē-or CHĂM-bĕr	
retrobulbar block rĕt-rō-BŬL-băr	
TobraDex TŌ-bră-dĕks	

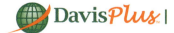

Visit the *Medical Terminology Systems* online resource center at Davis*Plus* to practice pronunciation and reinforce the meanings of the terms in this medical report.

OPERATIVE REPORT: PHACOEMULSIFICATION AND LENS IMPLANT

Physicians Day Surgery

1514 Ninth Avenue ■■ Sun City, USA 12345 ■■ (555) 936-1933

OPERATIVE REPORT

Date: 5/14/xx   Surgeon: Lewis Sloope, MD
Patient: Deetrick, Douglas   Patient ID#:   33422

PREOPERATIVE DIAGNOSIS: Right eye cataract.

POSTOPERATIVE DIAGNOSIS: Right eye cataract.

OPERATION: Phacoemulsification, right eye, with posterior chamber lens implantation.

COMPLICATIONS: None.

PROCEDURE: This 68-year-old male was brought to the operating suite on 8/4/xx as an outpatient. Intravenous anesthesia and retrobulbar block to the right eye were administered. The right eye was prepped in the usual manner. A blepharostat was inserted and a surgical microscope was positioned. Conjunctival peritomy was performed. Using a keratome, the anterior chamber was entered at the 12 o'clock position. A capsulorrhexis was performed. The cataract was removed by phacoemulsification.

After confirming the 20.5 diopters on the package, the implant was easily inserted into the capsular bag. The wound was observed and shown to be fluid tight. The incision required no sutures. TobraDex ointment was applied and a sterile patch was taped into place.

Patient was monitored until stable. Postoperative care was reviewed, and patient was released with instructions to return to the office the following day.

Lewis Sloope, MD
Lewis Sloope, MD

rk:bg

D: 5-14-20xx
T: 5-14-20xx

Analysis

Review the medical record *Operative Report: Phacoemulsification and Lens Implant* to answer the following questions.

1. What technique was used to destroy the cataract?

   _____

2. In what portion of the eye was the implant placed?

   _____

3. What anesthetics were used for surgery?

   _____

4. What was the function of the blepharostat?

   _____

5. What is a keratome?

   _____

6. Where was the implant inserted?

   _____

Answer Key

Chapter 1—Basic Elements of a Medical Word

Learning Activity 1-1
Understanding Medical Word Elements

1. word root *or* root, combining form, suffix, and prefix.
2. arthr
3. False—A combining vowel is usually an "o."
4. False—A word root links a suffix that begins with a vowel.
5. True
6. True
7. False—To define a medical word, first define the suffix or the end of the word. Second, define the first part of the word. Third, define the middle of the word.
8. True
9. <u>splen</u>/o
10. <u>hyster</u>/o
11. <u>enter</u>/o
12. <u>neur</u>/o
13. <u>ot</u>/o
14. <u>dermat</u>/o
15. <u>hydr</u>/o

Learning Activity 1-2
Identifying Word Roots and Combining Forms

1. <u>nephr</u>itis
2. <u>arthr</u>odesis
3. <u>dermat</u>itis
4. <u>dent</u>ist
5. <u>gastr</u>ectomy
6. <u>chondr</u>itis
7. <u>hepat</u>oma
8. <u>muscul</u>ar
9. <u>gastr</u>ic
10. <u>oste</u>oma
11. <u>nephr</u>
12. <u>hepat</u>/o
13. <u>arthr</u>
14. <u>oste</u>/o/<u>arthr</u>
15. <u>cholangi</u>/o

Learning Activity 1-3

Understanding Pronunciations

1. macron
2. breve
3. long
4. short
5. k
6. n
7. is
8. eye
9. second
10. separate

Learning Activity 1-4

Identifying Suffixes and Prefixes

1. -tomy
2. -scope
3. -itis
4. -ic
5. -ectomy
6. an-
7. hyper-
8. intra-
9. para-
10. poly-

Learning Activity 1-5

Defining Medical Words

Term	Definition
1. gastritis	inflammation of the stomach
2. nephritis	inflammation of the kidney(s)
3. gastrectomy	excision of the stomach
4. osteoma	tumor of bone
5. hepatoma	tumor of the liver
6. hepatitis	inflammation of the liver

Term	Rule	Summary of the Rule
7. arthr/itis	I	WR links a suffix that begins with a vowel.
8. scler/osis	I	WR links a suffix that begins with a vowel.
9. arthr/o/centesis	2	CF links a suffix that begins with a consonant.
10. colon/o/scope	2	CF links a suffix that begins with a consonant.
11. chondr/itis	I	WR links a suffix that begins with a vowel.
12. chondr/oma	I	WR links a suffix that begins with a vowel.
13. oste/o/chondr/ itis	3, I	CF links multiple roots to each other. This rule holds true even if the next word root begins with a vowel. WR links a suffix that begins with a vowel.
14. muscul/ar	I	WR links a suffix that begins with a vowel.
15. oste/o/arthr/itis	3, I	CF links multiple roots to each other. This rule holds true even if the next word root begins with a vowel. WR links a suffix that begins with a vowel.

Chapter 2—Suffixes

Learning Activity 2-1
Building Surgical Words

1. episiotomy
2. colectomy
3. arthrocentesis
4. splenectomy
5. colostomy
6. osteotome
7. tympanotomy
8. tracheostomy
9. mastectomy
10. lithotomy
11. hemorrhoidectomy
12. colostomy
13. colectomy
14. osteotome
15. arthrocentesis
16. lithotomy
17. mastectomy

18. tympanotomy

19. tracheostomy

20. splenectomy

Learning Activity 2-2
Building More Surgical Words

1. arthrodesis

2. rhinoplasty

3. tenoplasty

4. myorrhaphy

5. mastopexy

6. cystorrhaphy

7. osteoclasis

8. lithotripsy

9. enterolysis

10. neurotripsy

11. rhinoplasty

12. arthrodesis

13. myorrhaphy

14. mastopexy

15. cystorrhaphy

16. tenoplasty

17. osteoclasis

18. lithotripsy

19. enterolysis

20. neurotripsy

Learning Activity 2-3
Selecting a Surgical Suffix

1. lithotripsy

2. arthrocentesis

3. splenectomy

4. colostomy

5. dermatome

6. tracheostomy

7. lithotomy

8. mastectomy

9. hemorrhoidectomy

10. tracheotomy
11. mastopexy
12. colectomy
13. gastrorrhaphy
14. hysteropexy
15. rhinoplasty
16. arthrodesis
17. osteoclasis
18. neurolysis
19. myorrhaphy
20. tympanotomy

Learning Activity 2-4

Selecting Diagnostic, Pathological, and Related Suffixes

1. hepatoma
2. neuralgia
3. bronchiectasis
4. carcinogenesis
5. dermatosis
6. nephromegaly
7. otorrhea
8. hysterorrhexis
9. blepharospasm
10. cystocele
11. hemorrhage
12. lithiasis
13. hemiplegia
14. myopathy
15. dysphagia
16. osteomalacia
17. aphasia
18. leukemia
19. erythropenia
20. pelvimetry

Learning Activity 2-5

Building Pathological and Related Words

1. bronchiectasis
2. cholelith
3. carcinogenesis

4. osteomalacia

5. hepatomegaly

6. cholelithiasis

7. hepatocele

8. neuropathy

9. dermatosis

10. hemiplegia

11. dysphagia

12. aphasia

13. cephalodynia

14. blepharospasm

15. hyperplasia *or* hypertrophy

Learning Activity 2-6

Selecting Adjective, Noun, and Diminutive Suffixes

1. thoracic

2. gastric *or* gastral

3. bacterial

4. aquatic

5. axillary

6. cardiac *or* cardial

7. spinal *or* spinous

8. membranous

9. internist

10. leukemia

11. sigmoidoscopy

12. alcoholism

13. podiatry

14. allergist *or* allergy

15. mania

16. arteriole

17. ventricle

18. venule

Forming Plural Words

Singular	Plural	Rule
1. diagnosis	diagnoses	Drop *is* and add *es.*
2. fornix	fornices	Drop *ix* and add *ices.*
3. vertebra	vertebrae	Retain *a* and add *e.*
4. keratosis	keratoses	Drop *is* and add *es.*
5. bronchus	bronchi	Drop *us* and add *i.*
6. spermatozoon	spermatozoa	Drop *on* and add *a.*
7. septum	septa	Drop *um* and add *a.*
8. coccus	cocci	Drop *us* and add *i.*
9. ganglion	ganglia	Drop *on* and add *a.*
10. prognosis	prognoses	Drop *is* and add *es.*
11. thrombus	thrombi	Drop *us* and add *i.*
12. appendix	appendices	Drop *ix* and add *ices.*
13. bacterium	bacteria	Drop *um* and add *a.*
14. testis	testes	Drop *is* and add *es.*
15. nevus	nevi	Drop *us* and add *i.*

Chapter 3—Prefixes

Learning Activity 3-1
Identifying and Defining Prefixes

Word	Definition of Prefix
1. inter/dental	between
2. hypo/dermic	under, below, deficient
3. epi/dermis	above, upon
4. retro/version	backward, behind

Word	Definition of Prefix
5. sub/lingual	under, below
6. quadri/plegia	four
7. micro/scope	small
8. tri/ceps	three
9. an/esthesia	without, not
10. intra/muscular	in, within
11. supra/pelvic	above, excessive, superior
12. dia/rrhea	through, across
13. peri/odontal	around
14. brady/cardia	slow
15. tachy/pnea	rapid
16. dys/tocia	bad, painful, difficult
17. eu/pnea	good, normal
18. hetero/graft	different
19. mal/nutrition	bad
20. pseudo/cyesis	false

Learning Activity 3-2

Prefixes of Position, Number and Measurement, and Direction

1. retroversion
2. hypodermic
3. prenatal
4. subnasal
5. postoperative
6. intercostal
7. pseudocyesis
8. periodontal
9. diarrhea
10. ectogenous
11. suprarenal

12. hemiplegia
13. quadriplegia
14. macrocyte
15. polyphobia

Learning Activity 3-3
Other Prefixes

 1. dyspepsia
 2. heterograft
 3. panarthritis
 4. antibacterial
 5. bradycardia
 6. malnutrition
 7. amastia
 8. anesthesia
 9. eupnea
10. syndactylism
11. tachycardia
12. contraception
13. homograft
14. dystocia
15. homeoplasia

Chapter 4—Body Structure

Learning Activity 4-1
Body Cavity, Spine, and Directional Terms

 1. h. ventral cavity that contains digestive, reproductive, and excretory structures
 2. k. movement toward the median plane
 3. j. part of the spine known as the neck
 4. b. tailbone
 5. m. away from the surface of the body (internal)
 6. f. turning outward
 7. l. away from the head; toward the tail or lower part of a structure
 8. i. turning inward or inside out
 9. n. part of the spine known as the loin
10. a. pertaining to the sole of the foot
11. o. near the back of the body
12. e. lying horizontal with face downward
13. g. nearer to the center (trunk of the body)

14. d. toward the surface of the body (external)

15. c. ventral cavity that contains heart, lungs, and associated structures

Learning Activity 4-2
Word Elements

1. kary/o
2. dist/o
3. -graphy
4. -gnosis
5. leuk/o
6. viscer/o
7. jaund/o
8. hist/o
9. -genesis
10. infra-
11. ultra-
12. caud/o
13. dors/o
14. poli/o
15. eti/o
16. morph/o
17. xer/o
18. idi/o
19. ad-
20. somat/o

Learning Activity 4-3
Combining Forms, Suffixes, and Prefixes

1. cytometer
2. transabdominal
3. leukorrhea
4. cranioplasty
5. dorsalgia
6. gastromegaly
7. melanoma
8. infracostal
9. cytolysis
10. superior
11. erythrosis

12. etiology

13. diagnosis

14. sonography

15. cirrhosis

Learning Activity 4-4
Pathology, Diseases, and Conditions

1. etiology

2. diagnosis

3. adhesion

4. gangrene

5. hernia

6. ascites

7. sign

8. idiopathic

9. prognosis

10. inflammation

11. rupture

12. symptom

13. edema

14. mycosis

15. perforation

Learning Activity 4-5
Procedures and Abbreviations

1. percussion

2. excisional

3. CBC

4. ablation

5. endoscopy

6. fluoroscopy

7. Dx

8. cauterize

9. revision

10. MRI

11. anastomosis

12. nuclear scan

13. palpation

14. resection

15. computed tomography

Medical Record Activity 4-1

Radiological Consultation Letter: Cervical and Lumbar Spine

1. What was the presenting problem?

The patient had neck and lower back pain for more than 2 years' duration.

2. What were the three views of the radiologic examination of June 14, 20xx?

Anterior posterior (AP), lateral, and odontoid

3. Was there evidence of recent bony disease or injury?

There was no evidence of recent bony disease or injury.

4. Which cervical vertebrae form the atlantoaxial joint?

The first cervical vertebra (atlas) and the second cervical vertebra (axis)

5. Was the odontoid fractured?

No, the odontoid was intact.

6. What did the AP and lateral films of the lumbar spine demonstrate?

Apparent minimal spina bifida occulta of the first sacral segment.

Medical Record Activity 4-2

Radiology Report: Injury of Left Wrist, Elbow, and Humerus

1. Where are the fractures located?

Distal shafts of the radius and ulna

2. What caused the soft-tissue deformity?

A fracture caused deformity to surrounding soft tissue.

3. Did the radiologist take any side views of the left elbow?

The radiologist obtained a single view of the left elbow in the lateral projection.

4. In the AP view of the humerus, what structure was also visualized?

A portion of the elbow

5. What findings are causes for concern to the radiologist?

Lucency through the distal humerus on the AP view along its medial aspect and elevation of the anterior and posterior fat pads

Chapter 5—Integumentary System

Learning Activity 5-1

Combining Forms, Suffixes, and Prefixes

1. melanoma
2. hypodermic
3. dermatoplasty
4. lipocyte
5. pyoderma
6. dermatologist
7. xeroderma

8. anhidrosis
9. homograft
10. ichthyosis
11. scleroderma
12. mycosis
13. seborrhea
14. trichopathy
15. keratosis

Learning Activity 5-2
Building Medical Words

1. adipoma, lipoma
2. adipocele, lipocele
3. adipoid, lipoid
4. adipocyte, lipocyte
5. dermatitis
6. dermatomycosis
7. onychoma
8. onychomalacia
9. onychosis
10. onychomycosis
11. onychocryptosis
12. onychopathy
13. trichopathy
14. trichomycosis
15. dermatology
16. dermatologist
17. adipectomy *or* lipectomy
18. onychectomy
19. onychotomy
20. dermatoplasty *or* dermoplasty

Learning Activity 5-4
Burn and Oncology Terms

1. i. redness of skin
2. e. no evidence of primary tumor
3. h. cancerous; may be life-threatening

4. g. burn that heals without scar formation

5. f. determines degree of abnormal cancer cells compared with normal cells

6. a. develops from keratinizing epidermal cells

7. b. noncancerous

8. j. primary tumor size, small with minimal invasion

9. c. no evidence of metastasis

10. d. extensive damage to underlying connective tissue

Learning Activity 5-5
Pathology, Diseases, and Conditions

1. pediculosis
2. vitiligo
3. tinea
4. scabies
5. impetigo
6. urticaria
7. chloasma
8. ecchymosis
9. petechiae
10. alopecia
11. abscess
12. erythema
13. eschar
14. pruritus
15. verruca

Learning Activity 5-6
Procedures, Pharmacology, and Abbreviations

1. antifungals
2. fulguration
3. corticosteroids
4. dermabrasion
5. parasiticides
6. keratolytics
7. intradermal test
8. patch test
9. autograft
10. xenograft

Learning Activity 5-7
Medical Scenarios

1. erythematous

2. pruritic

3. dermatologist

4. metastasize

5. Mohs surgery

6. asymptomatic

7. biopsy

8. oncologist

9. lymphadenectomy

10. chemotherapy

Medical Record Activity 5-1
Pathology Report: Skin Lesion

1. In the specimen section, what does "skin on dorsum left wrist" mean?

Skin was obtained from the back, or posterior, surface of the left wrist.

2. What was the inflammatory infiltrate?

Lymphocytic inflammatory infiltrate in the papillary dermis

3. What was the pathologist's diagnosis for the left forearm?

Nodular and infiltrating basal cell carcinoma near the elbow

4. Provide a brief description of Bowen disease, the pathologist's diagnosis for the left wrist.

Bowen disease is a form of intraepidermal carcinoma (squamous cell) characterized by red-brown scaly or crusted lesions that resemble a patch of psoriasis or dermatitis.

Medical Record Activity 5-2
Patient Referral Letter: Onychomycosis

1. What pertinent disorders were identified in the past medical history?

History of hypertension and breast cancer

2. What pertinent surgery was identified in the past surgical history?

Mastectomy

3. Did the doctor identify any problems in the vascular system or nervous system?

Vascular and neurological systems were intact.

4. What was the significant finding in the laboratory results?

Alkaline phosphatase was elevated.

5. What treatment did the doctor use for the onychomycosis?

Debridement and medication or Sporanox PulsePak

6. What did the doctor recommend regarding the abnormal laboratory finding?

The doctor recommended a repeat of the liver enzymes in approximately 4 weeks.

Chapter 6—Digestive System

Learning Activity 6-1
Combining Forms, Suffixes, and Prefixes

1. gingivitis
2. colonoscope
3. gastroplasty
4. hypogastric
5. dyspepsia
6. sialolith
7. stomatopathy
8. perianal
9. jejunorrhaphy
10. pharyngitis
11. esophagoscope
12. anorexia
13. hematemesis
14. endoscopy
15. dysphagia

Learning Activity 6-2
Building Medical Words

1. esophagodynia *or* esophagalgia
2. esophagospasm
3. esophagostenosis
4. gastritis
5. gastrodynia *or* gastralgia
6. gastropathy
7. jejunectomy
8. duodenal
9. ileitis
10. jejunoileal
11. enteritis
12. enteropathy
13. enterocolitis
14. colitis
15. colorectal
16. coloptosis
17. colopathy
18. proctostenosis *or* rectostenosis

19. rectocele *or* proctocele
20. proctoplegia *or* proctoparalysis
21. cholecystitis
22. cholelithiasis
23. hepatoma
24. hepatomegaly
25. pancreatitis

Learning Activity 6-3
Building Surgical Words

1. gingivectomy
2. glossectomy
3. esophagoplasty
4. gastrectomy
5. gastrojejunostomy
6. esophagectomy
7. gastroenterocolostomy
8. enteroplasty
9. enteropexy
10. choledochorrhaphy
11. colostomy
12. hepatopexy
13. proctoplasty *or* rectoplasty
14. cholecystectomy
15. choledochoplasty

Learning Activity 6-4
Pathology, Diseases, and Conditions

1. hematemesis
2. dysphagia
3. fecalith
4. halitosis
5. anorexia
6. dyspepsia
7. cirrhosis
8. cachexia
9. obstipation
10. lesion
11. ascites
12. Crohn disease

13. steatorrhea
14. leukoplakia
15. flatus

Learning Activity 6-5
Procedures, Pharmacology, and Abbreviations

1. MRCP
2. ESWL
3. emetics
4. antispasmodics
5. choledochoplasty
6. lower GI series
7. gastroscopy
8. antiemetics
9. intubation
10. anastomosis
11. stool guaiac
12. endoscopy
13. laxatives
14. antacids
15. stool culture
16. liver function tests
17. bariatric
18. stat.
19. proctosigmoidoscopy
20. upper GI series

Learning Activity 6-6
Medical Scenarios

1. dysphagia
2. dyspepsia
3. gastric reflux
4. antacids
5. hiatal hernia
6. anorexia
7. nausea
8. sclerae
9. jaundice
10. hepatomegaly

Medical Record Activity 6-1
Chart Note: GI Evaluation

1. While referring to Figure 6-5, describe the location of the gallbladder in relation to the liver.

Posterior and inferior portion of the right lobe of the liver

2. Why did the patient undergo the cholecystectomy?

To treat cholecystitis and cholelithiasis

3. List the patient's prior surgeries.

Tonsillectomy, appendectomy, and cholecystectomy

4. How does the patient's most recent postoperative episode of discomfort (pain) differ from the initial pain she described?

The continuous, deep right-sided pain took a crescendo pattern and then a decrescendo pattern. Initially, it was intermittent and sharp epigastric pain.

Medical Record Activity 6-2
Operative Report: Esophagogastroduodenoscopy with Biopsy

1. What caused the hematemesis?

Etiology was unknown. Inflammation of the stomach and duodenum was noted.

2. What procedures were carried out to determine the cause of bleeding?

During x-ray tomography using the videoendoscope, biopsies were taken of the stomach and duodenum. It was also noted that previously the patient had esophageal varices.

3. How much blood did the patient lose during the procedure?

None

4. Were there any ulcerations or erosions found during the exploratory procedure that might account for the bleeding?

No

5. What type of sedation was used during the procedure?

Demerol and Versed administered intravenously

6. What did the doctors find when they examined the stomach and duodenum?

Diffuse, punctate erythema

Chapter 7—Respiratory System

Learning Activity 7-1
Combining Forms, Suffixes, and Prefixes

1. pleurocentesis
2. bronchoscope
3. tonsillectomy
4. bradypnea
5. dysphonia
6. cyanosis

7. oximeter

8. laryngoplegia

9. septoplasty

10. sinusotomy

11. hypercapnia

12. eupnea

13. bronchiectasis

14. rhinoplasty

15. pneumonia

Learning Activity 7-2
Building Medical Words

1. rhinorrhea

2. rhinitis

3. laryngoscopy

4. laryngitis

5. laryngostenosis

6. bronchiectasis

7. bronchopathy

8. bronchospasm

9. pneumothorax

10. pneumonitis

11. pulmonologist

12. pulmonary, pulmonic

13. dyspnea

14. bradypnea

15. tachypnea

16. apnea

17. rhinoplasty

18. thoracocentesis *or* thoracentesis

19. pulmonectomy *or* pneumonectomy

20. tracheostomy

Learning Activity 7-3
Pathology, Diseases, and Conditions

1. atelectasis

2. empyema

3. surfactant

4. hypoxia

5. exudate
6. anosmia
7. hypoxemia
8. tubercles
9. apnea
10. emphysema
11. hemoptysis
12. epistaxis
13. pulmonary edema
14. transudate
15. deviated septum
16. coryza
17. pneumonoconiosis
18. pleurisy
19. consolidation
20. pertussis

Learning Activity 7-4
Procedures, Pharmacology, and Abbreviations

1. sputum culture
2. polysomnography
3. CXR
4. antral lavage
5. antihistamine
6. antitussive
7. sweat test
8. oximetry
9. AFB
10. aerosol therapy
11. decongestant
12. Mantoux test
13. ABGs
14. expectorant
15. throat culture
16. pulmonary function tests
17. laryngoscopy
18. septoplasty
19. pneumectomy
20. rhinoplasty

Learning Activity 7-5

Medical Scenarios

1. dyspnea
2. coryza
3. deviated nasal septum
4. septoplasty
5. T&A
6. myalgia
7. cephalodynia
8. sinusitis
9. pharyngitis
10. antitussive

Medical Record Activity 7-1

SOAP Note: Respiratory Evaluation

1. What symptom caused the patient to seek medical help?

Shortness of breath

2. What was the patient's previous history?

Difficult breathing, high blood pressure, chronic obstructive pulmonary disease, and peripheral vascular disease

3. What were the abnormal findings of the physical examination?

Bilateral wheezes and rhonchi heard anteriorly and posteriorly

4. What changes were noted from the previous film?

Interstitial vascular congestion with possible superimposed inflammatory change and some pleural reactive change

5. What are the present assessments?

Acute exacerbation of chronic obstructive pulmonary disease, heart failure, hypertension, and peripheral vascular disease

6. What new diagnosis was made that did not appear in the previous medical history?

Heart failure

Medical Record Activity 7-2

SOAP Note: Chronic Interstitial Lung Disease

1. When did the patient notice dyspnea?

With activity

2. Other than the respiratory system, what other body systems are identified in the history of present illness?

Cardiovascular, urinary, and nervous system

3. What were the findings regarding the neck?

Supple and no evidence of thyromegaly or adenomegaly

4. What was the finding regarding the chest?

Basilar crackles without wheezing or rhonchi

5. What appears to be the likely cause of the chronic interstitial lung disease?

Combination of pulmonary fibrosis and heart failure

6. What did the cardiac examination reveal?

Trace of edema without clubbing or murmur

Chapter 8—Cardiovascular System

Learning Activity 8-1
Combining Forms, Suffixes, and Prefixes

1. cardiomegaly
2. atheroma
3. arteriorrhexis
4. endovascular
5. tachycardia
6. phlebectasis
7. aortogram
8. valvuloplasty
9. sclerosis
10. sclerotherapy
11. thrombolysis
12. arrhythmia
13. bradycardia
14. cardiodynia
15. aneurysmectomy

Learning Activity 8-2
Building Medical Words

1. atheroma
2. atherosclerosis
3. phlebitis
4. phlebothrombosis
5. venous
6. venospasm
7. cardiologist
8. cardiorrhexis
9. cardiotoxic
10. cardiomegaly
11. angiomalacia
12. angioma

13. thrombogen *or* thrombogenesis

14. thrombosis

15. aortostenosis

16. aortography

17. cardiocentesis

18. arteriorrhaphy

19. embolectomy

20. thrombolysis

Learning Activity 8-3
Pathology, Diseases, and Conditions

1. infarction

2. angina

3. insufficiency

4. tachycardia

5. varices

6. bruit

7. bradycardia

8. palpitation

9. thrombosis

10. aneurysm

11. embolism

12. arrhythmia

13. regurgitation

14. diaphoresis

15. arteriosclerosis

16. hypertension

17. hyperlipidemia

18. coarctation

19. ischemia

20. stenosis

Learning Activity 8-4
Procedures, Pharmacology, and Abbreviations

1. Holter monitor test

2. echocardiography

3. valvotomy

4. nitrates

5. statins

6. diuretics

7. cardiac enzymes studies

8. Doppler

9. stress test

10. catheter ablation

11. commissurotomy

12. biopsy

13. ICD insertion

14. stent placement

15. angioplasty

16. sclerotherapy

17. CABG

18. endarterectomy

19. PTCA

20. thrombolysis

Learning Activity 8-5
Medical Scenarios

1. angina pectoris

2. diaphoresis

3. palpitations

4. hypertension

5. edema

6. myocardial infarction

7. ischemia

8. angioplasty

9. catheter

10. stent

Medical Record Activity 8-1
Chart Note: Acute Myocardial Infarction

1. How long had the patient experienced chest pain before she was seen in the hospital?

Approximately 2 hours

2. Did the patient have a previous history of chest pain?

Yes

3. Initially, what medications were administered to stabilize the patient?

Streptokinase and heparin

4. What two laboratory tests will be used to evaluate the patient?

Partial thromboplastin time and cardiac enzymes

5. During the current admission, what part of the heart was damaged?

The lateral front side of the heart (anterior of the heart)

6. Was the location of damage to the heart for this admission the same as for the initial MI?

No, in the earlier admission, the damage was to the lower part of the heart.

Medical Record Activity 8-2

Operative Report: Right Temporal Artery Biopsy

1. Why was the right temporal artery biopsied?

To rule out arteritis

2. In what position was the patient placed?

Supine

3. What was the incision area?

Right preauricular area

4. How was the temporal artery located for administration of Xylocaine?

By palpation

5. How was the dissection carried out?

Down through the subcutaneous tissue and superficial fascia

6. What was the size of the specimen?

A segment of approximately 1.5 cm

Chapter 9—Blood, Lymph, and Immune Systems

Learning Activity 9-1

Combining Forms, Suffixes, and Prefixes

1. lymphangiitis
2. leukocytopenia
3. splenomegaly
4. thrombosis
5. embolectomy
6. thymoma
7. isochromic
8. anisocytosis
9. macrophagic
10. erythroblast
11. hemolysis
12. electrophoresis
13. adenoid
14. amorphic
15. leukocytopoiesis

Learning Activity 9-2
Building Medical Words

1. erythrocytosis
2. leukocytosis
3. lymphocytosis
4. reticulocytosis
5. leukopenia
6. erythropenia
7. thrombocytopenia *or* thrombopenia
8. lymphocytopenia
9. hemopoiesis *or* hematopoiesis
10. leukopoiesis *or* leukocytopoiesis
11. thrombocytopoiesis
12. immunologist
13. immunology
14. splenocele
15. splenolysis
16. splenectomy
17. thymectomy
18. thymolysis
19. splenotomy
20. splenopexy

Learning Activity 9-3
Pathology, Diseases, and Conditions

1. hemoglobinopathy
2. edema
3. lymphadenopathy
4. aplastic
5. anaphylaxis
6. opportunistic
7. Hodgkin disease
8. splenomegaly
9. erythropenia
10. multiple myeloma
11. mononucleosis
12. sepsis
13. myelogenous

14. Kaposi sarcoma
15. sickle cell
16. thrombocytopenia
17. hemolytic
18. thrombocythemia
19. hematoma
20. graft rejection

Procedures, Pharmacology, and Abbreviations

1. biological
2. lymphangiography
3. monospot
4. anticoagulants
5. WBC
6. homologous
7. ANA
8. lymphoscintigraphy
9. Shilling
10. lymphadenectomy
11. autologous
12. antimicrobials
13. RBC
14. thrombolytics
15. transfusion

Medical Scenarios

1. lymphadenopathy
2. splenomegaly
3. leukocytosis
4. erythropenia
5. hematologist
6. hemophilia
7. ecchymoses
8. arthralgia
9. hemarthrosis
10. hemostasis

Medical Record Activity 9-1
Discharge Summary: Sickle Cell Crisis

1. What blood product was administered to the patient?

Two units of packed red blood cells

2. Why was this blood product given to the patient?

The patient was anemic due to sickle cell anemia.

3. Why was a CT scan performed on the patient?

To determine the cause of abdominal pain

4. What were the three findings of the CT scan?

Ileus in the small bowel, dilated small bowel loops, and abnormal enhancement pattern in the kidney

5. Why should the patient see his regular doctor?

To follow up on the renal abnormality

Medical Record Activity 9-2
Discharge Summary: PCP and HIV

1. How do you think the patient acquired the HIV infection?

From her husband, who died of HIV

2. What were the two diagnoses of the husband?

Multifocal leukoencephalopathy and Kaposi sarcoma

3. What four disorders in the medical history are significant for HIV?

Several episodes of diarrhea, sinusitis, thrush, and vaginal candidiasis

4. What was the x-ray finding?

Diffuse lower lobe infiltrates

5. What two procedures are going to be performed to confirm the diagnosis of *pneumocystis* pneumonia?

Bronchoscopy and alveolar lavage

Chapter 10—Musculoskeletal System

Learning Activity 10-1
Combining Forms, Suffixes, and Prefixes

1. tenodesis
2. leiomyoma
3. synovitis
4. patellar
5. dystrophy
6. infracostal
7. ankylosis
8. craniomalacia
9. osteotome
10. arthritis

11. syndactylism
12. osteoclasia
13. craniotome
14. chondroma
15. fascioplasty

Learning Activity 10-2
Building Medical Words

1. osteocytes
2. ostealgia *or* osteodynia
3. osteoarthropathy
4. osteogenesis
5. cervical
6. cervicobrachial
7. cervicofacial
8. myeloma
9. myelosarcoma
10. myelocyte
11. myeloid
12. suprasternal
13. sternoid
14. chondroblast
15. arthritis
16. osteoarthritis
17. pelvimeter
18. myospasm
19. myopathy
20. myorrhexis
21. phalangectomy
22. thoracotomy
23. vertebrectomy
24. arthrodesis
25. myoplasty

Learning Activity 10-3
Pathology, Diseases, and Conditions

1. subluxation
2. rickets
3. spondylolisthesis

 4. claudication

 5. muscular dystrophy

 6. talipes

 7. sequestrum

 8. myasthenia gravis

 9. carpal tunnel

10. ganglion cyst

11. hypotonia

12. Ewing

13. greenstick fracture

14. kyphosis

15. osteoporosis

16. scoliosis

17. chondrosarcoma

18. comminuted fracture

19. spondylitis

20. gout

21. bunion

22. pyogenic

23. necrosis

24. ankylosis

25. phantom limb

Learning Activity 10-4
Procedures, Pharmacology, and Abbreviations

 1. myelography

 2. open reduction

 3. gold salts

 4. CTS

 5. laminectomy

 6. arthrography

 7. arthrodesis

 8. amputation

 9. HNP

10. salicylates

11. arthroscopy

12. sequestrectomy

13. ACL

14. relaxants

15. closed reduction

Learning Activity 10-5
Medical Scenarios

1. comminuted
2. clavicle
3. open fracture
4. femur
5. orthopedist
6. osteopenia
7. kyphosis
8. spondylalgia
9. osteoporosis
10. pathological fractures

Medical Record Activity 10-1
Operative Report: Right Knee Arthroscopy and Medial Meniscectomy

1. Describe the meniscus and identify its location.

The meniscus is the curved, fibrous cartilage in the knees and other joints.

2. What is the probable cause of the tear in the patient's meniscus?

The continuous pressure on the knees from jogging on a hard surface, such as the pavement

3. What does normal ACL and PCL refer to in the report?

The anterior and posterior cruciate ligaments appeared to be normal.

4. Explain the McMurray sign test.

Rotation of the tibia on the femur is used to determine injury to meniscal structures. An audible click during manipulation of the tibia with the leg flexed is an indication that the meniscus has been injured.

5. Because Lachman and McMurray tests were negative (normal), why was the surgery performed?

The medial compartment of the knee showed an inferior surface posterior and mid-medial meniscal tear that was flipped up on top of itself. The surgeon resected the tear, and the remaining meniscus was contoured back to a stable rim.

Medical Record Activity 10-2
Radiographic Consultation: Tibial Diaphysis Nuclear Scan

1. Where was the pain located?

Middle one-third of the left tibia

2. What medication was the patient taking for pain and did it provide relief?

He found no relief with NSAIDs.

3. How was the blood flow to the affected area described by the radiologist?

Focal, increased blood flow and blood pooling

4. How was the radiotracer accumulation described?

The radiotracer accumulation within the left mid-posterior tibial diaphysis was delayed.

5. What will be the probable outcome with continued excessive repetitive stress?
The rate of resorption will exceed the rate of bone replacement.

6. What will happen if resorption continues to exceed replacement?
A stress fracture will occur.

Chapter 11—Urinary System

Learning Activity 11-1

Combining Forms, Suffixes, and Prefixes

1. nephropathy
2. lithogenesis
3. pyeloplasty
4. anuria
5. glomerulosclerosis
6. cystoscopy
7. dialysis
8. hematuria
9. polyuria
10. ureterectasis
11. meatotome
12. azotemia
13. nephrocele
14. lithotripsy
15. cystogram

Learning Activity 11-2

Building Medical Words

1. nephrolith
2. nephropyosis *or* pyonephrosis
3. hydronephrosis *or* nephrohydrosis
4. pyelography
5. pyelopathy
6. ureterectasis *or* ureterectasia
7. ureterolith
8. ureteralgia
9. cystitis
10. cystoscope
11. cystoplegia
12. vesicocele
13. vesicourethral
14. urethrostenosis

15. urethrotome
16. urology
17. uropathy
18. dysuria
19. oliguria
20. pyuria
21. ureteroplasty
22. cystectomy
23. urethrorrhaphy
24. pyelostomy
25. cystopexy

Learning Activity 11-3

Pathology, Diseases, and Conditions

1. urgency
2. fistula
3. dysuria
4. anuria
5. azotemia
6. hydronephrosis
7. urolithiasis
8. hesitancy
9. oliguria
10. pyelonephritis
11. cystocele
12. enuresis
13. polycystic
14. neurogenic bladder
15. pyuria
16. nephrotic syndrome
17. nocturia
18. hypercalcemia
19. Wilms tumor
20. nephrolithiasis

Learning Activity 11-4

Procedures, Pharmacology, and Abbreviations

1. nephropexy
2. electromyography
3. cystoscopy

4. antibiotics

5. C&S

6. diuretics

7. stent insertion

8. ESWL

9. peritoneal

10. renal nuclear scan

11. hemodialysis

12. cystography

13. ultrasonography

14. potassium

15. UA

Learning Activity 11-5
Medical Scenarios

1. hematuria

2. pyuria

3. ureterolithiasis

4. hydronephrosis

5. lithotripsy

6. oliguria

7. hypertension

8. proteinuria

9. glomerulonephritis

10. prognosis

Medical Record Activity 11-1
Operative Report: Ureterocele and Ureterocele Calculus

1. What were the findings from the resectoscopy?

The prostate and bladder appeared normal but there was a left ureterocele.

2. What was the name and size of the urethral sound used in the procedure?

#26 French Van Buren

3. What is the function of the urethral sound?

To dilate the urethra

4. In what direction was the ureterocele incised?

Longitudinally

5. Was fulguration required? Why or why not?

Fulguration was not required because there was no bleeding.

Medical Record Activity 11-2

Operative Report: Extracorporeal Shock-Wave Lithotripsy

1. What previous procedures were performed on the patient?

ESWL and double-J stent placement

2. Why is this current procedure being performed?

To fragment the remaining calculus and remove the double-J stent

3. What imaging technique was used for positioning the patient to ensure that the shock waves would strike the calculus?

Fluoroscopy

4. In what position was the patient placed in the cystoscopy suite?

Dorsal lithotomy

5. How was the double-J stent removed?

Using grasping forceps and removing it as the scope was withdrawn

Chapter 12—Female Reproductive System

Learning Activity 12-1

Combining Forms, Suffixes, and Prefixes

1. colposcopy
2. prenatal
3. dystocia
4. hysterorrhexis
5. oophoroma
6. cervicitis
7. amniocentesis
8. perineorrhaphy
9. salpingoplasty
10. primigravida
11. pseudocyesis
12. hemosalpinx
13. multipara
14. menarche
15. galactopoiesis

Learning Activity 12-2

Building Medical Words

1. gynecopathy
2. gynecologist
3. cervicovaginitis

4. cervicovesical

5. colposcope

6. colposcopy

7. vaginitis

8. vaginocele

9. hysteromyoma

10. hysteropathy

11. hysterosalpingography

12. metrorrhagia

13. parametritis

14. uterocele

15. uterocervical

16. uterovesical

17. oophoritis

18. oophorosalpingitis

19. salpingocele

20. salpingography

21. oophoropexy *or* ovariopexy

22. hystero-oophorectomy

23. episiorrhaphy *or* perineorrhaphy

24. hysterosalpingo-oophorectomy

25. amniocentesis

Learning Activity 12-3
Pathology, Diseases, and Conditions

1. pyosalpinx

2. primipara

3. gestation

4. sterility

5. retroversion

6. trichomoniasis

7. dystocia

8. atresia

9. Down syndrome

10. septicemia

11. dyspareunia

12. metrorrhagia

13. menarche

14. fibroids

15. oligomenorrhea

16. breech

17. eclampsia
18. choriocarcinoma
19. pathogen
20. primigravida

Procedures, Pharmacology, and Abbreviations

1. Pap test
2. hysterosalpingography
3. amniocentesis
4. antifungals
5. colpocleisis
6. D&C
7. TAH
8. tubal ligation
9. OCPs
10. laparoscopy
11. episiotomy
12. PID
13. chorionic villus sampling
14. estrogens
15. oxytocins
16. cryocautery
17. IUD
18. cordocentesis
19. lumpectomy
20. prostaglandins

Learning Activity 12-5
Medical Scenarios

1. gravida 3, para 3
2. metrorrhagia
3. menorrhagia
4. dysmenorrhea
5. uterine fibroids
6. nullipara
7. menarche
8. menopause
9. mammography
10. needle biopsy

Medical Record Activity 12-1
SOAP Note: Primary Herpes I Infection

1. Did the patient have any discharge? If so, describe it.

Yes, a brownish discharge

2. What type of discomfort did the patient experience around the vulvar area?

She was experiencing severe itching (pruritus), fever, and blisters.

3. Has the patient been taking her oral contraceptive pills regularly?

Yes

4. Where was the viral culture obtained?

Ulcerlike lesion on the right labia

5. Even though her partner used a condom, how do you think the patient became infected with herpes?

She probably got infected from the cold sore when having oral-genital sex.

Medical Record Activity 12-2
Postoperative Consultation: Menometrorrhagia

1. How many pregnancies did this woman have? How many viable infants did she deliver?

Two pregnancies and one viable birth

2. What is a therapeutic abortion?

An abortion performed when the pregnancy endangers the mother's mental or physical health or when the fetus has a known condition incompatible with life

3. Why did the physician propose to perform a hysterectomy?

The patient desired definitive treatment for menometrorrhagia and had declined palliative treatment.

4. What is a vaginal hysterectomy?

Surgical removal of the uterus through the vagina

5. Did the surgeon plan to remove one or both ovaries and fallopian tubes?

The surgeon planned to perform a bilateral (pertaining to two sides) salpingo-oophorectomy.

6. Why do you think the physician planned to use the laparoscope to perform the hysterectomy?

To permit visualization of the abdominal cavity as the ovaries and fallopian tubes are removed through the vagina

Chapter 13—Male Reproductive System

Learning Activity 13-1
Combining Forms, Suffixes, and Prefixes

1. spermicide
2. varicocele
3. scrotoplasty
4. prostatomegaly
5. anorchism
6. gonadectomy
7. genitourinary

8. epididymectomy

9. brachytherapy

10. epispadias

11. balanitis

12. androgen

13. perineorrhaphy

14. vasectomy

15. vesiculography

Learning Activity 13-2
Building Medical Words

1. orchiditis

2. orchidoptosis

3. balanorrhea

4. balanocele

5. spermatocyte

6. spermatoblast

7. spermatocele

8. prostatalgia *or* prostatodynia

9. prostatorrhea

10. prostatomegaly

11. prostatolith

12. hypospadias

13. hyperspadias

14. vesiculitis

15. vesiculography

16. gonadopathy

17. balanoplasty

18. vasectomy

19. scrotoplasty

20. perineorrhaphy

Learning Activity 13-3
Pathology, Diseases, and Conditions

1. leukorrhea

2. genital herpes

3. cryptorchidism

4. hypospadias

5. phimosis

6. varicocele

7. epispadias

8. testicular torsion

9. condylomas

10. anorchidism

11. balanitis

12. priapism

13. prostatitis

14. cystitis

15. sterility

16. trichomoniasis

17. chlamydia

18. chancre

19. hesitancy

20. gynecomastia

Learning Activity 13-4
Procedures, Pharmacology, and Abbreviations

1. semen analysis

2. androgens

3. scrotal

4. GC

5. vasectomy

6. urethroplasty

7. vasovasostomy

8. antiandrogens

9. TURP

10. PSA

11. antivirals

12. orchiopexy

13. circumcision

14. HPV

15. BPH

Learning Activity 13-5
Medical Scenarios

1. leukorrhea

2. dysuria

3. pruritus

4. orchialgia

5. meatus

6. PSA

7. hesitancy

8. urgency

9. nocturia

10. prostatomegaly

Medical Record Activity 13-1
Consultation Report: Benign Prostatic Hyperplasia

1. What is the reason for the present admission?

Left inguinal hernia repair and right ventral hernia repair

2. What occurred when the Foley catheter was removed?

The patient complained of dysuria, frequency, and a feeling of incomplete emptying with weak stream.

3. What did his previous history indicate regarding these symptoms?

He had a history of hesitancy, weak stream, and voiding every 2 to3 hours.

4. Why was it difficult to assess for bladder distention?

The incision lies over the bladder area.

5. Was there a definitive diagnosis identified in the Impression?

The impression indicates questionable urine retention.

6. What procedure will be performed if the patient has difficulty voiding?

The doctor will catheterize the patient.

Medical Record Activity 13-2
Chart Note: Acute Epididymitis

1. What were the complaints of the patient?

Severe left-sided groin pain, scrotal pain, and urethritis with a clear urethral discharge

2. What procedure was performed regarding the urethral discharge?

The discharge was expressed upon compression of the glans and swabs were obtained for testing.

3. What information is provided regarding the left testicle?

Moderate pain and tenderness, which is alleviated with elevation of the testicles

4. How was the left epididymis described?

Palpable with significant induration and tenderness

5. What did the rectal examination reveal?

Mild prostatic hyperplasia and tenderness

Chapter 14—Endocrine System

Learning Activity 14-1
Combining Forms, Suffixes, and Prefixes

1. thymoma

2. glycolysis

3. polydipsia

4. pancreatolithectomy

5. endocrine

6. adipsia

7. exocrine

8. hyperglycemia

9. thymolysis

10. thyromegaly

11. adrenalitis

12. hypocalcemia

13. hyperkalemia

14. acromegaly

15. pancreatography

Learning Activity 14-2
Building Medical Words

1. hyperglycemia

2. hypoglycemia

3. glycogenesis

4. pancreatitis

5. pancreatolysis

6. pancreatopathy

7. thyroiditis

8. thyromegaly

9. parathyroidectomy

10. adrenalectomy

Learning Activity 14-3
Diseases and Conditions

1. acromegaly

2. myxedema

3. diuresis

4. hirsutism

5. cretinism

6. thyroid storm

7. Addison disease

8. exophthalmic goiter

9. hyperkalemia

10. pheochromocytoma

11. type 1 diabetes

12. hyponatremia

13. glycosuria

14. Cushing syndrome

15. type 2 diabetes

Learning Activity 14-4
Procedures, Pharmacology, and Abbreviations

1. FBS

2. RAIU

3. corticosteroids

4. growth hormone

5. thyroid scan

6. T_4

7. oral antidiabetics

8. GTT

9. antithyroids

10. hypophysectomy

11. T_3

12. MRI

13. exophthalmometry

14. CT scan

15. Humulin

Learning Activity 14-5
Medical Scenarios

1. polydipsia

2. polyuria

3. polyphagia

4. hyperglycemia

5. glycosuria

6. lethargy

7. constipation

8. bradycardia

9. hypopnea

10. triiodothyronine and thyroxine

Medical Record Activity 14-1
Consultation Note: Hyperparathyroidism

1. What is an adenoma?

Benign tumor of a gland

2. What does the physician suspect caused the patient's hyperparathyroidism?

Possible parathyroid adenoma

3. What type of laboratory findings revealed parathyroid disease?

Elevated calcium level

4. What is hypercalciuria?

Excessive amount of calcium in the urine

5. If the patient smoked 548 packs of cigarettes per year, how many packs did she smoke in an average day?

Approximately 1½ packs per day (365 days per year/548 packs = 1.5)

Medical Record Activity 14-2
SOAP Note: Diabetes Mellitus

1. How long has this patient been experiencing voracious eating?

For the past 10 days

2. Was the patient's obesity due to overeating or metabolic imbalance?

Overeating

3. Why did the doctor experience difficulty in examining the patient's abdomen?

Because she was so obese

4. Was the patient's blood glucose above or below normal on admission?

Above normal

5. What is the reference range for fasting blood glucose?

The range for fasting blood glucose is 70 to 110 mg/dL.

Chapter 15—Nervous System

Learning Activity 15-1
Combining Forms, Suffixes, and Prefixes

  1. ventriculostomy

  2. neuroma

  3. radiculalgia

  4. gangliitis

  5. narcolepsy

  6. unilateral

  7. meningitis

  8. quadriplegia

  9. hyperkinesia

10. myasthenia

11. cerebropathy

12. intrathecal

13. encephalocele

14. kinesiotherapy

15. myelorrhaphy

Learning Activity 15-2

Building Medical Words

1. encephalopathy
2. encephalocele
3. encephalography
4. cerebropathy
5. cerebritis
6. craniocele
7. craniometer
8. neuralgia *or* neurodynia
9. neurologist
10. neurotripsy
11. myelocele
12. myeloplegia
13. psychotic *or* psychic
14. psychosis
15. bradykinesia
16. dyskinesia
17. hemiplegia
18. quadriplegia
19. dysphasia
20. aphasia
21. neurolysis
22. craniotomy
23. cranioplasty
24. neurorrhaphy
25. encephalotomy

Learning Activity 15-3

Pathology, Diseases, and Conditions

1. hemiparesis
2. dementia
3. Alzheimer
4. bulimia
5. clonic
6. Guillain-Barrè
7. ataxia
8. bipolar disorder
9. epilepsies

10. ischemic
11. shingles
12. radiculopathy
13. paraplegia
14. poliomyelitis
15. convulsion
16. myelomeningocele
17. autism
18. Parkinson
19. multiple sclerosis
20. concussion

Learning Activity 15-4
Procedures, Pharmacology, and Abbreviations

1. NCV
2. psychostimulants
3. antipsychotics
4. general anesthetics
5. echoencephalography
6. cryosurgery
7. myelography
8. TIA
9. CSF analysis
10. electromyography
11. lumbar puncture
12. thalamotomy
13. tractotomy
14. hypnotics
15. trephination

Learning Activity 15-5
Medical Scenarios

1. neuralgia
2. sciatica
3. herniation
4. osteophyte
5. neuropathy
6. tremor
7. bradyphasia

8. bradykinesia
9. dysphagia
10. Parkinson disease

Medical Record Activity 15-1
Discharge Summary: Subarachnoid Hemorrhage

1. In what part of the head did the patient feel pain?

Occipital, the back part of the head

2. What imaging tests were performed, and what was the finding in each test?

CT scan showed blood in the cisterna subarachnoidalis and mild acute hydrocephalus. Cerebral angiogram and MRI showed no aneurysm.

3. What was the result of the lumbar puncture?

The results were consistent with recurrent subarachnoid hemorrhage.

4. What was the result of the repeat MRI?

It again showed no evidence of an aneurysm.

5. Regarding activity, what limitations were placed on the patient?

Avoid activity that could raise the pressure in the head, and perform no activity more vigorous than walking.

Medical Record Activity 15-2
Consultation Report: Acute-Onset Paraplegia

1. What was the original cause of the patient's current problems and what treatments were provided?

Fall at work about 15 to 20 years ago and four subsequent lumbar surgeries

2. Why was the patient admitted to the hospital?

Pain management

3. What medications did the patient receive and why was each given?

Clonidine for hypertension and methadone for pain

4. What was the cause of bladder retention?

Administration of clonidine

5. What occurred after the catheter was removed?

Subacute onset of paresis, paresthesias, and pain in the legs, approximately 2½ to 3 hours later

6. What three disorders were listed in the differential diagnosis?

Subarachnoid hemorrhage, epidural abscess, and transverse myelitis

Chapter 16—Special Senses

Learning Activity 16-1
Combining Forms, Suffixes, and Prefixes

1. amblyopia
2. phacocele

3. diplopia

4. blepharoptosis

5. goniometer

6. intraocular

7. keratotomy

8. otorrhea

9. audiometer

10. anacusia

11. labyrinthitis

12. otosclerosis

13. mastoiditis

14. myringoplasty

15. presbyacusia

Building Medical Words

1. ophthalmoplegia *or* ophthalmoparalysis

2. ophthalmology

3. pupilloscopy

4. keratomalacia

5. keratometer

6. scleritis

7. scleromalacia

8. iridoplegia *or* iridoparalysis

9. iridocele

10. retinopathy

11. retinitis

12. blepharoplegia

13. blepharoptosis

14. otopyorrhea

15. audiometer

16. myringotome

17. amblyopia

18. hyperopia

19. anacusis

20. hyperacusis

21. stapedectomy

22. labyrinthotomy

23. mastoidectomy

24. myringoplasty *or* tympanoplasty

25. keratotomy

Learning Activity 16-3
Pathology, Diseases, and Conditions

1. cataract
2. achromatopsia
3. nyctalopia
4. presbyacusis
5. anacusis
6. otitis externa
7. otosclerosis
8. otitis media
9. otopyorrhea
10. epiphora
11. hordeolum
12. otoencephalitis
13. neovascular
14. vertigo
15. exotropia
16. drusen
17. chalazion
18. amblyopia
19. retinoblastoma
20. tinnitus

Learning Activity 16-4
Procedures, Pharmacology, and Abbreviations

1. caloric stimulation
2. ophthalmoscopy
3. cochlear implant
4. fluorescein angiography
5. otoplasty
6. mydriatics
7. tonometry
8. visual acuity
9. evisceration
10. antiemetics
11. wax emulsifiers
12. enucleation
13. ST
14. ophthalmic decongestants
15. XT

16. gonioscopy
17. otoscopy
18. audiometry
19. radial keratotomy
20. otic analgesics

Learning Activity 16-5
Medical Scenarios

1. asymptomatic
2. tonometry
3. hyperopia
4. gonioscopy
5. trabeculoplasty
6. pediatrician
7. otalgia
8. pharyngalgia
9. otorrhea
10. tympanorrhexis

Medical Record Activity 16-1
Operative Report: Retained Foreign Bodies

1. Did the surgery involve one or both ears?

It was bilateral, involving both ears.

2. What was the nature of the foreign body in the patient's ears?

Retained tympanostomy tubes

3. What ear structure was involved?

Eardrum, or tympanum

4. What instrument was used to locate the tubes?

Operating microscope

5. What was the material in which the tubes were embedded?

Earwax, or cerumen

6. What occurred when the cerumen and tubes were removed?

It resulted in a large perforation.

7. How was the perforation treated?

The edges were freshened sharply with a pick, and a paper patch was applied.

Operative Report: Phacoemulsification and Lens Implant

1. What technique was used to destroy the cataract?

Phacoemulsification, an ultrasound technique

2. In what portion of the eye was the implant placed?

Posterior chamber

3. What anesthetics were used for surgery?

Intravenous and retrobulbar block

4. What was the function of the blepharostat?

To separate the eyelids during surgery

5. What is a keratome?

A knife used to incise the cornea

6. Where was the implant inserted?

In the capsular bag

Common Abbreviations and Symbols

Common Abbreviations

The table below lists common abbreviations used in health care and related fields, along with their meanings.

Abbreviation	Meaning	Abbreviation	Meaning
A		**AST**	angiotensin sensitivity test; aspartate aminotransferase
AAA	abdominal aortic aneurysm	**Ast**	astigmatism
A&P	auscultation and percussion	**ATN**	acute tubular necrosis
A, B, AB, O	blood types in ABO blood group	**AV**	atrioventricular; arteriovenous
AB, Ab, ab	antibody; abortion	**B**	
ABC	aspiration biopsy cytology	**Ba**	barium
ABG	arterial blood gas(es)	**baso**	basophil (type of white blood cell)
AC	air conduction	**BBB**	bundle branch block
Acc	accommodation	**BC**	bone conduction
ACE	angiotensin-converting enzyme (inhibitor)	**BCC**	basal cell carcinoma
ACL	anterior cruciate ligament	**BE**	barium enema; below the elbow
ACS	acute coronary syndrome	**BEAM**	brain electrical activity mapping
ACTH	adrenocorticotropic hormone	**BK**	below the knee
AD	Alzheimer disease	**BKA**	below-knee amputation
ADH	antidiuretic hormone (vasopressin)	**BM**	bowel movement
ADHD	attention deficit–hyperactivity disorder	**BMI**	body mass index
ad lib.	as desired	**BMR**	basal metabolic rate
ADLs	activities of daily living	**BMT**	bone marrow transplant
AE	above the elbow	**BNO**	bladder neck obstruction
AED	automatic external defibrillator	**BP, B/P**	blood pressure
AFB	acid-fast bacillus (TB organism)	**BPH**	benign prostatic hyperplasia; benign prostatic hypertrophy
AFib	atrial fibrillation	**BS**	blood sugar
AGN	acute glomerulonephritis	**BSE**	breast self-examination
AI	artificial insemination	**BUN**	blood urea nitrogen
AICD	automatic implantable cardioverter defibrillator	**Bx, bx**	biopsy
AIDS	acquired immune deficiency syndrome	**C**	
AK	above the knee	**C&S**	culture and sensitivity
ALL	acute lymphocytic leukemia	**c/o**	complains of, complaints
ALS	amyotrophic lateral sclerosis	**C1, C2, and so on**	first cervical vertebra, second cervical vertebra, and so on
ALT	alanine aminotransferase	**CA**	cancer; chronological age; cardiac arrest
AM, a.m.	in the morning or before noon	**Ca**	calcium; cancer
AML	acute myelogenous leukemia	**CABG**	coronary artery bypass graft
ANA	antinuclear antibody	**CAD**	coronary artery disease
ANS	autonomic nervous system	**CAH**	chronic active hepatitis; congenital adrenal hyperplasia
AOM	acute otitis media	**CAT**	computed axial tomography
AP	anteroposterior	**Cath**	catheterization; catheter
APC	antigen-presenting cell	**CBC**	complete blood count
APTT	activated partial thromboplastin time	**CC**	cardiac catheterization; chief complaint
ARDS	acute respiratory distress syndrome	**CCU**	coronary care unit
ARF	acute renal failure	**CDH**	congenital dislocation of the hip
ARMD, AMD	age-related macular degeneration	**CF**	cystic fibrosis
AS	aortic stenosis	**CHD**	coronary heart disease
ASD	atrial septal defect	**chemo**	chemotherapy
ASHD	arteriosclerotic heart disease		

Abbreviation	Meaning
CHF	congestive heart failure
Chol	cholesterol
CIS	carcinoma in situ
CK	creatine kinase (cardiac enzyme); conductive keratoplasty
CLL	chronic lymphocytic leukemia
cm	centimeter (1/100 of a meter)
CML	chronic myelogenous leukemia
CNS	central nervous system
CO	coccygeal nerves
CO_2	carbon dioxide
COLD	chronic obstructive lung disease
COPD	chronic obstructive pulmonary disease
CP	cerebral palsy
CPAP	continuous positive airway pressure
CPD	cephalopelvic disproportion
CPK	creatine phosphokinase (cardiac enzyme released into the bloodstream after a heart attack)
CPR	cardiopulmonary resuscitation
CRF	chronic renal failure
CRRT	continuous renal replacement therapy
CS, C-section	cesarean section
CSF	cerebrospinal fluid
CT	computed tomography
CTA	computed tomography angiography
CTS	carpal tunnel syndrome
CV	cardiovascular
CVA	cerebrovascular accident
CVD	cardiovascular disease
CVS	chorionic villus sampling
CWP	childbirth without pain
CXR	chest x-ray, chest radiograph
cysto	cystoscopy

D

Abbreviation	Meaning
D	diopter (lens strength)
D&C	dilatation (dilation) and curettage
Decub.	decubitus (lying down)
D.O.	Doctor of Osteopathy
D.P.M.	Doctor of Podiatric Medicine
Derm	dermatology
DES	diffuse esophageal spasm; drug-eluting stent
DEXA, DXA	dual energy x-ray absorptiometry
DI	diabetes insipidus; diagnostic imaging
DIC	disseminated intravascular coagulation
diff	differential count (white blood cells)
DJD	degenerative joint disease
DKA	diabetic ketoacidosis
DM	diabetes mellitus
DNA	deoxyribonucleic acid
DOE	dyspnea on exertion

Abbreviation	Meaning
DPI	dry powder inhaler
DPT	diphtheria, pertussis, tetanus
DRE	digital rectal examination
DSA	digital subtraction angiography
DUB	dysfunctional uterine bleeding
DVT	deep vein thrombosis; deep venous thrombosis
Dx	diagnosis

E

Abbreviation	Meaning
EBR	external beam radiation
EBT	external beam therapy
EBV	Epstein-Barr virus
ECCE	extracapsular cataract extraction
ECG, EKG	electrocardiogram; electrocardiography
ECHO	echocardiogram; echocardiography; echoencephalogram; echoencephalography
ECRB	extensor carpi radialis brevis (muscle or tendon)
ED	erectile dysfunction; emergency department
EEG	electroencephalography
EF	ejection fraction
EGD	esophagogastroduodenoscopy
ELT	endovenous laser ablation; endoluminal laser ablation
Em	emmetropia
EMG	electromyography
ENG	electronystagmography
ENT	ears, nose, and throat
EOM	extraocular movement
eos	eosinophil (type of white blood cell)
EPS	electrophysiology studies
ESR	erythrocyte sedimentation rate
ESRD	end-stage renal disease
ESWL	extracorporeal shock-wave lithotripsy
ETT	exercise tolerance test
EU	excretory urography

F

Abbreviation	Meaning
FBS	fasting blood sugar
FECG, FEKG	fetal electrocardiogram
FH	family history
FHR	fetal heart rate
FHT	fetal heart tone
FS	frozen section
FSH	follicle-stimulating hormone
FTND	full-term normal delivery
FVC	forced vital capacity
Fx	fracture

(continued)

Abbreviation	Meaning	Abbreviation	Meaning
G		**IDDM**	insulin-dependent diabetes mellitus
G	gravida (pregnant)	**Igs**	immunoglobulins
GB	gallbladder	**IM**	intramuscular; infectious mononucleosis
GBP	gastric bypass	**IMP**	impression (synonymous with diagnosis)
GBS	gallbladder series (x-ray studies)		
GC	gonococcus *(Neisseria gonorrhoeae)*	**INR**	international normalized ratio
GER	gastroesophageal reflux	**IVP**	intravenous pyelogram; intravenous pyelography
GERD	gastroesophageal reflux disease		
GH	growth hormone	**IOL**	intraocular lens
GI	gastrointestinal	**IOP**	intraocular pressure
GTT	glucose tolerance test	**IPPB**	intermittent positive-pressure breathing
GU	genitourinary	**IRDS**	infant respiratory distress syndrome
GVHD	graft-versus-host disease	**IS**	intracostal space
GVHR	graft-versus-host reaction	**IUD**	intrauterine device
GYN	gynecology	**IUGR**	intrauterine growth rate; intrauterine growth retardation
H		**IV**	intravenous
HAV	hepatitis A virus	**IVC**	intravenous cholangiogram; intravenous cholangiography
Hb, Hgb	hemoglobin		
HBV	hepatitis B virus	**IVF**	in vitro fertilization
HCG	human chorionic gonadotropin	**IVF-ET**	in vitro fertilization and embryo transfer
HCl	hydrochloric acid		
HCT, Hct	hematocrit	**IVP**	intravenous pyelogram; intravenous pyelography
HCV	hepatitis C virus		
HD	hemodialysis; hip disarticulation; hearing distance	**K**	
HDL	high-density lipoprotein	**K**	potassium (an electrolyte)
HDN	hemolytic disease of the newborn	**KD**	knee disarticulation
HDV	hepatitis D virus	**KUB**	kidney, ureter, bladder
HEV	hepatitis E virus	**L**	
HF	heart failure	**L1, L2, and so on**	first lumbar vertebra, second lumbar vertebra, and so on
HIV	human immunodeficiency virus		
H₂O	water	**LA**	left atrium
HMD	hyaline membrane disease	**LASIK**	laser-assisted in situ keratomileusis
HNP	herniated nucleus pulposus (herniated disk)	**LAT, lat**	lateral
HP	hemipelvectomy	**LBBB**	left bundle branch block
HPV	human papillomavirus	**LBW**	low birth weight
HRT	hormone replacement therapy	**LD**	lactate dehydrogenase; lactic acid dehydrogenase (cardiac enzyme)
HSG	hysterosalpingography		
HSV	herpes simplex virus	**LDL**	low-density lipoprotein
HSV-2	herpes simplex virus type 2	**LES**	lower esophageal sphincter
HTN	hypertension	**LFT**	liver function test
Hx	history	**LH**	luteinizing hormone
I, J		**LLQ**	left lower quadrant
IBD	irritable bowel disease	**LMP**	last menstrual period
I&D	incision and drainage	**LOC**	loss of consciousness
IBS	irritable bowel syndrome	**LP**	lumbar puncture
IC	interstitial cystitis	**LPR**	laryngopharyngeal reflux
ICD	implantable cardioverter-defibrillator	**LS**	lumbosacral spine
ICP	intracranial pressure	**LSO**	left salpingo-oophorectomy
ICU	intensive care unit	**lt**	left
ID	intradermal	**LUQ**	left upper quadrant

Abbreviation	Meaning
LV	left ventricle
lymphos	lymphocytes
M	
MDI	metered-dose inhaler
MEG	magnetoencephalography
MG	myasthenia gravis
mg	milligram (1/1,000 of a gram)
mg/dl, mg/dL	milligram per deciliter
MI	myocardial infarction
mix astig	mixed astigmatism
ml, mL	milliliters (1/1,000 of a liter)
mm	millimeter (1/1,000 of a meter)
mm Hg	millimeters of mercury
MNL	mononuclear leukocytes
MR	mitral regurgitation
MRA	magnetic resonance angiogram; magnetic resonance angiography
MRCP	magnetic resonance cholangiopancreatography
MRI	magnetic resonance imaging
MS	musculoskeletal; multiple sclerosis; mental status; mitral stenosis
MSH	melanocyte-stimulating hormone
MUGA	multiple-gated acquisition (scan)
MVP	mitral valve prolapse
Myop	myopia (nearsightedness)
N	
Na	sodium (an electrolyte)
NB	newborn
NCV	nerve conduction velocity
NG	nasogastric
NIDDM	non–insulin-dependent diabetes mellitus
NIHL	noise-induced hearing loss
NK cell	natural killer cell
NMT	nebulized mist treatment
NPH	neutral protamine Hagedorn (insulin)
NSAIDs	nonsteroidal antiinflammatory drugs
NSR	normal sinus rhythm
O	
O_2	oxygen
OB	obstetrics
OCG	oral cholecystography
OCPs	oral contraceptive pills
OD	overdose
O.D.	Doctor of Optometry
OM	otitis media
OP	outpatient; operative procedure
ORTH, ortho	orthopedics
OSA	obstructive sleep apnea

Abbreviation	Meaning
P	
P	phosphorus; pulse
p̄	after
PA	posteroanterior; pernicious anemia; pulmonary artery
PAC	premature atrial contraction
Pap	Papanicolaou (test)
para 1, 2, 3, and so on	unipara, bipara, tripara, and so on (number of viable births)
PAT	paroxysmal atrial tachycardia
PBI	protein-bound iodine
PCL	posterior cruciate ligament
PCNL	percutaneous nephrolithotomy
Pco_2	partial pressure of carbon dioxide
PCP	*Pneumocystis* pneumonia; primary care physician
PCTA	percutaneous transluminal coronary angioplasty
PCV	packed cell volume
PE	physical examination; pulmonary embolism; pressure-equalizing (tube)
PERRLA	pupils equal, round, and reactive to light and accommodation
PET	positron emission tomography
PFT	pulmonary function tests
PGH	pituitary growth hormone
pH	symbol for degree of acidity or alkalinity
PID	pelvic inflammatory disease
PIH	pregnancy-induced hypertension
PKD	polycystic kidney disease
PMH	past medical history
PMI	point of maximum impulse
PMP	previous menstrual period
PMN	polymorphonuclear
PMNL, poly	polymorphonuclear leukocyte
PMS	premenstrual syndrome
PND	paroxysmal nocturnal dyspnea
PNS	peripheral nervous system
Po_2	partial pressure of oxygen
post	posterior
PPV	pars plana vitrectomy
PRL	prolactin
PSA	prostate-specific antigen
PT	prothrombin time, physical therapy
pt	patient
PTCA	percutaneous transluminal coronary angioplasty
PTH	parathyroid hormone (also called parathormone)
PTT	partial thromboplastin time
PUD	peptic ulcer disease
PVC	premature ventricular contraction

(continued)

Abbreviation	Meaning
Q	
qEEG	quantitative electroencephalography
R	
RA	right atrium; rheumatoid arthritis
RAI	radioactive iodine
RAIU	radioactive iodine uptake
RBC, rbc	red blood cell
RD	respiratory distress
RDS	respiratory distress syndrome
RF	rheumatoid factor; radio frequency
RGB	Roux-en-Y gastric bypass
RK	radial keratotomy
RLQ	right lower quadrant
R/O	rule out
ROM	range of motion
RP	retrograde pyelogram; retrograde pyelography
RSO	right salpingo-oophorectomy
rt	right
RUQ	right upper quadrant
RV	residual volume; right ventricle
S	
S1, S2, and so on	first sacral vertebra, second sacral vertebra, and so on
SA, S-A	sinoatrial
SaO_2	arterial oxygen saturation
SD	shoulder disarticulation
segs	segmented neutrophils
SICS	small incision cataract surgery
SIDS	sudden infant death syndrome
SLE	systemic lupus erythematosus; slit-lamp examination
SNS	sympathetic nervous system
SOB	shortness of breath
sono	sonogram
SPECT	single photon emission computed tomography
sp. gr.	specific gravity
ST	esotropia
stat., STAT	immediately
STD	sexually transmitted disease
STI	sexually transmitted infection
Sx	symptom
T	
T&A	tonsillectomy and adenoidectomy
T1, T2, and so on	first thoracic vertebra, second thoracic vertebra, and so on
T_3	triiodothyronine (thyroid hormone)
T_4	thyroxine (thyroid hormone)

Abbreviation	Meaning
TAH	total abdominal hysterectomy
TB	tuberculosis
TFT	thyroid function test
THA	total hip arthroplasty
THR	total hip replacement
ther	therapy
TIA	transient ischemic attack
TKA	total knee arthroplasty
TKR	total knee replacement
TPR	temperature, pulse, and respiration
TRAM	transverse rectus abdominis muscle (flap)
TSE	testicular self-examination
TSH	thyroid-stimulating hormone
TURBT	transurethral resection of bladder tumor
TURP	transurethral resection of the prostate
TVH	total vaginal hysterectomy
Tx	treatment
U	
U&L, U/L	upper and lower
UA	urinalysis
UC	uterine contractions
UGI	upper gastrointestinal
UGIS	upper gastrointestinal series
ung	ointment
UPP	uvulopalatopharyngoplasty
URI	upper respiratory infection
US	ultrasound; ultrasonography
UTI	urinary tract infection
V	
VA	visual acuity
VC	vital capacity
VCUG	voiding cystourethrography
VD	venereal disease
VF	visual field
VSD	ventricular septal defect
VT	ventricular tachycardia
VUR	vesicoureteral reflux
W	
WBC, wbc	white blood cell
WD	well-developed
WN	well-nourished
WNL	within normal limits
X,Y,Z	
XP, XDP	xeroderma pigmentosum
XT	exotropia

Discontinued Abbreviations

The Joint Commission (JC) and the Institute for Safe Medication Practices (ISMP) report that the following abbreviations are commonly misinterpreted and have resulted in harmful medical errors. Both organizations have compiled a comprehensive "Do Not Use" list (available on their websites) for health-care providers.

To prevent harmful medical errors from occurring, both organizations recommend discontinuance of those abbreviations. Instead the abbreviations should be written out. Nevertheless, some of the abbreviations on the "Do Not Use" list are still used by health-care providers. A selected number are listed below.

Abbreviation	Meaning
AD	right ear
AS	left ear
AU	both ears
dc, DC	discharge; discontinue
OD	right eye
OS	left eye
OU	both eyes

Common Symbols

The table below lists common symbols used in health care and related fields, along with their meanings.

Symbol	Meaning	Symbol	Meaning
@	at	Ø	no
aa	of each	#	number; following a number, pounds
'	foot	÷	divided by
"	inch	/	divided by
Δ	change; heat	×	multiplied by; magnification
℞	prescription, treatment, therapy	=	equals
→	to, in the direction of	≈	approximately equal
↑	increase(d), up	°	degree
↓	decrease(d), down	%	percent
+	plus, positive	♀	female
−	minus, negative	♂	male
±	plus or minus; either positive or negative; indefinite		

Glossary of Medical Word Elements

Medical Word Elements

Element	Meaning	Element	Meaning
A		**arteri/o**	artery
		arteriol/o	arteriole
a-	without, not	**arthr/o**	joint
-a	noun ending	**-ary**	pertaining to
ab-	from, away from	**asbest/o**	asbestos
abdomin/o	abdomen	**-asthenia**	weakness, debility
abort/o	to miscarry	**astr/o**	star
-ac	pertaining to	**-ate**	having the form of, possessing
acid/o	acid	**atel/o**	incomplete; imperfect
acous/o	hearing	**ather/o**	fatty plaque
acr/o	extremity	**-ation**	process (of)
acromi/o	acromion (projection of the scapula)	**atri/o**	atrium
-acusia	hearing	**audi/o**	hearing
-acusis	hearing	**audit/o**	hearing
-ad	toward	**aur/o**	ear
ad-	toward	**auricul/o**	ear
aden/o	gland	**auto-**	self, own
adenoid/o	adenoids	**ax/o**	axis, axon
adip/o	fat	**azot/o**	nitrogenous compounds
adren/o	adrenal glands		
adrenal/o	adrenal glands	**B**	
aer/o	air		
af-	toward	**bacteri/o**	bacteria (singular, bacterium)
agglutin/o	clumping, gluing	**balan/o**	glans penis
agora-	marketplace	**bas/o**	base (alkaline, opposite of acid)
-al	pertaining to	**bi-**	two
albin/o	white	**bil/i**	bile, gall
albumin/o	albumin (protein)	**bi/o**	life
-algesia	pain	**-blast**	embryonic cell
-algia	pain	**blast/o**	embryonic cell
allo-	other, differing from the normal	**blephar/o**	eyelid
alveol/o	alveolus; air sac	**brachi/o**	arm
ambly/o	dull, dim	**brachy-**	short
amni/o	amnion (amniotic sac)	**brady-**	slow
an-	without, not	**bronch/o**	bronchus (plural, bronchi)
an/o	anus	**bronchi/o**	bronchus (plural, bronchi)
ana-	against; up; back	**bronchiol/o**	bronchiole
andr/o	male	**bucc/o**	cheek
aneurysm/o	aneurysm (widened blood vessel)		
angi/o	vessel (usually blood or lymph)	**C**	
angin/o	choking pain		
aniso-	unequal, dissimilar	**calc/o**	calcium
ankyl/o	stiffness; bent, crooked	**calcane/o**	calcaneum (heel bone)
ante-	before, in front of	**-capnia**	carbon dioxide (CO_2)
anter/o	anterior, front	**carcin/o**	cancer
anthrac/o	coal, coal dust	**cardi/o**	heart
anti-	against	**-cardia**	heart condition
aort/o	aorta	**carp/o**	carpus (wrist bones)
append/o	appendix	**cata-**	down
appendic/o	appendix	**caud/o**	tail
aque/o	water	**cauter/o**	heat, burn
-ar	pertaining to	**cec/o**	cecum
-arche	beginning	**-cele**	hernia, swelling

Medical Word Elements—cont'd

Element	Meaning	Element	Meaning
-centesis	surgical puncture	cruci/o	cross
cephal/o	head	cry/o	cold
-ceps	head	crypt/o	hidden
-ception	conceiving	culd/o	cul-de-sac
cerebell/o	cerebellum	-cusia	hearing
cerebr/o	cerebrum	-cusis	hearing
cervic/o	neck; cervix uteri (neck of uterus)	cutane/o	skin
chalic/o	limestone	cyan/o	blue
cheil/o	lip	cycl/o	ciliary body of the eye; circular; cycle
chem/o	chemical; drug	-cyesis	pregnancy
chlor/o	green	cyst/o	bladder
chol/e	bile, gall	cyt/o	cell
cholangi/o	bile vessel	-cyte	cell
cholecyst/o	gallbladder		
choledoch/o	bile duct	**D**	
chondr/o	cartilage		
chori/o	chorion	dacry/o	tear; lacrimal apparatus (duct, sac, or gland)
choroid/o	choroid	dacryocyst/o	lacrimal sac
chrom/o	color	dactyl/o	fingers; toes
chromat/o	color	de-	cessation
-cide	killing	dendr/o	tree
circum-	around	dent/o	teeth
cirrh/o	yellow	derm/o	skin
-cision	a cutting	-derma	skin
-clasia	to break; surgical fracture	dermat/o	skin
-clasis	to break; surgical fracture	-desis	binding, fixation (of a bone or joint)
-clast	to break; surgical fracture	di-	double
clavicul/o	clavicle (collar bone)	dia-	through, across
clon/o	clonus (turmoil)	dipl-	double
-clysis	irrigation, washing	dipl/o	double
coccyg/o	coccyx (tailbone)	dips/o	thirst
cochle/o	cochlea	-dipsia	thirst
col/o	colon	dist/o	far, farthest
colon/o	colon	dors/o	back (of body)
colp/o	vagina	duct/o	to lead; carry
condyl/o	condyle	-duction	act of leading, bringing, conducting
coni/o	dust	duoden/o	duodenum (first part of the small intestine)
conjunctiv/o	conjunctiva		
-continence	to hold back	dur/o	dura mater; hard
contra-	against, opposite	-dynia	pain
cor/o	pupil	dys-	bad; painful; difficult
core/o	pupil		
corne/o	cornea	**E**	
coron/o	heart		
corp/o	body	-eal	pertaining to
corpor/o	body	ec-	out, out from
cortic/o	cortex	echo-	repeated sound
cost/o	ribs	-ectasis	dilation, expansion
crani/o	cranium (skull)	ecto-	outside, outward
crin/o	secrete	-ectomy	excision, removal
-crine	secrete	-edema	swelling

(continued)

Medical Word Elements—cont'd

Element	Meaning	Element	Meaning
ef-	away from	gest/o	pregnancy
electr/o	electricity	gingiv/o	gum(s)
-ema	state of; condition	glauc/o	gray
embol/o	embolus (plug)	gli/o	glue; neuroglial tissue
-emesis	vomiting	-glia	glue; neuroglial tissue
-emia	blood condition	-globin	protein
emphys/o	to inflate	glomerul/o	glomerulus
en-	in, within	gloss/o	tongue
encephal/o	brain	glott/o	glottis
end-	in, within	gluc/o	sugar, sweetness
endo-	in, within	glucos/o	sugar, sweetness
enter/o	intestine (usually small intestine)	glyc/o	sugar, sweetness
eosin/o	dawn (rose-colored)	glycos/o	sugar, sweetness
epi-	above, upon	gnos/o	knowing
epididym/o	epididymis	-gnosis	knowing
epiglott/o	epiglottis	gonad/o	gonads, sex glands
episi/o	vulva	goni/o	angle
erythem/o	red	gon/o	seed (ovum or spermatozoon)
erythemat/o	red	-grade	to go
erythr/o	red	-graft	transplantation
eschar/o	scab	-gram	record, writing
-esis	condition	granul/o	granule
eso-	inward	-graph	instrument for recording
esophag/o	esophagus	-graphy	process of recording
esthes/o	feeling	-gravida	pregnant woman
-esthesia	feeling	gyn/o	woman, female
eti/o	cause	gynec/o	woman, female
eu-	good, normal		
ex-	out, out from	**H**	
exo-	outside, outward		
extra-	outside	hallucin/o	hallucination
		hedon/o	pleasure
F		hem/o	blood
		hemangi/o	blood vessel
faci/o	face	hemat/o	blood
fasci/o	band, fascia (fibrous membrane supporting and separating muscles)	hemi-	one half
		hepat/o	liver
femor/o	femur (thigh bone)	hetero-	different
-ferent	to carry	hidr/o	sweat
fibr/o	fiber, fibrous tissue	hist/o	tissue
fibul/o	fibula (smaller bone of the lower leg)	histi/o	tissue
		home/o	same, alike
fluor/o	luminous, fluorescence	homeo-	same, alike
		homo-	same
G		humer/o	humerus (upper arm bone)
		hydr/o	water
galact/o	milk	hyp-	under, below, deficient
gangli/o	ganglion (knot or knotlike mass)	hyper-	excessive, above normal
gastr/o	stomach	hyp/o	under, below, deficient
-gen	forming, producing, origin	hypn/o	sleep
gen/o	forming, producing, origin	hypo-	under, below, deficient
-genesis	forming, producing, origin	hyster/o	uterus (womb)
genit/o	genitalia		

Medical Word Elements—cont'd

Element	Meaning	Element	Meaning
I		**kerat/o**	horny tissue; hard; cornea
		kern/o	kernel (nucleus)
-ia	condition	**ket/o**	ketone bodies (acids and acetones)
-iac	pertaining to	**keton/o**	ketone bodies (acids and acetones)
-iasis	abnormal condition (produced by something specified)	**kinesi/o**	movement
		-kinesia	movement
iatr/o	physician; medicine; treatment	**kinet/o**	movement
-iatry	medicine; treatment	**klept/o**	to steal
-ic	pertaining to	**kyph/o**	humpback
-ical	pertaining to		
-ice	noun ending	**L**	
ichthy/o	dry, scaly		
-ician	specialist	**labi/o**	lip
-icle	small, minute	**labyrinth/o**	labyrinth (inner ear)
-icterus	jaundice	**lacrim/o**	tear; lacrimal apparatus (duct, sac, or gland)
idi/o	unknown, peculiar		
-ile	pertaining to	**lact/o**	milk
ile/o	ileum (third part of the small intestine)	-lalia	speech, babble
		lamin/o	lamina (part of the vertebral arch)
ili/o	ilium (lateral, flaring portion of the hip bone)	**lapar/o**	abdomen
		laryng/o	larynx (voice box)
im-	not	**later/o**	side, to one side
immun/o	immune, immunity, safe	**lei/o**	smooth
in-	in, not	**leiomy/o**	smooth muscle (visceral)
-ine	pertaining to	-lepsy	seizure
infer/o	lower, below	**lept/o**	thin, slender
infra-	below, under	**leuk/o**	white
inguin/o	groin	**lex/o**	word, phrase
insulin/o	insulin	**lingu/o**	tongue
inter-	between	**lip/o**	fat
intra-	in, within	**lipid/o**	fat
-ion	the act of	-listhesis	slipping
-ior	pertaining to	-lith	stone, calculus
irid/o	iris	**lith/o**	stone, calculus
-is	noun ending	**lob/o**	lobe
isch/o	to hold back; block	**log/o**	study of
ischi/o	ischium (lower portion of the hip bone)	-logist	specialist in the study of
		-logy	study of
-ism	condition	**lord/o**	curve, swayback
iso-	same, equal	-lucent	to shine; clear
-ist	specialist	**lumb/o**	loins (lower back)
-isy	state of; condition	**lymph/o**	lymph
-itic	pertaining to	**lymphaden/o**	lymph gland (node)
-itis	inflammation	**lymphangi/o**	lymph vessel
-ive	pertaining to	-lysis	separation; destruction; loosening
-ization	process (of)		
		M	
J, K			
		macro-	large
jaund/o	yellow	**mal-**	bad
jejun/o	jejunum (second part of the small intestine)	-malacia	softening
		mamm/o	breast
kal/i	potassium (an electrolyte)	-mania	state of mental disorder, frenzy
kary/o	nucleus		

(continued)

Medical Word Elements—cont'd

Element	Meaning	Element	Meaning
mast/o	breast	neur/o	nerve
mastoid/o	mastoid process	neutr/o	neutral; neither
maxill/o	maxilla (upper jaw bone)	nid/o	nest
meat/o	opening, meatus	noct/o	night
medi-	middle	nucle/o	nucleus
medi/o	middle	nulli-	none
mediastin/o	mediastinum	nyctal/o	night
medull/o	medulla		
mega-	enlargement	**O**	
megal/o	enlargement		
-megaly	enlargement	obstetr/o	midwife
melan/o	black	ocul/o	eye
men/o	menses, menstruation	odont/o	teeth
mening/o	meninges (membranes covering the brain and spinal cord)	-oid	resembling
		-ole	small, minute
		olig/o	scanty
meningi/o	meninges (membranes covering the brain and spinal cord)	-oma	tumor
		omphal/o	navel (umbilicus)
ment/o	mind	onc/o	tumor
meso-	middle	onych/o	nail
meta-	change, beyond	oophor/o	ovary
metacarp/o	metacarpus (hand bones)	-opaque	obscure
metatars/o	metatarsus (foot bones)	ophthalm/o	eye
-meter	instrument for measuring	-opia	vision
metr/o	uterus (womb); measure	-opsia	vision
metri/o	uterus (womb)	-opsy	view of
-metry	act of measuring	opt/o	eye, vision
mi/o	smaller, less	optic/o	eye, vision
micr/o	small	or/o	mouth
micro-	small	orch/o	testis (plural, testes)
mono-	one	orchi/o	testis (plural, testes)
morph/o	form, shape, structure	orchid/o	testis (plural, testes)
muc/o	mucus	-orexia	appetite
multi-	many, much	orth/o	straight
muscul/o	muscle	-ory	pertaining to
mut/a	genetic change	-ose	pertaining to; sugar
my/o	muscle	-osis	abnormal condition; increase (used primarily with blood cells)
myc/o	fungus (plural, fungi)		
mydr/o	widen, enlarge	-osmia	smell
myel/o	bone marrow; spinal cord	oste/o	bone
myos/o	muscle	ot/o	ear
myring/o	tympanic membrane (eardrum)	-ous	pertaining to
myx/o	mucus	ovari/o	ovary
		ox/i	oxygen
N		ox/o	oxygen
		-oxia	oxygen
narc/o	stupor; numbness; sleep	oxy-	quick, sharp
nas/o	nose		
nat/o	birth	**P**	
natr/o	sodium (an electrolyte)		
necr/o	death, necrosis	pachy-	thick
neo-	new	palat/o	palate (roof of the mouth)
nephr/o	kidney		

Medical Word Elements—cont'd

Element	Meaning	Element	Meaning
pan-	all	-plasia	formation, growth
pancreat/o	pancreas	-plasm	formation, growth
-para	to bear (offspring)	-plasty	surgical repair
para-	near, beside; beyond	-plegia	paralysis
parathyroid/o	parathyroid glands	pleur/o	pleura
-paresis	partial paralysis	-plexy	stroke
patell/o	patella (kneecap)	-pnea	breathing
path/o	disease	pneum/o	air; lung
-pathy	disease	pneumon/o	air; lung
pector/o	chest	pod/o	foot
ped/i	foot; child	-poiesis	formation, production
ped/o	foot; child	poikil/o	varied, irregular
pedicul/o	lice	poli/o	gray; gray matter (of the brain or spinal cord)
pelv/i	pelvis		
pelv/o	pelvis	poly-	many, much
pen/o	penis	polyp/o	small growth
-penia	decrease, deficiency	-porosis	porous
-pepsia	digestion	post-	after, behind
per-	through	poster/o	back (of body), behind, posterior
peri-	around		
perine/o	perineum (area between the scrotum [or vulva in the female] and anus)	-potence	power
		-prandial	meal
		pre-	before, in front of
		presby/o	old age
peritone/o	peritoneum	primi-	first
-pexy	fixation (of an organ)	pro-	before, in front of
phac/o	lens	proct/o	anus, rectum
phag/o	swallowing, eating	prostat/o	prostate gland
-phage	swallowing, eating	proxim/o	near, nearest
-phagia	swallowing, eating	pseudo-	false
phalang/o	phalanges (bones of the fingers and toes)	psych/o	mind
		-ptosis	prolapse, downward displacement
pharmaceutic/o	drug, medicine	ptyal/o	saliva
pharyng/o	pharynx (throat)	-ptysis	spitting
-phasia	speech	pub/o	pelvis bone (anterior part of the pelvic bone)
phe/o	dusky, dark		
-phil	attraction for	pulmon/o	lung
phil/o	attraction for	pupill/o	pupil
-philia	attraction for	py/o	pus
phim/o	muzzle	pyel/o	renal pelvis
phleb/o	vein	pylor/o	pylorus
-phobia	fear	pyr/o	fire
-phonia	voice		
-phoresis	carrying, transmission	**Q, R**	
-phoria	feeling (mental state)		
phot/o	light	quadri-	four
phren/o	diaphragm; mind	rachi/o	spine
-phylaxis	protection	radi/o	radiation, x-ray; radius (lower arm bone on the thumb side)
-physis	growth		
pil/o	hair	radicul/o	nerve root
pituitar/o	pituitary gland	rect/o	rectum
-plakia	plaque	ren/o	kidney
plas/o	formation, growth	reticul/o	net, mesh

(continued)

Medical Word Elements—cont'd

Element	Meaning	Element	Meaning
retin/o	retina	-spasm	involuntary contraction, twitching
retro-	backward, behind	sperm/i	spermatozoa, sperm cells
rhabd/o	rod-shaped (striated)	sperm/o	spermatozoa, sperm cells
rhabdomy/o	rod-shaped (striated) muscle	spermat/o	spermatozoa, sperm cells
rhin/o	nose	sphygm/o	pulse
rhytid/o	wrinkle	-sphyxia	pulse
roentgen/o	x-rays	spin/o	spine
-rrhage	bursting forth (of)	spir/o	breathe
-rrhagia	bursting forth (of)	splen/o	spleen
-rrhaphy	suture	spondyl/o	vertebrae (backbone)
-rrhea	discharge, flow	squam/o	scale
-rrhexis	rupture	staped/o	stapes
-rrhythm/o	rhythm	-stasis	standing still
rube/o	red	steat/o	fat
		sten/o	narrowing, stricture
S		-stenosis	narrowing, stricture
		stern/o	sternum (breastbone)
sacr/o	sacrum	steth/o	chest
salping/o	tube (usually the fallopian or eustachian [auditory] tube)	sthen/o	strength
		stigmat/o	point, mark
-salpinx	tube (usually the fallopian or eustachian [auditory] tube)	stomat/o	mouth
		-stomy	forming an opening (mouth)
sarc/o	flesh (connective tissue)	sub-	under, below
-sarcoma	malignant tumor of connective tissue	sudor/o	sweat
		super-	upper, above
scapul/o	scapula (shoulder blade)	super/o	upper, above
-schisis	a splitting	supra-	above; excessive; superior
schiz/o	split	sym-	union, together, joined
scler/o	hardening; sclera (white of the eye)	syn-	union, together, joined
scoli/o	crooked, bent	synapt/o	synapsis, point of contact
-scope	instrument for examining	synov/o	synovial membrane, synovial fluid
-scopy	visual examination		
scot/o	darkness	**T**	
seb/o	sebum, sebaceous		
semi-	one half	tachy-	rapid
semin/o	semen; seed	tax/o	order, coordination
semin/i	semen; seed	-taxia	order, coordination
sept/o	septum	ten/o	tendon
sequestr/o	separation	tend/o	tendon
ser/o	serum	tendin/o	tendon
sial/o	saliva, salivary gland	-tension	to stretch
sider/o	iron	test/o	testis (plural, testes)
sigmoid/o	sigmoid colon	thalam/o	thalamus
silic/o	flint	thalass/o	sea
sin/o	sinus, cavity	thec/o	sheath (usually referring to the meninges)
sinus/o	sinus, cavity		
-sis	state of; condition	thel/o	nipple
-social	society	therapeut/o	treatment
somat/o	body	-therapy	treatment
somn/o	sleep	therm/o	heat
son/o	sound	thorac/o	chest
-spadias	slit, fissure	-thorax	chest

Medical Word Elements—cont'd

Element	Meaning	Element	Meaning
thromb/o	blood clot	ungu/o	nail
thym/o	thymus gland	uni-	one
-thymia	mind; emotion	ur/o	urine, urinary tract
thyr/o	thyroid gland	ureter/o	ureter
thyroid/o	thyroid gland	urethr/o	urethra
tibi/o	tibia (larger bone of the lower leg)	-uria	urine
-tic	pertaining to	urin/o	urine, urinary tract
ill/o	to pull	-us	condition; structure
-tocia	childbirth, labor	uter/o	uterus (womb)
tom/o	to cut	uvul/o	uvula
-tome	instrument to cut		
-tomy	incision	**V, W**	
ton/o	tension	vagin/o	vagina
tonsill/o	tonsils	valv/o	valve
tox/o	poison	valvul/o	valve
-toxic	pertaining to poison	varic/o	dilated vein
toxic/o	poison	vas/o	vessel; vas deferens; duct
trabecul/o	trabecula (supporting bundles of fibers)	vascul/o	vessel (usually blood or lymph)
trache/o	trachea (windpipe)	ven/o	vein
trans-	across, through	ventr/o	belly, belly side
tri-	three	ventricul/o	ventricle (of the heart or brain)
trich/o	hair	-version	turning
trigon/o	trigone (triangular region at the base of the bladder)	vertebr/o	vertebrae (backbone)
		vesic/o	bladder
-tripsy	crushing	vesicul/o	seminal vesicle
-trophy	development, nourishment	vest/o	clothes
-tropia	turning	viscer/o	internal organs
-tropin	stimulate	vitr/o	vitreous body (of the eye)
tubercul/o	a little swelling	vitre/o	glassy
tympan/o	tympanic membrane (eardrum)	vol/o	volume
		voyeur/o	to see
U		vulv/o	vulva
-ula	small, minute	**X, Y, Z**	
-ule	small, minute	xanth/o	yellow
uln/o	ulna (lower arm bone on the opposite side of the thumb)	xen/o	foreign, strange
		xer/o	dry
ultra-	excess, beyond	xiph/o	sword
-um	structure, thing	-y	condition; process
umbilic/o	umbilicus, navel		

English Terms

Meaning	Element	Meaning	Element
A		attraction for	-phil
			phil/o
abdomen	abdomin/o		-philia
	lapar/o	away from	ef-
abnormal condition (produced by something specified)	-iasis	axis, axon	ax/o
		B	
abnormal condition; increase (used primarily with blood cells)	-osis	back (of body)	dors/o
		back (of body), behind, posterior	poster/o
above, upon	epi-	backward, behind	retro-
above; excessive; superior	supra-	bacteria (singular, bacterium)	bacteri/o
acid	acid/o		
acromion (projection of the scapula)	acromi/o	bad	mal-
		bad; painful; difficult	dys-
across, through	trans-	band, fascia (fibrous membrane supporting and separating muscles)	fasci/o
act of leading, bringing, conducting	-duction		
act of measuring	-metry	base (alkaline, opposite of acid)	bas/o
adenoids	adenoid/o		
adrenal glands	adren/o	to bear (offspring)	-para
	adrenal/o	before, in front of	ante-
after, behind	post-		pre-
against	anti-		pro-
against, opposite	contra-	beginning	-arche
against; up; back	ana-	belly, belly side	ventr/o
air	aer/o	below, under	infra-
air; lung	pneum/o	between	inter-
	pneumon/o	bile duct	choledoch/o
albumin (protein)	albumin/o	bile vessel	cholangi/o
all	pan-	bile, gall	bil/i
alveolus; air sac	alveol/o		chol/e
amnion (amniotic sac)	amni/o	binding, fixation (of a bone or joint)	-desis
aneurysm (widened blood vessel)	aneurysm/o		
angle	goni/o	birth	nat/o
anterior, front	anter/o	black	melan/o
anus	an/o	bladder	cyst/o
anus, rectum	proct/o		vesic/o
aorta	aort/o	blood	hem/o
appendix	append/o		hemat/o
	appendic/o	blood clot	thromb/o
appetite	-orexia	blood condition	-emia
arm	brachi/o	blood vessel	hemangi/o
around	circum-	blue	cyan/o
	peri-	body	corp/o
arteriole	arteriol/o		corpor/o
artery	arteri/o		somat/o
asbestos	asbest/o		
atrium	atri/o		

English Terms—cont'd

Meaning	Element	Meaning	Element
bone	oste/o	cochlea	cochle/o
bone marrow; spinal cord	myel/o	cold	cry/o
brain	encephal/o	colon	col/o
to break; surgical fracture	-clasia		colon/o
	-clasis	color	chrom/o
	-clast		chromat/o
breast	mamm/o	conceiving	-ception
	mast/o	condition	-esis
breathe	spir/o		-ia
breathing	-pnea		-ism
bronchiole	bronchiol/o	condition; process	-y
bronchus (plural, bronchi)	bronch/o	condition; structure	-us
	bronchi/o	condyle	condyl/o
bursting forth (of)	-rrhage	conjunctiva	conjunctiv/o
	-rrhagia	cornea	corne/o
		cortex	cortic/o
C		cranium (skull)	crani/o
		crooked, bent	scoli/o
calcaneum (heel bone)	calcane/o	cross	cruci/o
calcium	calc/o	crushing	-tripsy
cancer	carcin/o	cul-de-sac	culd/o
carbon dioxide (CO_2)	-capnia	curve, swayback	lord/o
carpus (wrist bones)	carp/o	to cut	tom/o
to carry	-ferent	a cutting	-cision
carrying, transmission	-phoresis		
cartilage	chondr/o	**D**	
cause	eti/o		
cecum	cec/o	darkness	scot/o
cell	cyt/o	dawn (rose-colored)	eosin/o
	-cyte	death, necrosis	necr/o
cerebellum	cerebell/o	decrease, deficiency	-penia
cerebrum	cerebr/o	deficient, under, below	hypo-
cessation	de-	development, nourishment	-trophy
change, beyond	meta-	diaphragm; mind	phren/o
cheek	bucc/o	different	hetero-
chemical; drug	chem/o	digestion	-pepsia
chest	pector/o	dilated vein	varic/o
	steth/o	dilation, expansion	-ectasis
	thorac/o	discharge, flow	-rrhea
	-thorax	disease	path/o
childbirth, labor	-tocia		-pathy
choking pain	angin/o	double	di-
chorion	chori/o		dipl-
choroid	choroid/o		dipl/o
ciliary body of the eye;	cycl/o	down	cata-
circular; cycle		drug, medicine	pharmaceutic/o
clavicle (collar bone)	clavicul/o	dry	xer/o
clonus (turmoil)	clon/o	dry, scaly	ichthy/o
clothes	vest/o	dull, dim	ambly/o
clumping, gluing	agglutin/o	duodenum (first part of the	duoden/o
coal, coal dust	anthrac/o	small intestine)	
coccyx (tailbone)	coccyg/o	dura mater; hard	dur/o

(continued)

English Terms—cont'd

Meaning	Element	Meaning	Element
dusky, dark	phe/o	foot; child	ped/i
dust	coni/o		ped/o
		foreign, strange	xen/o
E		form, shape, structure	morph/o
ear	aur/o	formation, growth	plas/o
	auricul/o		-plasia
	ot/o		-plasm
electricity	electr/o	formation, production	-poiesis
embolus (plug)	embol/o	forming an opening (mouth)	-stomy
embryonic cell	-blast	forming, producing, origin	-gen
	blast/o		gen/o
enlargement	mega-		-genesis
	megal/o	four	quadri-
	-megaly	from, away from	ab-
epididymis	epididym/o	fungus (plural, fungi)	myc/o
epiglottis	epiglott/o		
esophagus	esophag/o	**G**	
excess, beyond	ultra-	gallbladder	cholecyst/o
excessive, above normal	hyper-	ganglion (knot or knotlike mass)	gangli/o
excision, removal	-ectomy		
extremity	acr/o	genetic change	mut/a
eye	ocul/o	genitalia	genit/o
	ophthalm/o	gland	aden/o
eye, vision	opt/o	glans penis	balan/o
	optic/o	glassy	vitre/o
eyelid	blephar/o	glomerulus	glomerul/o
		glottis	glott/o
F		glue; neuroglial tissue	gli/o
face	faci/o		-glia
false	pseudo-	to go	-grade
far, farthest	dist/o	gonads, sex glands	gonad/o
fat	adip/o	good, normal	eu-
	lip/o	granule	granul/o
	lipid/o	gray	glauc/o
	steat/o	gray; gray matter (of the brain or spinal cord)	poli/o
fatty plaque	ather/o		
fear	-phobia	green	chlor/o
feeling	esthes/o	groin	inguin/o
	-esthesia	growth	-physis
feeling (mental state)	-phoria	gum(s)	gingiv/o
femur (thigh bone)	femor/o		
fiber, fibrous tissue	fibr/o	**H**	
fibula (smaller bone of the lower leg)	fibul/o	hair	pil/o
			trich/o
fingers; toes	dactyl/o	hallucination	hallucin/o
fire	pyr/o	hardening; sclera (white of the eye)	scler/o
first	primi-		
fixation (of an organ)	-pexy	having the form of, possessing	-ate
flesh (connective tissue)	sarc/o		
flint	silic/o	head	cephal/o
foot	pod/o		-ceps

English Terms—cont'd

Meaning	Element	Meaning	Element
hearing	acous/o	irrigation, washing	-clysis
	-acusis	ischium (lower portion	ischi/o
	audi/o	of the hip bone)	
	audit/o		
	-cusia	**J, K**	
	-cusis	jaundice	-icterus
heart	cardi/o	jejunum (second part of the	jejun/o
	coron/o	small intestine)	
heart condition	-cardia	joint	arthr/o
heat	therm/o	kernel (nucleus)	kern/o
heat, burn	cauter/o	ketone bodies (acids and	ket/o
hernia, swelling	-cele	acetones)	keton/o
hidden	crypt/o	kidney	nephr/o
to hold back	-continence		ren/o
to hold back; block	isch/o	killing	-cide
horny tissue; hard; cornea	kerat/o	knowing	gnos/o
humerus (upper arm bone)	humer/o		-gnosis
humpback	kyph/o		
		L	
I		labyrinth (inner ear)	labyrinth/o
ileum (third part of	ile/o	lacrimal sac	dacryocyst/o
the small intestine)		lamina (part of the vertebral	lamin/o
ilium (lateral, flaring	ili/o	arch)	
portion of the hip bone)		large	macro-
immune, immunity, safe	immun/o	larynx (voice box)	laryng/o
in, not	in-	to lead; carry	duct/o
in, within	en-	lens	phac/o
	end-	lice	pedicul/o
	endo-	life	bi/o
	intra-	light	phot/o
incision	-tomy	limestone	chalic/o
incomplete; imperfect	atel/o	lip	cheil/o
increase (used primarily with	-osis	lip	labi/o
blood cells); abnormal		liver	hepat/o
condition		lobe	lob/o
inflammation	-itis	loins (lower back)	lumb/o
to inflate	emphys/o	lower, below	infer/o
instrument for examining	-scope	luminous, fluorescence	fluor/o
instrument for measuring	-meter	lung	pulmon/o
instrument for recording	-graph	lymph	lymph/o
instrument to cut	-tome	lymph gland (node)	lymphaden/o
insulin	insulin/o	lymph vessel	lymphangi/o
internal organs	viscer/o		
intestine (usually small	enter/o	**M**	
intestine)		male	andr/o
involuntary contraction,	-spasm	malignant tumor of	-sarcoma
twitching		connective tissue	
inward	eso-	many, much	multi-
iris	irid/o	marketplace	agora-
iron	sider/o	mastoid process	mastoid/o

(continued)

English Terms—cont'd

Meaning	Element	Meaning	Element
maxilla (upper jaw bone)	maxill/o	nipple	thel/o
meal	-prandial	nitrogenous compounds	azot/o
mediastinum	mediastin/o	none	nulli-
medicine; treatment	-iatry	nose	nas/o
medulla	medull/o		rhin/o
meninges (membranes	mening/o	not	im-
covering the brain and	meningi/o	noun ending	-a
spinal cord)			-ice
menses, menstruation	men/o		-is
metacarpus (hand bones)	metacarp/o	nucleus	kary/o
metatarsus (foot bones)	metatars/o		nucle/o
middle	medi-		
	medi/o	**O**	
	meso-		
midwife	obstetr/o	obscure	-opaque
milk	galact/o	old age	presby/o
milk	lact/o	one	mono-
mind	ment/o		uni-
	psych/o	one half	hemi-
mind; emotion	-thymia		semi-
to miscarry	abort/o	opening, meatus	meat/o
mouth	or/o	order, coordination	tax/o
	stomat/o		-taxia
movement	kinesi/o	other, differing from the	allo-
	-kinesia	normal	
	kinet/o	out, out from	ec-
mucus	muc/o		ex-
	myx/o	outside	extra-
muscle	muscul/o	outside, outward	ecto-
	my/o		exo-
	myos/o	ovary	oophor/o
muzzle	phim/o		ovari/o
		oxygen	ox/i
N			ox/o
			-oxia
nail	onych/o		
	ungu/o	**P**	
narrowing, stricture	sten/o		
	-stenosis	pain	-algesia
navel (umbilicus)	omphal/o		-algia
near, beside; beyond	para-		-dynia
near, nearest	proxim/o	palate (roof of the mouth)	palat/o
neck; cervix uteri (neck of	cervic/o	pancreas	pancreat/o
uterus)		paralysis	-plegia
nerve	neur/o	parathyroid glands	parathyroid/o
nerve root	radicul/o	partial paralysis	-paresis
nest	nid/o	patella (kneecap)	patell/o
net, mesh	reticul/o	pelvis	pelv/i
neutral; neither	neutr/o		pelv/o
new	neo-	pelvis bone (anterior part of	pub/o
night	noct/o	the pelvic bone)	
	nyctal/o	penis	pen/o

English Terms—cont'd

Meaning	Element	Meaning	Element
perineum (area between the scrotum [or vulva in the female] and anus)	perine/o	pupil	cor/o core/o pupill/o
peritoneum	peritone/o	pus	py/o
pertaining to	-ac	pylorus	pylor/o
	-al		
	-ar	*Q, R*	
	-ary	quick, sharp	oxy-
	-eal	radiation, x-ray; radius (lower arm bone on the thumb side)	radi/o
	-iac		
	-ic		
	-ical	rapid	tachy-
	-ile	record, writing	-gram
	-ine	rectum	rect/o
	-ior	red	erythem/o
	-itic		erythemat/o
	-ive		erythr/o
	-ory		rube/o
	-ous	renal pelvis	pyel/o
	-tic	repeated sound	echo-
pertaining to poison	-toxic	resembling	-oid
pertaining to sugar	-ose	retina	retin/o
phalanges (bones of the fingers and toes)	phalang/o	rhythm	-rrhythm/o
		ribs	cost/o
pharynx (throat)	pharyng/o	rod-shaped (striated)	rhabd/o
physician; medicine; treatment	iatr/o	rod-shaped (striated) muscle	rhabdomy/o
		rupture	-rrhexis
pituitary gland	pituitar/o	*S*	
plaque	-plakia	sacrum	sacr/o
pleasure	hedon/o	saliva	ptyal/o
pleura	pleur/o	saliva, salivary gland	sial/o
point, mark	stigmat/o	same	homo-
poison	tox/o	same, alike	home/o
	toxic/o		homeo-
	-porosis	same, equal	iso-
potassium (an electrolyte)	kal/i	scab	eschar/o
power	-potence	scale	squam/o
pregnancy	-cyesis	scanty	olig/o
	gest/o	scapula (shoulder blade)	scapul/o
pregnant woman	-gravida	sea	thalass/o
process (of)	-ation	sebum, sebaceous	seb/o
	-ization	secrete	crin/o
process of recording	-graphy		-crine
prolapse, downward displacement	-ptosis	to see	voyeur/o
prostate gland	prostat/o	seed (ovum or spermatozoon)	gon/o
protection	-phylaxis	seizure	-lepsy
protein	-globin	self, own	auto-
to pull	ill/o	semen; seed	semin/o
pulse	sphygm/o		semin/i
	-sphyxia		

(continued)

English Terms—cont'd

Meaning	Element	Meaning	Element
seminal vesicle	vesicul/o	a splitting	-schisis
separation	sequestr/o	standing still	-stasis
separation; destruction; loosening	-lysis	stapes	staped/o
		star	astr/o
septum	sept/o	state of mental disorder, frenzy	-mania
serum	ser/o		
sheath (usually referring to the meninges)	thec/o	state of; condition	-ema
			-isy
to shine; clear	-lucent		-sis
short	brachy-	to steal	klept/o
side, to one side	later/o	sternum (breastbone)	stern/o
sigmoid colon	sigmoid/o	stiffness; bent, crooked	ankyl/o
sinus, cavity	sin/o	stimulate	-tropin
	sinus/o	stomach	gastr/o
skin	cutane/o	stone, calculus	-lith
	derm/o		lith/o
	-derma	straight	orth/o
	dermat/o	strength	sthen/o
sleep	hypn/o	to stretch	-tension
	somn/o	stroke	-plexy
slipping	-listhesis	structure, thing	-um
slit, fissure	-spadias	study of	log/o
slow	brady-		-logy
small	micr/o	stupor; numbness; sleep	narc/o
	micro-	sugar, sweetness	gluc/o
small growth	polyp/o		glucos/o
small, minute	-icle		glyc/o
	-ole		glycos/o
	-ula	surgical puncture	-centesis
	-ule	surgical repair	-plasty
smaller, less	mi/o	suture	-rrhaphy
smell	-osmia	swallowing, eating	phag/o
smooth	lei/o		-phage
smooth muscle (visceral)	leiomy/o		-phagia
society	-social	sweat	hidr/o
sodium (an electrolyte)	natr/o		sudor/o
softening	-malacia	swelling	-edema
sound	son/o	a little swelling	tubercul/o
specialist	-ician	sword	xiph/o
	-ist	synapsis, point of contact	synapt/o
specialist in the study of	-logist	synovial membrane, synovial fluid	synov/o
speech	-phasia		
speech, babble	-lalia		
spermatozoa, sperm cells	sperm/i	T	
	sperm/o		
	spermat/o	tail	caud/o
spine	rachi/o	tear; lacrimal apparatus (duct, sac, or gland)	dacry/o
	spin/o		
spitting	-ptysis		lacrim/o
spleen	splen/o	teeth	dent/o
split	schiz/o		odont/o

English Terms—cont'd

Meaning	Element	Meaning	Element
tendon	ten/o	two	bi-
	tend/o	tympanic membrane	myring/o
	tendin/o	(eardrum)	tympan/o
tension	ton/o		

U

Meaning	Element	Meaning	Element
testis (plural, testes)	orch/o		
	orchi/o	ulna (lower arm bone on the	uln/o
	orchid/o	opposite side of the thumb)	
	test/o	umbilicus, navel	umbilic/o
thalamus	thalam/o	under, below	sub-
the act of	-ion	under, below, deficient	hyp-
thick	pachy-		hyp/o
thin, slender	lept/o		hypo-
thing, structure	-um	unequal, dissimilar	aniso-
thirst	dips/o	union, together, joined	sym-
	-dipsia		syn-
three	tri-	unknown, peculiar	idi/o
through	per-	upper, above	super-
through, across	dia-		super/o
thymus gland	thym/o	ureter	ureter/o
thyroid gland	thyr/o	urethra	urethr/o
	thyroid/o	urine	-uria
tibia (larger bone of the	tibi/o	urine, urinary tract	ur/o
lower leg)			urin/o
tissue	hist/o	uterus (womb)	hyster/o
	histi/o		metri/o
tongue	gloss/o		uter/o
	lingu/o	uterus (womb); measure	metr/o
tonsils	tonsill/o	uvula	uvul/o
toward	-ad		
	ad-		

V

Meaning	Element	Meaning	Element
	af-		
trabecula (supporting	trabecul/o	vagina	colp/o
bundles of fibers)			vagin/o
trachea (windpipe)	trache/o	valve	valv/o
transplantation	-graft		valvul/o
treatment	therapeut/o	varied, irregular	poikil/o
	-therapy	vein	phleb/o
			ven/o
tree	dendr/o	ventricle (of the heart or	ventricul/o
trigone (triangular region at	trigon/o	brain)	
the base of the bladder)		vertebrae (backbone)	spondyl/o
tube (usually the fallopian or	salping/o		vertebr/o
eustachian [auditory] tube)	-salpinx	vessel (usually blood or	angi/o
tumor	-oma	lymph)	vascul/o
	onc/o	vessel; vas deferens; duct	vas/o
turning	-tropia	view of	-opsy
	-version		

(continued)

English Terms—cont'd

Meaning	Element	Meaning	Element
vision	-opia	white	albin/o
	-opsia		leuk/o
visual examination	-scopy	widen, enlarge	mydr/o
vitreous body (of the eye)	vitr/o	without, not	a-
voice	-phonia		an-
volume	vol/o	woman, female	gyn/o
vomiting	-emesis		gynec/o
vulva	episi/o	word, phrase	lex/o
	vulv/o	wrinkle	rhytid/o
		x-rays	roentgen/o
W, X, Y, Z		yellow	cirrh/o
			jaund/o
water	aque/o		xanth/o
	hydr/o		
weakness, debility	-asthenia		

Index of Genetic Disorders

Index of Clinical, Laboratory, and Imaging Procedures

CLINICAL

LABORATORY

IMAGING

Index of
Pharmacology

A

Aerosol therapy, Chapter 7, Respiratory System, 186

Analgesics, Chapter 16, Special Senses, 565t

Androgens, Chapter 13, Male Reproductive System, 444t

Anesthetics
Chapter 5, Integumentary System, 103t
Chapter 15, Nervous System, 524t

Angiotensin converting enzymes (ACE) inhibitors, Chapter 8, Cardiovascular System, 237t

Antacids, Chapter 6, Digestive System, 150t

Antiandrogens, Chapter 13, Male Reproductive System, 444t

Antiarrhythmics, Chapter 8, Cardiovascular System, 237t

Antibiotics
Chapter 7, Respiratory System, 192t
Chapter 11, Urinary System, 371t
Chapter 16, Special Senses, 565t

Anticoagulants, Chapter 9, Blood, Lymph, and Immune Systems, 281t

Anticonvulsants, Chapter 15, Nervous System, 524t

Antidepressants, Chapter 15, Nervous System, 525t

Antidiarrheals, Chapter 6, Digestive System, 150t

Antidiuretics, Chapter 14, Endocrine System, 483t

Antiemetics
Chapter 6, Digestive System, 150t
Chapter 16, Special Senses, 565t

Antifibrinolytics, Chapter 9, Blood, Lymph and Immune Systems, 281t

Antifungals
Chapter 5, Integumentary System, 102t
Chapter 12, Female Reproductive System, 412t

Antiglaucoma agents, Chapter 16, Special Senses, 565t

Antihistamines
Chapter 5, Integumentary System, 102t
Chapter 7, Respiratory System, 193t

Anti-impotence agents, Chapter 13, Male Reproductive System, 444t

Antimicrobials, Chapter 9, Blood, Lymph and Immune Systems, 281t

Antiparasitics, Chapter 5, Integumentary System, 102t

Antiparkinsonian agents, Chapter 15, Nervous System, 524t

Antipsychotics, Chapter 15, Nervous System, 525t

Antiseptics, Chapter 5, Integumentary System, 102t

Antispasmodics
Chapter 6, Digestive System, 150t
Chapter 11, Urinary System, 371t

Antithyroids, Chapter 14, Endocrine System, 483t

Antitussives, Chapter 7, Respiratory System, 193t

Antivirals,
Chapter 9, Blood, Lymph, and Immune Systems, 281t
Chapter 13, Male Reproductive System, 444t

B

Beta-blockers, Chapter 8, Cardiovascular System, 237t

Bronchodilators, Chapter 7, Respiratory System, 193t

C

Calcium supplements, Chapter 10, Musculoskeletal System, 335t

Calcium channel blockers, Chapter 8, Cardiovascular System, 237t

Corticosteroids,
Chapter 5, Integumentary System, 102t
Chapter 7, Respiratory System, 193t
Chapter 14, Endocrine System, 483t

D

Decongestants, Chapter 7, Respiratory System, 193t

Diuretics,
Chapter 8, Cardiovascular System, 237t
Chapter 11, Urinary System, 371t

E

Estrogens, Chapter 12, Female Reproductive System, 412t

Expectorants, Chapter 7, Respiratory System, 193t

F

Fat-soluble vitamins, Chapter 9, Blood, Lymph, and Immune Systems, 281t

G

Gold Salts, Chapter 10, Musculoskeletal System, 335t

Growth hormone replacements, Chapter 14, Endocrine System, 484t

H

Hormone replacement therapy (HRT), Chapter 12, Female Reproductive System, 391, 400, 412

Hypnotics, Chapter 15, Nervous System, 525t

I, J

Insulins, Chapter 14, Endocrine System, 484t

K

Keratolytics, Chapter 5, Integumentary System, 103t

L

Laxatives, Chapter 6, Digestive System, 150t

M

Miotics, Chapter 16, Special Senses, 552, 564

Muscle relaxants, Chapter 10, Musculoskeletal System, 335t

Mycostatics, Chapter 12, Female Reproductive System, 400

Mydriatics, Chapter 16, Special Senses, 565t

N

Nitrates, Chapter 8, Cardiovascular System, 238t

Nonsteroidal anti-inflammatory drugs (NSAIDs), Chapter 10, Musculoskeletal System, 335t

Index of Oncological Terms

Index

Rules for Singular and Plural Suffixes

This table presents common singular suffixes, the rules for forming plurals, and examples of each.

Rule		Example	
Singular	**Plural**	**Singular**	**Plural**
-*a*	Retain *a* and add *e*.	pleur*a*	pleur*ae*
-*ax*	Drop *x* and add *ces*.	thor*ax*	thora*ces*
-*en*	Drop *en* and add *ina*.	lum*en*	lum*ina*
-*is*	Drop *is* and add *es*.	diagnos*is*	diagnos*es*
-*ix*	Drop *ix* and add *ices*.	append*ix*	append*ices*
-*ex*	Drop *ex* and add *ices*.	ap*ex*	ap*ices*
-*ma*	Retain *ma* and add *ta*.	carcino*ma*	carcino*mata*
-*on*	Drop *on* and add *a*.	gangli*on*	gangli*a*
-*um*	Drop *um* and add *a*.	bacteri*um*	bacteri*a*
-*us*	Drop *us* and add *i*.	bronch*us*	bronch*i*
-*y*	Drop *y* and add *ies*.	deformit*y*	deformit*ies*